Blackwell's Five-Minute
Veterinary Consult
Clinical Companion

Equine Theriogenology

Blackwell's Five-Minute
Veterinary Consult
Clinical Companion

Equine Theriogenology

Edited by

Carla L. Carleton, DVM, MS

Diplomate, American College of Theriogenologists

Equine Theriogenologist

Department of Large Animal Clinical Sciences

College of Veterinary Medicine

Michigan State University

East Lansing, Michigan

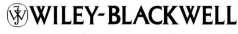

A John Wiley & Sons, Inc., Publication

Library of Congress Cataloging-in-Publication Data
Blackwell's five-minute veterinary consult clinical companion. Equine theriogenology / [edited by] Carla L. Carleton.
    p. ; cm. – (Blackwell's five-minute veterinary consult series)
  Other title: Five-minute veterinary consult clinical companion
  Other title: Equine theriogenology
  Includes bibliographical references and index.
  ISBN 978-0-7817-7670-7 (pbk. : alk. paper) 1. Horses–Generative organs–Diseases–Handbooks, manuals, etc. 2. Theriogenology–Handbooks, manuals, etc. I. Carleton, Carla L. II. Title: Five-minute veterinary consult clinical companion. III. Title: Equine theriogenology. IV. Series: Five minute veterinary consult.
  [DNLM: 1. Horse Diseases–Handbooks. 2. Fetal Diseases–veterinary–Handbooks. 3. Genital Diseases, Female–veterinary–Handbooks. 4. Genital Diseases, Male–veterinary–Handbooks. 5. Pregnancy Complications–veterinary–Handbooks. SF 959.U73]
  SF959.U73B63 2011
  636.1'0898–dc22
                                   2010026414

A catalogue record for this book is available from the British Library.

Set in 10.5/13 pt Berkeley by Toppan Best-set Premedia Limited

Printed and bound in Singapore by Markono Print Media Pte Ltd

1 2011

With family, encouragement, and good humor, all things can be accomplished. To Walter and Lillie Carleton, Cher and Con—you make it all worthwhile.

Carla L. Carleton

Contents

section 2 Stallion

section 3   Fetal/Neonatal

Contributors

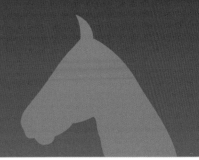

Jane E. Axon, BVSc, MACVSc, ACVIM,
    LAIM
Scone Veterinary Hospital
Head, Equine Medicine Department
Scone, New South Wales, Australia

Jane A. Barber, DVM, PhD, DACT
Veterinary Specialties Hospital at the
    Lake
Sherrills Ford, NC

Stefania Bucca, MV (DVM)
The Irish Equine Centre
Johnstown, NAAS
County Kildare, Ireland

Carla L. Carleton, DVM, MS, DACT
Michigan State University
College of Veterinary Medicine
East Lansing, MI

Andrea Carli, MV (DVM)
Somerton Equine Hospital
Friarstown, Kildare
County Kildare, Ireland

Maria E. Cadario, MV (DVM), DACT
Private Practice, Consultant
    Theriogenologist
Gainesville, FL

Alfred B. Caudle, DVM, DACT
Caudle Veterinary Practice
Watkinsville, GA

Sandra Curran, DVM, MS
Ultrascan, Inc.
Madison, WI

Timothy J. Evans, DVM, PhD, DACT,
    DABVT
University of Missouri, VM Diagnostic
    Lab
College of Veterinary Medicine
Columbia, MO

Kathryn T. Graves, PhD
Director, Animal Genetic Testing and
    Research Lab
University of Kentucky, Gluck Equine
    Research Center
Lexington, KY

Rolf E. Larsen, DVM, MS, DACT
St. George's University
School of Veterinary Medicine
St. Georges, Granada

Patrick M. McCue, DVM, PhD, DACT
Colorado State University
College of Veterinary Medicine
Ft. Collins, CO

Margo Macpherson, DVM, MS, DACT
University of Florida
College of Veterinary Medicine
Gainesville, FL

Judith V. Marteniuk, DVM, MS
Michigan State University
College of Veterinary Medicine
East Lansing, MI

Carole Miller, DVM, PhD, DACT
Director, Veterinary Technology Program
Athens Technical College
Athens, GA

Peter R. Morresey, BVSc, MACVSc,
   DACT, DACVIM
Rood & Riddle Equine Hospital
Lexington, KY

Gary J. Nie, DVM, MS, PhD, DACT,
   DACVIM, DABVP, cVMA
World Wide Veterinary Consultants, LLC
Springfield, MO

Philip E. Prater, DVM, DACT
Morehead State University
Veterinary Technology
Morehead, KY

Sarah L. Ralston, VMD, PhD, DACVN
Rutgers University
Howell, NJ

Jacobo Rodriguez, MV (DVM), MS
Washington State University
College of Veterinary Medicine
Pullman, WA

Walter R. Threlfall, DVM, MS, PhD,
   DACT
College of Veterinary Medicine
The Ohio State University
Columbus, OH

Ahmed Tibary, DVM, PhD, DACT
Washington State University
College of Veterinary Medicine
Pullman, WA

Dirk K. Vanderwall, DVM, PhD, DACT
New Bolton Center
University of Pennsylvania
Kennett Square, PA

Karen E. Wolfsdorf, DVM, DACT
Hagyard, Davidson & McGee
Lexington, KY

Gordon L. Woods (dec.), DVM, PhD,
   DACT
Colorado State University
College of Veterinary Medicine
Ft. Collins, CO

Foreword

The concept of the Five-Minute format goes back to an idea developed by Carroll Cann, a veteran of medical and veterinary publishing, having worked with Saunders, Lea & Febiger, and Williams & Wilkins. Following multiple mergers and acquisitions, the concept has survived, and this attests to the value that practitioners have found in the content and format. This contribution in the series will undoubtedly be of value to all who work with breeding horses and foals, and I congratulate Dr. Carleton and her colleagues on their achievement.

Chris Brown, Dean, Michigan State University College of Veterinary Medicine

Preface

Blackwell's Five-Minute Veterinary Consult Clinical Companion: Equine Theriogenology is a quick reference text designed mainly for clinicians, but it may also be of use for students of veterinary medicine.

There are many worthy texts of theriogenology, but this was written to take advantage of the Five-Minute format, which allows authors to make relatively concise, focused comments on topics of particular interest to those for whom theriogenology is a practice component. When included, images should assist the reader in appreciating the content, making it yet more user friendly. Unlike more comprehensive texts that have the luxury of providing comprehensive lists of references, the Five-Minute format targets literature that will serve as key supplemental reading.

Because their linkage is inseparable and overlaps are unavoidable in clinical medicine, the three primary sections encompass topics under the headings of mare, stallion, and neonate. Each section is primarily alphabetical by topic to assist the reader in more quickly identifying needed reference material. When topics might easily fit into more than one section, a heading appears in the remaining sections to direct the reader to that topic's location, e.g., cloning resides in the mare section, but its presence is also acknowledged in the stallion section and the reader is directed to the mare section.

Each chapter in the text is organized into sections of Definition/Overview, Etiology/Pathophysiology, Signalment/History, Clinical Features, Differential Diagnosis, Diagnostics, Therapeutics, and Comments. References can be found at the end of each chapter and certain chapters contain images where it helps further illuminate the topic being discussed.

Individual authors were allowed some leeway in their specific format, more prose, or bullets, wherein lay their comfort zone, or how they felt the material could best be presented for the benefit of the reader.

The purpose of this book was to provide a concise version of key topics relevant to the practice of theriogenology for a quick reference. The size and cost of the text are intended to make it accessible and *portable* for daily use.

Carla L. Carleton

Acknowledgments

To the authors, my colleagues in theriogenology who readily agreed to assist in this project as it first began to materialize, who provided great content and good images to bring the material to life, I extend my sincere gratitude. The challenges encountered with the shifting sands and names of publishing companies and editors made the eventual partnership with Erica Judisch, Nancy Simmerman, and Carrie Horn at Wiley-Blackwell all the more appreciated. The enormity of such an undertaking is not completed without the efforts of the *dedicated many*. To all, "Thank you."

Introduction

It is an adventure—a pleasure—combined with a small dose of trepidation and accompanied by a steep learning curve, when one first attempts to accept the lead role in a project of this sort. It is similar to clerkship training of residents and veterinary students: one proposes an idea, listens for novel suggestions, consideration is given to the innovative and substantive contributions, and from that evolves something that is much better than one could have created alone. This truly is better because of the sum of its parts.

It is also in no small measure a reflection of those who have shared their knowledge with me and encouraged me through difficult times: Drs. John Noordsy (Kansas State), Stephen J. Roberts (dec., Cornell and private practice), Walter R. Threlfall (Ohio State), C. J. Bierschwal (Univ. MO, ret.), Peter J. Timoney and Roberta M. Dwyer (Gluck Equine Research Center, Lexington, KY), Beverly L. Roeder (BYU), and many Michigan State colleagues. Essential to creating an honest tome are my clients, who have trusted me with caring for their horses. They have taught me how *to read a horse* and understand the economics and impact of industry practices on their survival.

Theriogenology remains a critical component of large animal general practice. A solid foundation in basic science, coupled with good clinical skills, a questioning mind, and an appreciation for the joy of working with clients to solve a reproductive mystery—what a treat. I hope many of you will come to share this passion and my love of theriogenology.

Carla L. Carleton

Blackwell's Five-Minute
Veterinary Consult

Clinical Companion

Equine Theriogenology

Mare

chapter 1

Abnormal Estrus Intervals

DEFINITION/OVERVIEW

Estrus is the period of sexual receptivity by the mare for the stallion. Estrus is abnormal when overt sexual behavior is displayed for longer or shorter periods than is considered normal for the species or the individual. Abnormal interestrus intervals can result from short or long estrus or diestrus intervals.

ETIOLOGY/PATHOPHYSIOLOGY

The mare is seasonally polyestrous, with estrous cycles in spring and summer months. The length of the average estrous cycle is 21 days (range: 19–22 days), which is defined as the period of time between ovulations that coincides with progesterone levels of less than 1 ng/mL. Estrus and estrous cycle lengths are quite repeatable in individual mares from cycle to cycle.

Key Hormonal Events in the Equine Estrous Cycle

- FSH (pituitary origin) causes ovarian follicular growth.
- Estradiol (follicular origin) stimulates increased GnRH (hypothalamic origin) pulse frequency to increase LH (pituitary origin) secretion.
- The surge of LH causes ovulation; estradiol returns to basal levels 1 to 2 days post-ovulation.
- Progesterone (CL origin) rises from basal levels (less than 1 ng/mL) at ovulation to greater than 4 ng/mL by 4 to 7 days post-ovulation.
- Progesterone causes a decrease in GnRH pulse frequency that results in an increase in FSH secretion to stimulate a new wave of ovarian follicles to develop during diestrus.
- Natural prostaglandin ($PGF_2\alpha$) of endometrial origin is released 14 to 15 days post-ovulation causing luteolysis and a concurrent decline in progesterone levels.

Length of Estrus

Averages from 5 to 7 days in normal, cycling mares, but it can range from 2 to 12 days.

Length of Diestrus

It averages 15 ± 2 days, with diestrual length exhibiting less variation than estrus in normal, cycling mares.

Sexual Behavior

- The absence of progesterone allows the onset of estrus behavior even if estrogens are present in only small quantities.
- Conditions that eliminate progesterone or increase estrogen concentrations are likely to induce estrus behavior. Persistence of these conditions results in abnormal estrus periods or interestrus intervals. The converse is also true.

Systems Affected

- Reproductive
- Endocrine

 # SIGNALMENT/HISTORY

- Mares of any breed may be affected.
- Geriatric mares (older than 20 years) tend to have prolonged transition periods, longer estrus duration, and fewer estrous cycles per year.
- Ponies may regularly have longer estrous cycles than horses (an average of 25 days).

Historical Findings

- Chief complaint: Infertility, failure to show estrus, prolonged estrus, split estrus, or frequent estrus behavior may be reported.
- Teasing records: The teasing methods used should be critically reviewed, to include: frequency, teaser type (e.g., pony, horse, or gelding), stallion behavior (e.g., aggressive/passive, vocalization, proximity), and handler experience.
- Seasonal influences: Normal individual variation in the onset, duration, and termination of cyclicity can be mistaken for estrus irregularity.
- Individual reproductive history: Estrous cycle length, response to teasing, foaling data, and previous injuries or infections of the genital tract may be related to current clinical abnormalities.
- Pharmaceuticals: Current and historical drug administration may be related to current clinical abnormalities.

 # CLINICAL FEATURES

- Body condition: Poor body condition or malnutrition may contribute to abnormal estrous cycles.

- Perineal conformation: Poor perineal conformation can result in pneumovagina, ascending infection, or urine pooling, which may result in symptoms consistent with behavioral estrus.
- Clitoral size: Clitoral enlargement may be related to prior treatment with anabolic steroids, progestational steroids, or intersex conditions.
- TRP: Essential when evaluating mares with abnormal cycles. To be meaningful and allow full assessment of a mare, all three of the primary anatomical components of the mare's genital tract must be described: uterine size and tone; ovarian size, shape, and location; and degree of cervical relaxation. Serial examination three times per week over the course of several weeks may be necessary to completely define the patient's estrous cycle.
- U/S: Useful to define normal or abnormal features of the uterus or ovaries.
- Vaginal examination: Inflammation, urine pooling, cervical competency, or conformational abnormalities may be identified. May also be used to help identify the stage of the estrous cycle (e.g., appearance, degree of external cervical os relaxation).
- When determining the cause of abnormal estrus intervals, it is helpful first to classify the abnormality in one of four categories and then to consider the common causes in each category as outlined here.

Shortened Estrus Duration

- Seasonality: Estrus duration tends to decrease in the height of the breeding season. This change may relate to more efficient folliculogenesis later in the breeding season (a normal physiologic shift).
- Silent estrus: Normal cyclic ovarian activity is occurring, but minimal or no overt signs of sexual receptivity are displayed. This is often a behavior-based problem associated with nervousness, a foal-at-side, or a maiden mare. Silent estrus has also been associated with previous anabolic steroid use.

Lengthened Estrus Duration

- Seasonality: Erratic estrus behavior associated with the transition period is common. Sexual receptivity can be short or long during vernal transition, but protracted estrus behavior is most common.
- Ovarian neoplasia (GCT, GTCT): Affected mares may chronically be in anestrus, exhibit persistent or frequent estrus behavior, or develop stallion-like behavior.
- Congenital disorders: Gonadal dysgenesis due to chromosomal defects (e.g., XO [Turner's syndrome], XXX) may be the underlying cause of anestrus, erratic estrus, or prolonged estrus.
- Hormone imbalance: Older mares may fail to ovulate and exhibit prolonged estrus, presumably due to ineffective LH release.

Shortened Interestrus Interval

- Uterine disease: Uterine inflammation (e.g., endometritis, pyometra) can result in atypical endometrial $PGF_2\alpha$ release, luteolysis, and an early return to estrus.

- Systemic illness: Endotoxin-induced PGF$_2\alpha$ release can lead to premature luteolysis and a shortened interestrus period.
- Iatrogenic/Pharmaceutical: PGF$_2\alpha$ administration, intrauterine infusions, and uterine biopsy procedures can also result in early regression of the CL and premature return to estrus.

Lengthened Interestrus Interval

- Prolonged luteal activity: Can occur with a normal, but diestrual, ovulation that results in the formation of a CL insufficiently mature to respond to endogenous PGF$_2\alpha$ release during a cycle that would otherwise be of normal length; severe uterine disease (pyometra) that prevents release of uterine PGF$_2\alpha$; EED after maternal recognition of pregnancy has already occurred; a CL that is persistent (i.e., its function is prolonged beyond the normal range); or subsequent to an ovarian hematoma, a prolonged period may be necessary to achieve luteinization that it may respond to PGF$_2\alpha$.
  - Persistent CLs have also been associated with consumption of fescue forages.
- Pregnancy: Luteal function persists in the presence of a conceptus. Estrus behavior during pregnancy is a normal occurrence and can be confused with abnormal interestrus intervals.
- Iatrogenic/Pharmaceutical:
  - Administration of progestin compounds to suppress behavioral estrus.
  - NSAIDs can potentially interfere with endometrial PGF$_2\alpha$ release and result in prolonged luteal activity. There is no evidence that chronic administration at recommended therapeutic dosages inhibits the spontaneous formation and release of PGF$_2\alpha$ from the endometrium.
  - GnRH agonist (deslorelin) implants used to stimulate ovulation have been associated with prolonged interovulatory intervals. At this time, deslorelin implants are unavailable in the United States but are still on the market in Canada and other countries. Their effect is more profound if PGF$_2\alpha$ is used during the diestrus period in an attempt to "short-cycle" the mare.

 DIFFERENTIAL DIAGNOSIS

Differentiating Conditions with Similar Symptoms

- Frequent urination caused by cystitis or urethritis, bladder atony, urine pooling, vaginitis, or pneumovagina may mimic submissive urination and thus be confused with behavioral estrus.
- Defensive or aggressive behavior can be confused with anestrus. Teasing methodologies should be reviewed or altered to clarify.

Differentiating Causes

- Minimum database: Complete medical and reproductive history (including teasing records), general physical examination, and reproductive examination (TRP and U/S [to distinguish pregnancy and pyometra], vaginal examination). Additional diagnostic samples that may aid in establishing a diagnosis include uterine cytology, culture, and endometrial biopsy.
- Silent estrus is often due to poor estrus detection (teasing). *Diagnosis*: TRP at least three times per week combined with frequent serum progesterone assays to allow detection of a short or inapparent estrus period.
- The transition period in the northern hemisphere typically extends from February through April, the period in which anestrus mares begin to develop follicles but have irregular estrous cycles. Mares may exhibit persistent estrus behavior, irregular estrus periods, or irregular diestrus intervals. *Diagnosis*: season, combined with results of serial TRP and U/S confirming the presence of numerous small to large follicles on both ovaries that fail to progress to ovulatory size.
- GCT/GTCT can occur at any age, but it is more typically is seen in the middle-age or older mare. The affected ovary is usually enlarged and often the ovulation fossa is obliterated. The contralateral ovary is usually small and inactive. U/S of the affected ovary often reveals a multilocular *honeycomb* appearance. *Diagnosis*: TRP and U/S; endocrine assays are also useful (*see* Large Ovary Syndrome).
- Gonadal dysgenesis may not be recognized until a mare enters the breeding herd and fails to have normal estrous cycles. *Diagnosis*: TRP and U/S confirm the absence of normal ovarian tissue and a juvenile reproductive tract. Karyotyping provides a definitive diagnosis.
- Ovulations can occur in diestrus. The CL that forms from a diestrus ovulation may not be sufficiently mature (responsiveness requires a minimum of 5 days post-ovulation) to be lysed by endogenous $PGF_2\alpha$ at the end of diestrus. Therefore, diestrual ovulations after day 10 of the estrous cycle result in persistent CL activity. *Diagnosis*: demonstration of a normal reproductive tract with failure of clinical estrus for more than 2 weeks post-ovulation and progesterone levels of greater than 4 ng/mL that last more than 2 weeks.
- The diagnosis of pregnancy, pyometra, endometritis, abortion, large ovary syndrome (including ovarian hematoma), and EED are discussed elsewhere.

 DIAGNOSTICS

- Serum progesterone concentrations: basal levels of less than 1 ng/mL indicate the absence of ovarian luteal tissue. Active CL function is associated with progesterone levels of more than 4 ng/mL.
- Serum testosterone and inhibin concentrations: mares typically have testosterone values less than 50 to 60 pg/mL and inhibin values less than 0.7 ng/mL. Hormone

levels suggestive of a GCT/GTCT (in a nonpregnant mare) are: testosterone greater than 50 to 100 pg/mL (produced if thecal cells are a significant tumor component) or inhibin greater than 0.7 ng/mL, with a progesterone level less than 1 ng/mL.

- Transrectal U/S is routinely used to evaluate the equine reproductive tract. The reader is referred to other texts for a comprehensive discussion on this technique.
- Uterine endoscopy is useful to diagnose intrauterine adhesions, glandular or lymphatic cysts, and polyps.
- Uterine cytology, culture, and endometrial biopsy techniques are discussed elsewhere.

 # THERAPEUTICS

- Evaluate teasing methods: silent estrus may be a reflection of poor teasing management.
- Monitor the problem mare, including TRP or U/S, three times weekly to better define the reproductive cycle.
- The treatment of pregnancy, pyometra, endometritis, abortion, large ovary syndrome (including ovarian hematoma), and EED are discussed elsewhere in this text.
- Artificial lighting (photo stimulation) is a management tool used to initiate ovarian activity earlier in the year. When successful, mares bred earlier in the season foal earlier the next year, to accommodate breed registries that use the January 1 equine "universal birth date." Photo stimulation does not eliminate vernal transition, but it merely shifts it to an earlier time of onset. Photo stimulation should begin no less than 90 days prior to the onset of early season breeding.

Drug(s) of Choice

- $PGF_2\alpha$ (Lutalyse® [Pfizer], 10 mg, IM) or its analogs, to lyse persistent CL tissue.
- Ovulation can be stimulated if a follicle is at least 30 mm by deslorelin, or equal to or greater than 35 mm by hCG (2,500 IU, IV).
- Altrenogest (Regu-Mate® [Intervet], 0.044 mg/kg, PO, SID, minimum 15 days) can be used to shorten the duration of vernal transition, providing follicles larger than 20 mm diameter are present and the mare is demonstrating behavioral estrus. $PGF_2\alpha$ on day 15 of the altrenogest treatment increases the reliability of this transition management regimen by lysing any late-to-luteinize (during the Regu-Mate treatment) transitional follicles.

Precautions/Interactions

Horses

- $PGF_2\alpha$ and its analogs are contraindicated in mares with asthma, COPD, or other bronchoconstrictive disease.
- Prostaglandin administration to pregnant mares can cause CL lysis and abortion. Carefully rule out pregnancy before administering this drug or its analogs.

- PGF$_2\alpha$ causes sweating and colic-like symptoms due to its stimulatory effect on smooth muscle cells. If cramping has not subsided within 1 to 2 hours, symptomatic treatment should be instituted.
- Antibodies to hCG can develop after treatment. It is desirable to limit its use to no more than two or three times during one breeding season, if possible. The half-life of these antibodies ranges from 30 days to several months; they typically do not persist from one breeding season to the next.
- Deslorelin implants have been associated with suppressed FSH secretion and decreased follicular development in the diestrus period immediately following its use, leading to a prolonged interovulatory period in nonpregnant mares. Implant removal within 1 to 2 days post-ovulation may decrease this possibility.
- Altrenogest, deslorelin, and PGF$_2\alpha$ should not be used in horses intended for food purposes.

Humans

- PGF$_2\alpha$ or its analogs should not be handled by pregnant women or people with asthma or bronchial disease. Any accidental exposure to skin should immediately be washed off.
- Altrenogest should not be handled by pregnant women or people with thrombophlebitis or thromboembolic disorders, cerebrovascular disease, coronary artery disease, breast cancer, estrogen-dependent neoplasia, undiagnosed vaginal bleeding or tumors that developed during the use of oral contraceptives, or estrogen-containing products. Any accidental exposure to skin should immediately be washed off.

Alternative Drugs

Cloprostenol sodium (Estrumate® [Schering-Plough Animal Health], 250 µg, IM), is a prostaglandin analog. This product is used in similar fashion as the natural prostaglandin, but it has been associated with fewer side effects. It is not currently approved but is widely used in horses.

Surgical Considerations

- Poor vulvar conformation should be addressed by performing a Caslick's vulvoplasty (e.g., episioplasty) of a portion of the dorsal vulvar commissure to control pneumovagina.
- GCT/GTCT ovarian tumors should be removed surgically (ovariectomy).
- Urine pooling, rectovaginal fistulas, or cervical tears should be corrected surgically.

 COMMENTS

Patient Monitoring

Until normal cyclicity is established or pregnancy has been confirmed, regular reproductive examinations are recommended.

Possible Complications

Unless corrected, abnormalities in estrus behavior frequently result in infertility.

Abbreviations

CL	corpus luteum
COPD	chronic obstructive pulmonary disease
EED	early embryonic death
FSH	follicle stimulating hormone
GCT	granulosa cell tumor
GnRH	gonadotropin releasing hormone
GTCT	granulosa theca cell tumor
hCG	human chorionic gonadotropin
IM	intramuscular
IV	intravenous
LH	luteinizing hormone
NSAID	nonsteroidal anti-inflammatory drug
$PGF_2\alpha$	natural prostaglandin
PO	per os (by mouth)
SID	once a day
TRP	transrectal palpation
U/S	ultrasound

See Also

- Aggression
- Anestrus
- Clitoral enlargement
- Disorders of sexual development
- Early embryonic death
- Endometritis
- Large ovary syndrome
- Ovulation failure
- Pneumovagina/Pneumouterus
- Prolonged diestrus
- Pseudopregnancy
- Pyometra
- Urine pooling/Urovagina
- Vaginitis and vaginal discharge
- Vulvar conformation

Suggested Reading

Daels PF, Hughes JP. 1993. The abnormal estrous cycle. In: *Equine Reproduction*. McKinnon AO and Voss JL (eds). Philadelphia: Lea & Febiger; 144–160.

Ginther OJ. 1992. *Reproductive Biology of the Mare: Basic and Applied Aspects*, 2nd ed. Cross Plains, WI: Equiservices.

Ginther OJ. 1995. *Ultrasonic Imaging and Animal Reproduction: Horses*. Cross Plains, WI: Equiservices.

Hinrichs K. 2007. Irregularities of the estrous cycle and ovulation in mares (including seasonal transition). In: *Current Therapy in Large Animal Theriogenology*. Youngquist RS and Threlfall WR (eds). St. Louis: Saunders Elsevier; 144–152.

McCue PM, Farquhar VJ, Carnevale EM, Squires EL. 2002. Removal of deslorelin (Ovuplant™) implant 48h after administration results in normal interovulatory intervals in mares. *Therio* 58: 865–870.

Author: Carole C. Miller

Abortion, Induction of (Elective Termination)

chapter

2

DEFINITION/OVERVIEW

- The mechanism of pregnancy maintenance is dependent on and alters with the stage of gestation.
  - Before 35 days (i.e., early pregnancy), maintenance is attributed to the primary CL.
  - Between 35 and 110 days, maintenance is by progesterone from the primary and secondary (or accessory) CL. Accessory CLs (luteinized follicles) develop after formation of the endometrial cups.
  - From 110 days to term gestation, maintenance is primarily by the feto-placental unit (the endocrine function of the placenta).

ETIOLOGY/PATHOPHYSIOLOGY

- Abortion may be induced if the primary mechanism of pregnancy maintenance is disrupted by:
  - Destruction of the CL (luteolysis)
  - Disruption of the feto-placental unit
  - Induction of hormonal changes similar to the mechanism of parturition.

Luteolysis

- Luteolysis is achieved by administration of an effective dose of $PGF_2\alpha$ or one of its analogues.
- A single treatment is usually sufficient prior to formation of endometrial cups (less than 35 days gestation).
- Several $PGF_2\alpha$ or analogue injections may be necessary if endometrial cups are present.
- Less than 80 days gestation: abortion occurs within 48 hours of treatment.
- More than 80 days gestation: abortion occurs 2 to 7 days after series of injections.

Mechanical Disruption of the Pregnancy

- Per rectum manual rupture (crushing) of the embryonic vesicle is possible up to 25 days gestation.

- Uterine flushing may result in abortion of an early pregnancy if done before the placenta is established.
- Transvaginal U/S-guided aspiration or injection of the conceptus is possible in the first 45 days of pregnancy.
- Per vagina manual cervical dilation and disruption of the uteroplacental unit (CA at the cervical star) is appropriate for terminating a gestation of more than 100 days.
- Transcutaneous abdominal intrafetal injection of procaine G penicillin.
- Surgical disruption (cervical dislocation of the fetus).
  - Not a common procedure for elective termination of pregnancy.

Induction of Uterine Contractions

- Uterine contractions may be induced with a series of injections of $PGF_2\alpha$ or one of its analogues, or oxytocin.
  - Treatment should not be instituted before manual cervical dilation has been achieved.

Systems Affected

Reproductive

 # SIGNALMENT/HISTORY

- Pregnancy diagnosis
- Abnormal pregnancies (e.g., twins, fetal hydrops: hydrops amnion or hydrops allantois).
- Health concerns for the dam
  Elective termination of pregnancy is indicated for medical or management reasons.
- Medical reasons include:
  - Compromised health of the mare or fetus
  - Twin pregnancies
  - Fetal hydrops
  - Rupture of the ventral abdominal wall
  - Herniation
  - Severe lameness
  - Respiratory or cardiac compromise
  - Chronic renal failure
  - Liver failure
- Management reasons include:
  - A mare bred to the wrong stallion (mismating)
  - Genetic fault or concern

CLINICAL FEATURES

- Sweating, colicky signs after treatment has begun.
- Vaginal discharge or presence of fetal membranes at the vulva.
- Presence of fetal membranes or fetus in the vagina.

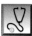

DIFFERENTIAL DIAGNOSIS

Spontaneous abortion (*see* also Infectious and Noninfectious Abortion).

DIAGNOSTICS

CBC/Biochemistry/Urinalysis

Unremarkable, unless complications develop due to dystocia, RFM, or retained fetus.

Other Laboratory Tests

Hormonal assays

Imaging

- Transrectal or transabdominal U/S to determine stage of pregnancy and to monitor progress of abortion.
- Hysteroscopy: to determine if fetal parts are present in the uterus or to identify endometrial cups.

THERAPEUTICS

Drug(s) of Choice

$PGF_2\alpha$ or its analogues, early in pregnancy.
- Single injection of dinoprost tromethamine (5 to 10 mg, IM only) or cloprostenol (250 to 500 µg, IM only) will reliably induce abortion in the first 35 days of gestation.
- Daily (multiple) injections of dinoprost tromethamine (5 mg, IM) or cloprostenol (100 to 250 µg, IM) may be necessary if 40 to 120 days gestation.
- Mid- to late-term pregnant mares may require higher doses of $PGF_2\alpha$ (1 mg/45 kg body weight).
- Late-term mares may respond to oxytocin (20 to 40 IU) after manual dilation of the cervix, but fetal malpresentation is a common complication (*see* Induction of Parturition).
- Intracervical application of PGE_2 may facilitate cervical dilation.

Appropriate Health Care

- Monitor mare for overt reaction to $PGF_2\alpha$.
- Monitor progress of abortion by U/S.
- Hysteroscopy: to determine if fetal parts are present in the uterus or to identify endometrial cups.
- Monitor mare for complications following abortion: RFM, uterine infection.
  - Treat accordingly: refer to RFM, endometritis, metritis.

Nursing Care

Depends on reason for induction of abortion and postabortion complications.

 COMMENTS

Client Education

- Proper management of mares to avoid twin pregnancies.
- Avoid accidental mating

Patient Monitoring

- Mares should be monitored until the fetus and placenta are delivered.
- U/S and vaginal examination.

Prevention/Avoidance

- Client education
- Mare evaluation before breeding

Possible Complications

- Mares with severely compromised respiratory system.
- Mares with acute abdominal pain.
- Delayed return to cyclicity or extended anestrus, if abortion is induced after endometrial cups have formed.
- Fetal mummification or maceration, if it is not eliminated after its death or the induction of abortion treatment.
- Uterine infection
- Cervical injury may be caused by aggressive manual dilation.
- Late-term induction of abortion increases the risk for dystocia and RFM.

Expected Course and Prognosis

- Good for early termination of pregnancy (gestation of less than 100 days).
- Fair to good for later-term termination of pregnancy.
- Guarded, if late-term termination of pregnancy (induction of abortion) was in response to concerns for the dam's health or because of fetal abnormalities.

Abbreviations

CA   chorioallantois
CBC   complete blood count
CL   corpus luteum
IM   intramuscular
PGE_2 prostaglandin E2
$PGF_2\alpha$ natural prostaglandin
RFM   retained fetal membranes, retained placenta
U/S   ultrasound, ultrasonography

Suggested Reading

Penzhorn BL, Bertschinger HJ, Coubrough RI. 1986. Reconception of mares following termination of pregnancy with prostaglandin F2α before and after day 35 of pregnancy. *Eq Vet J* 18: 215–217.
Volkmann DH, Bertschinger HJ, Schulman ML. 1995. The effect of prostaglandin E$_{(2)}$ on the cervices of dioestrous and prepartum mares. *Reproduction in Domestic Animals* 30: 240–244.
Volkman DH, DeCramer KGM. 1991. PGE$_2$ as an adjunct to the induction of abortion in mares. *J Reprod and Fert* (Supplement 44): 722–723.

Author: Ahmed Tibary

Abortion, Spontaneous, Infectious

DEFINITION/OVERVIEW

Fetal loss after 40 days of gestation (term *stillbirth* may apply at greater than 300 days) involving maternal, placental, or fetal invasion by microorganisms.

ETIOLOGY/PATHOPHYSIOLOGY

- Approximately 5% to 15% of abortions are infectious in nature.
- Abortion *storms* can occur, especially with EHV or in instances of MRLS when caterpillar populations are greatly increased.
- Spontaneous, infectious abortions can involve viruses, bacteria, Rickettsial organisms, protozoa, fungi, and in the case of MRLS, penetrating caterpillar setae contaminated with microorganisms, primarily bacteria.

Etiology

Some of the specific microorganisms associated with spontaneous, infectious equine abortions are listed here:

Viruses

- EHV-1 (1P and 1B strains); EHV-4; rarely EHV-2 (EHV abortions generally occur late in gestation; at more than 7 months).
- EVA (more than 3 months of gestation)
- EIA (direct causal relationship not yet established).
- Vesivirus (recent correlation between antibodies of vesivirus and equine abortions).

Bacteria

- Placentitis (Fig. 3.1) and possible, subsequent fetal infection by *Streptococcus* sp., *Actinobacillus* sp., *Escherichia coli*, *Pseudomonas* sp., *Klebsiella* sp., *Staphylococcus* sp., *Nocardioform actinomycetes*, such as *Amycolatopsis* sp., *Cellulosimicrobium* sp., *Crossiella* sp., and *Rhodococcus* sp. (Fig. 3.2), *Taylorella equigenitalis* (rare, reportable), and *Leptospira* serovars.

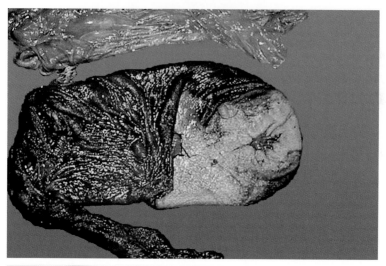

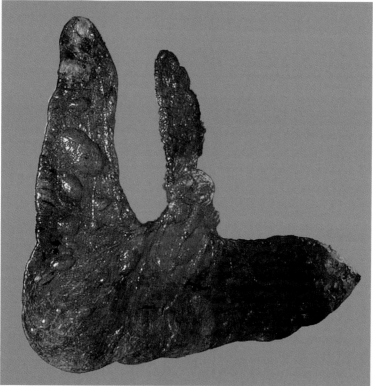

■ **Figure 3.1** Gross appearances of ascending placentitis *(top)* and nocardioform placentitis *(bottom)*. Images courtesy of D. Volkmann.

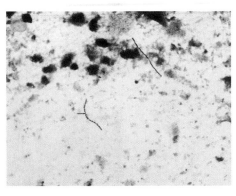 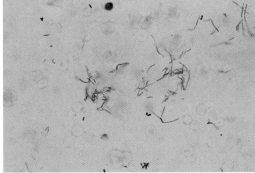

■ **Figure 3.2** Cytological appearance of nocardioform actinomycetes stained with Diff-Quick stain *(left)* and Gram stain *(right)*.
Images courtesy of D. Volkmann.

- Endotoxemia causes release of $PGF_2\alpha$ (especially at less than 80 days of gestation [day 60 in many mares]; may be a factor later in gestation, if there is repeated exposure).

Rickettsiae

- *Ehrlichia risticii* (PHF)
- Fungi
- Placentitis caused by *Aspergillus* sp., *Candida* sp., or *Histoplasma capsulatum*
- Protozoa
- Sarcocystis neurona or, possibly, *Neospora* sp. in aborted fetuses from mares affected by EPM.

MRLS

- Although generally only a major concern in years when caterpillar populations are greatly increased, the geographical distribution, financial impact, and unusual pathogenesis of this syndrome make it a topic worthy of discussion.
- Early (approximately 40–150 days of gestation) and late (more than 269 days of gestation) abortion syndromes.
- Associated with greatly increased populations of ETCs (Fig. 3.3).
- Oral exposure to ETC setae in conjunction with MRLS, which is currently theorized to be associated with microscopic bowel puncture and bacteremic spread to fetus or placenta (*see* penetrating septic setal emboli hypothesis in this chapter).

Pathophysiology

Depending on the specific infectious cause, the mechanisms of spontaneous infectious, abortions can involve the sequence of events outlined here:
- Fetal death by microorganisms.
- Fetal expulsion after placental infection, insufficiency, or separation.

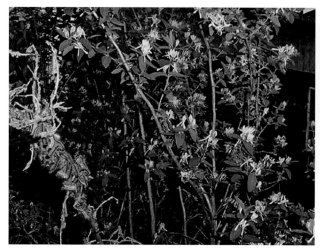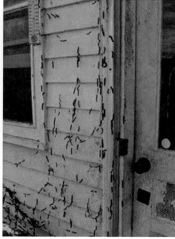

■ **Figure 3.3** Eastern tent caterpillars *(Malacosoma americanum)* observed on vegetation and buildings in central Kentucky.
Images courtesy of H. Q. Murphy.

- Premature parturition induced by microbial toxins, fetal stress, or a combination of mechanisms.
- Final result: Fetal death followed by absorption, maceration, or autolysis; fetal death during the stress of delivery (stillbirth) or birth of a live fetus incapable of extrauterine survival.
- Although some have suggested a caterpillar toxin-associated cause for the 2001 outbreak of MRLS in central Kentucky and surrounding areas, a unique pathogenesis for MRLS, involving *septic penetrating setal emboli*, has been proposed by Dr. Tom Tobin and his colleagues from the University of Kentucky, based on epidemiological and experimental data. This novel hypothesis requires the ingestion of ETC by pregnant mares and the subsequent penetration of the intestinal mucosa by bacteria-contaminated, barbed caterpillar setae, as well as their fragments, which migrate in blood vessels as *septic setal emboli* and are deposited in vascular, immunologically susceptible targets, such as the early and late-term fetus and placenta.

Systems Affected

- Reproductive
- Other organ systems can be affected if there is systemic maternal disease.

    SIGNALMENT/HISTORY

Risk Factors

- Pregnant mares intermixed with young horses or horses-in-training are susceptible to EHV-1, EVA, or *E. risticii*.

- Immunologically naïve mares brought to premises with enzootic EHV-1, EVA, *E. risticii*, or *Leptospira* infections.
- Pregnant mares traveling to horse shows or competitions.
- Poor perineal conformation predisposes mares to ascending bacterial or fungal placentitis and, possibly, subsequent fetal infection.
- Concurrent maternal GI disease or EPM.
- Large numbers ETCs in pastures with pregnant mares.
- Geographical location with respect to MRLS and nocardioform placentitis.

Historical Findings

One or more of the following:
- Vaginal discharge, which can potentially be mucopurulent, hemorrhagic, or serosanguineous.
- Premature udder development with dripping milk.
- Anorexia or colic; GI disease.
- Failure to deliver on expected due date.
- *Recent* (1–16 weeks before presentation) systemic infectious disease or, similarly, recent introduction of infected carrier horses to the premises.
- Other, recently aborting, mares.
- Inadequate EHV-1 prophylaxis.
- History of placentitis.
- Previous endometrial biopsy with moderate or severe endometritis or fibrosis.
- None or excessive abdominal distention consistent with gestation length.
- Behavioral estrus in a pregnant mare, which might be normal, depending on gestation length, time of year, gestation length at time of loss.
- Climactic and environmental conditions favoring increased populations of ETC (*Malacosoma americanum*) and development of MRLS in early and late pregnant mares (Fig. 3.3).
- Possibly geographical location if suspect MRLS and nocardioform placentitits.

 CLINICAL FEATURES

- Early pregnancy loss is frequently unobserved and is described as *asymptomatic*.
- Unless complications occur, abortion may occur rapidly, with the sole sign being a relatively normal, previously pregnant mare later found open.
- Signs range from none to multisystemic and life-threatening, especially if dystocia occurs during delivery or if maternal organs are infected.
- Depending on microorganisms involved, multiple animals can be affected.
- Most *symptomatic* spontaneous infectious abortions occur during the second half of gestation and are characterized by one or more of the following findings on physical examination:
  - Fetal parts and membranes protruding through vulvar lips; abdominal straining or discomfort.

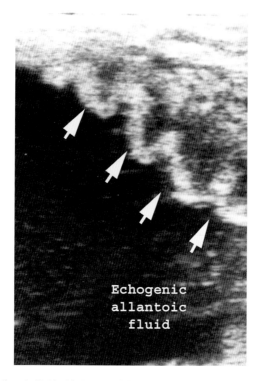

■ Figure 3.4 Echogenic allantoic fluid with increased thickness and possible detachment of the chorioallantoic membrane (arrows) associated with MRLS.
(Image courtesy of D. Volkmann).

- Premature placental separation (*red bag*).
- Vulvar discharge (variable appearance), premature udder development, dripping milk.
- A previously documented pregnancy is not detected at the next examination.
- Evidence of fetal death by palpation, transrectal or transabdominal U/S.
- Anorexia, fever, signs of concurrent systemic disease, especially with endotoxemia, dystocia, or RFM.
- Evidence of placental separation or echogenic allantoic fluid, especially in association with MRLS (Fig. 3.4), as observed using transrectal or transabdominal U/S.

DIFFERENTIAL DIAGNOSIS

Other Causes of Abortion (Spontaneous, Noninfectious)

- Twinning
- Fetal abnormalities, teratogenesis
- Umbilical cord abnormalities with excessive twisting and thrombosis
- Placental pathology

- Maternal malnutrition or other noninfectious systemic disease
- Old mare, history of EED or abortion
- Old mare, poor endometrial biopsy (inflammation or fibrosis)
- Maternal exposure to endophyte-infected tall fescue pasture, exposure to ergotized grasses, small cereal grains during last month of gestation with no mammary development (agalactia, if term is reached)
- Maternal exposure to phytoestrogens
- Maternal exposure to other xenobiotics
- Iatrogenic or inappropriately timed induction of labor

Other Causes Signs of Labor or Abdominal Discomfort

- Normal parturition
- Dystocia unassociated with abortion
- Prepartum uterine artery rupture
- Colic associated with uterine torsion
- Discomfort associated with hydrops of fetal membranes or prepubic tendon rupture
- Colic unassociated with reproductive disease

Other Causes of Vulvar Discharge

- Normal parturition
- Dystocia unassociated with abortion
- Normal estrus
- Endometritis
- Metritis or partial RFM
- Mucometra or pyometra

DIAGNOSTICS

- Except for placentitis, abortions secondary to endotoxemia, and fetal expulsion associated with dystocia, most abortions are *asymptomatic*. The expelled fetus and fetal membranes vary in condition from intact to autolytic in appearance.
- Definitive causative diagnosis of equine abortion is determined in approximately 50% to 60% of all cases.
- Excluding twins and EHV-1, the diagnostic rate may approach only 30%, especially if limited samples are submitted and are accompanied by moderate to severe fetal and placental autolysis with environmental contamination.
- Laboratory testing to determine the cause of a spontaneous, potentially infectious abortion includes the following procedures:
  - CBC with differential, as well as serum biochemical data to determine inflammatory or stress leukocyte response, as well as other organ system involvement.
  - With suspected endotoxemia, a maternal progesterone assay is indicated if the pregnancy is at risk prior to the determination of an infectious cause of an

impending abortion. ELISA or RIA analyses for progesterone may be useful at less than 80 days of gestation (normal levels vary from greater than 1 to greater than 4 ng/mL, depending on the reference laboratory). At more than 100 days gestation, RIA detects both progesterone (very low if more than day 150) and cross-reacting 5α-pregnanes of uterofetoplacental origin. Acceptable levels of 5α-pregnanes vary with stage of gestation and the laboratory used.

- A uterine swab from the mare may provide a useful sample for culture and cyto-logical examination and aid in establishing a diagnosis of abortion caused by placentitis.
- Analyses for other maternal hormones can also be performed (*see* Abortion, Spontaneous, Noninfectious).
- Maternal serological testing can be useful in the diagnosis of infectious abortion (diagnostic for abortions by *Leptospira* serovars; confirms EVA abortion). Serum samples should be collected in all cases of abortion in which cause is unknown (a paired sample collected 21 days later might be indicated).
- Imaging (transrectal and transabdominal) U/S can be used to evaluate fetal viabil-ity, placentitis, and alterations in the appearance of amniotic or allantoic fluids (*see* Fig. 3.4), as well as other gestational abnormalities.
- The following samples should collected from the fetus and the fetal membranes for histopathologic and cytological evaluations, as well as microbiological, serological, and molecular testing procedures:
  - If available, fresh/chilled fetal thoracic or abdominal fluid and serum from the fetal heart or cord blood.
  - Fetal stomach contents.
  - Ten percent formalin-fixed and chilled/frozen samples of fetal membranes (chorioallantois/allantochorion; amnion/allantoamnion), fetal heart, lung, thymus, liver, kidney, lymph nodes, thymus, spleen, adrenal, skeletal muscle, and brain.
  - Stained cytological smears collected from fetal membranes can be useful in diag-nosing some specific causes of infectious abortions (*see* Fig. 3.2).
  - Selected viral infections can be diagnosed using PCR and other molecular analyses of various biological samples.

Pathological Findings

Viruses

EHV

- Gross pleural effusion, ascites, fetal icterus, pulmonary congestion and edema; 1-mm, yellowish-white spots on enlarged liver; relatively fresh fetus.
- Histopathologic findings for EHV-1 and EHV-4 include: areas of necrosis, prominent, eosinophilic, intranuclear inclusion bodies in lymphoid tissue, liver, adrenal cortex, and lung, as well as a hyperplastic, necrotizing bronchiolitis.
- FA staining of fetal tissues.
- Virus isolation from aborted fetus.

EVA

- Few gross lesions
- Autolyzed fetus
- Placental/fetal vascular lesions

Vesivirus

- Nonspecific lesions

Bacteria and Fungi

Fetal Infection and Placentitis

- Gross pleural effusion, ascites with enlarged liver; rare plaques of mycotic dermatitis; placental edema and thickening with fibro-necrotic exudate on the chorionic surface (*see* Fig. 3.1), especially at *cervical star* in fungal infections.
- Histopathologic evidence of inflammatory disease; autolysis may make interpretation difficult.
- Leptospirosis
- Gross fetal icterus and autolysis.
- Nonspecific histologic changes; mild, diffuse placentitis.

Endotoxemia

- Fetus minimally autolyzed.

Rickettsiae

E. RISTICII

- Gross placentitis
- Typical histopathologic findings include colitis, periportal hepatitis, lymphoid hyperplasia, and necrosis.

Protozoa

- There are reports of sarcocystis neurona-associated abortions in EPM positive mares.

MRLS

- Histopathologic findings similar to bacterial infections.

 THERAPEUTICS

Drug(s) of Choice

- Altrenogest administered 0.044 to 0.088 mg/kg PO daily can be started later during gestation, continued longer, or used only for short periods of time, depending on serum progesterone levels during the first 80 days of gestation, clinical circumstances, risk factors, clinician preference. **NOTE:** Serum levels reflect only endogenous progesterone, not the exogenous, oral product.

- If near term, altrenogest frequently is discontinued 7 to 14 days before the foaling date unless indicated otherwise by fetal maturity/viability or the actual gestational age is in question.

Precautions/Interactions

- Altrenogest is only used to prevent abortion in cases of endotoxemia or placentitis (more than 270 days of gestation) if the fetus is viable.
- Altrenogest is absorbed through skin; wear gloves and wash hands.

Alternative Drugs

- Injectable progesterone (150–500 mg oil base) IM.
- Newer, repository forms of progesterone are occasionally introduced; however, some evidence of efficacy should be provided prior to use.

Appropriate Health Care

- Except late-gestational placentitis (more than 270 days) and endotoxemia, no therapy is indicated to preserve fetal viability with spontaneous, infectious abortion.
- For mares that abort, there is only prophylactic therapy for metritis or endometritis.
- Therapy is generally limited to intrauterine lavage with or without antibacterial therapy but might include a systemic component consisting of antibiotics, NSAIDs, or intravenous fluids, especially if septicemia, endotoxemia, or laminitis is suspected.
- Preexisting GI disease and complications, such as laminitis, may warrant hospitalization and intensive care.

Nursing Care

- Most affected horses require limited nursing care, except in instances of endotoxemia and gram-negative septicemia, dystocia, RFM, metritis, and laminitis.

Diet

- Feed and water intake, as well defecation and urination should be monitored, but no particular dietary changes should take place in the absence of GI disease or laminitis.

Activity

- There should be paddock exercise to permit observation, but this recommendation is subject to change if the mare exhibits clinical signs of laminitis.

Surgical Considerations

- Only indicated in instances of dystocia or GI disease requiring surgical intervention.

COMMENTS

Client Education

Inform owners of possible complications of abortion.

Patient Monitoring

- At 7 to 10 days post-abortion, TRP and U/S to monitor uterine involution
- Observation for any signs of systemic disease and laminitis.
- Assess genital tract health using vaginal speculum, uterine culture and cytology, and endometrial biopsy.
- Base treatment on clinical results.
- Uterine culture less than 14 days postpartum or post-abortion is affected by contamination of the uterus at the time of parturition (abortion).

Prevention/Avoidance

Vaccines

- A killed-virus EHV-1p and 1b vaccine, at 5, 7, and 9 months of gestation (some recommend vaccination at 3 months of gestation, as well); approved for abortion prevention in pregnant mares; 2-month interval due to short-lived vaccinal immunity.
- Other EHV vaccines have been used off-label for abortion prevention, and there are anecdotal reports of their efficacy for this purpose.
- EVA vaccine is not specifically labeled for abortion prevention It is a MLV, which should only be administered to open mares 3 weeks before anticipated exposure to infected semen or in enzootic conditions. First-time vaccinated mares should be isolated for 3 weeks after exposure to infected semen. **NOTE**: Some countries forbid importation of horses with titers to EVA.

Additional Prophylactic Steps

- Segregate pregnant mares from horses susceptible or exposed to infections.
- Isolate immunologically naïve individuals until immunity to enzootic infections is established or enhanced. Depending on the infectious agent, protection may only be accomplished postpartum.
- Limit transport of pregnant mares to exhibitions or competitions.
- Use appropriate biosecurity protocols and isolate aborting mares with proper disposal of contaminated fetal tissues.

- Proper diagnostics to identify an infectious cause of abortion.
- Correct poor perineal conformation, prevent placentitis.
- Prevent pregnant mare exposure to ETCs until 7 to 8 weeks after ETC death.
- Insecticides to control ETCs; consider toxicity of insecticide.

Possible Complications

Future fertility and reproductive value can be impaired by dystocia, RFM, endometritis, laminitis, septicemia, or trauma to genital tract.

Expected Course and Prognosis

- Most patients recover with appropriate treatment.
- Complications can involve significant impact on mare's survivability and her future fertility. Prognosis is guarded for pregnancy maintenance with endotoxemia and placentitis.

Synonyms and Closely Related Conditions

- Abortion
- Spontaneous abortion
- Infectious abortion
- Bacterial abortion
- Viral abortion
- Fungal abortion
- Mycotic abortion
- Protozoal abortion
- Rickettsial abortion

Abbreviations

CBC	complete blood count
EED	early embryonic death
EHV	equine herpes virus
EIA	equine infectious anemia
ELISA	enzyme-linked immunosorbent assay
EPM	equine protozoal encephalomyelitis
ETC	eastern tent caterpillar
EVA	equine viral arteritis
FA	fluorescent antibody
GI	gastrointestinal
IM	intramuscular
MRLS	mare reproductive loss syndrome
NSAIDS	nonsteroidal anti-inflammatory drugs
PCR	polymerase chain reaction
PHF	Potomac horse fever

PO   per os (by mouth)
RIA   radioimmunoassay
RFM   retained fetal membranes/placenta
TRP   transrectal palpation
U/S   ultrasound, ultrasonography

See Also

- Abortion, spontaneous, noninfectious
- Dystocia
- Endometrial biopsy
- Endometritis
- Fetal stress/viability
- High-risk pregnancy
- Metritis
- Placental insufficiency
- Placentitis
- Premature placental separation
- RFM

Suggested Reading

Christensen BW, Roberts JF, Pozor MA, et al. 2006. Nocardioform placentitis with isolation of Amycolatopsis spp in Florida-bred mare. *JAVMA* 228: 1234–1239.

Gluck Equine Research Center. Mare reproductive loss syndrome (MRLS). Available at: www.ca.uky.edu/gluck/MRLSindex.asp.

Kurth A, Skilling DE, Smith AW. 2006. Serologic evidence of vesivirus-specific antibodies associated with abortion in horses. *AJVR* 67: 1033–1039.

Tobin T, Harkins JD, Roberts JF, et al. 2004. The mare reproductive loss syndrome and eastern caterpillar II: a toxicokinetic/clinical evaluation and a proposed pathogenesis: septic penetrating setae. *Intern J Appl Res Vet Med* 2(2): 142–158.

Youngquist RS, Threlfall WR (eds). 2007. *Current Therapy in Large Animal Theriogenology*, 2nd ed. St. Louis: Elsevier-Saunders.

Author: Tim J. Evans

Abortion, Spontaneous, Noninfectious

chapter 4

DEFINITION/OVERVIEW

Fetal loss greater than 40 days (term *stillbirth* may apply if more than 300 days) associated with a variety of noninfectious conditions.

ETIOLOGY/PATHOPHYSIOLOGY

- Approximately 85% to 95% of abortions are noninfectious in nature.
- Some of the specific etiologies associated with spontaneous, noninfectious equine abortions are listed here.

Twins

For twin pregnancies that persist longer than 40 days, approximately 70% end in abortion/stillbirth (Fig. 4.1).

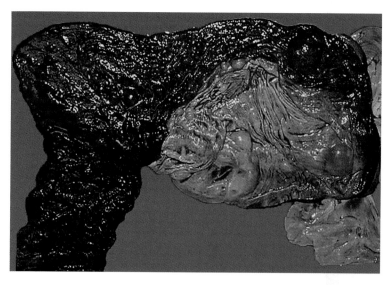

■ **Figure 4.1** Gross appearance of the avillous chorionic membrane at the point of contact between the fetal membranes of aborted twins.
Image courtesy of D. Volkmann.

Luteal Insufficiency/Early CL Regression

- Anecdotal, and somewhat controversial.
- Caused by decreased levels of luteal progesterone at fewer than 80 days of gestation.

Placental Abnormalities

- Although twists in the umbilical cord are normal, umbilical cord torsion, as evidenced by vascular compromise (e.g., cord thrombus,) can be associated with abortion
- Torsion of the amnion (Fig. 4.2)
- Long umbilical cord/cervical pole ischemia disorder
- Confirmed body pregnancy (Fig. 4.3)
- Placental separation.
- Villous atrophy, hypoplasia, or placental insufficiency (can also be associated with prolonged gestation)
- Hydrops

Fetal Abnormalities

- Developmental abnormalities, such as hydrocephalus (Fig. 4.4) or anencephaly
- Fetal trauma
- Chromosomal abnormalities

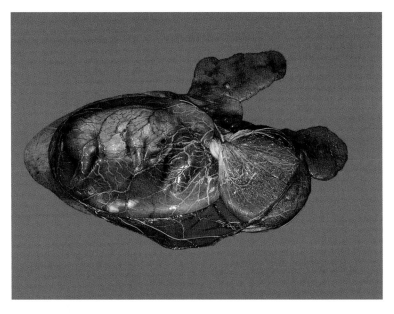

■ **Figure 4.2** Gross appearance of an amniotic torsion, which resulted in an abortion. Image courtesy of D. Volkmann.

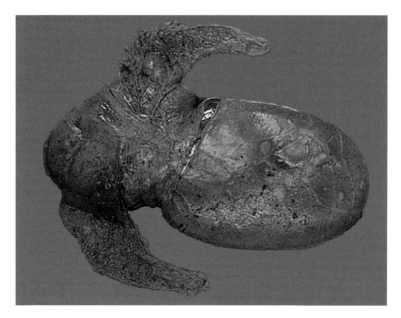

■ **Figure 4.3** Gross appearance of a body pregnancy, which resulted in placental insufficiency and subsequent abortion.
Image courtesy of D. Volkmann.

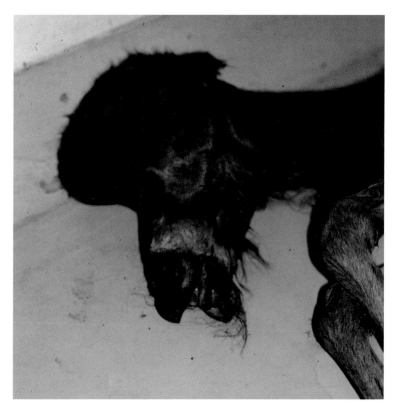

■ **Figure 4.4** Gross appearance of hydrocephalus in a neonate delivered at term.
Image courtesy of C. L. Carleton.

Maternal Abnormalities

- Concurrent maternal disease, maternal stress
- Trauma as related to maternal pain/stress
- Malnutrition, starvation; selenium deficiency
- Anecdotal reports of severe maternal anxiety are anecdotal
- Moderate to severe endometritis or endometrial periglandular fibrosis (*see* EED)
- Endometrial cysts, although this is subject to debate within the literature (*see* EED)
- Maternal chromosomal abnormalities

Xenobiotics

- Ergopeptine alkaloids associated with fescue toxicosis or ergotism can be associated with placental thickening and abortion, although prolonged gestation is more common (*see* Fetal Stress/Viability).
- Phytoestrogens have been associated with anecdotal instances of abortions in early spring
- Xenobiotics causing maternal disease, such as cardiac glycosides, taxine alkaloids, carbamates, organophosphates
- Xenobiotics causing placental or fetal disease were originally suspected with respect to MRLS, but this explanation is considered much less likely at the present time because of the *penetrating septic setal emboli* hypothesis (*see* Abortion, Spontaneous, Infectious).
- Possible deleterious effects of medications, such as EPM therapies, on pregnancy
- Repeated large doses of corticosteroids during late gestation

Iatrogenic Causes

- $PGF_2\alpha$ may require repeated injections if more than 40 days of gestation
- Procedures mistakenly done on a pregnant mare, such as AI, intrauterine infusions, samples taken for cytology, culture, or biopsy

Pathophysiology

Depending on the specific noninfectious cause, the pathophysiological mechanisms of spontaneous, noninfectious, abortions can involve the sequence of events outlined here:
- Fetal death/premature parturition from some intrinsic structural or functional defect or exposure to xenobiotics.
- Fetal expulsion at less than 80 days of gestation after CL loss as a result of endometritis or other factors.
- Fetal death or expulsion by placental insufficiency or separation.
- Fetal stress, dead twin fetus, maternal stress, or combination.
- Fetal reabsorption, maceration, mummification, autolysis, death during delivery (*stillbirth*) or delivery of live fetus incapable of extrauterine survival.

Systems Affected

- Reproductive
- Other organ systems can be affected if there is maternal systemic disease.

SIGNALMENT/HISTORY

Risk Factors

- Often nonspecific
- Manipulations of the cervix or perforation of the placental barrier
- Previous history of twins or abortion
- Family history of twinning or noninfectious spontaneous abortion
- Breeds, including Thoroughbred, draft mares, Standardbreds and related breeds predisposed to double ovulations, which can lead to twinning
- Maiden or barren mares which are also prone to double ovulations and twinning
- Mares more than 15 years old, especially those with endometrial periglandular fibrosis or endometriosis and, possibly, those with large numbers of endometrial cysts
- There are anecdotal reports of placental insufficiency in maiden American Miniature Horse mares
- Concurrent maternal disease
- Grazing endophyte-infected fescue pasture, ergotized grasses or grains, or plants producing phytoestrogens (anecdotal) late in gestation
- Exposure to xenobiotics
- Geographical location with respect to consumption of endophyte-infected fescue or ergotized grasses or grains

Historical Findings

One or more of the following:
- Signs consistent with labor at an unexpected stage of gestation
- Dystocia, birth of nonviable foal
- Previous history of abortion, dystocia, or birth of a nonviable foal
- Vaginal discharge, which is generally mucoid, hemorrhagic, or serosanguineous
- Premature udder development; dripping milk
- Anorexia or colic
- *Recent* systemic disease
- Moderate/severe endometritis or endometrial periglandular fibrosis
- Failure to deliver on expected due date
- None or excessive abdominal distention consistent with stage of gestation
- Behavioral estrus in pregnant mare, which might be normal for stage of gestation and is dependent on time of year and stage of pregnancy when the pregnancy is lost
- Geographical location, especially with relation to endophyte-infected fescue pastures, hay, or ergotized grasses or grains

CLINICAL FEATURES

- Depends on the cause, time of fetal death, stage of gestation, duration of the condition, and whether the pregnancy ended in dystocia or with RFM.
- Unless complications occur, abortion may occur rapidly, with the sole sign being a relatively normal, previously pregnant mare later found open.
- Signs range from none to multisystemic and life-threatening disease, especially if dystocia occurs during delivery, or if maternal organs are infected.
- Most *symptomatic*, spontaneous, noninfectious abortions occur during the second half of gestation and are characterized by one or more of the following findings on physical examination:
    - Fetal or placental structures protruding through vulvar lips; abdominal straining or discomfort
    - Premature placental separation (*red bag*)
    - Vulvar discharge (variable appearance), premature udder development, dripping milk
    - Previously diagnosed pregnancy is absent at the next examination; fetal death determined by TRP or transrectal or transabdominal U/S
    - Twin fetuses identified by TRP or transrectal or transabdominal U/S.
    - Evidence of placental separation or hydrops of fetal membranes during transrectal or transabdominal U/S.
    - Signs of concurrent, systemic disease, dystocia, or RFM.
    - NOTE: Signs are extremely variable. Mares pregnant at early check can remain *asymptomatic* but abort. Abortion can be unobserved early in gestation and may be rapid and without signs.

 DIFFERENTIAL DIAGNOSIS

Other Causes of Abortion

- Infectious, spontaneous abortion
- Placentitis, as determined by physical examination or by laboratory diagnostic procedures

Other Causes of Signs of Labor or Abdominal Discomfort

- Normal parturition
- Dystocia unassociated with abortion
- Prepartum uterine artery rupture
- Colic associated with uterine torsion
- Discomfort associated with hydrops of fetal membranes or prepubic tendon rupture
- Colic unassociated with reproductive disease

Other Causes of Vulvar Discharge

- Normal parturition
- Dystocia not associated with abortion
- Normal estrus
- Endometritis
- Metritis or RFM
- Mucometra or pyometra

 DIAGNOSTICS

- Except for placentitis, abortions secondary to endotoxemia, and fetal expulsion associated with twins or dystocia, most abortions are *asymptomatic*. The expelled fetus and fetal membranes vary in condition from intact to autolytic in appearance.
- Definitive causative diagnosis of equine abortion occurs in approximately 50% to 60% of all cases.
- Excluding twins and EHV-1, the diagnostic rate may approach only 30%, especially if limited samples are submitted and are accompanied by moderate to severe fetal and placental autolysis with environmental contamination.
- NOTE: Unless the cause of the abortion is obvious, such as twins or iatrogenic, it is necessary to rule out infectious causes of abortion, especially if multiple mares are affected or at risk (*see* Abortion, Spontaneous, Infectious).

Laboratory testing for specific causes of a spontaneous, noninfectious abortion includes the following procedures:

- CBC with differential, as well as serum biochemical data to determine inflammatory or stress leukocyte response, as well as other organ system involvement.
- ELISA or RIA analyses for maternal progesterone may be useful at less than 80 days of gestation (normal levels vary from greater than 1 to greater than 4 ng/mL, depending on the reference laboratory). At more than 100 days of gestation, RIA detects both progesterone (*very low* if more than 150 days gestation) and cross-reacting 5α-pregnanes of uterofetoplacental origin. Acceptable levels of 5α-pregnanes vary with stage of gestation and the laboratory used.
- Maternal estrogen concentrations can reflect fetal estrogen production and viability, especially conjugated estrogens (e.g., estrone sulfate).
- Decreased maternal relaxin concentration is thought to be associated with abnormal placental function.
- Decreased maternal prolactin secretion during late gestation is associated with fescue toxicosis and ergotism.
- Anecdotal reports of lower T_3/T_4 levels in mares with history of conception failure, EED, or abortion. The significance of low T_4 levels is unknown and somewhat controversial.
- Cytogenetic studies can be useful if maternal or fetal chromosomal abnormalities are suspected (difficult to do on the fetus if it is autolyzed).

- Endometrial biopsy procedures might be indicated to assess endometrial inflammation or fibrosis.
- Vaginal speculum examination and hysteroscopy might be indicated if structural abnormalities are suspected in the cervix or uterus.
- Maternal and fetal assays for xenobiotics might be indicated in cases of specific intoxications. Samples of the dam's whole blood, plasma, or urine can be collected and analyzed. Samples of fetal serum (from heart or umbilical blood), thoracic or abdominal fluid, and liver or kidney can also be collected and analyzed. These analyses might be expensive and not productive, if testing is not narrowed down to one or several potential xenobiotics.
- Feed or environmental analyses might be indicated for specific xenobiotics, ergopeptine alkaloids, phytoestrogens, heavy metals, or fescue endophyte (*Neotyphodium coenophialum*).
- Imaging with transrectal and transabdominal U/S can be used to evaluate fetal viability, placentitis, and alterations in appearance of amniotic or allantoic fluids, as well as other gestational abnormalities, such as hydrops.

As mentioned for spontaneous equine infectious abortions, the following samples should be collected from the fetus and the fetal membranes for histopathologic and cytological evaluations, as well as microbiological, serological, and molecular testing procedures:

- If available, fresh/chilled fetal thoracic or abdominal fluid and serum from the fetal heart or cord blood.
- Fetal stomach contents.
- Ten percent formalin-fixed and chilled/frozen samples of fetal membranes (chorioallantois/allantochorion; amnion/allantoamnion), fetal heart, lung, thymus, liver, kidney, lymph nodes, thymus, spleen, adrenal, skeletal muscle, and brain.

Pathological Findings

Twins

- Two fetuses, often dissimilar in size, with one mummified or severely autolytic.
- Avillous chorionic membrane at point of contact between the twins' fetal membranes (*see* Fig. 4.1).

Placental Abnormalities

- Umbilical cord torsion should be confirmed by evidence of vascular compromise
- Torsion of the amnion (*see* Fig. 4.2)
- Confirmation of a body pregnancy (*see* Fig. 4.3)
- Villous atrophy or hypoplasia might suggest endometrial periglandular fibrosis and/or endometrial cysts
- Placental edema, gross and histopathological, is consistent with equine fescue toxicosis (*see* Fetal Stress/Viability)
- Hydrops allantois and amnion can be diagnosed grossly, if the dam suffers prepartum death

Fetal Abnormalities

Developmental abnormalities, such as hydrocephalus (*see* Fig. 4.4) and anencephaly, can be diagnosed by U/S or grossly, with histopathologic confirmation.

 THERAPEUTICS

Drug(s) of Choice

- Altrenogest administered 0.044 to 0.088 mg/kg PO daily, can be started later during gestation, continued longer, or used only for short periods of time, depending on serum progesterone levels during the first 80 days of gestation, clinical circumstances, risk factors, clinician preference. NOTE: Serum levels reflect only endogenous progesterone, not the exogenous, oral product.
- If near term, altrenogest frequently is discontinued 7 to 14 days before foaling date, unless indicated otherwise by fetal maturity/viability, or the actual gestational age is in question.

Precautions/Interactions

- Altrenogest is only used to prevent abortion in cases of endotoxemia or placentitis (more than 270 days of gestation) if the fetus is viable.
- Altrenogest is absorbed through skin; wear gloves and wash hands.

Alternative Drugs

- Injectable progesterone (150–500 mg oil base) IM.
- Newer, repository forms of progesterone are occasionally introduced; however, some evidence of efficacy should be provided prior to use.

Appropriate Health Care

- Except in cases of late-gestational placentitis (more than 270 days gestation) and endotoxemia, no therapy is indicated to preserve fetal viability with spontaneous, infectious abortion.
- For mares which abort, there is only *prophylactic* therapy for metritis or endometritis.
- Therapy is generally limited to intrauterine lavage, with or without antibacterial therapy, but might include a systemic component consisting of antibiotics, NSAIDs, or intravenous fluids, especially if septicemia, endotoxemia, or laminitis are suspected subsequent to the abortion.
- Preexisting GI disease and complications, such as laminitis, might warrant hospitalization and intensive care.

Nursing Care

Affected horses require limited nursing care, except in instances of complications, such as septicemia, dystocia, RFM, metritis, and laminitis.

Diet

Feed and water intake, as well defecation and urination should be monitored, but no particular dietary changes should take place in the absence of GI disease or laminitis.

Activity

There should be paddock exercise to permit observation, but this recommendation is subject to change if the mare exhibits clinical signs of laminitis.

Surgical Considerations

- Generally indicated in instances of dystocia or GI disease requiring surgical intervention.
- Reduction of twin pregnancies can involve surgical approaches for selected fetal decapitation or other means for elimination of one twin.
- Hysteroscopic removal of endometrial cysts to prevent future abortions.

 COMMENTS

Client Education

- The increased survivability of twin foals has led some breeders and even veterinarians to be less concerned about twin pregnancies. However, the risk of abortion, dystocia and neonatal complications associated with twins still warrants prevention or management of this condition and discussion of the inherent risks related to a type of pregnancy ending in abortion or complicated delivery.
- Owners should be educated about the irreversible nature of endometrial periglandular fibrosis and the potential for abortion and neonatal complications.
- Embryo transfer should be discussed for mares with a history of abortion or those with severe endometrial periglandular fibrosis or severe structural abnormalities.
- Inform owners of the possible risks associated with the ingestion of endophyte-infected fescue or ergotized grasses and grains.
- Inform owners of the possible complications of abortion.

Patient Monitoring

- At 7 to 10 days post-abortion, TRP and U/S to monitor uterine involution.
- Observation for any signs of systemic disease and laminitis.
- Assess genital tract health using vaginal speculum, hysteroscopy, uterine culture and cytology, or endometrial biopsy.

- Base treatment on clinical results of these procedures.
- Uterine culture at less than 14 days postpartum or post-abortion is affected/compounded by contamination at the time of parturition (abortion).

Prevention/Avoidance

- Early recognition of at-risk mares.
- Records of double ovulations in prior estrous cycles or breeding seasons.
- Early twin diagnosis (at less than 25 days gestation, perhaps as early as day 14 or 15).
- Selective embryonic or fetal reduction involving transrectal, transvaginal or transabdominal U/S or, potentially, surgery and induced death of one fetus.
- Manage preexisting endometritis before next breeding to minimize inflammation.
- Careful observation of pregnant mares and monitoring of mammary gland development.
- Limit application of nitrogen-containing fertilizer to fescue pastures; mow pastures to remove seed heads.
- Remove mares from fescue pasture during last third of gestation (minimum 30 days prior to foaling date).
- Domperidone (1.1 mg/kg PO daily) at earliest signs of equine fescue toxicosis or 10 to 14 days prior to due date; continue until parturition and development of normal mammary gland is observed.
- Injection with fluphenazine (25 mg IM in pony mares) on day 320 of gestation has been suggested for prophylaxis of fescue toxicosis.
- Careful use of medications in pregnant mares.
- Avoiding exposure to known toxicants.

Possible Complications

- Future fertility and reproductive value can be impaired by dystocia, RFM, endometritis, laminitis, septicemia, or trauma to genital tract.
- Potential complications associated with twin reductions, which increase with duration of pregnancy.

Expected Course and Prognosis

- Most patients recover with appropriate treatment.
- Complications can involve significant impact on mare's survivability and future fertility.
- Prognosis is guarded for pregnancy maintenance with severe endometritis and endometrial periglandular fibrosis.

Synonyms/Closely Related Conditions

- Abortion
- Spontaneous abortion

- Noninfectious abortion
- Twin abortion

Abbreviations

AI   artificial insemination
CBC   complete blood count
CL   corpus luteum
EED   early embryonic death
EHV   equine herpes virus
ELISA   enzyme-linked immunosorbent assay
EPM   equine protozoal encephalomyelitis
GI   gastrointestinal
IM   intramuscular
NSAIDS   nonsteroidal anti-inflammatory drugs
PGF   natural prostaglandin
PO   per os (by mouth)
RIA   radioimmunoassay
RFM   retained fetal membranes/placenta
T3   triiodothyronine
T_4 thyroxine
TRP   transrectal palpation
U/S   ultrasound, ultrasonography

See Also

- Abortion, spontaneous, noninfectious
- Dystocia
- Endometrial biopsy
- Endometritis
- Fetal stress/viability
- High-risk pregnancy
- Metritis
- Placental insufficiency
- Placentitis
- Premature placental separation

Suggested Reading

Bain FT, Wolfsdorf KE. 2003. Placental hydrops. In: *Current Therapy in Equine Medicine 5*. Robinson NE (ed). Philadelphia: Saunders; 301–302.

Ball BA, Daels PF. 1997. Early pregnancy loss in mares: application for progestin therapy. In: *Current Therapy in Equine Medicine 4*. Robinson NE (ed). Philadelphia: WB Saunders; 531–533.

Evans TJ, Rottinghaus GE, Casteel SW. 2003. Ergopeptine alkaloid toxicoses in horses. In: *Current Therapy in Equine Medicine 5*. Robinson NE (ed). Philadelphia: Saunders; 796–798.

Fraser GS. 2003. Twins. In: *Current Therapy in Equine Medicine 5*. Robinson NE (ed). Philadelphia: Saunders; 245–248.

Smith KC, Blunden AS, Whitwell KE, et al. 2003. A survey of equine abortion, stillbirth and neonatal death in the UK from 1988 to 1997. *Equine Vet J* 35: 496–501.

Youngquist RS, Threlfall WR (eds). 2007. *Current Therapy in Large Animal Theriogenology*, 2nd ed. St. Louis: Elsevier-Saunders.

Author: Tim J. Evans

chapter 5

Agalactia/Hypogalactia

DEFINITION/OVERVIEW

Agalactia is the failure of lactation after parturition. Hypogalactia is milk production at volumes less than what is considered normal.

ETIOLOGY/PATHOPHYSIOLOGY

Estrogens produced by the fetoplacental unit in late pregnancy induce the development of mammary ducts, whereas progesterone stimulates lobulo-alveolar growth. Lactogenesis is triggered with the sharp decrease of progesterone and abrupt increase in PRL just prior to parturition. The increase in PRL production by the anterior pituitary gland is made possible by suppression of a PRL inhibitory factor (presumed to be dopamine) and possibly the release of a PRL-releasing factor (proposed to be serotonin) from the hypothalamus. Agalactia/hypogalactia can be the result of interference with these hormonal events (primary endocrinologic disease), a defect in the mammary tissue itself (primary mammary gland disease), or as a result of systemic illness or disease.

Systems Affected

- Reproductive, primary
- Endocrine/metabolic, secondary

SIGNALMENT/HISTORY

There is no age or breed predisposition.

Risk Factors

- Widespread use of tall fescue grass in pasture management in the central and southeastern United States has led to the recognition of "fescue syndrome." The most frequently reported clinical finding in this syndrome is agalactia at the time of parturition. The grazing of endophyte-infected fescue pastures is considered the most likely cause of lactation failure in mares in these areas. *See* Fescue Toxicosis.

- In South America, feeds infected with the fungus *Claviceps purpurea* (ergot) have been implicated as the cause of agalactia in mares.

Historical Findings

- Grazing of endophyte-infected tall fescue pastures or ergot-infected feedstuffs prepartum.
- Prolonged gestation, dystocia, thickened fetal membranes, RFM.
- Agalactia/hypogalactia or mammary gland disease at previous parturition.
- Clinical manifestations of systemic disease or known exposure to infectious disease.

 # CLINICAL FEATURES

- Weak or septicemic foals due to FPT or inadequate nutrition.
- A flaccid udder and secretion of a clear or thick, yellow-tinged fluid from the teats.
- Mastitis results in a swollen, painful udder that is warm to the touch, and secretion of visibly or microscopically abnormal milk.
- In the case of mammary abscessation or neoplasia, distinct masses may be palpable.

 # DIFFERENTIAL DIAGNOSIS

- Agalactia must be differentiated from the refusal of nursing associated with mare anxiety, pain, or udder edema. Direct physical examination of the udder and its secretions and observation of the interaction between mare and foal during attempts at nursing should allow differentiation.
- Failure of milk letdown can occur in mares. Parenteral oxytocin can stimulate milk letdown but does not stimulate milk secretion.
- Any debilitating systemic disease or stress-producing disorder, including malnutrition or nutritional deficiencies, may contribute to agalactia/hypogalactia; such disorders should be apparent upon physical examination.
- Mastitis, mammary fibrosis, neoplasia, abscessation, or traumatic injury and systemic illness should be apparent on physical examination and may contribute to agalactia/hypogalactia.
- A history of fescue ingestion, prolonged gestation, dystocia, RFM, thickened fetal membranes, and a weak, dysmature foal with agalactia is indicative of fescue syndrome. Ingestion of tall fescue grass infected with *Neotyphodium coenophialum* (formerly *Acremonium coenophialum*), an ergot alkaloid-producing fungus, or feedstuffs infected with *Claviceps purpurea* sclerotia, depress PRL secretion because they are dopamine DA2 receptor agonists and serotonin antagonists.
- Mid- to late-term abortions and premature births occur prior to the normal and necessary hormonal shifts (including progesterone, estrogen, and PRL) needed for lactation, leaving the mare unable to lactate normally.

DIAGNOSTICS

- Serum PRL levels are decreased in fescue-induced agalactia.
- If mastitis is suspected, cytologic evaluation or microbiologic culture of udder secretions should be conducted.
- If mammary neoplasia is suspected, fine-needle aspirates or biopsy specimens should be acquired and evaluated.

 # THERAPEUTICS

- Nutritional deficiencies or systemic illnesses must be addressed.
- Treat the mare's mastitis by administering lactating cow intramammary infusion products (can be difficult or impossible to deliver treatment through the multiple, smaller mare teat ducts) and systemic antibiotics based on culture/sensitivity results. Frequent stripping of the mammary gland and the use of hot packs or hydrotherapy are essential components of the treatment regimen. *See* Mastitis.
- Foals should be provided nutritional supplementation during periods of agalactia and should be administered plasma transfusions if suffering from FPT.

Drug(s) of Choice

- Domperidone (1.1 mg/kg, PO, SID), a selective DA2 dopamine receptor antagonist, to reverse the effects of fescue ingestion. This drug has not yet received approval from the FDA and is available only as an experimental product. There are no known side effects associated with treating pregnant mares. Ideally begin treatment at least 15 days prepartum and discontinue when or if lactation is observed at foaling. However, if mares are agalactic at foaling and were not treated prior to parturition, initiate treatment at the time of foaling and continue for 5 days or until lactation ensues.
- TRH, 2.0 mg, SC, BID for 5 days, beginning on day 1 postpartum. Increases serum PRL levels in agalactic mares, presumably due to its action as a PRL-release factor.

Alternative Drugs

- Acepromazine maleate (20 mg, IM, TID) has been used to address fescue agalactia for its dopamine antagonistic properties. There is at least one study in which this phenothiazine tranquilizer had no effect on lactation. Sedation is the primary side effect. Not FDA approved for this use.
- Reserpine (0.5 to 2.0 mg, IM, every 48 hours or 0.01 mg/kg, PO, every 24 hours) depletes serotonin, dopamine and norepinephrine in the brain and other tissues. Side effects can include increased GI motility causing profuse diarrhea and sedation. Not FDA approved for this use.

- Sulpiride (3.3 mg/kg, PO, SID) has been used as a dopamine antagonist to treat fescue-induced agalactia. Reported to be less effective than domperidone. Not FDA approved for this use.

  The use of the following drugs has been published, but cannot be recommended at this time:

- Perphenazine has been administered as a dopamine receptor antagonist. Severe side effects (e.g., sweating, colic, hyperesthesia, ataxia, posterior paresis) when used in horses, preclude its use for this condition.
- Metoclopramide has been reportedly used to treat equine agalactia of unknown origin. Significant risk for developing severe CNS side effects occurs when this drug has been used, precluding its use in the horse.

COMMENTS

Patient Monitoring

Most treatments stimulate milk production in 2 to 5 days if they are going to have an effect. In the absence of other related systemic signs, agalactia is not life-threatening. The foal may require intensive medical and nutritional management in cases of prolonged agalactia.

Prevention/Avoidance

- Remove pregnant mares from endophyte-infected fescue pastures at least 30 days, and preferably 60 to 90 days, prior to the expected date of parturition.
- If mares cannot be removed from endophyte-infected fescue pastures, treat mares with domperidone during the last 2 to 4 weeks of pregnancy.

Possible Complications

- Fescue agalactia is associated with prolonged gestation, abortion, dystocia, uterine rupture, thickened placental membranes, red bag, RFM, infertility, prolonged luteal function, EED, and weak and dysmature foals.
- Foals born to mares with hypogalactia or agalactia are at risk for FPT, malnutrition, and starvation.

Abbreviations

BID   twice a day
CNS   central nervous system
EED   early embryonic death
FDA   Food and Drug Administration
FPT   failure of passive transfer
GI   gastrointestinal

IM   intramuscular
PO   per os (by mouth)
PRL   prolactin
RFM   retained fetal membranes, retained placenta
SID   once a day
SC   subcutaneous
TID   three times a day
TRH   thyrotropin releasing hormone

See Also

- Dystocia
- Fescue toxicity
- Mammary gland, normal
- Mammary gland, mastitis
- Mammary gland, lactation
- Prolonged pregnancy
- Retained fetal membranes
- Failure of passive transfer

Suggested Reading

Chavatte P. 1997. Lactation in the mare. *Equine Vet Educ* 9(2): 62–67.

Cross DL. Fescue toxicosis in horses. 1997. In: *Neotyphodium/Grass interactions*. Bacon CW and Hill NS (eds). New York: Plenum Press; 289–309.

Evans TJ, Youngquist RS, Loch WE, Cross DL. 1999. A comparison of the relative efficacies of domperidone and reserpine in treating equine "fescue toxicosis." *Proc AAEP* 45: 207–209.

McCue PM. Lactation. 1993. In: *Equine Reproduction*. McKinnon AO and Voss JL (eds). Philadelphia, Lea & Febiger; 588–595.

Van Camp SD, Stanton MB. 2007. Abnormalities of lactation. In: *Current Therapy in Large Animal Theriogenology*, 2nd ed. Youngquist RS, Threlfall WR (eds). Louis: Saunders Elsevier; 131–134.

Author: Carole C. Miller

chapter 6

Anatomy of the Mare, Reproductive Review

DEFINITION/OVERVIEW

- A review of the normal reproductive anatomy of the mare.
- Knowledge of anatomy of the mare is important for all aspect of clinical examination, obstetrical manipulation in surgical considerations (Figs. 6.1A, 6.1B, and 6.1C).
- Anatomy will be described sequential from the caudal part to the cranial part.

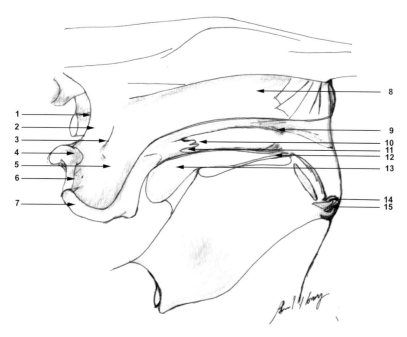

■ **Figure 6.1A** General anatomy of the reproductive tract: 1. suspensory ligament of the ovary; 2. mesovarium (part of the broad ligament); 3. round ligament of the uterus; 4. ovary; 5. mesometrium (part of the broad ligament); 6. mesosalpinx (part of the broad ligament); 7. uterine horn; 8. rectum; 9. vestibulo-vaginal sphincter (vestibular bulb); 10. cervix; 11. fornix; 12. urethral orifice; 13. urinary bladder; 14. clitoris; 15. ventral clitoral fossa.

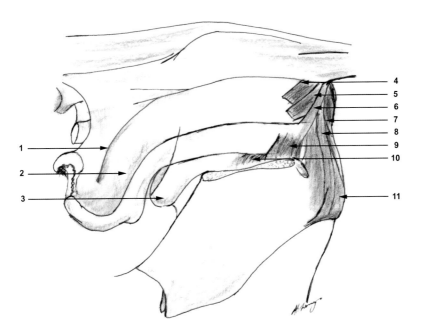

■ **Figure 6.1B** Detailed anatomy of the vulva and vagina: 1. round ligament of the uterus; 2. broad ligament; 3. urinary bladder; 4. coccygeus muscle; 5. levator ani muscle (coccygeal part); 6. levator ani muscle (anal part); 7. external anal sphincter muscle; 8. constrictor vaginae muscle; 9. constrictor vestibulae muscle; 10. urethralis muscle; 11. constrictor vulvae muscle.

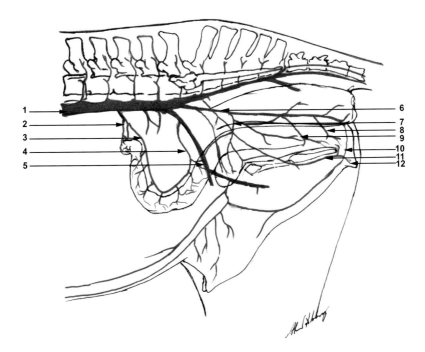

■ **Figure 6.1C** The main blood supply to the mare's genital tract: 1. aorta; 2. ovarian artery; 3. utero-ovarian branch of the ovarian artery; 4. uterine artery (branch of the external iliac artery); 5. external iliac artery; 6. internal pudendal artery; 7. vaginal artery; 8. vestibular bulb artery; 9. vestibular artery; 10. dorsal labial artery; 11. middle clitoral artery; 12. deep clitoral artery.

ETIOLOGY/PATHOPHYSIOLOGY

Systems Affected

- Reproductive

CLINICAL FEATURES

Vulva and perineal area (Figs. 6.2A *and* 6.2B)
- The embryonic origin of the vulvar labia is the urogenital fold.
- The embryonic origin of the clitoris is the phallus.
- The vulva should be located in a vertical alignment with the anal sphincter and is separated from it by the perineal body, which measures 3 to 5 cm.
- The two labia of the vulva form a dorsal pointed commissure and a ventral more rounded commissure.
- The clitoris (clitoral glans) is well-developed and enclosed within the fold of the ventral commissure.
- The clitoral sinus presents a central part (medial clitoral sinus is very deep, 1–1.5 cm) and two shallower lateral parts.
- The musculature is primarily formed by the vulvae constrictor muscle, an extension of the external anal sphincter, and the clitoral retractor muscle. Contractions of the vulvae constrictor muscle with the vestibular constrictor muscle causes eversion of the clitoris after urination or during estrus ("winking").
- Sebaceous glands within the clitoral fossa are responsible for production of smegma.
- The vulvar vasculature is provided by branches (dorsal perineal vessel) of the internal pudendal vessels.
- The clitoris is richly vascular, supplied by the dorsal and deep clitoral arteries and veins provided by the genitofemoral vessels of the internal iliac vessels.
- The perineum is innervated by the deep perineal nerve (motor) and superficial perineal nerve (sensory to the vulva and perineum) branches of the pudendal nerve.
- The peculiar arrangement of the vulvar muscle allows it to stretch during foaling.

Vestibule
- *See* Figures 6.2A, 6.2B, and 6.3.
- The embryonic origin of the vestibule is the urogenital sinus.
- The vestibule extends inward from the vulvar labia to the transverse fold (hymen in maiden or remnant of the hymen in parous mares).
- The depth and inclination of the vestibule depends on age, parity, and body condition.
- The urethral orifice is located ventral just caudal to the transverse fold.
- The vestibular mucosal surface is primarily stratified squamous epithelium. The vestibular mucosa contains branched tubular mucous vestibular glands that open laterally and ventrally in rows of orifices.

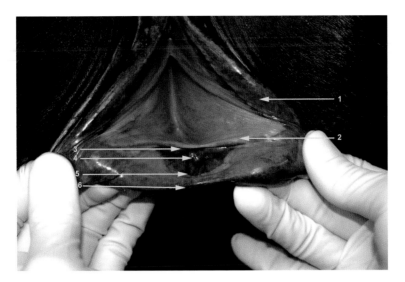

■ **Figure 6.2A** Detailed anatomy of the vulva and clitoris: 1. vulvar labia; 2. transverse fold forming the prepuce of clitoris; 3. clitoral sinuses; 4. glans clitoris; 5. clitoral fossa; 6. ventral commissure.

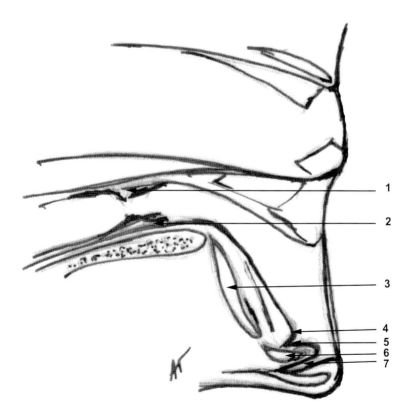

■ **Figure 6.2B** Detailed anatomy of the vulva and clitoris: 1. vestibular bulb (vestibulovaginal sphincter); 2. urethral orifice; 3. body of the clitoris; 4. prepuce of the clitoris; 5. sinus of the clitoris; 6. glans clitoris; 7. fossa of the clitoris.

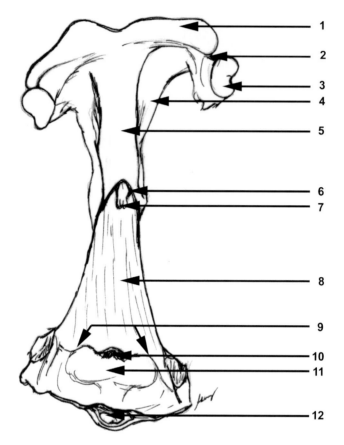

■ **Figure 6.3** Mare reproductive tract: 1. right uterine horn; 2. mesovarium; 3. ovary; 4. broad ligament; 5. uterine body; 6. fornix; 7. cervix (external os); 8. vagina; 9. hymen; 10. urethral orifice; 11. vestibulum; 12. clitoris.

■ The vestibular musculature is provided by a strong constrictor muscle (i.e., vestibular sphincter, vestibular bulb) that provides separation between the external genitalia and the vaginal cavity.

■ The vestibular area vasculature is provided by vessels of the vestibular bulb originating from the internal pudendal vessels.

Vagina
■ *See* Figure 6.3.
■ The embryonic origin of the cranial vagina is the paramesonephric duct, whereas the embryonic origin of the caudal vagina is the urogenital sinus.
■ The vagina extends cranially from the transverse fold or hymen to the cervix.
■ The vaginal cavity is normally completely collapsed (a *potential space*) and is formed by vaginal mucosal folds. Its tissue is elastic and limited only by the bony structures of the pelvis.
■ The vagina is covered internally by the visceral layer of the peritoneum.

- At the level of the cervix, the vagina forms a fornix, which is more prominent when the cervix is tight and the caudal portion of the cervix protrudes into the vagina.
- The vaginal mucosa is lined with stratified squamous epithelium and is devoid of glandular tissue.
- The vasculature of the vagina is provided primarily by branches from the internal pudendal artery and vein.

Cervix
- *See* Figure 6.3.
- The embryonic origin of the cervix is the paramesonephric duct.
- The cervix in the mare is an elastic and muscular structure that extends from the vagina to the body of the uterus. It varies in length from 4 to 8 cm.
- The cervical sphincter is formed by smooth muscle derived from the inner layer of the myometrium.
- Cervical tone and its morphology (shape) respond to variations in ovarian steroid hormones during the cycle: it is tight and firm during diestrus and relaxed and edematous during estrus.
- A frenulum is identified on the dorsal aspect of the cervix at the fornix.
- The cervical canal is formed by longitudinal mucosal folds, which continue into the uterus (uterine mucosal folds).
- The epithelial layer of the cervix presents ciliated and mucigenous cells. Tubular glands are present and produce large amount of mucus. The blood supply to the cervix is provided by small branches of the uterine and vaginal arteries.

Uterus
- *See* Figure 6.3.
- The embryonic origin of the uterus is the paramesonephric duct.
- The uterus is bicornuate. The body of the uterus is relatively long and varies in size from 12 to 20 cm and starts within the cranial part of the pelvic cavity and extends into the abdomen. The uterine horns are entirely located within the abdominal cavity and are 15 to 30 cm in length, becoming narrower as each progresses toward its rounded tip (terminal portion by the ovary).
- On its external surface, cranial aspect, the intercornual ligament is evident but rudimentary compared with that of a cow's uterus. Internally, the uterine horns are separated by an internal bifurcation made of a short septum.
- The uterus is suspended by the mesometrium (portion of the broad ligament) extending from the tip of the uterine horn to the cervix on either side.
- Uterine tone and tubularity vary during the different phases of the estrous cycle (estrus versus diestrus) and pregnancy and provide important clinical information to the examiner to determine normalcy of a mare's cycle during TRP.
- Histologically, the uterine wall is composed of a serosa, muscularis (inner longitudinal and outer circular smooth muscle layers), and the endometrium.
- The endometrial epithelium is simple columnar during diestrus and pseudostratified during estrus. The epithelial cells vary from cuboidal to tall depending on the stage of the cycle with some ciliated and nonciliated cells present.

- Endometrial histology is extremely important for the evaluation of reproductive function.
- The blood supply to the uterus is provided primarily by the uterine artery, a branch of the external iliac artery. This artery anastomoses cranially with the uterine branch of the ovarian artery and caudally with the uterine branch of the vaginal artery.
- The uterus is drained by a rich network of lymphatic vessels.

The uterine tube (Oviduct, Salpinx, and Fallopian tube)
- *See* Figures 6.4A and 6.4B.
- The oviduct is a tubular structure suspended by the mesosalpinx (portion of the broad ligament). It measures 20 to 30 cm in length. It starts near the ovary with the infundibulum, continuing portions as it leads to the uterus are called the ampulla and, ending at the uterus, the isthmus.
- The infundibulum is a richly vascularized funnel-shaped structure with thin irregular fimbria partly attached to the cranial boarder of the ovary with a free border covering the ovulation fossa on the ventral aspect of the ovary. The epithelial lining of the fimbria is ciliated. The centrally located ostium is wide (6 mm in diameter) and can easily be catheterized.
- The ampulla is poorly defined.

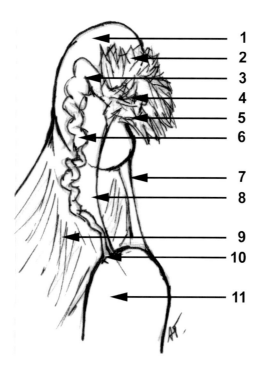

■ **Figure 6.4A** Detailed anatomy of the ovary and uterine tube: 1. ovary; 2. fimbria of the infundibulum; 3. ampulla of the salpinx; 4. infundibulum of the salpinx with its ostium; 5. ovulation fossa; 6. uterine tube (also known as oviduct, Fallopian tube, salpinx); 7. proper ligament of the ovary; 8. ovarian bursa formed by the mesosalpinx; 9. mesometrium; 10. uterotubal junction (UTJ); 11. uterine horn.

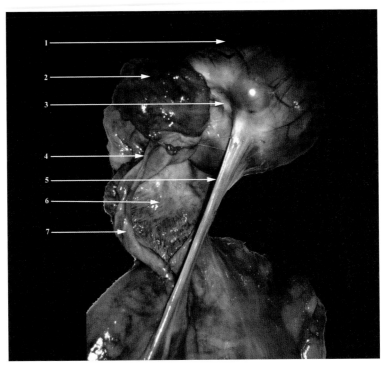

■ **Figure 6.4B** Detailed anatomy of the ovary and salpinx: 1. ovary; 2. infundibulum; 3. ovulation fossa; 4. ampulla; 5. proper ligament of the ovary; 6. mesosalpinx; 7. uterine tube. Image courtesy of C. L. Carleton.

- The isthmus makes up the majority of the oviduct and ends as a projection within the uterine lumen, on the papilla of the uterotubal junction. The thickness of the muscularis of the uterine tube increases from the ovarian end as it approaches the uterine end. It terminates with a strong muscular sphincter of the papilla at the UTJ. The uterine ostium is 2 to 3 mm in diameter.

The Ovary
- *See* Figures 6.4A and 6.4B.
- The equine ovary is large and kidney shaped. It is located about 10 cm caudal to the kidney at the level of the fifth lumbar vertebrae, cranio ventral to the tuber coxae.
- The ovary is suspended by the mesovarium (proper ovarian ligament), which splits off the mesosalpinx laterally. The ovary is surrounded by a shallow bursa formed with the medial wall of the mesosalpinx.
- The equine ovary presents several distinct characteristics compared to other domestic species:
- With the exception of the ovulation fossa, the entire ovarian surface is covered with the visceral peritoneum (mesothelial cells).
- The ventral free border presents an indentation: the ovulation fossa where the germinal epithelium is concentrated.

- The dorsal convex portion is richly vascularized.
- Follicles tend to change the shape and regularity of the ovarian surface, but CL are internal and do not project on or above the surface of the ovary as in other species.
- Blood supply to the ovary is provided by the ovarian artery directly from the aorta.

Abbreviations

CL   corpus luteum
TRP   transrectal palpation
UTJ   uterotubal junction

See Also

- Breeding soundness examination
- Estrous cycle
- Ultrasonography
- Transrectal palpation
- Endometrial biopsy

Suggested Reading

Budras KD, Sack WO, Rock S, et al. 2009. *Anatomy of the horse*, 5th ed. Frankfurt, Germany: Schlutersche; 80–84.
Ginther OJ. 1992. *Reproductive Biology of the Mare*. Basic and applied aspects, 2nd ed, Cross Plains, WI: Equiservices.

Authors: Ahmed Tibary and Jacobo Rodriguez

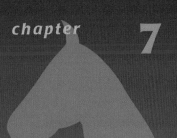

Anestrus

DEFINITION/OVERVIEW

Anestrus is the period of reproductive inactivity. The ovaries are small and inactive with no follicular activity. It is characterized by the mare's behavioral indifference in the presence of the stallion.

ETIOLOGY/PATHOPHYSIOLOGY

The mare is seasonally polyestrous, with estrous cycles in the spring and summer months. Cyclicity is primarily regulated by photoperiod, which begins a cascade of events:

- Increasing day length decreases secretion of melatonin (pineal gland origin).
- Decreasing melatonin allows increased production and release of GnRH (hypothalamic origin).
- Increased GnRH stimulates gonadotropin release (FSH, LH; pituitary origin).
- FSH promotes folliculogenesis and ultimately the onset of estrus behavior.
- When sufficient LH is present, ovulation occurs (the end of vernal transition arrives with the first ovulation of the season [e.g., the onset of cyclicity]).

The length of the average estrous cycle is 21 days (range: 19–22 days) and is defined as the period of time between ovulations that coincides with progesterone levels of less than 1 ng/mL. Estrus and estrous cycle lengths are quite repeatable in individual mares from cycle to cycle. Key hormonal events or sequence of the equine estrous cycle are:

- FSH (pituitary origin) causes ovarian follicular growth.
- Estradiol (follicular origin) stimulates increased GnRH (hypothalamic origin) pulse frequency, resulting in secretion of LH (pituitary origin).
- LH surge causes ovulation; estradiol returns to basal levels 1 to 2 days post-ovulation.
- Progesterone (CL origin) rises from basal levels (less than 1 ng/mL) at ovulation to greater than 4 ng/mL by 4 to 7 days post-ovulation.
- Progesterone causes a decrease in GnRH pulse frequency that results in an increase in FSH secretion to stimulate a new wave of ovarian follicles to develop during diestrus.

- Natural prostaglandin ($PGF_2\alpha$) of endometrial origin is released 14 to 15 days post-ovulation causing luteolysis and a concurrent decline in progesterone levels.

Systems Affected

- Reproductive
- Endocrine

 # SIGNALMENT/HISTORY

Mares of any age and any breed may be affected.

Risk Factors

Postpartum anestrus tends to occur more often in mares that foal early in the year, those that are in poor body condition at the time of parturition, and in aged mares.

Historical Findings

- Chief complaint: Failure to accept the stallion is the usual complaint. Rarely, stallion-like behavior is reported.
- Teasing records: The teasing methods used should be critically reviewed, to include: frequency, teaser type (e.g., pony, horse, or gelding), stallion behavior (e.g., aggressive/passive, vocalization, proximity), and handler experience.
- Seasonal influences: Normal individual variation in the onset, duration, or termination of cyclicity can be mistaken for anestrus.
- Individual reproductive history: Estrous cycle length, response to teasing, foaling data, and previous injuries or infections of the genital tract may be related to current clinical abnormalities.
- Pharmaceuticals: Current and historical drug administration may be related to current clinical abnormalities.

 # CLINICAL FEATURES

- Body condition: Poor condition or malnutrition may contribute to anestrus.
- Perineal conformation: Poor conformation can result in pneumovagina, ascending infections, or urine pooling, which may contribute to anestrus or infertility.
- Clitoral size: Enlargement may be related to prior treatment with anabolic steroids, progestational steroids, or intersex conditions.
- TRP: Essential when evaluating mares with abnormal cycles. To be meaningful and allow full assessment of a mare, all three of the primary anatomical components of the mare's genital tract must be described: uterine size and tone, ovarian size, shape and location, and cervical relaxation. Serial examination three times per week

over the course of several weeks may be necessary to completely define the patient's status.

- Transrectal U/S: Useful to define normal or abnormal features of the uterus or ovaries.
- Vaginal examination: Inflammation, urine pooling, cervical competency, or conformational abnormalities may be identified. May also be used to help identify the stage of the estrous cycle (e.g., appearance, degree of external cervical os relaxation).

 # DIFFERENTIAL DIAGNOSIS

General Comments

- Critically review teasing records.
- Review general and reproductive history for foaling data and evidence of infections, injuries, or medications that may affect current reproductive health.
- Every-other-day TRP with or without U/S over the course of 2 to 3 weeks time should be sufficient to differentiate transitional anestrus, behavioral anestrus, and pregnancy from hypoplastic ovaries, LOS/ovarian neoplasia, and pyometra.
- Anestrus due to EED after the formation of endometrial cups may cause pseudopregnancy. *See* Pregnancy Diagnosis for a discussion of eCG assays.

Normal Physiologic Variation

- Winter anestrus: Approximately 20% of mares continue to cycle during the winter months (November to January in the northern hemisphere), whereas the majority enter a period of ovarian quiescence. This is the time of year when failure to cycle is considered normal. Two transitional phases occur for the mare each year. Autumnal (fall), as the mare moves into anestrus, and vernal (spring), during which the mare progresses from anestrus through transition to resume cyclicity. Behavioral patterns vary during these transition periods. Individual variation in the onset and length of these phases is normal.
- Behavioral anestrus (silent heat): These mares have normal estrous cycles as determined by serial TRP but do not demonstrate estrus (*see* Abnormal Estrus Intervals).
- Pregnancy: After maternal recognition of pregnancy, CL function and progesterone production continue. The majority of pregnant mares demonstrate anestrus behavior.
- Pseudopregnancy: Embryonic death after maternal recognition of pregnancy or the formation of endometrial cups results in persistent CL activity and behavioral anestrus. Equine eCG produced by the endometrial cups between 35 and 150 days of pregnancy is luteotropic and plays a role in maintenance of the primary CL as well as stimulating formation of secondary CLs during pregnancy.
- Postpartum anestrus: Most mares (greater than 95%) reestablish cyclic activity within 20 days of parturition. Some fail to continue to cycle after the first postpartum ovulation (foal heat), due either to prolonged CL function or ovarian inactivity.

- Age-related conditions: Puberty generally occurs between 12 to 24 months of age. Individual variations occur in response to age, weight, nutrition, and season. Aged mares tend to have protracted seasonal anestrus, and mares older than 25 years of age may stop cycling completely.

Congenital Abnormalities

- Gonadal dysgenesis and intersex conditions should be suspected based on history (e.g., anestrus, irregular estrus), TRP and U/S findings (e.g., small ovaries, flaccid uterus and cervix), repeated low serum progesterone concentrations (less than 1 ng/mL, every 7 days for 5 weeks), and karyotype analysis.
- Gonadal dysgenesis: The absence of functional ovarian tissue can result in anestrus, erratic estrus, or prolonged estrus. Behavioral estrus has been attributed to adrenal-origin steroid production in these mares in the absence of progesterone. Mares typically have a flaccid, often infantile uterus and hypoplastic endometrium in addition to small, nonfunctional ovaries. The most common chromosomal abnormality in these cases is XO monosomy (Turner's syndrome).
- Intersex conditions: XY sex reversal chromosomal abnormalities.

Endocrine Disorders

- Cushing's disease (hyperadrenocorticism): An adenomatous hyperplasia of the intermediate pituitary gland can lead to destruction of FSH- and LH-secreting cells or the overproduction of glucocorticoids. This may be accompanied by increased levels of adrenal-origin androgens causing suppression of the normal hypothalamic-pituitary-ovarian axis. Primary hypothalamic-pituitary-ovarian axis interference has been proposed as a cause of anestrus in mares.

Ovarian Abnormalities

- Ovarian hematoma: *See* LOS.
- Ovarian neoplasia: GCT/GTCT, cystadenoma, and germ cell tumors. Affected mare behavior may be reflected as anestrus, stallion-like, or continuous estrus. *See* LOS.

Uterine Abnormalities

Pyometra: Severe uterine infections can destroy the endometrium and prevent the formation and release of $PGF_2\alpha$ essential to CL regression. Clinically, this appears as prolonged diestrus or anestrus.

Iatrogenic/Pharmaceutical

- Anabolic steroids: Affected mares may behave as if in anestrus or become more aggressive (stallion-like).
- Progesterone/progestin: Continued administration effectively inhibits the expression of estrus.

- NSAIDs: These compounds could potentially interfere with endometrial $PGF_2\alpha$ release and result in prolonged luteal activity. There is no evidence that chronic administration at recommended therapeutic dosages inhibits the spontaneous formation and release of $PGF_2\alpha$ from the endometrium.

DIAGNOSTICS

- Serum progesterone concentrations: basal levels of less than 1 ng/mL indicate no ovarian luteal tissue. Active CL function is associated with levels of greater than 4 ng/mL.
- Serum testosterone and inhibin concentrations: mares typically have testosterone values less than 50 to 60 pg/mL and inhibin values less than 0.7 ng/mL. Hormone levels suggestive of a GCT/GTCT (in a nonpregnant mare) are: testosterone greater than 50 to 100 pg/mL (produced if thecal cells are a significant tumor component), inhibin greater than 0.7 ng/mL, and progesterone less than 1 ng/mL.
- Serum eCG levels: eCG is measured by an ELISA assay. *See* Pregnancy Diagnosis.
- GnRH stimulation test: may be useful to identify primary hypothalamic or pituitary dysfunction.
- Karyotype analysis is indicated for suspected gonadal dysgenesis or intersex conditions.
- Transrectal U/S is routinely used to evaluate the equine reproductive tract. The reader is referred to other texts for a comprehensive discussion on this technique.
- Uterine cytology, culture, and biopsy techniques are useful in the diagnosis and treatment of pyometra and endometritis. *See* Endometritis, Pyometra.

THERAPEUTICS

- Behavioral anestrus may be solved simply by altering management techniques (e.g., varying teasing methods to elicit a response from a mare and/or basing the timing of AI on serial TRP and U/S findings).
- Artificial lighting can hasten the onset of vernal transition through manipulation of photoperiod. Whether by natural light or supplemental lighting, the period of time to progress from winter anestrus through transition to the first ovulation is a minimum of 60 to 90 days. Mares are kept in lighted conditions for 14.5 to 16 hours a day (supplemental light added prior to dusk each day to complete needed hours of light exposure), or alternatively, by adding 1 to 2 hours of light 10 hours after dusk (flash lighting) for 60 days. As 60 days (minimum) of supplemental lighting are required for the progression from anestrus to cyclicity, light supplementation is typically initiated by December 1 in the northern hemisphere.
- Mares due to foal early in the year may be placed under artificial lighting 2 months prior to parturition to improve postpartum cyclicity and decrease the potential for lactational anestrus.

- Progesterone by itself is not recommended to treat mares in deep anestrus. Artificial lighting for 60 days, then coupled with progesterone, is an effective means to achieve the onset of early, regular estrous cycles.
- Ovarian tumors/ovariectomy: removal of a GCT/GTCT allows the opposite ovary to recover from the effects of inhibin suppression by the tumor. Dependent on the season when the tumor is removed, there could be a longer latent period for ovarian activity to return. If an ovariectomy is done in the autumn and the mare is exposed and can respond to the normal increase in day length after the winter solstice, she will more quickly return to normal estrous activity. Rarely, in cases of long-present (years) ovarian tumors, the remaining ovary may remain quiescent for the mare's life.
- The management of pyometra and endometritis is discussed elsewhere.

Drug(s) of Choice

- $PGF_2\alpha$ (Lutalyse® [Pfizer], 10 mg, IM) or its analogs to lyse persistent CL tissue. Multiple injections may be needed in cases of pseudopregnancy.
- Deslorelin, a GnRH analog, is used to induce ovulation within 48 hours in mares with a follicle(s) larger than 30 mm in diameter.
- hCG (2,500 IU, IV) is used to induce ovulation in mares with a follicle(s) larger than 35 mm in diameter.
- Altrenogest (Regu-Mate® [Intervet], 0.044 mg/kg, PO, SID, minimum 15 days) can be used to shorten the duration of vernal transition, providing multiple follicles, bigger than 20 mm diameter are present and the mare is demonstrating behavioral estrus. $PGF_2\alpha$ on day 15 of the altrenogest treatment increases the reliability of this transition management regimen. Its use in mares deep in seasonal anestrus or with follicles smaller than 15 to 20 mm in diameter, is not recommended and may result in further ovarian suppression.

Precautions/Interactions

Horses

- $PGF_2\alpha$ and its analogs are contraindicated in mares with asthma, COPD, or other bronchoconstrictive disease.
- Prostaglandin administration to pregnant mares can cause CL lysis and abortion. Carefully rule out pregnancy before administering this drug or its analogs.
- $PGF_2\alpha$ causes sweating and colic-like symptoms due to its stimulatory effect on smooth muscle cells. If cramping has not subsided within 1 to 2 hours, symptomatic treatment should be instituted.
- Antibodies to hCG can develop after treatment. It is desirable to limit its use to no more than two to three times during one breeding season. The half-life of these antibodies ranges from 30 days to several months. These antibodies typically do not persist from one breeding season to the next.
- GnRH agonist (deslorelin) implants used to stimulate ovulation have been associated with prolonged interovulatory intervals, due to suppression of FSH secretion and decreased follicular development in the diestrus period immediately following use.

This results in a prolonged interovulatory period in non-pregnant mares. Implant removal within 1 to 2 days post-ovulation decreases this possibility. At this time, deslorelin implants are unavailable in the United States, but they are still on the market in Canada and other countries. The response to deslorelin is more reliable, if $PGF_2\alpha$ is used during the diestrus period in an attempt to "short-cycle" the mare. A deslorelin injectable product is available from Canada and some U.S. pharmacies (compounding).

- Progesterone supplementation has been associated with decreased uterine clearance. Its use may be contraindicated in mares with a history of uterine infection.
- Altrenogest, deslorelin, and $PGF_2\alpha$ should not be used in horses intended for food purposes.

Humans

- $PGF_2\alpha$ or its analogs should not be handled by pregnant women or people with asthma or bronchial disease. Any accidental exposure to skin should immediately be washed off.
- Altrenogest should not be handled by pregnant women or people with thrombophlebitis or thromboembolic disorders, cerebrovascular disease, coronary artery disease, breast cancer, estrogen-dependent neoplasia, undiagnosed vaginal bleeding or tumors that developed during the use of oral contraceptives, or estrogen-containing products. Any accidental exposure to skin should immediately be washed off.

Alternative Drugs

Cloprostenol sodium (Estrumate® [Schering-Plough Animal Health], 250 μg, IM), is a prostaglandin analog. This product is used in similar fashion as the natural prostaglandin, but it has been associated with fewer side effects. It is not currently approved, but it is widely used in horses.

 COMMENTS

Patient Monitoring

- Serial evaluation (three times weekly) of the reproductive tract during the physiologic breeding season is necessary to establish a tentative diagnosis for the cause of anestrus behavior.
- Pseudopregnant mares return to normal cyclic activity when the endometrial cups regress and eCG levels decrease. Serum eCG may persist for up to 150 days following an early pregnancy loss. In cases when embryonic death has been confirmed, intervention in the early months post-loss may be ineffective until the cups regress.

Possible Complications

Infertility may result in cases of intractable persistent anestrus.

Synonyms

- Postpartum anestrus, lactational anestrus
- Gonadal dysgenesis, gonadal hypoplasia

Abbreviations

AI	artificial insemination
CL	corpus luteum
COPD	chronic obstructive pulmonary disease
eCG	equine chorionic gonadotropin
EED	early embryonic death
ELISA	enzyme linked immunosorbent assay
FSH	follicle stimulating hormone
GCT/GTCT	granulosa cell tumor/granulosa-theca cell tumor
GnRH	gonadotropin releasing hormone
hCG	human chorionic gonadotropin
IM	intramuscular
LH	luteinizing hormone
LOS	large ovary syndrome
NSAIDs	nonsteroidal anti-inflammatory drugs
PGF	natural prostaglandin
PO	per os (by mouth)
SID	once a day
TRP	transrectal palpation
U/S	ultrasound

See Also

- Abnormal estrus intervals
- Aggression
- Cushing's syndrome
- Disorders of sexual development
- Early embryonic death
- Endometritis
- Large ovary syndrome
- Ovarian hypoplasia
- Ovulation failure
- Prolonged diestrus
- Pyometra

Suggested Reading

Bowling AT, Hughes JP. 1993. Cytogenetic abnormalities. In: *Equine Reproduction*. McKinnon AO and Voss JL (eds). Philadelphia: Lea & Febiger; 258–265.

Daels PF, Hughes JP. 1993. The abnormal estrous cycle. In: *Equine Reproduction*. McKinnon AO and Voss JL (eds). Philadelphia: Lea & Febiger; 144–160.

Hinrichs K. 2007. Irregularities of the estrous cycle and ovulation in mares (including seasonal transition). In: *Current Therapy in Large Animal Theriogenology*, 2nd ed. Youngquist RS and Threlfall WR (eds). St. Louis: Saunders Elsevier; 144–152.

McCue PM, Farquhar VJ, Carnevale EM, et al. 2002. Removal of deslorelin (Ovuplant™) implant 48 h after administration results in normal interovulatory intervals in mares. *Therio* 58: 865–870.

Nie G, Sharp D, Robinson G, et al. 2007. Clinical aspects of seasonality in mares. In: *Current Therapy in Large Animal Theriogenology*. Youngquist RS and Threlfall WR (eds). St. Louis: WB Saunders, Elsevier; 68–73.

Author: Carole C. Miller

chapter 8

Artificial Insemination

DEFINITION/OVERVIEW

- Extended fresh, cooled, frozen semen introduced into the mare's uterus using aseptic technique.
- Standard AI: deposition of a minimum of 300 to 1,000 (average: 500) $\times 10^6$ PMS into the uterine body.
- DHI or low-dose AI: 1 to 25×10^6 PMS deposited into the tip of a uterine horn (ipsilateral to dominant follicle/side of ovulation).

ETIOLOGY/PATHOPHYSIOLOGY

- Efficient use of semen.
- Ejaculate can be divided into several AI doses, to breed a greater number of mares in a season (120 by AI; 40 to 80 by live cover) by a stallion.
- Wider use of genetically superior stallions.
- Eliminate cost and risk of transport, mares with foals at side.
- Antibiotics in semen extenders prevent many genital infections.
- Fewer breeding injuries.
- Continued use of stallions with problems (musculoskeletal and behavioral).
- Protect mares with genital tract impairments or a recent surgical repair from further breeding-related trauma.
- Semen quality can be assessed before AI.
- Low-dose AI is for stallions with limited availability or costly semen due to:
  - Excessive size of book.
  - Low sperm cell production or high percentage of dead sperm.
  - Use of sex-sorted sperm.
  - Epididymal spermatozoa collected at the time of castration or stallion's death.

Systems Affected

- Reproductive

SIGNALMENT/HISTORY

- Thoroughbred breed allows only live cover.
- All other breed registries allow AI; may impose restrictions.

Historical Findings

Records of mare's prior cycles help predict days in heat and time of ovulation.

CLINICAL FEATURES

Teasing and Physical Examination

- Ovulation timing is critical.
  - Predict by mare's history, teasing response, and results of genital tract TRP and U/S.
  - During estrus, teased daily; not less than every other day.
  - On second day of estrus, begin daily or every-other-day TRP.
  - Perform U/S, as needed, to determine optimal time to breed.
- TRP: Record dominant follicle (35+mm), uterine edema, percent of cervical relaxation, follicle size and its growth (serial TRPs), increasing uterine estrual edema (cartwheel appearance) evident with U/S.
- Preovulatory follicle may become irregular/pear-shaped 12 to 24 hours pre-ovulation.
- Estrual edema peaks at 96 to 72 hours, decreases to light or absent by 36 hours, pre-ovulation in young, normal mares.
- Identification of an OVD, CH, or CL is evidence that ovulation has occurred.

DIAGNOSTICS

Timing and Frequency of Breeding

- Depends on semen longevity affected by stallion idiosyncrasy and semen preservation method (fresh, cooled, frozen).
- Equine ova have a short period of viability (reported as short as 6 to 10 hours, may be to 12 hours in some mares, occasionally [less likely] to 18 hours) post-ovulation.

Teasing and Examinations

- GnRH analog or hCG can be administered when preovulatory follicle is equal to or greater than 35mm to induce ovulation within 36 to 42 hours. AI as close to the time of ovulation as possible.

- U/S 4 to 6 hours post-AI for presence of intrauterine fluid (especially new/DUC mare, or if bred with frozen semen) and for ovulation.
- Evaluate normal, fertile mares 24 to 48 hours after AI for ovulation.

Fresh (Raw or Extended) Semen

- Routine breeding every other day:
  - Begin day 2 to 3 of estrus until the mare teases out, or
  - When a large preovulatory follicle is detected by TRP and U/S.
- Inseminate within 48 hours pre-ovulation to achieve acceptable pregnancy rates.

Cooled Transported Semen

- More intense management; fertility of cooled semen from some stallions decreases markedly if it is inseminated more than/older than 24 hours post-collection.
- Deslorelin (a GnRH analogue) or hCG when pre-ovulatory follicle is at least 35 mm to induce ovulation within 36 to 42 hours; order semen for overnight shipment.
- Inseminate within 12 to 24 hours pre-ovulation for acceptable conception rates.
- Semen with poor post-cooling fertility should be sent *counter to counter* (i.e., airline transport).
  - Administer deslorelin or hCG 24 to 36 hours before expected semen arrival to ensure ovulation is very close to time of AI.
- No advantage to keeping a second AI dose to rebreed next day. The mare's uterus is the best incubator for sperm, not a chilled shipper that was opened to remove one dose; the coolant curve has been disturbed. If client insists on using a second dose the next day, the isothermalizer may be wrapped in a towel and placed in a refrigerator (low and near the back of the compartment) to maintain the second dose nearer to 5°C to 6°C overnight.

Frozen Thawed Semen

- Precise timing of AI: post-thaw longevity is reduced to less than or equal to 12 to 24 hours.
- Mare management: serial, daily teasing, TRP, and U/S.
- Deslorelin or hCG when dominant follicle is at least 35 mm.
- TRP and U/S: TID to QID, ensure AI is as close before ovulation as possible; either before, but most importantly, within narrow window of time of no more than 6 to 8 hours post-ovulation.
- New frozen semen strategy for AI if have multiple doses:
  - Deslorelin or hCG when dominant follicle is at least 35 mm.
  - AI at 24 hours and again at 40 hours after injection; ensures viable sperm are available during the ovulatory period.
  - Treat the mare if intrauterine fluid is present 4 to 6 hours after first AI.
  - Pregnancy rate is equivalent to a one-time AI done by 6 hours post-ovulation, but minus the intensive labor and requires fewer veterinary examinations.

Low-Dose Insemination

- Allows use of a reduced dose of semen (fresh, cooled, frozen).
- Varies with semen quality:
  - DHI dose has been decreased to as few as 14×10^6 motile, frozen-thawed sperm.
  - Average of 60 to 150×10^6 PMS for DHI.
  - Semen is deposited at the UTJ, tip of uterine horn ipsilateral to dominant follicle.
- DHI can be either hysteroscopically guided or transrectally guided (with or without U/S). *See* Figs. 8.1 and 8.2.
- Mare management varies according to method of semen preservation.

General Comments

If ovulation has not occurred within the recommended times for fresh (48 hours), cooled (24 hours), or frozen (6 to 12 hours) semen, rebreed the mare.

Diagnostic Procedures

Semen Analysis

- Minimum parameters to be evaluated: volume, motility, concentration.
- Morphology: optional, but of particular use if a stallion has fertility problems.
- Small sample of cooled or frozen semen should be saved and warmed (at 37°C) to evaluate immediately after AI.
- Slide, coverslip, and pipette: pre-warm; stallion semen is susceptible to cold shock.
- The total number of sperm should be at least 300 to 1000×10^6 PMS (concentration [in millions of sperm per mL] × volume used).

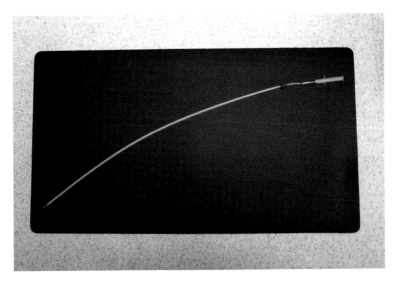

■ **Figure 8.1** Flexible catheter to deliver semen for artificial insemination by deep horn insemination. Image courtesy of Ahmed Tibary.

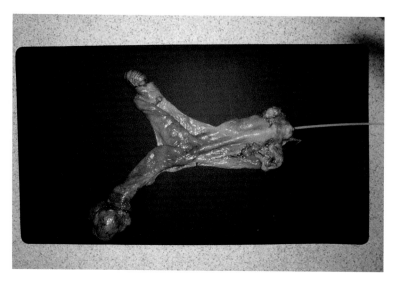

■ **Figure 8.2** Dissected tract showing the arc of the pipet carrying it through the uterine body into the uterine horn to its tip for deposition of semen.
Image courtesy of Ahmed Tibary.

Stallion's Disease Status

Should be negative for EIA, EVA, CEM, and venereal diseases.

Mare Selection

- Her fertility takes on special significance if using frozen semen or the quality of the semen is less than optimal.
- Include reproductive history, ± normal estrous cyclicity, results of uterine culture and cytology, and presence of intrauterine fluid during estrus.

Prebreeding Uterine Culture and Cytology of Mare

- All, except young maiden mares, should have at least one negative uterine culture and cytology pre-breeding.
  - Avoid transmitting infections to the stallion.
  - Early identification of possible mare problems.
  - Maximize the likelihood of first-cycle conception.
- Pregnancy rates are lower and EED higher for mares treated for uterine infections during the same cycle as the AI.

AI Technique

- Sterile and disposable equipment. Mares are restrained and the perineal area thoroughly cleansed with a mild detergent, antiseptic solution or soap; then any residue is completely removed (minimum three rinses).

- Sterile sleeve on arm and nonspermicidal lubricant applied to dorsum of the gloved hand.
  - A 50- to 56-cm (20- to 22-in) AI pipet is carried in the gloved hand.
  - Index finger is first passed through the cervical lumen. It serves as a guide by which the pipet can readily be advanced (advanced to a position no more than 2.5 cm into the uterine body).
  - Syringe with a nonspermicidal plastic plunger (e.g., Air-tite) containing the extended semen is attached to the pipet, and the semen is slowly deposited into the uterus. The remaining semen in the pipet is delivered by using a small bolus of air (1 mL) in the syringe.

Fresh Extended Semen

- Perform AI immediately after collection.
- Semen can be mixed with an appropriate extender for immediate insemination, with semen-to-extender ratio of 1:1 or 1:2, if the ejaculate volume is small and of high concentration.

Cooled Transported Semen

- Semen is collected, diluted in semen extender, and cooled to 5°C to 6°C for 24 to 48 hours. With transport, there can be a modest decrease of fertilizing capacity (stallion fertility dependent).
- A semen-to-extender ratio of 1:3 or 1:4 is acceptable; may be as high as 1:19.
- Semen longevity optimized by extending the ejaculate to a final sperm concentration of 25 to 50×10^6 sperm/mL.

Frozen Thawed Semen

- Frozen semen is packed in 0.5 to 5 mL straws and stored in liquid N_2.
- A 5-mL straw contains from 600 to 1000×10^6 sperm cells.
  - Dependent on postfreeze viability of the spermatozoa, only one straw may be needed.
- A 0.5 mL straw contains 200 to 800×10^6 sperm cells.
  - Number of straws needed depends on post-thaw motility and method of AI.
  - Thawing protocols vary and are reported ideally paired with a particular freezing method. Seek specific information regarding thawing. In the absence of a recommended protocol, 37°C for 30 to 60 seconds may provide an acceptable alternative.
- If details are not provided with frozen semen received, seek instructions regarding thawing before the day of AI to ensure proper handling.
- Post-thawing, semen should be in the mare within 5 minutes.
- Post-AI uterine treatment is strongly recommended. The high concentration of sperm cells in a thawed straw and absence of seminal plasma (provides a natural protective effect in the uterus) may induce an acute PMIE.

Low-Dose Insemination Procedures

- Sedation of the mare is recommended. Procedure should be performed quickly (less than or up to 10 minutes) and avoid inducing uterine trauma.
- Hysteroscopic AI: introduction of an endoscope into the mare's uterus:
  - Approach and visualize the UTJ ipsilateral to the dominant follicle.
  - Small catheter is passed through the endoscope's channel and semen deposited at or on the UTJ (Fig. 8.3).
- DHI: Pass a flexible AI pipet through the cervix toward the tip of the uterine horn ipsilateral to the dominant follicle.
  - Pipet is guided by either TRP or U/S (*see* Figs. 8.1 and 8.2).
  - Semen is deposited close to or onto the UTJ.
  - Manual TRP elevation of the tip of the uterine horn may help pass the pipet.

 # THERAPEUTICS

Pre-Breeding

- If the presence of 2 cm or more (height) of prebreeding uterine fluid has been observed (U/S), a LRS uterine lavage immediately before AI is advisable.
- Does not affect fertility.

Post-Breeding

- U/S examination 4 to 6 hours after AI for presence of intrauterine fluid.
  - If present, lavage uterus with sterile saline or LRS, followed by oxytocin beginning 4 to 6 hours after AI.
  - Repeat oxytocin at 2- to 4-hour intervals until 8 to 10 hours post-AI, and again at 12 to 24 hours until the inflammation resolves.

Drug(s) of Choice

- Ovulation induction most effective if follicle is at least 35 mm.
  - Within 36 to 42 hours with hCG (1,500 to 3,000 IU IV); response range is 12 to 72 hours.
  - Within 36 to 42 hours with deslorelin 1.5 mg IM.
- Ecbolic drugs may be used to treat PMIE and DUC.
- Prostaglandin analogs: Misoprostol (PGE1 analog 2,000 mcg/3 mL) or cloprostenol (PGE2 analog 2 mg mixed with 2 to 4 mL lubricant jelly) deposited in the cervical canal for relaxation 2 to 4 hours: before deep AI (only with good-quality semen).

Precautions/Interactions

See Endometritis.

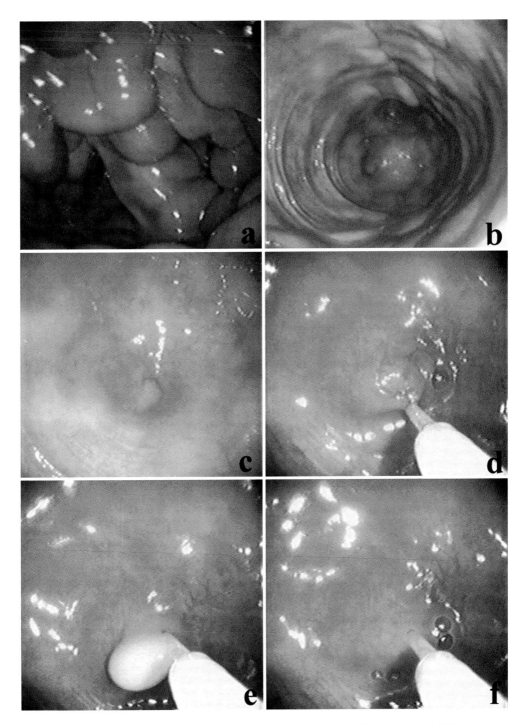

■ **Figure 8.3** Endoscopic delivery of semen onto the uterotubal junction (UTJ). *A*, endometrial folds in uterine body and horns; *B*, and *C*, ostium is evident near the tip of the uterine horn; *D*, pipet placed on or near the ostium; *E*, and *F*, semen is deposited onto the ostium or UTJ.
Images courtesy of A. Tibary.

COMMENTS

Patient Monitoring

- Begin teasing by 11 days post-ovulation.
  - Early detection of endometritis: indicated by a shortened cycle due to endogenous prostaglandin release.
- U/S for pregnancy 14 to 15 days post-ovulation, includes ruling-out potential twins versus lymphatic cyst.
- Follow-up TRP and U/S: 24 to 30 days; confirm the presence of a heartbeat in the embryo.
- Serial TRP pregnancy examinations: 45, 60, 90, and 120 days.

Possible Complications

- AV preparation, handling, maintenance.
- Semen evaluation at collection: ship adequate AI dose or send correct number of semen straws.
- Shipping methods: Equitainer (24 to 72 hours dependent on semen quality, number of coolant cans in shipper, and so on), reusable box cooling containers (maximum 24 hours holding, less reliable and shorter holding time if shipped to or in extreme hot ambient temperatures), or vapor tank.
  - With cooled shipments, entire breeding program is at the mercy of airlines or couriers.
- Operator skill and experience to manipulate and place semen through the cervix, into the uterine lumen or to the tip of the horn, in a proper and timely manner.
- Misidentification of stallions or mares.

Expected Course and Prognosis

Cooled Semen

Per cycle pregnancy rates equivalent to on-farm AI with fresh semen (60%–75%) if semen quality remains good after cooling period of 24 hours at 5°C to 6°C.

Frozen Semen

- Pregnancy rates decrease for most stallions.
- Spermatozoa suffer many stresses; anticipate attrition rate of approximately 50% with freezing and thawing.
- First-cycle pregnancy rates: 30% to 40% (range: 0%–70%); wide range between stallions.
  - Intense breeding management and good quality of semen have a positive impact on the pregnancy rate.

- Candidate selection for frozen semen breeding:
  - Most fertile: young, maiden and normal pluriparous mares.
  - Least fertile: old, maiden or barren and abnormal pluriparous mares.
- Older eggs or semen
  - Due to poor timing; Pregnancy rate decreased by 30 days; increased EED.

Synonyms

Artificial breeding

Abbreviations

AI	artificial insemination
AV	artificial vagina
CEM	contagious equine metritis
CH	corpus hemorrhagicum
CL	corpus luteum
DHI	deep horn insemination
DUC	delayed uterine clearance
EIA	equine infectious anemia
EED	early embryonic death
EVA	equine viral arteritis
GnRH	gonadotropin-releasing hormone
hCG	human chorionic gonadotropin
IM	intramuscular
IV	intravenous
LRS	lactated Ringer's solution
OVD	ovulation depression
PMIE	persistent mating-induced endometritis
PMS	progressively motile sperm
QID	four times a day
TID	three times a day
TRP	transrectal palpation
U/S	ultrasound, ultrasonography
UTJ	utero-tubal junction

See Also

- Conception failure
- Delayed uterine clearance
- Early embryonic death
- Endometritis
- Semen evaluation, abnormal
- Semen evaluation, normal
- Venereal diseases

Suggested Reading

Blanchard TL, Varner D, Schumacher J. 1998. Semen collection and artificial insemination. In: *Manual of Equine Reproduction*. St. Louis: Mosby-Year Book; 111–125.

Brinsko SP. 2006. Insemination doses: how low can we go? *Therio* 66: 543–550.

Morris LH. 2004. Low dose insemination in the mare: an update. *Anim Reprod Sci* 82–83: 625–632.

Author: Maria E. Cadario

chapter 9

Behavior: Estrus Scoring System

DEFINITION/OVERVIEW

- Understanding the relationship between a mare's estrual behavior, dominant follicle characteristics, and U/S images is key to breeding a mare at the proper time, as few times as possible within an estrus period, to maximize the likelihood of achieving pregnancy.
- Variations in fertility and pregnancy rates are not solely determined by the presence of a dominant follicle and estrual edema. Pregnancy rate may also be affected by breed differences or selection characteristics used for breeding.
- The intent is to breed a mare when she is either behaviorally receptive (necessitates good records of teasing, cycle length, and estrus/diestrus responses) or characteristic signs are present based on the findings of TRP or U/S.

ETIOLOGY/PATHOPHYSIOLOGY

Systems Affected

- Reproductive
- Neuroendocrine

SIGNALMENT/HISTORY

Risk Factors

- Estrus detection can be made more difficult if a mare shows either equivocal or weak signs of estrus.
- Difference in teasing response may be due to age (very young or old mare), a foal-at-side (maternal protection), maiden mare, fear response to a vocal/aggressive stallion, season (winter anestrum or transitional period), breed of the mare, and gonadal pathology.

Historical Findings

- Clinical study (Górecka, 2005) comparing native Polish ponies and thoroughbreds found differences attributable to breed that affected reproductive efficiency and thus pregnancy rate.
- The scoring scale used in the study has merit for individuals wishing to monitor and improve record keeping of teasing responses, to understand the shifts in their mare's behavior, and its relationship to the time of ovulation.

- Estrus signs are associated with larger follicles up to the time of ovulation. There is a good correlation with development of endometrial fold edema in relationship to follicular estradiol production.
- In the 2005 study, the behavioral responses of thoroughbred mares were muted compared with native ponies.
  - Native ponies were more obvious in their teasing responses, had only single ovulations, and were gauged less affected by stress compared with thoroughbred mares.
  - Hypotheses for thoroughbred mare's higher percentage of silent heats included their increased emotional reactivity (impact on endogenous GnRH, leading to decreased gonadotropins, and subsequent decreased follicular estradiol) and the impact of double ovulations on overall fertility (the increase of progesterone from the first ovulation, muting the estrus behavior of the second follicle).
- If thoroughbreds could be bred by AI, the significance of some mares failing to exhibit more exuberant estrus would be less an issue. Timing of breeding could be based on TRP and U/S findings and appropriately timed AI.
- Teasing behavior provides invaluable information regarding the synchronous nature of a mare's cycle. Coupled with TRP and U/S, the pregnancy rate of those mares bred at the appropriate time should be maximized.

CLINICAL FEATURES

Scoring of mare teasing behavior (Górecka, 2005):
1 Nonreceptive behavior (i.e., tail switching, mare moves, squealing, ears back, attempts to kick; she attacks or kicks the teaser stallion).
2 Nonreceptive behavior (i.e., tail switching, moves, squealing, ears back, attempts to kick; no severe attack toward the teaser stallion).
3 Nonreceptive behavior (i.e., tail switching, squealing, ears back, attempts to kick, but stands still).
4 Stands indifferently; neither receptive nor nonreceptive behavior.
5 Exhibits estrus behavior: stands, tail raised, winking; some nonreceptive behavior.
6 Exhibits estrus behavior: stands, tail raised, winks; no nonreceptive behavior.
7 Full estrus behavior: stands, tail raised, winks, urinates in small increments, lowers pelvis (breaks down); some nonreceptive behavior (± tail switching, squealing, ears back, attempts to kick).
8 Full estrus behavior: stands, tail raised, winks, urinates, breaks down; no nonreceptive behavior.

COMMENTS

Client Education

- Teasing mares can be difficult, boring, and downright unpleasant early in the year in cold climates, but the time spent and the consistency of a regular teasing program can offset the need for many veterinary examinations and help identify the best days to breed a mare.

- Ovulation occurs 24 to 48 hours prior to the end of estrus. Knowing the length of each mare's prior period of receptivity helps determine when best to breed each one on the subsequent cycle.

Patient Monitoring

An appropriate interval for teasing all mares during the ovulatory period ranges from daily to every other day. Less frequent observations will result in missing some mares either coming into heat or identifying mares that have undergone EED.

Abbreviations

AI   artificial insemination
EED   early embryonic death
GnRH   gonadotropin-releasing hormone
TRP   transrectal palpation
U/S   ultrasound, ultrasonography

See Also

- Abnormal estrus intervals
- Anestrus
- Breeding soundness examination, components, mare
- Clitoral enlargement
- Conception failure
- Early embryonic death
- Endometritis
- Estrous cycle, manipulation of
- Estrus detection, fundamentals
- Ovulation failure
- Ovulation induction
- Ovulation, synchronization of
- Transrectal palpation

Suggested Reading

Ginther OJ. 1992. *Reproductive Biology of the Mare. Basic and Applied Aspects*, 2nd ed. Cross Plains, WI: Equiservices.

Górecka A, Jezierski TA, Słoniewski K. 2005. Relationships between sexual behaviour, dominant follicle area, uterus ultrasonic image and pregnancy rate in mares of two breeds differing in reproductive efficiency. *An Reprod Sci* 87: 283–293.

Pryor P, Tibary A. 2005. Management of estrus in the performance mare. In: *Current Techniques in Equine Practice*. Philadelphia: Elsevier Saunders; 197–209.

Author: Carla L. Carleton

chapter 10

Behavior of Mares, Poor Reproductive Performance

DEFINITION/OVERVIEW

- Mares are seasonally polyestrous with the ovulatory period during times of increasing or long day light. The average estrous cycle is 21 days. The duration of diestrus (luteal activity) averages 14 to 15 days. The interval allocated to estrus can be significantly longer earlier in the breeding season (e.g., 12 days) compared with as short as 3 to 4 days during the middle of the physiologic breeding season (mid to late summer).
- Recognizing and properly addressing problems related to the estrous cycle are essential to effective broodmare practice. Problem behaviors of mares may be linked with different stages of the estrous cycle or season or mimic particular stages of the estrous cycle.
- Collecting specific details related to behavior, a thorough physical examination, and determining if there are associations with TRP and U/S findings, can provide a path to identifying an appropriate solution or resolution.

ETIOLOGY/PATHOPHYSIOLOGY

- Behavior and performance problems may be in response to estrous cycle activity.
- Different breeds exhibit signs of estrus less obviously than others.
- The tunic surrounding the mare's ovary is well innervated. A rapidly growing dominant follicle can be a source of discomfort for a mare, not just during TRP, and may present as cyclic colic. This includes broader manifestations of pawing, abdominal discomfort, tail swishing, and so on. Even in the most stoic mare, reports abound of attitude changes during estrus, an inability to focus (fillies in race training becoming more difficult), frequent urination (whether or not in the presence of colts), kicking, or more excitable, squealing.
- With symptoms of general pain, it is critical to determine which are related to reproductive cycle activity and which are not.

Systems Affected

- Reproductive
- Endocrine

SIGNALMENT/HISTORY

Risk Factors

An intact mare capable of estrous cyclic activity during late winter, spring/summer, or early autumn.

Historical Findings

- To distinguish pain from reproductive activity, a thorough history is essential: details of the problem, its onset, duration, season, increasing or decreasing frequency or intensity (i.e., investigate common threads with her environment or personnel involved in her management).
- Assessment of a mare's ovarian cycle may identify problematic factors associated with either estrus or diestrus, or problems unrelated to the genital tract that mimic estrous cycle activity. Knowledge of normal estrous cycle activity and a thorough history serves to pare down the list of potential rule-outs.
- TRP and U/S findings are important to establishing the normalcy of a mare's estrous cycle activity. More difficulties are reported for estrus than diestrus problems (e.g., split estrus, silent heats, or prolonged estrus).
- A comprehensive listing of medications, including doses, duration, treatment frequencies; prior diagnoses; supplements, changes of trainers (aggression, fear), training schedules, and training beyond current fitness level, can all be pertinent.
- If specific behaviors are repeated, videotaping of them and gathering knowledge of the "when, where, how, and why" can provide invaluable knowledge. Problems of nonreproductive origin can still have reproductive repercussions (i.e., lameness, pain, over-medication).

 CLINICAL FEATURES

- Establish a cause-effect relationship between identified behavior and stage of the estrous cycle. All individuals involved with and working around the horse become partners in identifying what exacerbates the problem, time of day, or stage of cycle when the problem is most prominent. If multiple problems are identified, pick and choose which to address first.
  - During an episode when the perceived problem is present, partner with the mare owner or trainer and establish baseline normals: TRP, U/S, or hormonal assays.
- Treatment to suppress estrus in a mare:
  - Ovariectomy: last resort to control estrus suppression. Elect this procedure only with caution. If a mare is later successful in a particular arena of performance, her ability to reproduce is gone. Emphasize the finality of this to owners. A thorough history should report whether the mare's undesirable behavior was absent when she was in winter anestrus. If she was aggressive during a period of ovarian quiescence, ovariectomy will not solve the problem she may be exhibiting.

- Hormonal treatment for estrus suppression: progesterone and progestagens administered either PO or IM can suppress estrus. *See* Drug(s) of Choice below.
- Induce a state of false pregnancy:
  - IUD
  - Some 35- to 37-mm balls (i.e., usually large glass marbles, may be hard rubber or other substances) placed *in utero* prevent luteolysis and maintenance of a CL. A few instances have been reported of glass balls breaking/cracking into shards *in utero*. Use meticulous wash and prep of mare, and sterile placement or sterilized marble.
  - Effective to 90 days in approximately 40% of mares.
  - Effect can be longer in a small subset.
- Suppression of ovarian activity:
  - Immunization against GnRH to induce formation of GnRH antibodies. Antibody response varies widely between mares.
  - Stimulus for gonadotropin secretion is inhibited resulting in decreased ovarian activity and, in some mares, anestrus. Some mares with completely inactive ovaries continued to show signs of estrus (irregular intervals and duration).
  - More reliable response in young mares than adults, but still not a reliable means of preventing estrus.
  - Equity™ oestrous control, CSL Animal Health in Australia, is one of first licensed products. Duration is variable, but reversible over time (6–15 months).

 DIFFERENTIAL DIAGNOSIS

Problems Unrelated to the Estrous Cycle

- Lameness
- Neurologic
- Pain, orthopedic, or soft tissue (distinguish back pain from ovarian discomfort).
- Abdominal pain unrelated to large, rapidly growing follicles or ovulation.
- Human-animal interaction (e.g., horse becomes sour on training or has an aversion to a particular trainer and performance suffers).

Behaviors Resembling Estrus Behavior

- Poor VC resulting in vaginitis, pneumovagina: raised tail, frequent urination, or winking.
- Cystitis, uroliths.
- A mare kicking at her abdomen: GI colic versus colic associated with estrous cycle activity. Ovarian pain rarely elicits a kicking response.
- In response to a threatening situation (e.g., submissive cowering, passive urination).

Stallion-like Behavior

- Need to distinguish aggression from diestrus rejection of stallion during teasing.
- Rule-outs include medications administered (supplements during training, anabolic steroids) or possibly a hormone-producing tumor (GTCT).

THERAPEUTICS

Drug(s) of Choice

- Synthetic progestagens are less than ideal at suppressing estrus in the mare because of their failure to bind to equine progesterone receptors.
    - Altrenogest (0.044 mg/kg per day) PO: generally suppresses estrus behavior within 2 to 3 days of treatment onset, but follicular activity continues and ovulation may still occur.
    - Progesterone in oil (50 mg IM, SID) treatment started during diestrus will prevent demonstration of estrus behavior during the next ovulation. A larger dose (100–200 mg IM, SID) is necessary to suppress estrus if treatment is begun during the follicular phase of the estrous cycle.
    - Injection reactions are possible with the daily administration of progesterone in oil.
- Other formulations of progesterone, including long-acting formulations, are not yet FDA approved, but are being used in some practices for estrus suppression as well as reported for maintenance of pregnancy.
- PRID or CIDR are finding some use in mares, but are not yet a common option.

Precautions/Interactions

Bovine hormonal implants (SC) are ineffective in suppressing estrus because of the failure to absorb progesterone in sufficient quantity.

- The implants are designed for sustained release of a small amount of progesterone over a period of several months.
- Eight implants of Synovex-S contain a total of 200 mg of progesterone and 20 mg of estradiol benzoate. All mares receiving Synovex-S returned to estrus at the predicted time. It did not block ovulation.
- Up to 80 implants administered 5 days post-ovulation failed to maintain progesterone levels about 0.5 ng/mL. Progesterone concentrations less than 1 ng/mL are insufficient to suppress estrus.

Surgical Considerations

Ovariectomy to suppress estrus, refer to Clinical Features.

COMMENTS

Abbreviations

CIDR   controlled internal drug release device
CL   corpus luteum
FDA   Food and Drug Administration

GI   gastrointestinal
GnRH   gonadotropin-releasing hormone
GTCT   granulosa thecal cell tumor
IM   intramuscular
IUD   intrauterine device
PO   per os (by mouth)
PRID   progesterone releasing intravaginal device
SC   subcutaneous
SID   once a day
TRP   transrectal palpation
U/S   ultrasound, ultrasonography
VC   vulvar conformation

See Also

- Abnormal estrus intervals
- Anestrus
- Breeding soundness examination, components, mare
- Clitoral enlargement
- Conception failure
- Endometritis
- Estrous cycle, manipulation of
- Estrus detection, fundamentals
- Large ovary syndrome
- Ovulation failure
- Ovulation induction
- Ovulation, synchronization of
- Transrectal palpation

Suggested Reading

Carleton CL. 2007. Clinical examination of the nonpregnant equine female reproductive tract. In: *Current Therapy in Large Animal Theriogenology*, 2nd ed. Youngquist RS, Threlfall WR (eds). Philadelphia: Elsevier Saunders; 74–90.

McCue PM, Lemons SS, Squires EL, et al. 1997. Efficacy of Synovex-S® implants in suppression of estrus in the mare. *J Eq Vet Sci* 17: 327–329.

Pryor P, Tibary A. 2005. Management of Estrus in the Performance Mare. In: *Current Techniques in Equine Practice*. Philadelphia: Elsevier Saunders; 197–209.

Author: Carla L. Carleton

chapter 11

Broad Ligament Hematoma

DEFINITION/OVERVIEW

A rupture of the utero-ovarian, middle uterine, or external iliac arteries near the time of parturition can lead to a hematoma of the broad ligament. The broad ligament is actually two layers of thin tissue apposed to each other; hemorrhage into this area separates the layers but confines the blood. If the broad ligament tissue is too weak to maintain the amount of blood from the ruptured artery, the blood will enter the abdominal cavity and the mare will die. Mares with a hematoma may appear to be in shock, with pale mucous membranes, but death rarely occurs if the broad ligament layers remain intact.

ETIOLOGY/PATHOPHYSIOLOGY

With aging, the walls of the utero-ovarian and middle uterine arteries undergo degenerative processes believed to result in loss of elasticity. This loss in elasticity combined with the increased size or stretching increases the likelihood the arteries will rupture. Preexisting damage to the intima and underlying media of the external iliac arteries (e.g., parasites) may result in necrosis and accumulation of material, predisposing them to rupture.

Systems Affected

- Reproductive
- Cardiovascular
  The reproductive system is ultimately affected, but the vascular component of the cardiovascular system is the actual problem as described previously. The loss of blood into the broad ligament may decrease the speed of the sequential stages of parturition and result in delivery of a dead fetus. A rupture of the ligament, releasing blood into the abdominal cavity, may result in the mare's death prior to delivery of the fetus and therefore also its death. The loss of blood from the cardiovascular system will cause an increase in HR and respiration. The mucous membranes will become pale depending on the amount of the blood lost from the vascular system.

SIGNALMENT/HISTORY

Risk Factors

- The biggest risk factor is pregnancy or delivery of an offspring within minutes before the condition becomes apparent.
- A genetic component of this condition is not known but is not believed to be a factor.
- Rupture of the broad ligament can occur at any age but is most commonly reported in mares older than 12 years of age. Personal history includes witnessing a 7-year-old mare rupture the vessels within the broad ligament during her first gestation.
- Rolling of the mare near term has been suggested as a possible inciting cause but has not been proven. Also, movement of the fetus within the uterus has been speculated as a cause.

Historical Findings

There are no specific historical comments characteristic of this condition other than pregnancy and exhibiting the clinical signs listed previously. Increased respirations and HR observed by the owner in a mare at term and possibly in labor are not unusual. Pale mucous membranes observed by the client would be of major significance. Following rupture of an artery within the broad ligament and with accumulation of blood, some mares may exhibit colicky pain associated with stretching of the affected portion of the mesometrium (broad ligament attached to the uterus).

CLINICAL FEATURES

- The first assessment to make is of the mucous membranes. They will be pale to white depending on the amount of blood loss. This will be true whether there is bleeding into the broad ligament or bleeding into the abdominal cavity. Clinical signs suggestive of hemorrhagic shock (e.g., tachycardia, delayed CRT, sweating) may also appear. The mare may appear anxious or frightened with eyelids wide open.
- If these signs are present, a TRP should be performed very carefully. The palpation of an enlarged structure within the area of the broad liganent should be an immediate cause for concern and further palpation *should cease*. Although the swelling can be bilateral, it usually is restricted to one side.

DIFFERENTIAL DIAGNOSIS

There is no other cause other than external trauma with obvious blood loss that would account for the history and signs observed with this condition. Colicky signs may occur with rupture of the broad ligament vessels and may create uncomfortable signs, sweating, increased respiration and HR, but they will not account for the pale mucous membranes. Abscesses in the area of the vagina may occur, but these would have developed after the previous parturition and should have been diagnosed prior to the current parturition.

DIAGNOSTICS

- Careful TRP of the area adjacent to the uterus is the preferred diagnostic method to confirm this diagnosis. U/S equipment can be used to confirm the enlarged area is indeed caused by the presence of blood, but this is rarely necessary. Both of these techniques should be performed with care.
- If the fetus has not been delivered at the time clinical signs develop, attention should be directed toward maintaining its life while attempting to do no further damage to the mare's vessel wall or broad ligament.

THERAPEUTICS

Two major considerations involved with broad ligament hematoma:
- First: avoid transporting the mare anywhere until she is medically stable. That would be based on clinical indications that the hematoma has clotted, contracted, and begun noticeably to reduce in size.
- Secondly, prevent the mare from rolling, running, or becoming excited in any manner that might result in further bleeding from the weakened vessel or terminal rupture of the broad ligaments or mesometrium, permitting blood to escape into the abdomen.
- IV fluids can be administered, as can whole blood, if available.
- Medications that would further lower blood pressure or increase cardiac activity should be avoided. Agents to enhance clotting have little or no value because the primary problem is hemorrhage and not failure to form clots. The increased pressure within the broad ligament(s), if the broad ligament remains intact, can prevent the further accumulation of blood.
- Oxytocin administration is ill-advised because the bleeding is occurring in the broad ligament and further stimulation of uterine contractions may cause additional hemorrhage from the vessels leading to it.

Appropriate Health Care

Immediately upon diagnosis, in addition to restricting the mare's movement and maintaining her in a quiet environment, take care to avoid activity of the foal or overly vigorous nursing activity, which is behavior that would excite the mare and have a negative impact on the hematoma.

Activity

The mare's activity should be restricted for at least 2 weeks; longer is preferable. Slow hand-walking for exercise is indicated, if necessary.

Surgical Considerations

Surgery to ligate a ruptured vessel usually is impossible without transporting the mare to a surgical facility. The act of transporting the mare to such a facility increases her risk of further bleeding, so it is contraindicated. It is always advisable to maintain the mare in a quiet environment with conservative therapy.

 COMMENTS

Client Education

Clients should be made aware that the likelihood of broad ligament hematomas increases with age. Any aged mare to be bred can rupture a uterine vessel. This conversation with the owner may determine if the mare remains a broodmare or is removed from production to become a *family member*. The possibility of recurrence is obvious because the inciting cause appears to be loss of elasticity of the vessels and owners should be cautioned regarding rebreeding mares that have had this condition.

Patient Monitoring

- The owner should monitor the mucous mebranes and activity of the mare. Note should be taken of her appetite and defecations, as well as lactation.
- Once a hematoma has been confirmed, subsequent TRP should be avoided to reduce the possibility of iatrogenic rupture of a broad ligament that is stretched or under great pressure.

Prevention/Avoidance

The only definite way to avoid this condition is not to breed the mare.

Possible Complications

- Mares with this condition frequently die following blood loss into the abdominal cavity.
- The second possible complication is a broad ligament hematoma that becomes infected and develops into a large abscess.
- The third possibility is the scar tissue that remains after hemorrhage, clot formation, and contraction reduces the size of the pelvic canal, making future deliveries more difficult or requiring a C-section.

Expected Course and Prognosis

- The best outcome would be bleeding confined to the broad ligament, in the absence of infection, and the size of the birth canal after complete healing, is not reduced.
- It may take months for the hematoma to reduce to its final size. Once affected, mares are at increased risk of future rupture.

Synonyms

- Mesometrial hematoma
- Utero-ovarian artery rupture
- Middle uterine artery rupture
- Iliac artery rupture

Abbreviations

CRT capillary refill time
HR heart rate
IV intravenous
TRP transrectal palpation
U/S ultrasound, ultrasonography

See Also

- Dystocia

Suggested Reading

Asbury AC. 1993. Care of the mare after foaling. In: *Equine Reproduction.* McKinnon AO and Voss JL (eds). Philadelphia: Lea & Febiger; 979.

Pascoe RR. 1979. Rupture of the utero-ovarian or middle uterine artery in the mare at or near parturition. *Vet Rec* 104: 77–82.

Rooney JR. 1966. Internal hemorrhage related to gestation. In: *Progress in Equine Practice.* Catcott EJ and Smithcors JF (eds); Wheaton, IL: American Veterinary Publications; 360–361.

Author: Walter R. Threlfall

chapter 12

Breeding Soundness Examinations of Mares

 DEFINITION/OVERVIEW

- A BSE looks at the *big picture*. It takes into consideration more information than a prebreeding examination. Its intent is to define and prognosticate about a mare's current state of reproductive soundness.
- A BSE is designed to evaluate the mare for her potential to conceive, carry a pregnancy to term, and deliver a healthy foal.

 ETIOLOGY/PATHOPHYSIOLOGY

Systems Affected

- All body systems are evaluated for general health.
- Reproductive system receives specific attention for its soundness.

 SIGNALMENT/HISTORY

Indications for a BSE

- Pre-breeding, particularly if the mare is new to the owner and little is known about the mare's history.
- Pre-purchase
- Post-purchase (if not possible before sale).
- Barren mares
- Maiden mares
- Foaling problems
- Mares reproductively idle for an extended period.
- Candidates for ET (donor and recipients).
- Any problems detected during a routine prebreeding examination.
- Any other situation in which it would be beneficial to have a more complete understanding of a mare's reproductive soundness.

Risk Factors

- Risks of injury to the horse, handler, or examiner are associated with the BSE procedures.

Risks for the Horse

- Age
- Gender
- Breed
- Inadequate or improper restraint
- Inadequate examiner experience
- Poor technique
- Prior or current damage to the rectal wall

Risks for the Handler or Examiner

- Inadequate or improper restraint

Historical Findings

- Frequently employed in reproductive practice, although often broadly applied by name to less thorough reproductive examinations conducted on mares for a variety of reasons.
- Mare of breeding age, regardless of breed or use; for a specific breeding related evaluation.

History

- Consider the three key factors of the fertility equation (i.e., mare, stallion, and management) and gather as much information about each as is available.
- The following is a minimum list of areas in which to gather information. These lists are by no means exhaustive for every mare or circumstance.

Mare Factors

- Signalment of mare (i.e., breed, age, parity, etc.)
- General reproductive history
- Recent reproductive history
- Reproductive treatments
- Results of previous PBE or BSE
- Preventive health program
- Previous disease
- Other information pertinent to the individual mare or circumstances

Stallion Factors

- Type of semen being used (preparation: fresh, raw or extended; chilled; frozen)
- Semen quality

- Per cycle conception rate
- Breedings per conception
- Pregnancy rate
- Foaling rates
- Health status
- Other information pertinent to the individual mare or circumstances.

Management Factors

- Breeding season (type of cover, live (natural) or AI)
- Teasing (frequency and procedures)
- Breeding technique
- Farm reproductive efficiency (i.e., conception, foaling, and abortion rates, etc.)
- Preventive treatments (reproductive and general health maintenance)
- Vaccination programs (reproductive and general health maintenance)
- Nutritional program
- Other information pertinent to the individual mare or circumstances.

 CLINICAL FEATURES

Supplies and Equipment Necessary to Conduct a Routine BSE:

- Shoulder length palpation sleeve
- Palpation lubricant (e.g., carboxymethylcellulose)
- Ultrasound unit with a 5- or 7.5-MHz linear probe
- Tube or mechanical vaginoscope, sterilized
- Focused light source (to illuminate the vaginal cavity)
- Endometrial culture swabs
- Endometrial cytology swab (or brush)
- Endometrial biopsy instrument
- Fixative for endometrial tissue (10% BNF/formalin or Bouin's solution)
- Sterile sleeves
- Sterile lubricant
- Clean bucket with disposable liner
- Clean water source
- Liquid soap (preferably antiseptic)
- Roll cotton (or other suitable material for meticulous cleaning of the perineum)
- Tail wrap
- Tail tie
- Halter
- Lead rope

Optional Materials

- Recommended to be available, may be necessary in some situations:
  - Transport media or culture plates for endometrial culture

- Microscope slides and stain for cytology
- Stocks
- Twitch
- Sedation
- Anticholinergic agent
- Local anesthetic

 DIAGNOSTICS

Timing of a BSE

- A mare should be in her ovulatory season (so her reproductive tract is under the alternating influence of the steroid hormones, estrogen and progesterone) when a BSE is performed. Information obtained from a BSE is of less value if performed outside of the ovulatory season.
- A BSE can be performed during estrus or diestrus, the cervix does not present a physical barrier to performing the intrauterine procedures. Some theriogenologists feel it is contraindicated to perform a BSE during diestrus when the cervix is closed and progesterone concentrations are elevated. Others do not feel diestrus is a limitation and, in fact, find it may yield more valuable information, particularly from the uterine culture and endometrial biopsy.

Procedures/Techniques

- The most benefit is gained when a BSE is conducted in a systematic fashion, but it is of particular importance that the components of the basic examination of the reproductive organs be conducted in the sequence that will be discussed.
- Performing the procedures out of sequence may, at best, interfere with your ability to derive a meaningful interpretation from the information gathered and, at worst, abort a previously undiagnosed pregnancy.

Identify the Mare

- Record and maintain a permanent description of the mare that can be used in the future, if needed, to verify the identity of the mare examined.
- Particularly important in prepurchase situations.
- This may include a written record and description of permanent markings, a photograph, or a microchip.
- Also make note of her dental age.

General Physical Examination

- Initially, step back and take a general look at the mare to gain an overall impression.
- Record the mare's BCS.
- Evaluate her general conformation and soundness.

- Record her temperature, pulse, and respiratory rate.
- Conduct a general examination of her nonreproductive body systems.
- Note and investigate further any signs of systemic illness.

Mammary Gland

- Visually inspect the gland for size, symmetry, or discharge.
- Palpate the gland for consistency, signs of inflammation, or secretions.

Vulvar and Perineal Conformation

- Evaluate the perineum for overall conformation, orientation, symmetry and structure (Figs. 12.1 and 12.2).
- Examine for lesions, vulvar discharge and apposition of the vulvar labia (Fig. 12.3).
- Determine if a Caslick's vulvoplasty is in place or if there is evidence one was present in the past.
- Evaluate the size, position, and orientation of the vulva.

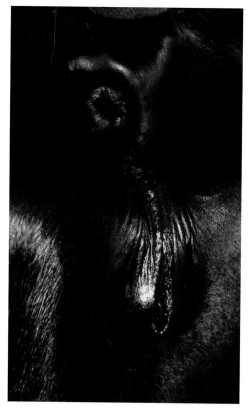

■ **Figure 12.1** Perineal assessment of vulvar conformation. Example of severe cranial slant of vulvae, poor vulvular conformation.

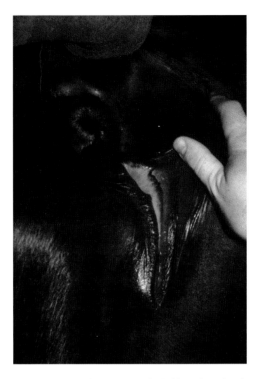

■ **Figure 12.2** Poor vulvar conformation. With one vulvar lip held to the side, the degree of slant, location of the dorsal commissure, and portion of the vulvar cleft lying dorsal to the floor of the pubis are very evident.

- Dorsal commissure of the vulva should not incline more than 10 degrees cranially from a vertical plane.
  - This declination is referred to as the *AS*.
  - Ideally the dorsal commissure should be even with or slightly below the floor of the pubis; certainly no more than 2–4 cm above the pelvic floor.
  - Minimally 70% of the vulvar cleft (opening) should be below a horizontal plane extended caudally from the floor of the mare's pubis (ischial arch) (Fig. 12.4).
  - The portion (in cm) of vulvar cleft above the horizontal plane is referred to as dorsal displacement.
- Determine and record a CI
  - Record the DD of the vulva (in cm).
  - Record the AS of the vulva (degrees of displacement).
  - Calculate the CI by multiplying the DD × AS. For example, if the dorsal commissure is 2 cm above the pubic floor and the AS is 20 degrees, 2 × 20 = 40. Not ideal but adequate. An almost perpendicular vulva (less than or equal to 5 degrees AS) typical of most warm-blooded and draft breeds of horses) with at most 1 cm above the pubic floor, would be: 5 × 1 = a CI of 5.

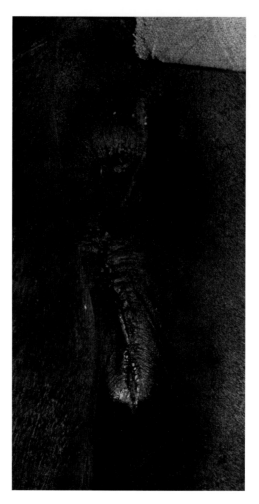

■ **Figure 12.3** Cranial slant to the vulvae, compounded by a poor seal between the vulvar lips. In addition, one-third of the vulvar cleft lay above the floor of the pubis.

- ■ CI of less than 50 reflects adequate or good perineal conformation.
- ■ CI of 50 to 150 is a grey zone; the impact of VC depends on the contribution of each individual factor (i.e., AS, DD) to the index, although a CI over 100 usually has some related reproductive problems.
- ■ A mare with a CI over 150 is highly likely to have reproductive problems related to perineal conformation.
- ■ Note: Theriogenologists often employ yet more rigid standards, anticipating that the dorsal commissure lie no less than 2.5 cm *below* or lower than the pubic floor. This ensures that even late in gestation, when the weight of the uterus, placenta, fetus, and fetal fluids is greatest, and the vulvae are drawn forward (maximal AS), that the dorsal commissure of the vulvar lips remains at least marginally protective against ascending infections late in gestation (preferably closed so that the dorsal

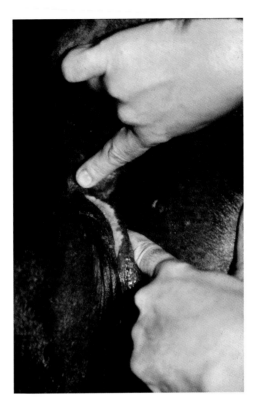

■ **Figure 12.4** Demonstration of the minimum limit of vulvoplasty required to protect the mare from ascending contamination (to the floor of the pubis, plus an additional 2.5 cm, as long as sufficient ventral vulvar cleft remains to allow urination in a free stream).

commissure is still at least 1 to 2 cm lower than the floor of the pubis). If a mare has terrible VC there may be insufficient vulvar cleft remaining to attain protection with a Caslick's vulvoplasty.
■ In extreme cases, an alternative procedure (e.g., the Pouret) may be necessary. The Pouret technique involves a division of the perineal body (horizontal dissection, caudal to cranial), separating the tubular genital tract from the rectum. The perineal body dissection allows the genital tract to "slide" caudally, bringing the vulvar cleft to a more ventral position. Closure involves none of the deeper tissue, only the skin incision. This procedure must be done with proper restraint and anesthetic. Dissection of the perineal body must be careful and deliberate to avoid incising into either the rectum (dorsally) or the vestibule or vagina (ventrally).

TRP of the Internal Reproductive Tract

Examine the *ovaries* for size, shape, symmetry. and structures (Fig. 12.5):
■ Evaluate follicular structures for size, number, location, and consistency.
■ The CL is not palpable in mares more than 5 days post-ovulation.

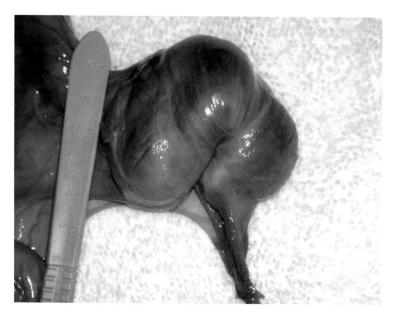

■ **Figure 12.5** Dominant follicles on middle and caudal pole of mare's ovary.

- Ovulation fossa (Fig. 12.6).
- Record the presence of any paraovarian cysts that are larger than 10 mm. Less experienced veterinarians may mistake a large paraovarian cyst for a follicle. With a thorough, methodical palpation, it is evident that they are para-ovarian and not *of the ovary*.

Examine the *uterus* for size, shape, symmetry, and consistency (Fig. 12.7):

- Expect some degree of muscular relaxation (decreased uterine tone) and edema of the endometrial folds during estrus (Fig. 12.8); estradiol (follicular origin) is the dominant hormone responsible for edema. Decreased uterine tone is primarily a reflection of the *absence of* progesterone.
- Expect increased muscular tone during diestrus when progesterone is the dominant ovarian contribution (CL origin).
- Expect an atonic (or flaccid) uterus during anestrus.
- Rule-out pregnancy, especially in the presence of increased uterine tone.

Examine the *cervix* for size and consistency:

- Helps to determine the stage of her estrous cycle.
- In estrus the cervix relaxes, becomes softer and wider up to the time of ovulation. A normal cervix will generally close within 48 hours following ovulation under the influence of progesterone.
- In diestrus the cervix will be found to be toned and tight (closed). The proportions of the cervix may become even more dramatic in early pregnancy (15 to 21–22 days): closed and narrow (CN), or closed, narrow, and elongated (CNE, essentially the approximate proportions of a #2 pencil).

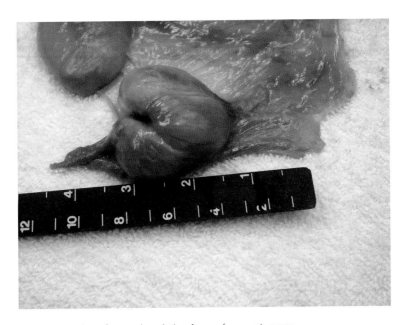

■ **Figure 12.6** Demonstration of normal ovulation fossa of a mare's ovary.

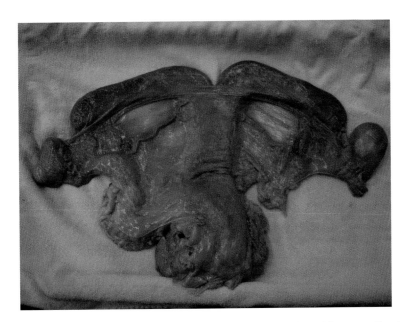

■ **Figure 12.7** Dorsal view of a normal mare uterus, cervix, ovaries, and broad ligament. The characteristic blunt ends of the mare's uterine horns make their identification during transrectal palpation easy. The proper ligaments extend from the dorsal tip of the uterine horn to the pole of the ipsilateral ovary, maintaining a constant relationship between ovary and uterine horn throughout the mare's reproductive life, in contrast to the stretching of the broad ligament with increasing parity.

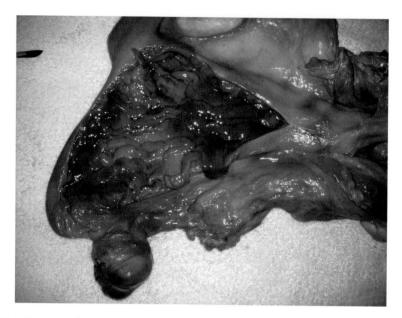

■ **Figure 12.8** Dissection of a mare's tract to reveal the linear, endometrial folds. The folds are most prominent during estrus with the presence of edema due to elevated levels of follicular estradiol.

Transrectal U/S of the Internal Reproductive Tract

Examine the *ovaries* for:
- The presence, size, shape, and number of follicles, as well as periovulatory signs.
- CL
- Abnormalities (e.g., hematomas, tumors, AHF)

Examine the uterus for:
- Size, particularly the diameter of each horn and body. Usually the uterine horn diameter of barren or maiden mares will be similar, within 5 mm, left to right.
- Character of the lumen and wall (i.e., look for edema, fluid, cysts, masses).
- Rule out pregnancy.

Vaginoscopy

- At this point in the BSE, the perineum should be meticulously cleansed and prepared for the remaining *clean techniques.*
- Tips on technique:
  - Use a powerful, focused light source.
  - Inserting the speculum beyond the VVJ prevents examination of areas caudal to the cranial end of the speculum and introduces contaminants further into the vagina.
  - Maiden mares may have a hymen at the VVJ that will need to be broken down before passing the speculum.

Visually examine the vaginal cavity for:

- Color
- Lesions
- Content (e.g., urine, inflammatory fluid)

Visually examine the cervix for:

- Color, position, shape, discharge, lacerations, adhesions, or lesions. Note: cervical lacerations are often missed when diagnosis is solely attempted via vaginal speculum. A digital evaluation is essential to adequately describe loss or compromise of cervical integrity (percentage involvement of the cervical lumen, depth, and thickness of a tear or tears). After a meticulous perineal prep/washing, using a sterile glove and lubricant, place an index finger into the cervical lumen, thumb remains around the perimeter of the external cervical os, to examine it thoroughly for defects/tears.
- In estrus the cervix is moist, glistening, pink and relaxed, and usually in contact with the vaginal floor (described as "melted").
- In diestrus the cervix appears dry, pale pink or nearly blanched, toned and is usually up, off the vaginal floor and appears as a *rosette*.
- Note: The cervix may not relax under estrogen dominance in maiden mares regardless of age.
- Note: Do not confuse the dorsal or ventral cervical frenulum with an abnormality (Fig. 12.9). It can be quite prominent during periods of progesterone dominance (i.e., diestrus or pregnancy) when the cervix is toned and off the vaginal floor.

Endometrial Culture

Most Common Sampling Procedure

- Use a uterine culture swab, preferably double guarded, although other models are available.
- Using clean technique the swab is passed (protected in the palm of the sterile gloved hand) through the vagina to the cervix (Fig. 12.10).
- The swab alone is passed through the cervix to sample the endometrium of the uterine body. Note: A less often practiced option is the use of a speculum and cervical forceps to avoid the need for carrying the swab into the vaginal cavity with a sleeved hand.
- The lumen of the cervical canal may not be straight and easy to traverse. Slight diversions (dorsal or ventral, left or right) mid-way through the lumen, can certainly occur. If technique is meticulous, one's finger may serve as a stylette to first traverse the entire cervical lumen and the culture rod advanced alongside the finger to the depth of the internal cervical os. Only at that time is the culture rod advanced an additional 2 to 2.5 cm into the uterine body to ensure the swab will obtain a representative sample from the uterus.
- After obtaining the sample, immediately transport the swab to a microbiology laboratory, place it in appropriate transport media, or streak the swab on a plate/agar in the examination area.

Another Sampling Procedure

- A piece of endometrial tissue can also be used to inoculate a culture plate.

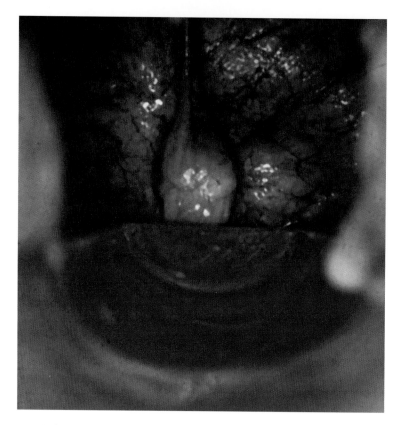

■ **Figure 12.9** Vaginal speculum examination of the diestrus external cervical os; described as a "rosette," high and dry off of the vaginal floor. Note the normal, dorsal frenulum above the external cervical os.

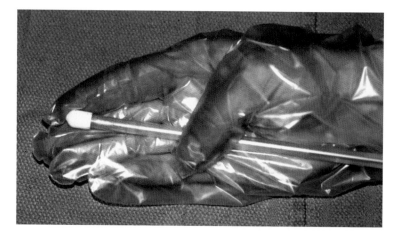

■ **Figure 12.10** Double guarded culture swab ready to be carried into the mare's genital tract to swab the uterine lumen.

Interpretation

- Interpret culture results in conjunction with endometrial cytology.
- False-positive results are common.
- It is unlikely a positive culture is significant without evidence of endometrial inflammation.
- Negative culture results do not rule-out a uterine infection, particularly if evidence of endometrial inflammation is present.

Most Commonly Isolated Reproductive Pathogens in Mares

- B-hemolytic *Streptococci equi* (var. *zooepidemicus* or *S. equisimilis*)
- *Pseudomonas aeruginosa*
- *Klebsiella pneumoniae*
- *Escherichia coli* (a primary fecal contaminant)

Endometrial Cytology

- Used to identify the presence of inflammation on the endometrial surface.
- Cytology does not determine the status of deeper endometrial layers.

Most Common Sampling Procedure

- Proper technique is critical to achieving useful information.
- An endometrial culture swab is typically used to obtain a sample for cytology.
- Note: It is advisable to use a second swab for cytology after obtaining a sample for culture. Using the same swab for both procedures is less likely to yield meaningful results.
- Similar to the procedure for uterine culture, using clean technique, the swab is passed (protected in the palm of the hand) through the vagina to the cervix.
- The swab alone is passed through the cervix to sample the endometrium of the uterine body.
- After obtaining the sample, gently roll the swab on a clean glass microscope slide and air-dry or spray the slide with fixative.
- The slide can be examined later after staining with a number of stains, but Diff Quik is one of the most commonly used.
- Tip: Moistening the cotton swab with sterile saline or PBS before sampling the endometrium helps preserve cell architecture and prevents smudging, streaking and rupturing the cells when preparing the slide.

Other Sampling Procedures

- A cytology brush is used to collect a sample from the endometrium and smear a slide.
- Effluent from a low-volume lavage of the uterus is centrifuged and the pellet used to smear a slide.
- Endometrial biopsy tissue is used to create an impression smear on a glass slide.

Interpretation

- A "normal" or noninflammatory cytology contains plenty of healthy appearing endometrial cells, but no inflammatory cells, debris, or microbes.
- An "abnormal" or inflammatory cytology sample often contains unhealthy appearing endometrial cells and inflammatory cells (primarily neutrophils), along with microbial organisms (particularly if engulfed by the inflammatory cells), or debris.
- Note: Because the concentration of cells on a slide may vary with the technique used to obtain the sample and prepare the slide, it is advisable to use a ratio of neutrophils to endometrial cells or a percentage of neutrophils of the overall cell count on the slide to diagnose inflammation.
- Between 0.5% and 5% of neutrophils on a cytology slide is generally considered indicative of acute endometrial inflammation.

Endometrial Biopsy

- Used to evaluate all layers of the endometrium (Fig. 12.11).
- The biopsy is classified based on pathologic changes present in the endometrium.
- The classification is predictive of the endometrium's ability to support a pregnancy to term.
- It can also be used to develop treatment strategies and monitor response.

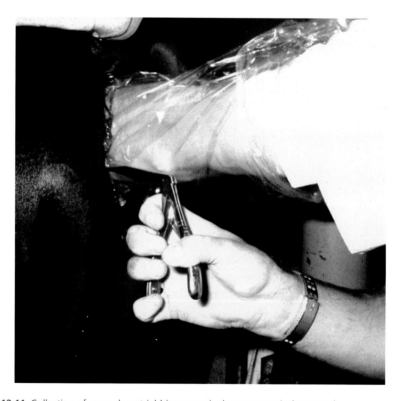

■ **Figure 12.11** Collection of an endometrial biopsy, vaginal or transcervical approach.

Sampling Procedure

- Using clean technique an endometrial biopsy forceps is passed through the cervix and a tissue sample taken near the uterine horn-body junction.
- A single specimen is usually sufficient if enough tissue (preferably 1–2 linear cm) is obtained, but representative samples from two sites may be desirable.
- The endometrial tissue specimen is fixed in Bouin's solution or 10% buffered neutral formalin before shipping it to a histology lab for processing. Note: If the tissue is fixed in Bouin's solution, it should be transferred to 70% ethanol after 4 to 24 hours; otherwise, the sample will become brittle (makes cutting the tissue and preparation of a good slide for interpretation difficult).
- A synopsis of the BSE findings, especially the TRP findings and estimation of the stage of the mare's estrous cycle, should be sent with the tissue sample to aid the pathologist or theriogenologist with evaluation and interpretation of the findings.

Interpretation

- Category I mares have at least an 80% chance of conceiving and carrying a fetus to term (Fig. 12.12).
- Category IIa mares conceive and carry a fetus to term 50% to 80% of the time.
- Category IIb mares are expected to conceive and carry a fetus to term 10% to 50% of the time.
- Category III mares have a less than 10% chance of conceiving and carrying a fetus to term due to the severity of their endometrial changes (Fig. 12.13).

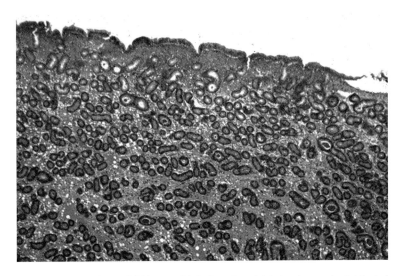

■ **Figure 12.12** Category I endometrial biopsy with lush endometrial glands, evenly distributed and uniform in appearance.

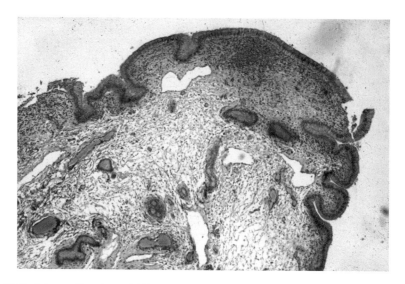

■ **Figure 12.13** Category III endometrial biopsy. Note the dearth of endometrial glands and inflammatory cell locus in the stratum compactum (bluish locus near the luminal epithelium).

Direct (Manual) Cervical Examination

- Direct examination of the cervix can be performed anytime after the sample for endometrial culture is taken.
- Digitally palpate the external os and as much of the cervical canal as can easily be accessed.
- Examine the cervix (its lumen, external os and internal cervical os) for scar tissue, adhesions, masses, and lacerations.
  - The ideal stage of the estrous cycle in which a suspected cervical tear can be identified is diestrus. During diestrus, the cervix is under the influence of progesterone and is most toned or closed.
  - Immediately postpartum, it is often difficult, if not impossible, to distinguish between a cervical tear and the loose, sloppy folds of the postpartum, uninvoluted cervix.

Endoscopy

- Technique used less often with the advent of U/S. If all other examination modalities fail to identify a cause of infertility, endoscopy may yield additional information otherwise missed.
- Intraluminal adhesions will not be evident by TRP or U/S (Fig. 12.14).

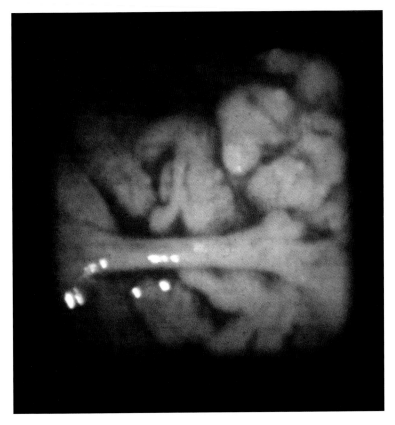

■ **Figure 12.14** Uterine endoscopy and luminal adhesion. When severe the potential arises to interfere with transuterine migration of the early conceptus and/or maintenance of a pregnancy.

 THERAPEUTICS

Drug(s) of Choice

- Sedation or administration of an anticholinergic agent may be necessary to facilitate proper restraint and safe conditions for TRP and other BSE procedures.
- After all BSE procedures are completed it may be advisable to administer an ecbolic or luteolytic agent (i.e., prostaglandin) to aid uterine clearance or ensure the mare returns to estrus. If an endometrial biopsy has been taken, the mare may return to heat subsequent to the release of prostaglandin from the endometrium. Mention to the owner that he or she may see a small amount of blood at the vulvar lips post-biopsy (5 to 15 mL) the day of or following day, to avoid their worry post-procedure.
  - If a mare is in early diestrus when the BSE is performed, an additional dose of prostaglandin may be dispensed for administration 3 to 5 days later.

Sedation

- Xylazine (0.2–1.1 mg/kg), IV.
- Xylazine (0.33–0.44 mg/kg) and butorphanol (0.033–0.066 mg/kg), IV.
- Detomidine (0.01–0.02 mg/kg), IV.
- Detomidine (0.01–0.02 mg/kg) and butorphanol (0.044–0.066 mg/kg), IV.

Alternative Drugs

Anticholinergics

- N-butylscopolammonium bromide or Buscopan® (0.3 mg/kg), IV.
- Propantheline bromide (0.014–0.07 mg/kg), IV.

Local Anesthetic

- 2% Lidocaine (50 mL) infused into the rectum. This may help with palpation of mares or colicky males (stallions, geldings) that pose particular difficulty when trying to achieve relaxation (lateral or dorso-ventral mobility within the rectum).

Ecbolic/Luteolytic Agent

- Dinoprost tromethamine (10 mg) IM.
- Cloprostenol (250 μg) IM.

Appropriate Health Care

General health care appropriate for the region in which the horse is located.

Nursing Care

It is advisable to rinse and wipe any remaining lubricant off the perineum following all BSE procedures to avoid skin irritation.

Diet

No special dietary accommodations are necessary.

Activity

No limit on activity unless complications develop from the procedures.

Surgical Considerations

Poor perineal conformation may necessitate surgical repair. Refer to chapter on Caslick's vulvoplasty.

 COMMENTS

Client Education

- Inform the owner of the risks associated with the BSE procedures, particularly TRP.

- Advise the owner to observe the horse within a few hours following the BSE procedure for signs associated with a rectal tear.

Patient Monitoring

- TRP and U/S are associated with some risk of damage to the rectal wall, therefore the horse should be observed within a few hours of the examination for clinical signs consistent with a rectal tear.
- The owner may also observe a low volume (5 to 15 mL) bloody discharge from the vulva for a couple of days following a uterine biopsy. Although not a problem, for the owner should be advised to avoid undue concern.

Prevention/Avoidance

- Many of the BSE procedures cannot be performed in young mares that have not reached sufficient body size to permit a safe examination.

Possible Complications

- Rectal tear
- Pregnancy should be ruled-out early in the BSE to avoid an iatrogenic abortion from the intrauterine procedures.
- Avoid attempting a BSE on a mare that is too young or small to safely perform the procedures.
- Although sedation may be necessary to make the horse more tractable to the BSE procedures, over-sedation can cause instability and increase the risk to horse, handler, and examiner.
- Some horses may display signs of abdominal discomfort due to the generalized effects of propantheline bromide on the GI tract.

Expected Course and Prognosis

- In the vast majority of cases, the BSE procedures are minimally invasive and progress without incident or complication.
- A written report should be prepared for the owner summarizing findings from all aspects of the BSE, including diagnosis, recommended treatment, and prognosis.

Abbreviations

AHF   anovulatory hemorrhagic follicle
AS   anterior slope
BCS   body condition score
BNF   buffered neutral formalin
BSE   breeding soundness examination
CI   Caslick's index
CL   corpus luteum
DD   dorsal displacement
ET   embryo transfer

GI   gastrointestinal
IM   intramuscular
IV   intravenous
PBE   prebreeding examination
PBS   phosphate buffered saline
TRP   transrectal palpation
U/S   ultrasound, ultrasonography
VC   vulvar conformation
VVJ   vestibulo-vaginal junction

See Also

- Anestrus
- Broad ligament hematoma
- BSE Stallion
- Cervical lesions
- Clitoral enlargement
- Conception failure
- Delayed uterine involution
- Endometrial biopsy
- Endometritis
- History, mare
- Large ovary syndrome
- Pneumovagina/pneumouterus
- Postpartum metritis
- Prolonged diestrus
- Rectal tears
- TRP of the reproductive tract
- Urine pooling, urovagina
- Vaginal prolapse
- Vaginitis and vaginal discharge
- Vulvar conformation

Suggested Reading

Blanchard TL, Varner DD, Schumacher J, et al. 2003. Breeding soundness examination of the mare. In: *Manual of Equine Reproduction*. St. Louis: Mosby; 31–42.

Carleton CL. 1988. Basic techniques for evaluating the subfertile mare. *Vet Med* 83: 1253–1261.

Carleton CL. 2007. Clinical examination of the non-pregnant female reproductive tract. In: Youngquist RS and Threlfall WR (eds). *Current Therapy in Large Animal Theriogenology*, 2nd ed. Philadelphia: Saunders Elsevier; 74–90.

McKinnon AO, Voss JL (eds). 1993. *Equine Reproduction*. Philadelphia: Lea & Febiger; 196–303.

Authors: Carla L. Carleton and Gary J. Nie

chapter 13

Cervical Abnormalities

DEFINITION/OVERVIEW

- Most common cervical problems encountered are inflammation, lacerations, and adhesions and the inability to dilate during estrus.
- Congenital abnormalities and neoplasia of the cervix are rare.

ETIOLOGY/PATHOPHYSIOLOGY

- The thick circular muscular layer and the elastic fibers of the cervix, when normal, are responsible for relaxation (opening) and contraction (closure) (Fig. 13.1).
- Progesterone, either from diestrus or pregnancy, is responsible for keeping the cervix closed and tight.

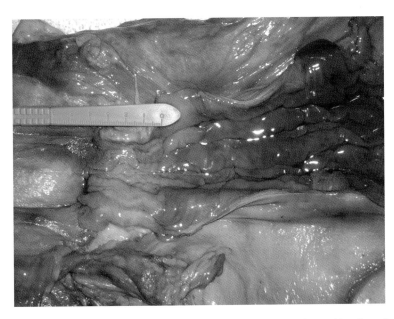

■ **Figure 13.1** Dissected mare tract. Easy to distinguish between the smooth transition from linear, cervical folds (0–3.5 cm next to the shaft of the scalpel handle) onto endometrial folds that continue to the right. Image courtesy of C. L. Carleton

- Lesions may impair normal cervical function and competency, leading to infertility, repeated uterine infections, and possible pregnancy loss.

Systems Affected

Reproductive

SIGNALMENT/HISTORY

- Old (mean age, 12–13 years), pluriparous mares (mean parity before surgery, 6.2 years) after either an apparently normal parturition (85% of cervical lacerations) or dystocia.
- Old, pluriparous mares are more predisposed to cervicitis caused by pneumovagina, urovagina, or DUC.
- Young or old, nervous, maiden mares.

Risk Factors

- Pluriparous and old mares.
- Prolonged natural or assisted parturition.
- More than 2 to 3 cuts with the fetotome.
- Young or old maiden mares.
- Aggressive uterine therapy.
- Concurrent acute and chronic endometritis.

Historical Findings

- Infertility, recurrent uterine infections and pregnancy loss; most commonly associated with cervical lacerations:
  - EED is generally the result of a large laceration present. The cervix is too incompetent, incapable of even short-term pregnancy maintenance.
  - Late gestation problems or pregnancy loss is more often associated with less extensive, medium size lacerations or disruptions.
- Pyometra: associated with cervical adhesions.

CLINICAL FEATURES

Infectious

- Associated with anatomic abnormalities: vaginitis and endometritis can be linked with pneumovagina.
- Severe acute cervicitis develops after inoculation or infection with *Taylorella equigenitalis* (CEM).
- *See* also Endometritis and Ascending Placentitis.

Noninfectious

Cervical Trauma

- A frequent occurrence, resulting in full- or partial-thickness lacerations, during unassisted, prolonged parturition or dystocia (assisted, difficult foaling).
- Prolonged manipulation and traction aggravate the outcome.
  - Extended fetal pressure against the cervical walls can lead to necrosis associated with loss of mucosa.
  - Use of a fetotome: mucosal cuts due to malposition of the obstetric wire (i.e., insufficient guarding of saw-wire within the fetotome channels or the wire portion extending around a fetal part for transection).
- Lacerations most frequently occur in the vaginal portion of the cervix but may extend cranially toward the uterus; partial to full-length, at its most extreme include the internal cervical os.
- Two types of lacerations
  - Overstretching or partial-thickness laceration of the muscular layer with intact mucosa.
  - Full-thickness laceration.

Adhesions

- Frequently present when or with cervical lacerations.
- Fibrous bands of variable thickness extending across the cervical lumen (intraluminal) or from external cervical os to vaginal wall (peri-cervical).
- Location/position of the damage affects cervical opening/patency (intraluminal) or ability to close under the influence of progesterone (peri-cervical).
- May be a sequel to cervical trauma, inadequate relaxation (maiden mare, excessively nervous mare) during parturition, or may have originated subsequent to the use of irritating solutions for uterine therapy, pyometra, and rarely, chronic endometritis.
- May obliterate the cervical lumen and prevent it from opening and closing properly.

Cervicitis

- May be iatrogenic (e.g., chemical substances) or secondary to trauma (e.g., parturition, dystocia, obstetric manipulation) or infection (e.g., vaginitis, endometritis).
- Individual sensitivity exists to the use of diluted iodine, chlorhexidine, or acetic acid. These products may produce mucosal irritation, ulceration, and necrosis, even at low dilutions.
- May occur following the use of nonbuffered aminoglycosides, antibiotics, or antimycotics for endometritis.
- Pneumovagina and urovagina may result in vaginal, cervical, and uterine irritation.

Idiopathic Failure to Dilate

- Some maiden mares (young or old) show impaired cervical relaxation during estrus.
- More evident in older maiden mares where collagen is progressively replaced by fibrous tissue.
- No associated adhesions are evident.
- Affects ability to conceive by natural breeding (vaginal versus uterine deposition of the ejaculate).
- Routinely results in DUC. The closed/indurated cervix prevents active removal of uterine glandular secretions, debris, residual content of the ejaculate, and so on that would otherwise be eliminated during estrus (as through a normal, relaxed cervix during estrus); further compounds an existing endometritis.
- Once affected mares conceive, the cervix dilates normally at parturition.

Neoplasia

- Very rare
- Uterocervical leiomyoma has been reported.

Developmental Abnormalities

- Rare: Cervical aplasia, hypoplasia, and double cervix (Fig. 13.2).
- Congenital incompetency

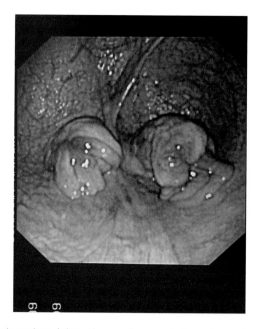

■ **Figure 13.2** Double cervix as viewed through an endoscope. Each cervix was found to be completely developed with a complete lumen.
Image courtesy of C. L. Carleton.

DIFFERENTIAL DIAGNOSIS

Other causes of vaginal discharge:
- Endometritis
- Pyometra
- Placentitis

DIAGNOSTICS

U/S

First determine if the mare is pregnant. A digital evaluation is contraindicated and may result in termination of an existing pregnancy. Fluid accumulation in the uterine lumen can be caused by a tight cervix (e.g., failure to relax while in estrus, preventing normal fluid clearance after breeding) or adhesions.

Cervical Examination

- The cervix is examined by TRP, direct visualization with a speculum (Fig. 13.3), and direct vaginal/digital palpation. The latter is recommended over speculum examination.

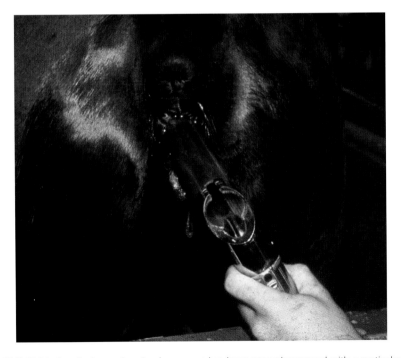

■ **Figure 13.3** Lighted vaginal speculum in place; mare has been properly prepped with a meticulous perineal wash prior to beginning vaginal procedures.
Image courtesy of W. R. Threlfall.

- TRP: only determines the size, tone, and degree of cervical relaxation. Cervical tears cannot be identified transrectally.
- Vaginoscopy: provides information regarding cervical and vaginal color (e.g., hyperemia), presence of edema, secretions (e.g., pus, urine), cysts, varicose veins, adhesions between the external cervical os and the vaginal fornix and/or walls, and an approximation of relaxation as the mare approaches estrus (Figs. 13.4 and 13.5).
- Digital palpation of the cervix is essential to evaluate lacerations or intraluminal adhesions. It is performed by placing the index finger into the cervical lumen and the thumb on the vaginal side of the cervix, feeling carefully for defects around its full perimeter.
- To assess the cervix' ability to relax and the presence and consequences of intraluminal adhesions, perform cervical evaluation during estrus using sterile glove and lubrication.
- To evaluate cervical closure and tone and for the presence and extent of lacerations, conduct the assessment during diestrus.
- During the noncycling phase of the year, mares can be placed on exogenous progesterone for 4 days to evaluate cervical tone, competency, and its ability to close.

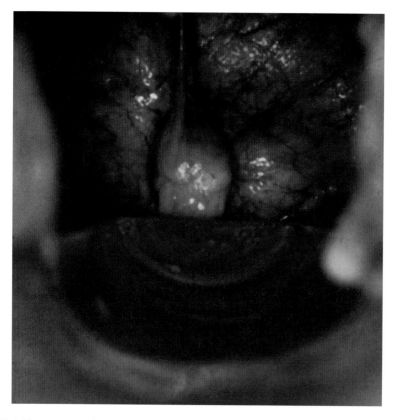

■ **Figure 13.4** Diestrus external cervical os, oft described as a rosette. Its dorsal frenulum is readily apparent.

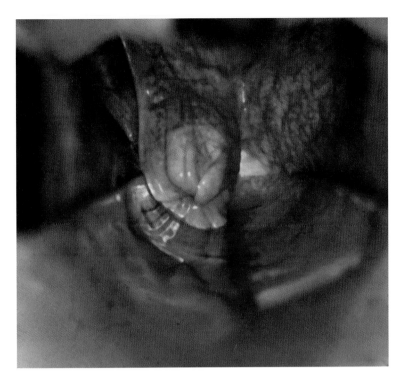

■ **Figure 13.5** A relaxing external cervical os as the mare enters estrus.

- Only mayor defects can be detected in postpartum mares. Allow at least 7 days for substantial involution, reduction in size, and for normal postpartum inflammation to subside.

Pathological Findings

- Vaginal examination: pneumovagina or urovagina; vaginal discharge; purulent material coming through the cervix; cervical and vaginal mucosal irritation; cervical lacerations or mucosal roughness; adhesions between the cervix and vaginal fornix or in the cervical lumen; intrauterine fluid accumulation, with or without cervical adhesions.
- Intrauterine fluid accumulation after breeding.

 THERAPEUTICS

Cervical Lacerations

- Surgical repair may not be necessary if or when less than 50% of the vaginal portion of the cervix (the cervical lumen) is affected (i.e., stretching, partial- or full-thickness lacerations that don't compromise the competency of the internal cervical os).

- Progesterone supplementation, beginning prior to the embryo's arrival and migration into the uterus, may provide sufficient benefit by increasing cervical tone, such that surgery is not required to overcome minor anatomic/functional damage.
- Cervical repair may be warranted for small cervical lacerations if coupled with a history of infertility.
- Surgical repair is required:
  - for longitudinal, full- or partial-thickness lacerations within the cervical muscle if they encompass more than 50% of the length of the cervical lumen, progressing cranially
  - or that involve the junction of the external portion of the cervix with the vagina (the vaginal fornix) and therefore affect the ability of the cervix to close.
- An extensive, wide laceration or multiple lacerations will increase surgical complexity and aggravate the prognosis for fertility.
- With a successful surgical repair, prognosis is fair to good for delivering a term foal.
- Mild intraluminal adhesions are usually found after surgery. Apply ointment with antibiotics and steroids if the mare is not pregnant.
- Perform endometrial biopsy before surgery to evaluate endometrial well-being (determine the mare's current biopsy category). Unnecessary repair and expense can be avoided if it is found that surgery cannot improve the mare's ability to carry a fetus to term.

Adhesions

- Mucosal and submucosal lacerations are treated daily with antimicrobial/steroidal anti-inflammatory ointment to avoid cervical adhesions.
- Recently formed adhesions are manually debrided daily, and ointment is applied BID to avoid recurrence.
- If some cervical lumen remains, mature cervical adhesions may be circumvented by AI or be reduced surgically, with a guarded prognosis for fertility. They are difficult to resolve completely.
- Chronic pyometra resulting from cervical adhesions: control with lavage, oxytocin, and ET.
- Begin treatment of cervical lacerations immediately postpartum to prevent adhesions and infection.

Cervicitis

- Anatomic defects resulting in cervical inflammation, such as pneumovagina and urovagina, should be corrected surgically.
- Infection: *see* Endometritis and Ascending Placentitis.

Idiopathic

- AI and treatment for DUC. If natural breeding is necessary, dilate the cervix manually or use prostaglandin E1 analog.

Drug(s) of Choice

Progestin Supplementation

- Altrenogest: Double dose (0.088 mg/kg PO daily) during and after surgery (for 7–10 days).
- Altrenogest: Single dose (0.044 mg/kg PO daily) until 90 to 110 days gestation.
- Bio-release progesterone every 10 days.

Systemic and Oral Antibiotics

See Endometritis.

NSAIDs

- Flunixin meglumine: anti-inflammatory dose, 1 mg/kg IV or IM BID.
- Phenylbutazone: 2.2 to 4.4 mg/kg IV or PO BID.

Prostaglandin E1 and E2 Analogs for Cervical Relaxation

- Prostaglandin E1 analog, misoprostol 2,000 μg/3 mL tube or Prostaglandin E2 analog, closprostenol 2 mg mixed with 2 to 4 mL lubricating jelly, intracervically 2 to 4 hours before breeding. Cervix will be dilated for 8 hours. Less effective in older mares with previous cervical trauma. Frequent application produces irritation.

Local Therapy

- Panalog ointment (anti-inflammatory, antibiotic, and antifungal). Frequency of application is based on severity of lesion or adhesions, from three times to once daily.

Precautions/Interactions

- Be careful using antiseptics or nonbuffered antibiotics to treat infections of the vagina, cervix, or uterus.
- Minimize forced extraction during dystocia, use ample lubrication, and consider Caesarean-section in cases with intractable cervical induration, poor dilation of the birth canal, as well as with large, deformed fetuses, or a fetus with contracted tendons.

Nursing Care

- Treatment-induced inflammation: When using antiseptics or nonbuffered antibiotics, check for signs of acute mucosal irritation before administering subsequent treatments.
- If inflammation is present, it may be preferable to cease additional intrauterine therapy and change to systemic treatment.

Surgical Considerations

- Wait 30 to 60 days after cervical injury for inflammation and edema to subside.
- Perform outpatient standing surgery, general sedation, and epidural anesthesia.

- The mare should be on progesterone treatment. The effect of progesterone (whether diestrual or exogenous) will increase cervical tone and permit better apposition of cervical layers during surgery.
- If more than one laceration is present, the success of the repair may be enhanced if sites of damage are repaired 3 to 4 weeks apart.

Timing of Repair in Postpartum Mares

- Postpartum mares may be evaluated for surgical readiness if at least 30 days after foaling (i.e., after the 30-day heat); allows for normal cervical involution.
- Alternatively, if a mare has foaled normally, apart from its recurrent cervical tear, breeding earlier can readily be accomplished: skip foal heat, short-cycle, and AI on the next estrus, with daily or every-other-day serial TRP and U/S to determine the day of ovulation.
  - Surgical repair is ideally accomplished within 24 to 48 hours after ovulation.
  - It must be done by or within no more than 72 hours after ovulation, such that inflammation induced by the surgical procedure will have abated before entry of the embryo into the uterus by 5.5 to 6 days post-ovulation.
  - The use of progesterone supplementation, even double dose, is recommended during surgery and, single dose, for a longer period, if the mare is pregnant.
  - NSAIDs and antibiotics are also warranted in the peri-surgical time period.
  - There is no need, nor should one attempt, to evaluate the repair before the mare's 14 to 16 day pregnancy check and not later than 30 days.
  - If the repair has been unsuccessful, considerations to terminate the pregnancy before endometrial cups develop may be appropriate.
  - If normal cervical tone and competency have been restored and the mare is found to be pregnant, further cervical examination is unnecessary.

 COMMENTS

Client Education

- Routine postpartum evaluation of the reproductive tract of the mare is recommended, especially when there is a history of assisted, prolonged manipulation, or unassisted, traumatic parturition.
- Postpartum evaluation increases the likelihood of early identification of traumatic injury and avoids loss of the breeding season.

Patient Monitoring

- Do not examine the cervix for competency or patency until at least 2 to 4 weeks after surgical repair.
- Thirty days of sexual rest is recommended before AI or natural breeding. If live cover is necessary (i.e., thoroughbreds), the use of a stallion roll is advised to restrict or prevent full intromission by the stallion during cover.

Prevention/Avoidance

Unnecessary manipulation during parturition.
- Use of irritants.
- Check for normalcy of anatomic barriers that protect the genital tract (i.e., perineum, vulva, vestibulovaginal sphincter, and cervix) especially postpartum. Repair any defects identified.

Possible Complications

- The scar/site of repair lacks the elasticity of normal cervical tissue. A high percentage will tear again at the next foaling and require annual surgical repair after foaling.
- The decision to perform subsequent surgeries is based on the degree of cervical damage after the most recent foaling, assessment of surgical cost, value of the broodmare and breeding/treatment expenses versus the potential value of an additional foal.
- Minor adhesions may develop postoperatively. They can generally be broken down digitally.
- Uterine contamination is possible during repair. Instillation of antibiotics (uterine lumen) postoperatively may be indicated.

Expected Course and Prognosis

- Fair to good for maintenance of pregnancy after successful repair of cervical lacerations.
- Guarded prognosis if laceration was extensive or repair unsuccessful.

Abbreviations

AI	artificial insemination
BID	twice a day
CEM	contagious equine metritis
DUC	delayed uterine clearance
EED	early embryonic death
ET	embryo transfer
IM	intramuscular
IV	intravenous
NSAIDs	nonsteroidal anti-inflammatory drugs
PO	per os (by mouth)
TRP	transrectal palpation
U/S	ultrasound/ultrasonography

See Also

- Artificial insemination
- Dystocia

- Endometritis
- Delayed uterine clearance
- Pyometra

Suggested Reading

Blanchard TL, Varner D, Schumacher J. 1998. Surgery of the mare reproductive tract. In: *Manual of Equine Reproduction*. St. Louis: Mosby-Year Book; 165–167.

Embertson RM, Henderson CE. 2007. Cervical tears. In: *Current Therapy in Equine Reproduction*. Samper JC, Pycock JF, McKinnon AO (eds). St. Louis: Saunders/Elsevier; 130–133.

Sertich PL. Cervical problems in the mare. 1993. In: *Equine Reproduction*. McKinnon AO and Voss JL (eds). Philadelphia: Lea & Febiger; 404–407.

Sertich PL. 2007. Cervical adhesions. In: *Current Therapy in Equine Reproduction*. Samper JC, Pycock JF, McKinnon AO (eds). St. Louis: Saunders/Elsevier; 137–139.

Author: Maria E. Cadario

chapter 14

Clitoral Enlargement

DEFINITION/OVERVIEW

The clitoris appears larger than normal and may appear to protrude through the vulvar lips at the ventral commissure. The clitoris is a complex structure of distinct components.

- Corpus cavernosum clitoris: erectile tissue.
- Corpus clitoris: body of the clitoris regularly around 5 cm in length.
- Crura: fibrous projections attached to the ischial arch.
- Glans clitoris: bulbous structure at the distal extremity of the clitoral body that is approximately 2.5 cm in diameter. The glans clitoris is situated in the clitoral fossa at the ventral commissure of the vulva. A well-developed median sinus and lateral sinuses may be present.

ETIOLOGY/PATHOPHYSIOLOGY

During sexual differentiation of the fetus, the clitoris develops from the embryonic genital tubercle in the absence of testicular testosterone production or its conversion to the active form 5α-dihydrotestosterone. The clitoris is considered to be the female homologue of the penis. Abnormalities of genetic or gonadal sex, or exogenous compounds may affect this process.

Systems Affected

Reproductive: concurrent abnormalities of the genital tract may be present.

SIGNALMENT/HISTORY

- Female offspring of a mare treated with a known causative drug, are at risk.
- A genetic basis may be present with abnormalities of sexual development.

Risk Factors

- Administration of anabolic steroids.
- Progestin (altrenogest) usage for estrus control, behavior modification, and pregnancy maintenance can lead to female progeny having an associated alteration in gonadotropin secretion and increased clitoral size to 21 months of age. However, no effect on reproductive function has been reported.

- Aberrant endogenous sex-steroid production during gestation (e.g., granulosa theca cell tumor present in the dam during gestation).

Historical Findings

- Congenital lesion: female offspring of a treated mare or the presence of intersex conditions.
- Iatrogenic, following hormone administration to female.

 CLINICAL FEATURES

- Enlargement of the glans clitoris may be visible externally as a swelling of the ventral vulvar commissure or may protrude from the clitoral sinus between the labia.
- May be associated with other genital tract anomalies: internal (tubular genitalia, gonadal) or external (ambiguous genitalia).

 DIFFERENTIAL DIAGNOSIS

Intersex Conditions

- Pseudohermaphrodite: associated with clitoral enlargement (Fig. 14.1).

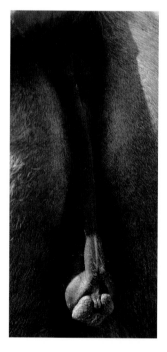

■ **Figure 14.1** Pseudohermaphrodite. Note the extended raphé along midline in place of a normal vulvar cleft; penile homologue is protruding at ventral aspect.
Image courtesy of C. L. Carleton.

Hypospadia Penis

- Hypoplastic penis with incomplete closure of embryonic urethral folds.
- Associated with a prominent perineal median raphe, ventrally displaced vulva, and caudad direction of penis.
- Most common presentation is 64,XX male.

 DIAGNOSTICS

Hormonal Assay

- Testosterone/hCG challenge: collect a baseline serum sample, administer 3000 IU of hCG, then collect additional blood samples at 3 and 24 hours. Increased testosterone indicates testicular tissue is present (i.e., Leydig cell production).
- Estrone sulfate: produced by Sertoli cells in the testicle; couple with hCG challenge to improve diagnostic accuracy.

Immunology

- Test for presence of 5α-reductase or cytosolic receptor.
- Use labial skin only, because the receptors are site specific.

Karyotyping

- Determine presence of correct type and number of sex chromosomes.

Imaging

- U/S coupled with TRP of internal genitalia may detect ovarian pathology or an internal genital anomaly suggestive of an intersex condition.

Pathological Findings

- Increased clitoral size

 THERAPEUTICS

Treatment involves elimination of exposure to the causative therapeutic agents. Intersex conditions result in permanent genital alteration.

Appropriate Health Care

- If genital abnormalities are present, monitor health and function of the urogenital system.

Activity

▪ Remove intersex animals from breeding programs.

Surgical Considerations

▪ Establish patency or removal of tubular genitalia if a segmental obstruction is present.

 COMMENTS

Because iatrogenic cases will spontaneously resolve with cessation of exposure to responsible agents, client should be informed that reproductive potential is not proven to be compromised.

Client Education

▪ Use of progestagens (altrenogest) in pregnant mares can be responsible for this condition.
▪ If a genetic basis is proven, parent stock should be removed from breeding programs.

Prevention/Avoidance

▪ Rational causative drug usage.
▪ If genetic, elimination of parent stock from breeding pool.

Possible Complications

▪ If associated with an intersex condition, reproductive failure will be present.

Expected Course and Prognosis

▪ In iatrogenic cases, cessation of exposure to causative agents will allow resolution.
▪ With intersex conditions, condition may be seen to progress.

Abbreviations

hCG   human chorionic gonadotropin
TRP   transrectal palpitation
U/S   ultrasound, ultrasonography

See Also

▪ Disorders of sexual development

Suggested Reading

Hughes JP. 1993. Developmental anomalies of the female reproductive tract. In: *Equine Reproduction.* McKinnon AO and Voss JL (eds). Philadelphia: Lea & Febiger; 409–410.
Noden J, Squires EL, Nett TM. 1990. Effect of maternal treatment with altrenogest on age at puberty, hormone concentrations, pituitary response to exogenous GnRH, oestrous cycle characteristics and fertility of fillies. *J Reprod Fertil* 88: 185–195.

Author: Peter R. Morresey

15

Cloning

DEFINITION/OVERVIEW

- Clones are genetically identical animals.
- Clones can develop when an embryo spontaneously splits during early gestation to produce identical offspring (extremely rare in horses).
- Clones can be produced by mechanically splitting (i.e., bisecting) an early embryo (e.g., morula or blastocyst) to produce identical offspring (successfully done in horses in the 1980s).
- Clones can be produced through the use of SCNT, a technique that was first successful with the cloning of Dolly the sheep in 1996.

ETIOLOGY/PATHOPHYSIOLOGY

- Although equine cloning has been successful, it is an inefficient process.
  - Currently, less than 3% of cloned equine embryos result in the birth of live offspring, which is similar to other species.
- The primary problem contributing to the inefficiency of cloning has been referred to as "cloned offspring syndrome," which is characterized by a high incidence of embryonic, fetal, or placental developmental abnormalities that result in extremely high rates of embryonic loss, abortion and stillbirths during gestation, and compromised neonatal health after birth.
- The embryonic/fetal and/or placental developmental abnormalities that result in these gestational/neonatal problems are thought to reflect incomplete or abnormal genetic reprogramming of the donor cell nucleus, specifically related to imprinted genes (genes in which only one parental allele is expressed).

Systems Affected

- Potentially, cells from any organ system may provide source material for a clone.

SIGNALMENT/HISTORY

- Cloning mammals using SCNT has been recognized as a major scientific milestone.
  - It demonstrated that a fully differentiated somatic cell can be genetically "reprogrammed" back to the undifferentiated state of a one-cell embryo that can undergo complete embryonic/fetal development resulting in the birth of an animal that is genetically identical to the original somatic cell donor.
- Nuclear transfer cloning is performed by micromanipulating and fusing two cells.
  - One cell (the nuclear donor) is derived from the animal to be cloned.
  - The other cell is a mature, unfertilized oocyte from the same (or closely related) species.
  - The chromosomal genetic material is removed from the oocyte resulting in a structure called a cytoplast.
- The cytoplast is then fused with the nuclear donor cell resulting in a one-celled cloned embryo.
- The cytoplast contains numerous cellular factors (mRNA, proteins, etc.) that play an important role in the genetic reprogramming of the nuclear donor cell, which enables the resulting cloned embryo to initiate and complete embryonic/fetal development.
- The cloned embryo uses the donor cell DNA as the template for gene expression resulting in a genetic clone of the original cell donor animal.

Risk Factors

- In cloned lambs and calves, neonatal health complications that have been observed include lung dysmaturity; pulmonary hypertension; respiratory distress; hypoxia; hypothermia; hypoglycemia; metabolic acidosis; enlarged umbilical veins and arteries; or development of sepsis in either umbilical structures or lungs.
- To date, similar problems have been observed in neonatal equine clones.

Historical Findings

- Equine cloning using nuclear transfer was first successful in 2003 when three cloned mules (Fig. 15.1) and one cloned horse were produced.
- For the equine industry, nuclear transfer is one of several new assisted reproductive techniques (e.g., oocyte transfer, ICSI, etc.) being developed for clinical use.
- Potential uses of equine cloning include:
  - Preservation of genetics from individual animals that would otherwise not be able to reproduce (e.g., geldings).
  - Preservation of genetic material of endangered or exotic species such as the Mongolian Wild Horse (Przewalski's horse).
  - Emotional links of owner's to their companion animals. Horses fill that role for some individuals. It is likely that some owners will have individual horses cloned for emotional fulfillment.

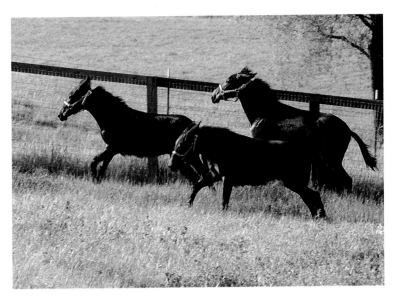

■ Figure 15.1 Identical cloned mules *(left to right)* Idaho Star, Utah Pioneer, and Idaho Gem running in their pasture when they were approximately 1 year of age in 2004.
Image courtesy of the University of Idaho.

- Of these, cloning geldings to produce intact males for breeding purposes has been the first direct clinical application of equine cloning.
- Although some breed associations (e.g., The Jockey Club, AQHA) do not currently allow the registration of cloned animals, for some equine sporting activities (dressage, show-jumping, etc.) breed registry status is irrelevant, which eliminates that regulatory impediment to the utilization of cloning technology.

 CLINICAL FEATURES

- As described previously, all of the chromosomal genetic material in nuclear transfer clones is provided by the nuclear donor cell; however, the cytoplast does contribute mitochondrial DNA to the resulting offspring.
- The effect of the mitochondrial DNA on the resulting phenotype of a clone is not known.

 COMMENTS

Client Education

- Veterinarians can assist their clientele to prepare for cloning of individual animals (if so desired) by "banking" tissue from those animals.

- In North America, ViaGen, Inc. (www.viagen.com) provides commercial equine tissue banking and cloning services.
- ViaGen provides the veterinarian with a tissue collection and transport kit; the procedure involves aseptically collecting a small skin (or gum tissue) biopsy, which is placed in tissue culture medium and returned to the company where cells are grown in tissue culture.
- Once the cells have grown in culture, they can be used immediately for cloning or they can be harvested and stored frozen in LN2 for use in the future.
- Ideally, tissue should be collected from a live animal; however, in an emergency it may be possible to collect a suitable sample after death.
- To maximize the likelihood of recovering viable cells, tissue from the deceased animal should be kept refrigerated between and 3°C and 8°C (37°F and 47°F).
- The chance of recovering viable cells diminishes when the tissue has been frozen or stored at temperatures above 10°C (50°F).

Synonyms

SCNT

Abbreviations

AQHA   American Quarter Horse Association
ICSI   intra-cytoplasmic sperm injection
LN2   liquid nitrogen
SCNT   somatic cell nuclear transfer

Suggested Reading

Galli C, Lagutina I, Crotti G, et al. 2003. Pregnancy: a cloned horse born to its dam twin. *Nature* 424: 635.

Galli C, Lagutina I, Duchi R, et al. 2008. Somatic cell nuclear transfer in horses. *Reprod Dom Anim* 43 (Suppl 2): 331–337.

Hinrichs K. 2005. Update on equine ICSI and cloning. *Therio* 64: 535–541.

Johnson AK, Clark-Price SC, Choi YH, et al. 2010. Physical and clinicopathological findings in foals derived by use of somatic cell nuclear transfer: 14 cases (2004–2008). *JAVMA* 236: 983–990.

Vanderwall DK, Woods GL, Sellon DC, et al. 2004. Present status of equine cloning and clinical characterization of embryonic, fetal, and neonatal development of three cloned mules. *JAVMA* 225: 1694–1699.

Vanderwall DK, Woods GL, Roser JF, et al. 2006. Equine cloning: applications and outcomes. *Reprod Fertil Dev* 18: 91–98.

Woods GL, White KL, Vanderwall DK, et al. 2003. A mule cloned from fetal cells by nuclear transfer. *Science* 301: 1063.

Authors: Dirk K. Vanderwall and Gordon L. Woods (deceased)

chapter 16

Conception Failure in Mares

DEFINITION/OVERVIEW

Maternal structural or functional defects that prevent:
- The fertilized ovum from normal embryonic development.
- Transport of the embryo into the uterus on day 6 after ovulation.
- Embryonic survival until pregnancy is diagnosed by transrectal U/S at 14 or more days after ovulation.

ETIOLOGY/PATHOPHYSIOLOGY

- The *normal* rate of conception failure is approximately 30%, but it approaches 50% to 70% in older, subfertile mares.
- Some of the specific causes of failure of conception are listed here.

Defective Embryos (Fig. 16.1)

- Old mares
- Seasonal effects

Unsuitable or Hostile Uterine Environment

- Endometritis (Fig. 16.2) can result in early regression of the CL and failure of *maternal recognition of pregnancy*.
- Endometrial periglandular fibrosis (Fig. 16.3).
- Endometrial lymphatic cysts of sufficient size to impede embryonic mobility (transuterine migration) resulting in the failure of *maternal recognition of pregnancy* (Figs. 16.3 and 16.4).
- Inadequate secretion of histotrophs.

Xenobiotics

- Equine fescue toxicosis and ergotism (Fig. 16.5).
- Phytoestrogens—anecdotal.

Oviductal Disease

- Unsuitable/hostile environment for embryonic development.
- Oviductal blockage.

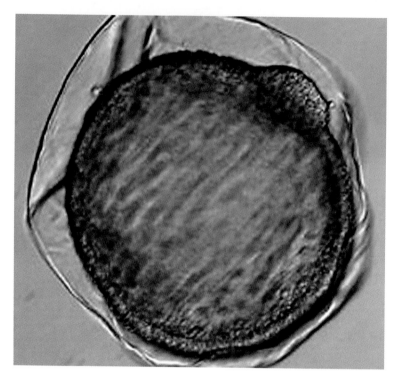

■ **Figure 16.1** Appearance of a poorer quality (Grade 3) equine embryo, exhibiting some shrinkage with extruded blastomeres.
Image is courtesy of R. Foss.

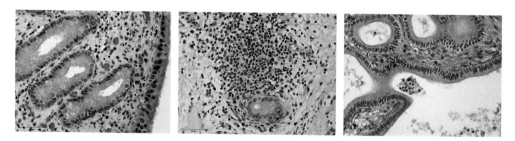

■ **Figure 16.2** *Left:* Evidence of superficial endometritis involving neutrophils, eosinophils, and mononuclear cells in an endometrial biopsy sample collected from an older mare. *Middle:* Evidence of deeper inflammatory changes, involving primarily mononuclear cells, as well as one or two eosinophils, in the same endometrial biopsy sample. *Right:* Evidence of neutrophils in the glandular lumina of an endometrial biopsy sample collected from another older mare (bars = 50 μm).

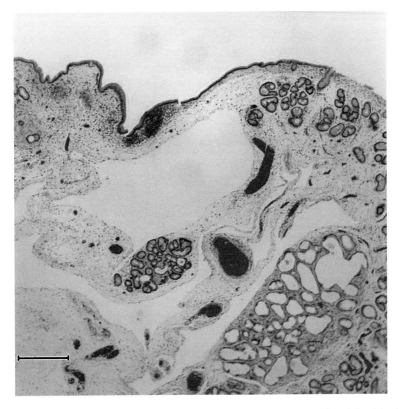

■ **Figure 16.3** Evidence of mild endometritis, with moderately severe endometrial periglandular fibrosis and large lymphatic lacunae, observed as endometrial cysts by hysteroscopy or transrectal ultrasound (bar = 300 μm).

Endocrine Disorders

- Hypothyroidism—anecdotal
- Luteal insufficiency—anecdotal

Maternal Disease

- Fever
- Pain—anecdotal

Pathophysiology

Depending on the specific cause, the pathophysiological mechanisms for conception failure can involve one or more of the following:

- Defective embryo which cannot continue to develop (*see* Fig. 16.1).
- Unsuitable oviductal or uterine environment which prevents fertilization or embryonic development (*see* Figs. 16.2, 16.3, and 16.4).

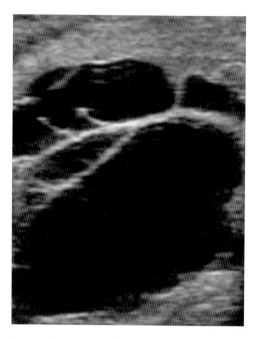

■ **Figure 16.4** Transrectal ultrasound appearance of a large complex of multiple endometrial cysts, approximately 2.5 to 3 inches in diameter.
Image is courtesy of D. Volkmann.

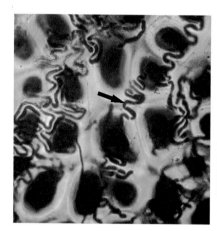 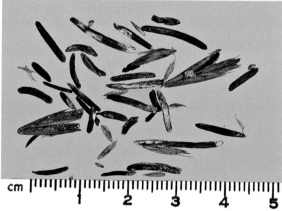

■ **Figure 16.5** The microscopic appearance of the intercellular mycelia *(arrow)* of the tall fescue endophyte, *Neotyphodium coenophialum* is shown on the left, and the gross appearances of ergotized grains is on the right.
Image of fescue endophyte courtesy of D. Cross.

- Oviductal blockage or impaired function.
- Failure of maternal recognition of pregnancy.
- Early CL regression.
- Luteal insufficiency—anecdotal

Systems Affected

Reproductive

SIGNALMENT/HISTORY

Risk Factors

- Older mares (more than 15 years of age), especially those with moderate/severe endometritis, endometrial periglandular fibrosis, and/or endometrial cysts (*see* Figs. 16.2, 16.3, and 16.4).
- Anatomical defects predisposing the genital tract to endometritis.
- Seasonal effects.
- Foal heat breeding: anecdotal and somewhat controversial.
- Inadequate nutrition.
- Exposure to xenobiotics: fescue toxicosis and ergotism.
- Some heterospecific matings: stallion x jenny.
- Susceptibility to PMIE.

Historical Findings

One or more of the following:
- Diagnosis of failure of conception (embryonic vesicle absent) by transrectal U/S at 14 or more days after ovulation, following an appropriately timed breeding with semen of normal fertility.
- Diagnosis of failure of conception (embryonic vesicle absent) by TRP at 25 or more days after ovulation, following an appropriately timed breeding with semen of normal fertility.
- History of PMIE.
- History of abortion or dystocia.
- Return (possibly early) to estrus after an appropriately timed breeding with semen of normal fertility.
- Previous exposure to endophyte-infected fescue or ergotized grasses and grains.
- Recent systemic disease.
- Geographical location, especially with relation to endophyte-infected fescue pastures/ hay or ergotized grasses or grains.

CLINICAL FEATURES

- Nonpregnant uterus, possibly with edema of endometrial folds or accumulation of intrauterine (luminal) fluid.
- Absence of a CL.
- Mucoid or mucopurulent vulvar discharge.

 ## DIFFERENTIAL DIAGNOSIS

Mistiming of Insemination or Breeding

- Monitor follicular development and ovulation by TRP or U/S.
- Appropriate timing of insemination or breeding.
- Ovulation induction to complement timing of insemination or breeding.

EED

- Transrectal U/S detects pregnancy at 14 or more days, but the pregnancy is absent on subsequent examination at less than 40 days of gestation.

Pregnancy Undetected by Transrectal U/S

- Careful, systematic visualization of the entire uterus—horns, body, and region near cervix. A slow sweep, twice per examination to include the entire tract, will reduce likelihood of missing a pregnancy.

Ovulation Failure

- TRP or U/S (preferred) to confirm ovulation and formation of a CL.
- Serum progesterone level 6 to 7 days after ovulation or at end of estrus.

Poor Semen Quality

- Monitoring/examination of ejaculate for adequate number and assessment of progressive motility and normal morphology of spermatozoa.

Ejaculation Failure

- Observe *flagging* of stallion's tail.
- Palpate ventral penile surface during live cover or collection of semen in an AV. Confirm ejaculation is complete: 6 to 10 pulses of the urethra.
- Examine dismount semen sample for motile spermatozoa.

Mishandling of Semen

- Systematically review all procedures and examine semen collection equipment, extenders, incubator temperature, and any containers coming into contact with semen that may be causing death of spermatozoa.

Impaired Spermatozoal Transport

- Transrectal U/S: ensure absence of intrauterine fluid at insemination or breeding.
- Vaginal speculum and digital cervical examination: assess cervical patency and rule-out urovagina.

 DIAGNOSTICS

- CBC with differential, as well as serum biochemical data: determine if there is an inflammatory or stress leukocyte response, as well as other organ system involvement; usually not indicated unless the mare has been ill recently.
- ELISA or RIA analyses for maternal progesterone: may be useful at if less than 80 days of gestation (normal levels vary from greater than 1 to greater than 4 ng/mL, depending on the reference laboratory). Maternal estrogen concentrations can reflect fetal estrogen production and viability, especially conjugated estrogens (e.g., estrone sulfate).
- Anecdotal reports of lower T_3/T_4 levels in mares with history of conception failure, EED, or abortion. The significance of low T_4 levels is unknown and somewhat controversial.
- Cytogenetic studies: to detect chromosomal abnormalities.
- Endometrial cytology, culture, and biopsy procedures: to assess endometrial inflammation and/or fibrosis.
- Vaginal speculum examination and hysteroscopy if structural abnormalities are suspected in the cervix or uterus.
- Feed or environmental analyses for specific xenobiotics, ergopeptine alkaloids, phytoestrogens, heavy metals, or fescue endophyte (*Neotyphodium coenophialum*).
- Transrectal U/S: essential to confirm ovulation and early pregnancy, as well as to detect intrauterine fluid and endometrial cysts.
- A thorough reproductive evaluation (i.e., transrectal U/S, vaginal speculum, endometrial cytology, culture, and biopsy) is indicated pre-breeding for individuals predisposed to conception failure (e.g., barren, older mares with history of conception failure, EED, or endometritis).
- Transrectal U/S, if performed at 10 days post-ovulation (earlier than normal), can determine the presence of an embryo; however, there can be confusion between embryonic vesicles and endometrial cysts. Reexamination in 2 to 4 or 6 days is generally required to determine whether the structure identified is indeed rapidly increasing in size (a conceptus versus a cyst).
- Embryo recovery, using the same procedures as for ET, to detect embryonic transport into the oviduct (2 to 4 days after ovulation) or into the uterus (6 to 8 days after ovulation). The flushing procedure might be therapeutic as well.
- Hysteroscopy of uterine lumen and uterotubal junctions.
- Oviductal patency: assessed by starch granules or microspheres deposited on the ovarian surface, followed by uterine lavage. Lavage fluid is evaluated to determine if starch granules have been recovered.

- Laparoscopy can be used to evaluate normal structure and function and ovarian-oviductal interactions.

Pathological Findings

- An endometrial biopsy can demonstrate the presence of moderate to severe, chronic endometritis, endometrial periglandular fibrosis, and/or lymphatic lacunae (*see* Figs. 16.2, 16.3, and 16.4).

 THERAPEUTICS

Drug(s) of Choice

Altrenogest

- Mares with a history of conception failure or moderate to severe endometritis (i.e., no active, infectious component) or fibrosis can be administered altrenogest (0.044–0.088 mg/kg PO, SID) beginning 2 to 3 days after ovulation or upon diagnosis of pregnancy. Altrenogest is continued until at least day 100 of gestation (taper daily dose over a 14-day period at the end of treatment).
- Altrenogest administration can be started later during gestation, continued longer, or used for only short periods of time, depending on serum progesterone levels during the first 80 days of gestation (may range from greater than 1 to greater than 4 ng/mL, depending on the reference lab), clinical circumstances, risk factors, and clinician preference.
- If used near term, altrenogest frequently is discontinued 7 to 14 days before the expected foaling date, depending on the case, unless otherwise indicated by assessment of fetal maturity/viability or by questions regarding the accuracy of gestational length.

Oxytocin

- IM administration of 10 to 20 IU, 4 to 8 hours post-mating for PMIE.

Cloprostenol

- IM administration of 250 μgm 12 to 24 hours post-mating for PMIE.

Precautions/Interactions

- Use altrenogest only to prevent conception failure of noninfectious endometritis.
- Care should be taken in the administration of cloprostenol or other prostaglandins following ovulation to prevent interference with CL formation and function.
- Iatrogenic administration of oxytocin and cloprostenol to pregnant mares: adverse effects are dependent on the stage of pregnancy.
- Use transrectal U/S to diagnose pregnancy if at least 14 to 16 days after ovulation to identify intrauterine fluid or pyometra early in the disease course for appropriate treatment.

- If pregnancy is diagnosed, frequent monitoring (weekly initially) may be indicated to detect EED.
- Altrenogest is absorbed through the skin. Persons handling this preparation should wear gloves and wash their hands.
- Cloprostenol can be absorbed through the skin, so persons handling this preparation should wear gloves and wash their hands after treating mares.
- Supplemental progestins are in common and wide use for treating cases of conception failure, but their efficacy is controversial.
- Primary, age-related embryonic defects do not respond to supplemental progestin treatment.

Alternative Drugs

- Injectable progesterone (150–500 mg/day, oil base) can be administered IM, SID instead of the oral formulation. Variations, contraindications, and precautions are similar to those associated with altrenogest.
- Other injectable and implantable progestin preparations are available commercially for use in other species. Any use in horses of these products is off-label and little scientific data is available regarding their efficacy.
- Newer, repository forms of progesterone are occasionally introduced; however, some evidence of efficacy should be provided prior to use.
- T_4 supplementation has been successful (anecdotally) for treating mares with histories of subfertility. Its use remains controversial, however, and it is considered deleterious by some clinicians.
- Other prostaglandin products (e.g., $PGF_2\alpha$) have been used to prevent PMIE, but their efficacy has been suggested to be less than that of cloprostenol, with a greater risk for interference with subsequent CL formation and function.

Appropriate Health Care

- Treat preexisting endometritis before insemination or breeding mares during the physiologic breeding season.
- Mares being bred should have adequate body condition.
- Inseminate or breed foal heat mares if ovulation occurs more than 9 to 10 days postpartum and no intrauterine fluid is present.
- Uterine lavage 4 to 8 hours post-mating with administration of oxytocin or cloprostenol to treat PMIE.
- Progestin supplementation: remains somewhat controversial.
- Anecdotal reports of oviductal flushing to resolve oviductal occlusion.
- Depending on breed restrictions, various forms of advanced reproductive technologies (e.g., manipulations involving the zygote, embryo) are used to retrieve embryos from the oviduct (about days 2 to 4 after ovulation) or uterus (days 6 to 8 after ovulation) for ET. Oocyte retrieval and successful IVF with subsequent ET have been used in some instances.
- Primary, age-related embryonic defects are refractory to treatment.
- Most cases of conception failure can be handled in an ambulatory situation.

- Increased frequency of U/S monitoring of follicular development and ovulation, to permit insemination closer to ovulation, as well as more technical diagnostic procedures, may need to be performed in a hospital setting. Adequate restraint and optimal lighting might not be available in the field to permit quality U/S examination.

Nursing Care

- Generally requires none.
- Minimal nursing care might be necessary after more invasive diagnostic and therapeutic procedures.

Diet

- Generally no restriction, unless indicated by concurrent maternal disease or nutritional problems (e.g., under- or over-nourished).

Activity

- Generally no restriction of broodmare activity, unless contraindicated by concurrent maternal disease or diagnostic or therapeutic procedures.
- Preference may be to restrict activity of mares in competition because of the impact of stress on cyclicity and ovulation.

Surgical Considerations

- Indicated for repair of anatomical defects predisposing mares to endometritis.
- Certain diagnostic and therapeutic procedures discussed previously might also involve some surgical intervention.

    COMMENTS

Client Education

- Emphasize the *aged* mare's susceptibility to conception failure and her refractoriness to treatment.
- Inform clients regarding the cause, diagnosis, and treatment of endometritis.
- Inform clients regarding the seasonal aspects and nutritional requirements needed for successful conception.
- Inform clients regarding the role that endophyte-infected fescue and certain heterospecific breedings might play in conception failure.

Patient Monitoring

- Accurate teasing records.
- Reexamine mares treated for endometritis before breeding.

- Early examination for pregnancy by transrectal U/S.
- Monitor embryonic and fetal development with transrectal or transabdominal U/S.

Prevention/Avoidance

- Recognition of at-risk mares.
- Management of endometritis before breeding.
- Removal of mares from fescue-infected pasture and ergotized grasses and grains after breeding and during early gestation.
- Prudent use of medications in bred mares.
- Avoid exposure to known toxicants.

Possible Complications

- Later EED
- High-risk pregnancy.
- Abortion: infectious or noninfectious, depending on the circumstances.

Expected Course and Prognosis

- Young mares with resolved cases of endometritis can have a fair to good prognosis for conception and completion of pregnancy.
- Older mares (more than 15 years of age) with a history of chronic, moderate to severe endometritis, endometrial periglandular fibrosis, or endometrial cysts, as well as conception failure or EED, have a guarded to poor prognosis for conception success, safe completion of pregnancy, and delivery of a healthy foal.

Synonyms/Closely Related Conditions

- EED
- Infertility
- Sterility
- Subfertility

Abbreviations

AV   artificial vagina
CBC   complete blood count
CL   corpus luteum
EED   early embryonic death
ELISA   enzyme-linked immunosorbent assay
ET   embryo transfer
IM   intramuscular
IVF   in vitro fertilization

PGF	natural prostaglandin
PMIE	post-mating induced endometritis
PO	per os (by mouth)
RIA	radioimmunoassay
SID	once a day
T_3	triiodothyronine
T_4	thyroxine
TRP	transrectal palpation
U/S	ultrasound, ultrasonography

See Also

- Abortion, spontaneous, infectious or noninfectious
- Conception failure, stallions
- EED
- Embryo transfer
- Endometrial biopsy
- Endometritis
- Metritis
- Ovulation failure

Suggested Reading

Evans TJ, Rottinghaus GE, Casteel SW. 2003. Ergopeptine alkaloid toxicoses in horses. In: *Current Therapy in Equine Medicine 5*. Robinson NE (ed). Philadelphia: Saunders; 796–798.

LeBlanc MM. 2003. Persistent mating-induced endometritis. In: *Current Therapy in Equine Medicine 5*. Robinson NE (ed). Philadelphia: Saunders; 234–237.

Paccamonti D. 2003. Endometrial cysts. In: *Current Therapy in Equine Medicine 5*. Robinson NE (ed). Philadelphia: Saunders; 231–234.

Youngquist RS, Threlfall WR (eds). 2007. *Current Therapy in Large Animal Theriogenology*, 2nd ed. St. Louis: Elsevier-Saunders.

Author: Tim J. Evans

chapter 17

Contagious Equine Metritis

DEFINITION/OVERVIEW

CEM is a reportable, highly contagious disease. The causative agent is *Taylorella equigenitalis*. The organism is primarily spread by coitus. Genital infection of stallions and mares also occurs as a result of transmission by contaminated equipment and other fomites.

ETIOLOGY/PATHOPHYSIOLOGY

Two strains of *T. equigenitalis* have been identified: streptomycin resistant and streptomycin sensitive.

In addition to coitus, transmission by contaminated equipment (e.g., specula, artificial insemination) and handling personnel (e.g., gloves) has been reported.

Stallions

- The organism is transmitted primarily by coitus.
- Stallions are asymptomatic carriers, with the organism harbored in the fossa glandis, urethral sinus, and smegma. It is also recoverable from the terminal urethra, preputial surface, and preejaculatory fluid.

Mares

- Clinical signs only occur in mares and range from inapparent infection to acute endometritis with overt purulent discharge.
- Initially, the organism is found in the endometrium and cervix. The organism is less frequently found in the vagina, vulva, clitoris, and oviducts. Between 3 weeks to 4 months following infection, the organism is occasionally recoverable from the ovarian surface, oviduct, uterus, cervix, and vagina.
- The organism is more reliably isolated from and can persist within the clitoral fossa and sinuses.
- Mares may be mechanical carriers via the smegma of the clitoral fossa.

- The organism also is recoverable from the placenta of positive mares and the genitalia of colts and fillies with infections being acquired *in utero* or at parturition.

Systems Affected

Reproductive

SIGNALMENT/HISTORY

Risk Factors

- Horses of breeding age from countries identified as CEM-affected.
- Coitus with an inapparently infected carrier stallion is the main cause of mare infection.
- Equipment or personnel contaminated during genital examinations or procedures act as fomites and readily spread infection.
- No lifelong immunity has been demonstrated in previously affected and cleared animals. Previous exposure does not afford absolute protection against subsequent challenge.

Historical Findings

Stallions

- Inapparent infection

Mares

- Within 2 to 7 days of infection, mares develop varying amount of odorless, grayish, mucopurulent discharge.
- No systemic involvement.

CLINICAL FEATURES

Stallions

Inapparent infection

Mares

- Severe diffuse endometritis and cervicitis: becomes severe and plasmacytic by 14 days, then declines and persists as mild, diffuse, and multifocal inflammation for as long as 2 weeks.
- Shortened diestrus period because of premature luteolysis.
- Temporary infertility

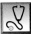 ## DIFFERENTIAL DIAGNOSIS

- Bacterial endometritis: *Klebsiella* and *Pseudomonas* spp.
- Fungal endometritis
- Vaginitis: local irritation, aspiration of air.
- Cervicitis: intrauterine infection, extension of vaginitis, aspiration of air.
- Urine pooling: poor vulvar conformation, urethral damage.
- Pyometra: cervical adhesions or incompetence.
- Urinary tract infection: urethral compromise, urinary calculus.
- Persistent hymen: detected on speculum examination.
- Neoplasia of the uterus or vagina: secondary bacterial infection of affected tissues.
- *Taylorella asinigenitalis* sp. nov: a nonpathogenic gram-negative bacterium phenotypically indistinguishable from *T. equigenitalis*. Recently isolated from the genital tract of male donkeys and a stallion.

 ## DIAGNOSTICS

CBC/Biochemistry/Urinalysis

- Unremarkable

Speculum Examination

- Females: cervicitis, purulent cervical discharge, grayish mucopurulent material pooling in vagina.

Imaging

- U/S: intrauterine fluid suggestive of endometritis.

Bacterial Cultures

- Stallions: urethral fossa and urethral sinus, distal urethra, penile skin, and preputial folds.
- Mares: clitoral sinus and fossa; endometrium, vaginal fluid, and cervix of estrus mare.
- Culture requirements for *T. equigenitalis* are exacting: immediately place swabs in Amies charcoal medium and maintain at 4°C for transport. Plate samples within 24 hours of collection.
- Colonies usually form in 2 to 3 days. The streptomycin-sensitive strain may take as long as 6 days to become apparent.
- Reportable disease that requires a federally approved laboratory for identification.

Cytology (Mares)

- Presence of PMN indicating endometritis.
- Presence of morphologically suggestive bacteria, either free or phagocytized.

Serology

- Detectable antibody in acute cases: mares only.
- No value in stallions because contamination is surface only and a measurable systemic immune response is not generated.

Test Breeding (Stallions)

- Breed to known uninfected mares.

PCR

- Used in conjunction with culture. Allows more rapid detection of causative agent.

Pathological Findings

Characteristic finding of endometritis (female). No lesions in the male.

 THERAPEUTICS

Under federal supervision at approved quarantine station. Treatment recommendations are subject to change at any time. Consult current governmental regulations before initiating treatment.

Mares

- Intrauterine antibiotics: crystalline penicillin, 5 to 10 million IU, for 5 to 7 days.
- Cleansing of the clitoral fossa and sinuses with 2% chlorhexidine scrub to remove all smegma for 5 consecutive days.
- Pack with nitrofurazone ointment.

Stallions

- Completely extrude and wash penis in 2% chlorhexidine scrub for 5 consecutive days.
- Remove all smegma, especially from the urethral fossa and skin folds of prepuce.
- Nitrofurazone dressing for 5 days.

Drug(s) of Choice

- Chlorhexidine 2%: recommended 2% as higher concentrations can lead to penile irritation.
- Nitrofurazone (0.2% ointment).

Activity

Quarantine in federally approved facility until treatment has been completed.

Surgical Considerations

Mares: clitoral sinusectomy or clitorectomy has previously been practiced for intractable cases. Due to efficacy of aforementioned treatment protocols this is no longer advocated.

 COMMENTS

Patient Monitoring

Culture (Timing)

- Culture 7 days after the last day of treatment for three consecutive sets of negatives.
- Stallions: every 2 days for three sets.
- Mares: three consecutive estrus periods.

Culture (Locations)

- Mares: swab the clitoris and endometrium at estrus before breeding; swab during abnormal estrous intervals.
- Stallions: swabs from teaser and breeding stallions before season begins.

Culture (Equipment)

- Disposable gloves, sleeves, and speculum.
- Use AI when feasible or permitted by breed-society rules and regulations.

Prevention/Avoidance

- All horses older than 2 years entering the United States from CEM-affected countries must follow treatment and testing protocol.
- Mares: test three times in 7 days (days 1, 4, and 7), then treat for 5 days; if three negative cultures are obtained, the mare is released.
- Stallions: require negative culture and negative test breeding to two mares; if positive, repeat cycle until three consecutive, negative culture results are obtained.

Possible Complications

Infertility of the mare, repeat breedings.

Expected Course and Prognosis

Recovery is anticipated with treatment protocol as described previously.

Synonyms

Causative organism formerly known as *Haemophilus equigenitalis.*

Abbreviations

AI artificial insemination
CEM contagious equine metritis
PCR polymerase chain reaction
PMN polymorphonuclear
U/S ultrasound, ultrasonography

See Also

- Venereal diseases

Suggested Reading

Blanchard TL, Kenney RM, Timoney PJ. 1992. Venereal disease. *Vet Clin North Am Equine Pract* 8: 193–195.

Timoney PJ. 1998. Aspects of the occurrence, diagnosis and control of selected venereal diseases of the stallion. In: *Proc of the Stallion Symposium*, Sponsored by the ACT/SFT, Hastings, Nebraska, December, 76–78.

Watson ED. 1997. Swabbing protocols in screening for contagious equine metritis. *Vet Rec* 140: 268–271.

Author: Peter R. Morresey

chapter 18

Contraception in the Mare

DEFINITION/OVERVIEW

- By definition contraception aims at preventing conception or fertilization or the maintenance of pregnancy.
- Contraception is an important step in the management of wild or feral equids and management/welfare issues surrounding unwanted horses.
- Contraception may be achieved by elimination of normal ovarian activity or prevention of normal sperm-oocyte interaction.
- The ideal contraception technique should be safe for the patient, practical, efficacious and economically viable.
- Means of prevention of fertilization include:
  - Hormonal manipulation
  - Surgical manipulation
  - Immunological

ETIOLOGY/PATHOPHYSIOLOGY

- Contraception can be achieved by altering the normal ovarian activity and the mares behavior, or by preventing fertilization.
- Suppression of ovarian activity can be reversible (hormonal manipulation) or definitive (ovariectomy).

Short-term Alteration of Normal Estrus Behavior

- The aim of these techniques is to eliminate estrus behavior and therefore receptivity to the stallion during the breeding season
- Estrus behavior may be eliminated by:
  - Maintaining/prolonging luteal function
  - By simulating diestrus.
- Maintenance of luteal function can be achieved by placing glass, plastic or metal marbles in the uterine cavity following ovulation. Response rate is variable 12% to 75% and mares may maintain their CL for up to 90 days.

- The effect of the marbles is thought to be due to inhibition of $PGF_2\alpha$ from the endometrium and prevention of luteolyis.
- Simulation of luteal phase is accomplished by chronic administration of progesterone or altrenogest.

Alteration of Normal Ovarian Function

- The aim of these techniques is to eliminate normal follicular development and ovulation. Two main techniques are used
  - Elimination of follicular development
  - Permanent surgical ablation of the ovary (ovariectomy).
- Normal follicular activity is controlled by FSH and LH which are primarily under the control of pulsatile secretion of GnRH from the hypothalamus.
- Immunization against endogenous GnRH reduces circulating GnRH and the subsequent pituitary response; leads to a state of anestrus.
- The efficacy of the treatment depends on the level and persistence of circulating anti-GnRH antibodies.
- Duration of inhibition of ovarian activity presents great individual variability.
- Ovarian activity can be reduced by down-regulation with GnRH agonists.
- Repeated administration of a GnRH agonist (25 mg per day for 30 days) has been shown to cause a down-regulatory effect on ovarian function and cause anestrus.
  - A single implant of deslorelin acetate, a potent GnRH analogue, suppressed follicular development for 22 days. However, with three implants, this interovulatory period was reported yet longer, 36.8 days.
  - Cyclicity was suspended in 80% of the mares treated with 20 mg of deslorelin acetate. Complete inactivity of the ovaries (anestrus) is not easily and reliably obtained, even with three deslorelin implants.
- Ovarian atrophy was not achieved in any mare with these implants.
- GnRH antagonist, Antarelix, administered (0.01 mg/kg IV twice per day) for 3 days postpones ovulation in mares by approximately 10 days and increases the interovulatory interval.
- Chronic administration of a GnRH antagonist could be considered as an option for suppression of ovarian activity.

Prevention of Normal Sperm-Oocyte Interaction

- Three techniques have been used to prevent conception or early embryo development in the mare:
  - Surgical: tubal ligation.
  - Derangement of the uterine environment: IUD.
  - Prevention of sperm-egg attachment: immunization against the zona pellucida.
- Surgical methods are very efficacious but present two main disadvantages: they can be costly and are irreversible.
- Tubal ligation could be simplified by the use of standing laparoscopy.

- IUDs have been used in the mare and have been shown to be very efficacious in preventing fertilization, although mares continue to cycle.
- IUDs are silastic rings placed into the uterine cavity.
- IZP is currently the most commonly used technique for contraception in feral/wild horses.
- IZP uses vaccine based on purified PZP or purified ZP3.
- IZP has been shown to be safe and reversible.
- Immunized mares show an increase in anti-zona pellucida antibodies, which bind to the ovulated egg and prevent sperm attachment, thus preventing fertilization.
- Although reversible, IZP has been associated with development of oophoritis and reduced fertility after multiple uses.
- A new improved delivery system of the PZP vaccine provides two years of contraception (infertility) following a single inoculation.

Systems Affected

- Reproductive
- Central nervous system

SIGNALMENT/HISTORY

Management Reason

- Feral or wild population of equids.
- Horse rescue ranches; reducing population of surplus horses.

Physical Examination Findings

- Return to estrus in feral population.
- Chronic endometritis with IUD.
- Long lasting anestrus with immunization against GnRH.
- Loss of ovarian function with immunization against PZP.

Historical Findings

- Increased population
- Welfare concerns

DIFFERENTIAL DIAGNOSIS

- Anestus
- Infertility

DIAGNOSTICS

Other Laboratory Tests

Hormonal Assays

■ Low estradiol and progesterone in mares immunized against GnRH.

Antibodies levels

■ Level of antibodies against GnRH or PZP may be used to determine the efficacy of the immunization.

Imaging

■ Transrectal U/S to determine ovarian activity and pregnancy status.

Pathologic Findings

■ Chronic endometritis due to irritation by IUD.
■ Oophoritis in mares immunized against PZP.

THERAPEUTICS

Drug(s) of Choice

Progestogen treatments

■ Progesterone in oil may be administered daily (150 mg IM).
■ Progesterone Long Acting: every 8 to 10 days (1500 mg IM).
■ Altrenogest daily (0.044 mg/kg PO).
■ Compounded Altrenogest injectable every 10 days (225 mg IM), 15 days (450 mg IM) or 30 days (500 mg IM).

GnRH Downregulation

■ GnRH antagonist, Antarelix (0.01 mg/kg IV twice per day).
■ Deslorelin, implants.
■ Deslorelin, 25 mg/day for 30 days.

IUDs

■ Sterile glass, metal or plastic marbles (diameter 25–35 mm) are placed into the uterine cavity following ovulation. Plastic marbles seems to give better results.
■ IUD (flexible silastic O-ring®, 5 mm in thickness and 40 mm external diameter) placed in the uterine cavity.

IZP

- PZP vaccine delivered by darting or IM injection. Original treatment required a primary inoculation and one or two boosters 1 month apart. New vaccines are delivered in a single IM injection as a polymer microsphere and carbomer adjuvant.

Immunization against GnRH

- GnRH or LHRH vaccines are produced by conjugation of the peptide with a protein carrier such as serum albumin and adjuvant. The vaccine is given IM twice at a 4-week interval.
- Commercial GnRH vaccines are available, but not in the USA (Equity® Pfizer Animal Health P/L, West Ryde, NSW, Australia; Improvac®, Pfizer Animal Health, Sandton, South Africa).

Appropriate Health Care

- Monitor mare for injection site reaction (usually not very severe).
- Surgical procedures requires postsurgical care.

Surgical Considerations

- Complications from ovariectomy.
- Laparoscopic ovariectomy or tubal ligation has less complications.

 COMMENTS

Client Education

- Public education regarding population control.

Patient Monitoring

- Mares should be monitored for resumption of ovarian activity when using nonpermanent techniques.

Possible Complications

- Delayed return to cyclicity or extended anestrus.
- Long-term effect on the ovary (PZP).
- Uterine infection for IUD.
- Surgical complications for ovariectomy or tubal ligation.
- Behavioral problems within the herd.

Expected Course and Prognosis

Good

Abbreviations

CL   corpus luteum
FSH   follicle stimulating hormone
GnRH   gonadotropin releasing hormone
IM   intramuscular
IV   intravenous
IUD   intrauterine device
IZP   immunization against zona pellucida
LH   luteinizing hormone
LHRH   luteinizing hormone releasing hormone
PGF   natural prostaglandin
PZP   Porcine zona pellucida
U/S   ultrasound, ultrasonography
ZP3   purified zona pellucida protein 3

See Also

- Manipulation of estrus
- Estrus supression

Suggested Reading

Botha AE, Schulman ML, Bertschinger HJ, Guthrie AJ, Annandale CH, Hughes SB. 2008. The use of a GnRH vaccine to suppress mare ovarian activity in a large group of mares under field conditions. *Wildlife Research* 35: 548–554.

Burns PJ, Thompson DL, Strorer WA, Gilley RM. 2008. Evaluation of sustained release progestin formulations in mares. *Proc of the 7th International Symposium on Equine Embryo Transfer*, Cambridge, UK; 71–72.

Daels PF, Hughes JP. 1995. Fertility control using intrauterine devices: an alternative for population control in wild horse. *Therio* 44: 629–639.

Elhay M, Newbold A, Britton A, Turley P, Dowsett K, Walker J. 2007. Suppression of behavioural and physiological oestrus in the mare by vaccination against GnRH. *Australian Vet J* 85: 39–45.

Nie GJ, Johnson KE, Braden TD, et al. 2003. Use of an intra-uterine glass ball protocol to extend luteal function in mares. *J Eq Vet Sci* 23: 266–273.

Pryor P, Tibary A. 2005. Management of estrus in the performance mare. *Clin Tech Eq Pract* 4:197–209.

Rivera del Alamo, Reilas T, Kindhal H, et al. 2008. Mechanism behind intrauterine device-induced luteal persistence in mares. *Anim Reprod Sci* 107: 94–106.

Turner JW, Liu IK, Flanagan DR, et al. 2007. Immunocontraception in wild horses: One Inoculation Provides Two Years of Infertility. *J Wildlife Mgt* 71: 662–667.

Authors: Jacobo Rodriguez and Ahmed Tibary

chapter 19

Delayed Uterine Involution

DEFINITION/OVERVIEW

- Any delay in the return of the uterus to its prepartum state. Delays may be demonstrated as abnormalities of size, tone, endometrial regeneration, or elimination of bacteria from the uterine lumen. In normal mares, endometrial involution is complete by 13 to 25 days, with the exception of returning to prepartum size, which may require 35 days or longer. Some mares, especially primiparous mares, never fully return to prepartum size.

ETIOLOGY/PATHOPHYSIOLOGY

- The origin of delayed uterine involution can be mechanical (decreased muscular contractions), inflammatory (neutrophil influx), or immunologic.
- It may, but does not necessarily follow dystocia or RFM, and is characterized by a compromised ability to eliminate postpartum debris and bacteria from the uterus.
- Some individual mares have a predisposition to slower postpartum uterine involution.
- Greater contamination at the time of parturition may increase the time needed to complete involution.

Systems Affected

- Reproductive
- Other systems may play a role in delaying the process.

SIGNALMENT/HISTORY

- All breeds can be affected with delayed uterine involution.
- Mares of any breeding age may be affected but it is more prevalent in older mares.
- A vulvar discharge that persists past 3 days postpartum is abnormal.

Risk Factors

- Increased incidence occurs in older mares, postdystocia mares, mares with a severely contaminated uterus at parturition, mares with decreased oxytocin release, and mares with a uterus that fails to respond to oxytocin (endogenous or exogenous).

Historical Findings

- A history of postpartum delayed involution may be suspected with failure to conceive when bred during an early foal heat (especially with an ovulation occurring at less than 9 days postpartum) or at any foal heat breeding.

 CLINICAL FEATURES

- Because foal heat and rebreeding can occur within 5 to 18 days postpartum, it is extremely important for the uterus to return rapidly to a normal prepartum diameter (or close to it).
- Evaluation of uterine size and tone are as important as is recording the presence of any luminal fluid. Notation of any abnormal discharge from the vulva should also be made. Any of the aforementioned signs may indicate delayed uterine involution.

 DIFFERENTIAL DIAGNOSIS

- It is important to distinguish metritis from delayed uterine involution. Delayed uterine involution may accompany infection or inflammation of the uterus, but these are not necessarily co-dependent.

 DIAGNOSTICS

- Endometrial cytology is an excellent method to determine the characteristics of any accumulated uterine fluid. U/S examination revealing fluid within the postpartum uterine lumen indicates delayed uterine involution if present past the fifth day postpartum. The presence or absence of other findings (e.g., decreased uterine tone, increased uterine size) that are linked with delayed involution also aid in its diagnosis. The absence of WBC is a good indication that uterine fluid, if present, is not of an inflammatory nature.

THERAPEUTICS

Appropriate Health Care

- Delayed uterine involution may accompany uterine infections or inflammation. Differentiate inflammatory delayed involution from infectious delayed involution. Delayed involution is not the result of a systemic infection, so systemic antibiotics are not necessary. Unless infection of the uterus is present, antibiotic therapy is not indicated. Local intrauterine instillation of antibiotics may be contraindicated if not needed, but is of value if uterine infection is present.
- Uterine flushes or the use of hormonal uterine stimulants (e.g., oxytocin, $PGF_2\alpha$) may be more appropriate therapy for noninfectious conditions. Oxytocin (20 IU IV or 20 IU IM, every 2 hours for the first 24 hours postpartum) and $PGF_2\alpha$ (10 mg IM) or prostaglandin analogue (cloprostenol, 250 micrograms IM), are the hormones of choice for aiding involution of the uterus. Uterine flushes, with warm sterile saline or water, when indicated, may aid involution. Instillation of irritants or antiseptics (e.g., dilute Lugol solution) sometimes has value to stimulate further uterine involution. Antibiotics locally should only be used if a bacterial pathogen has been identified.

Activity

- Mares should be permitted normal exercise as it may enhance uterine contractility.

Surgical Considerations

- Mares with poor VC should have a Caslick's vulvoplasty (a minor surgical procedure) immediately postpartum to reduce contamination of the uterus. Contaminants, *windsucking* further retards uterine involution.

 # COMMENTS

Client Education

- Not all mares will have sufficient uterine involution by the onset of foal heat and will not be ready to breed at foal heat. Once a mare has been bred on two to three foal heats (two to three parturitions) and has failed to conceive, it would be best to skip her subsequent foal heats, short cycle her, and breed during the next estrus.

Patient Monitoring

- Serial TRP or U/S examinations may be necessary to determine the degree of uterine involution and helpful in selecting those mares with the highest probability of conceiving if bred on foal heat.

Prevention/Avoidance

- Clean foaling conditions and clean techniques, if assistance is necessary, reduce uterine contamination and thereby possibly aid in a more rapid return of the uterus to its normal prepartum size.
- The mare's stall should be bedded with clean straw for foaling.
- Diligence to maximize stall hygiene (for the health of the mare and foal) during the first several days postpartum is essential.
- The expense of bedding and labor is offset by improved reproductive health.
- Light exercise during late gestation and postpartum can aid uterine contractions and involution.

Possible Complications

- Do not over-treat delayed uterine involution with unnecessary antibiotics or other local or systemic medications.
- Treatment may further retard the uterus' return to normal, costing the owner additional expense in the absence of measurable benefit.

Prevention/Avoidance

- The cleanliness of the foaling area is of major importance in reducing uterine contamination.
- Attention to cleanliness during obstetrical manipulations will yield benefits by decreasing the number of infected mares.

Possible Complications

- The major complications observed with delayed uterine involution are failure to conceive, EED, and lost reproductive time.

Expected Course and Prognosis

- The majority of mares return to normal without treatment but require longer than normal for complete uterine involution.
- In some cases, involution remains incomplete throughout the breeding season and may prevent conception or pregnancy maintenance. These mares obviously need assistance to aid in conception and pregnancy maintenance.
- Delayed uterine involution may or may not be coupled with a uterine infection. There is an increased occurrence in old mares.

Abbreviations

EED   early embryonic death
IM   intramuscular
PGF   natural prostaglandin
RFM   retained fetal membranes, retained placenta

TRP   transrectal palpation
U/S   ultrasound, ultrasonography
WBC   white blood cells

See Also

- Dystocia
- Postpartum problems
- RFM
- Uterine infection
- Vaginitis
- Vulvar discharge

Suggested Reading

McKinnon AO, et al. 1988. Ultrasonographic studies on the reproductive tract of mares after parturition: effect of involution and uterine fluid on pregnancy rates in mares with normal and delayed first postpartum ovulatory cycles. *JAVMA* 192: 350–353.

Roberts SJ. 1986. *Veterinary obstetrics and genital diseases (Theriogenology)*, 3rd ed. Woodstock, VT: Author; 584.

Stewart DR, et al. 1984. Concentrations of 15-keto-13,14-dihydroprostaglandin $PGF_2\alpha$ in the mare during spontaneous and oxytocin induced foaling. *Eq Vet J* 16: 270–274.

Vandeplassche M, et al. 1983. Observations on involution and puerperal endometritis in mares. *Irish Vet J* 37: 126–132.

Author: Walter R. Threlfall

chapter 20

Donkey Reproduction

DEFINITION/OVERVIEW

- Donkey, *Equus asinus*, is a separate species of equid that presents several peculiarities in its reproductive patterns compared to horses.
- Male donkeys are called jacks, jackasses, or donkey stallions.
- Female donkeys are called jennies, jennets, or donkey mares.
- Horses and donkeys can interbreed, the product of which is infertile and known as a:
  - Mule (*E. asinus* × *Equus caballus*, a jennet crossed with a stallion), or a
  - Hinny (*Equus caballus* × *E. asinus*, a mare crossed with a jack).
  - However, pregnancy and live births have been reported in mules.
- There are many breeds of donkeys. The most commonly studied are the Mammoth, Pega, Sardinian, Catalonian, Poitou, and Miniature breeds. Some breeds are on the verge of becoming extinct.

ETIOLOGY/PATHOPHYSIOLOGY

General

- Donkey karyotype: 62 chromosomes.
- Donkeys have distinct reproductive anatomical, physiological and behavioral characteristics when compared to horses.

Female Reproduction

Seasonality and Estrous Cycle

- Onset of ovarian activity is generally present between 8 and 24 months of age, dependent on breed, season, nutrition, and health.
- Jennets reproductive seasonality is similar to that of horses, however many jennets continue to cycle year-round.
- Seasonality is more marked in harsh desert and arid zones due to a shortage of adequate nutrition and loss of body condition.
- The estrous cycle is slightly longer than that of the mare (23 to 24 days).
- Estrus lasts 3 to 15 days.

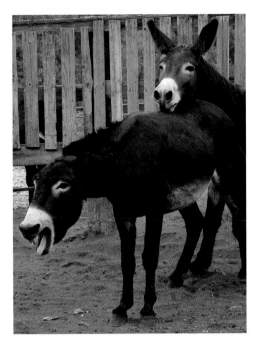

■ **Figure 20.1** Typical behavior of the jenny in heat: jaw clapping, yawing, or jawing.
Photo courtesy Pr. G. Catone, Dept Therio, Faculty Vet Med, Messina, Italy.

- Signs of estrus include:
  - Tail raising, urination stance, winking of the clitoris, ears back, mounting other females, receptivity to the male, and vulvar edema.
  - Extension of the neck and yawing reflex (repetitive jaw clamping) is a characteristic behavior of estrus females when mounted by the jack (Fig. 20.1).
- Follicular dominance is established at a diameter of 25 mm.
  - Dominant follicle grows approximately 2.7 mm per day.
- Ovulation takes place in the last 24 hours of estrus.
  - Females remain receptive for an average of 18 hours post-ovulation.
- Size of the preovulatory follicle varies according to breed:
  - Poitou: 30 to 33 mm.
  - Pega and Mammoth: 35 to 40 mm.
  - North African: 32 to 35 mm.
  - Miniature donkey: 30 to 40 mm.
- Some breeds (Mammoth and some European breeds) have a high incidence of double ovulation (37%). Triple ovulations are not rare, but most are asynchronous.
- The average life span of the CL (15 to 20 days) is longer than that of the mare.
- Endocrinology of the estrous cycle is similar to that of the mare.

Pregnancy

- Endocrinology of pregnancy is not well studied in the donkey.

- Serum P4 level increases during the first 19 days of gestation, to approximately 20 ng/mL, and then decreases by day 30 to approximately 12 ng/mL.
  - Another increase is observed between days 30 and 40.
  - A gradual decline occurs between 110 and 160 days.
- Secondary CL are formed between 38 and 46 days post-ovulation.
- Chorionic gonadotropin is secreted after Day 36 of pregnancy.
- The incidence of twinning is high in some breeds.
  - Strategies to reduce twin pregnancies are similar to those used in horses.
- Gestation length is longer than that of the mare; ranging from 340 to 396 days (average 355 days).

Parturition

- Mammary gland development and predicting the time of foaling is based on changes of mammary gland secretion similar to the mare (Fig. 20.2). Calcium concentration is greater than 500 ppm 24 hours prior to foaling.
- Stages of parturition are similar to the mare.
  - Jennets tend to be more discrete and isolate themselves from observers.
  - Foals are delivered within 10 to 25 minutes of *breaking water*.
  - The placenta is delivered within one hour of foaling.

Postpartum

- Uterine involution is complete by 3 weeks.
- Lochia is present for up to 7 days postpartum, but intrauterine fluid may be visible by U/S for up to 10 days.

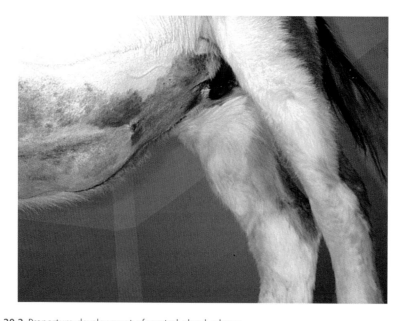

■ **Figure 20.2** Prepartum development of ventral gland edema.

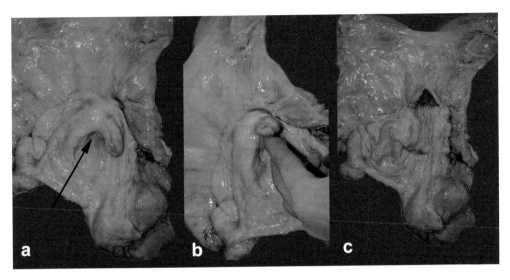

■ **Figure 20.3** Long cervix anatomy. Note the deep fornix *(arrow)* and long narrow cervical canal.

- Foal heat occurs 8 to 9 days after foaling and most females ovulate 13 to 17 days postpartum.
- Extended periods of postpartum ovarian inactivity (lactational anestrus) have been reported, particularly under harsh climactic conditions.
- Lactation usually lasts 10 months.

Reproductive Loss

- The pathophysiology of infertility and pregnancy loss in donkeys is poorly studied.
- Uterine infections tend to be more prevalent in the postpartum period.
- Abnormal perineal conformation is less frequent than in horses. The vulva commonly appears small and tight.
- Donkeys are more prone to cervical laceration during parturition due to their long, tight cervix (Fig. 20.3).
- Infectious causes of infertility and abortion are similar to those affecting horses.
  - Some strains of EAV appear to be poorly transmissible to horses.
  - CEM organisms isolated from donkeys (*Taylorella asinigenitalis*) are different from *Taylorella equigenitalis* and may cause a CEM-like syndrome in the mare.

Male Reproduction

- Reproductive organs in the jack are larger than those of the horse (Fig. 20.4).
  - The scrotum is more pendulous.
  - The testicles are large and the tail of the epididymis is more prominent (Fig. 20.5).
  - Testicular size of adult males of medium-size breeds:
    - Height: 6 to 7.5 cm

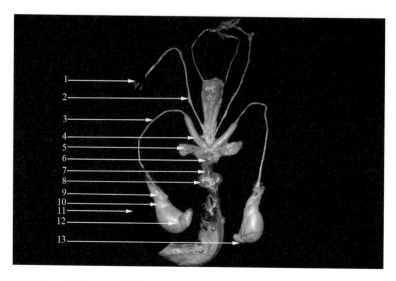

■ **Figure 20.4** Anatomy of the urogenital system anatomy in the male: 1. kidney; 2. ureter; 3. ductus (aka vas) deferens; 4. ampulla of the vas deferens; 5. seminal vesicle; 6. prostate; 7. pelvic portion of the penis; 8. bulbourethral gland; 9. testicular/spermatic cord; 10. head of the epididymis; 11. glans penis; 12. testis; 13. tail of the epididymis.

- ■ Length: 9 to 10.5 cm
- ■ Width: 4.8 to 6 cm
- ■ Sperm production parameters have been established for some breeds.
  - ■ Spermatogenic efficiency increases until 6 years of age then plateaus.
  - ■ Sperm production and quality is affected by season.
- ■ Reproductive behavior of the jack is distinct from that of the stallion.
  - ■ Jacks are more territorial.
  - ■ Interaction with jennets occurs in brief episodes.
  - ■ Sexually active females tend to seek out the male.
  - ■ Precopulatory behavior sequence includes naso-nasal contact, nibbling or sniffing the head, neck, back of the knee, body, flank, perineal area, and flehmen response.
  - ■ First mount occurs without erection. Spontaneous erection and masturbation is common.
  - ■ Season affects reproductive behavior and libido.
- ■ With in-hand mating, and in particular when mating horse mares, the erection and mounting latency is prolonged (up to 90 minutes).
- ■ In mule production systems, jacks need to be conditioned to mount mares. This is done by rearing them as young colts with horse fillies. Mares tend to exhibit less outwards signs of estrus to a jack than to a stallion.

Artificial Breeding

- ■ Estrus, ovulation synchronization techniques used in mares are effective for the jennet.

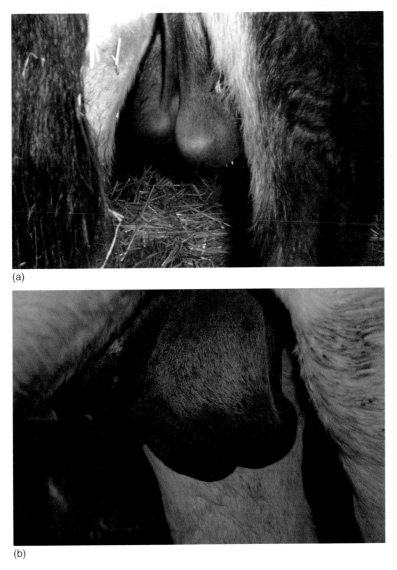

(a)

(b)

■ **Figure 20.5** Caudal *(a)* and lateral *(b)* views of the donkey's pendulous scrotum with its obvious tail of the epididymis.

- Techniques used for horse semen preservation are applicable to jackass semen.
  - Motility is maintained in skim milk extenders at 5°C for up to 96 hours and fertility remains good for up to 48 hours. Preservation at 15°C causes less membrane damage.
  - Lactose/egg yolk extender is better than Kenny's extender for cooled storage.
  - Daily AI with 250 million spermatozoa produces excellent conception rates.
- Freezability of donkey semen can be improved by using only the sperm-rich fraction of the ejaculate, adding L-glutamine to the extender, and replacing hen's egg-yolk with that of quail egg-yolk.

- ET techniques are similar to those used in the horse. However, pregnancy rates are low following nonsurgical transfer probably due to PGF$_2\alpha$ release caused by cervical manipulation.

Genetics

- Breed affect on cyclicity, follicular size, twinning rate.
- Age of puberty in the male is breed dependent.
- Miniature donkeys are predisposed to genetic abnormalities (e.g., hydrocephalus, domed head, spontaneous abortion).

Causes

- Female-specific causes of infertility and abortion are similar to those of horses.
- Male infertility is often due to severe testicular degeneration.

Systems Affected

Reproductive

 SIGNALMENT/HISTORY

Physical Examination Findings

Examination of the open female

- The perineal area and vulva are small and tight. Overt edema may be present when the female is in estrus.
- TRP is performed as for the mare.
  - Some breeds of donkey (i.e., North African and miniature donkey) may offer some challenges due to smallness of the tract and pelvis.
- Vaginal examination is best performed with a small Polanski speculum.

Examination of the Pregnant and Parturient Female

- Diagnosis of pregnancy by TRP is similar to horses. However, if more than 4 months of gestation, the fetus is often out of reach of the palpator.
- Sick pregnant females should always be checked for hyperlipidemia.
- Dystocia is more common in donkeys than in horses.
  - Highest rate of the dystocia is found in miniature donkeys.
  - Dystocia risk increases from breeding a jennet to a horse stallion.
- Obstetrical management is similar to that used in the mare, but C-section is often preferable to fetotomy.
  - Excessive manipulation within the narrow pelvis often results in severe vaginal adhesions.

Examination of the Male

- The protocol for examination of a stud jack is similar to that used for a stallion.
- Semen is best collected by an AV.
- Large equine AVs should be used for large and medium breeds.
  - Chemical induction of ejaculation has not been very rewarding.
- Semen volume varies by breed:
  - Miniatures: 25 to 115 mL.
  - Small breeds: 12.5 to 140 mL.
  - Large breeds: 25 to 250 mL.
  - The gel fraction can be copious.
- Total number of spermatozoa per ejaculate ranges from 5 to 18 billion.
- Evaluation of semen quality is similar to that used for horse semen.

DIFFERENTIAL DIAGNOSIS

- The clinical work-up of common reproductive problems is similar to those used to assess horses.
- Donkeys are more prone to hyperlipidemia.
- Donkeys are more prone to pre- and postpartum hypocalcemia.

DIAGNOSTICS

CBC/Biochemistry/Urinalysis

- Indications are similar to horses for specific conditions.
- Blood lipids should be determined in sick pregnant females.
- Hypocalcemia is common in females with:
  - RFM
  - Pre- or postpartum depression
  - Muscle fasciculations

Other Laboratory Test

Microbiology

Similar to horses

Cytology

- Similar to horses

Imaging

U/S of the female reproductive tract

- U/S characteristics of the uterus during estrus and diestrus are similar to those of the mare. Transrectal U/S in miniature donkeys is similar to that of miniature horses (*see* Reproduction in Miniature Horses).

- Pregnancy diagnosis:
  - By transrectal U/S at 10 to 12 days post-ovulation.
  - Mean embryonic vesicle growth is 3 to 3.5 mm per day until 18 days, then 0.5 mm/day until 29 days.
  - Fetal heart beat can be detected at 23 to 25 days.
- Fetal well-being and utero-placental thickness are evaluated in the same manner as in the mare. CTUP measurement is smaller, 1 to 1.5 mm less, than in the mare.
- In late pregnancy, the fetus extends cranially, deep into the abdomen.
- Asinine fetuses are less active than horse fetuses during examination.

U/S of the Male Genital Organs

- Examination technique is similar to that of stallion.
  - Testicles present a large tortuous central vein (Fig. 20.6).
  - The epididymal tail is prominent (*see* Fig. 20.6).
  - The accessory sex glands are larger than those of the stallion (Fig. 20.7).

Other Diagnostic Procedures

- Endometrial biopsy technique is similar to that used in mares.
- Endoscopic examination of the jennet's uterus and the jack's urethra and accessory sex glands, are similar to those of horses.
- Cryptorchidism: endocrine diagnosis by *hCG stim-test*:
  - Collect a sample for baseline testosterone level, and additional samples at 2 and 24 hours after administration of hCG (6,000 to 10,000 IU, IV). One additional sample collected yet later has been shown of value in horse stallions, that occasionally demonstrate a latent rise of testosterone 48 to 72 hours following administration of hCG.
  - A minimum of a twofold increase of testosterone is indicative of testicular tissue.
  - Estrone sulfate levels are not satisfactory to differentiate geldings from cryptorchids.

 THERAPEUTICS

Drug(s) of Choice

Hormone Therapy

Oxytocin

- RFM treatment: 30 IU in LRS, IV drip-rate of 1 IU every 2 minutes.
- Induction of parturition: repeated doses of 2.5 IU when gestation length exceeds 340 days, and the cervix is relaxed.

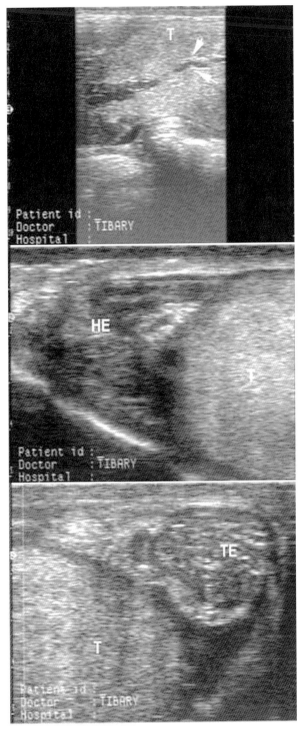

■ Figure 20.6 Ultrasound of the normal testis and epididymis. *T*, testicular parenchyma with a hypoechoic central vein *(arrows)*; *HE*, head of the epididymis; *TE*, tail of the epididymis.

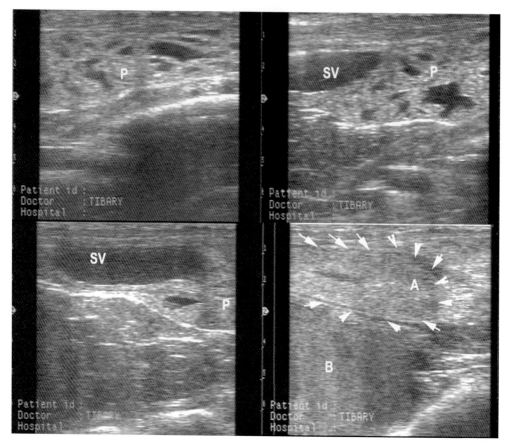

■ **Figure 20.7** Ultrasound of the accessory sex glands. *p*, prostate; *SV*, seminal vesicle; *A*, ampulla (delineated by arrows); *B*, urinary bladder.

hCG

- Induction of ovulation: 1,500 to 2,000 IU when the follicle is larger than 32 mm in diameter and the jennet is in estrus.
- Techniques for synchronization of estrus and ovulation are similar to those used in mares.

Appropriate Health Care

- Similar to horses.
- Pregnant donkeys should be carefully monitored for hyperlipidemia, if off-feed.

Surgical Considerations

- C-section is preferable to fetotomy in complicated obstetrical cases.
- Flank approach for C-section has been used successfully in the field.

COMMENTS

Abbreviations

AI	artificial insemination
AV	artificial vagina
CEM	contagious equine metritis
CL	corpus luteum
CTUP	combined thickness of the uterus and placenta
EAV	equine arteritis virus
ET	embryo transfer
hCG	human chorionic gonadotropin
IM	intramuscular
IV	intravenous
LRS	lactated Ringer's solution
P4	progesterone
PGF	natural prostaglandin
RFM	retained fetal membranes
TRP	transrectal palpation
U/S	ultrasound, ultrasonography

See Also

- See specific conditions in mares.

Suggested Reading

Blanchard TL, Taylor TS, Love CL. 1999. Estrous cycle characteristics and response to estrus synchronization in mammoth asses (*Equus asinus americanus*). *Therio* 52: 827–834.

Dadarwal D, Tandon SN, Purohit GN, et al. 2004. Ultrasonographic evaluation of uterine involution and postpartum follicular dynamics of French Jennies (*Equus asinus*). *Therio* 62: 257–264.

McDonnell SM. 1998. Reproductive behavior of donkeys (*Equus asinus*). *Applied Anim Behaviour Sci* 60: 277–282.

Purdy SR. 2005. Ultrasound examination of the female miniature donkey reproductive tract. In: *Veterinary Care of Donkeys*, Matthews NS and Taylor TS (eds). New York: International Veterinary Information Service (IVIS), www.ivis.org. Last updated: 11 May; A2925.0505.

Tibary A, Sghiri A, Bakkoury A. 2008. Chapter 17: Reproduction. In: *The Professional Handbook of the Donkey*, 4th ed, Svenden ED, Duncan J and Hardill D (eds). The Donkey Sanctuary, Whittet Books; 314–342.

Author: Ahmed Tibary

chapter 21

Dystocia

DEFINITION/OVERVIEW

- Dystocia is defined as any difficult delivery with or without assistance.
- Usually due to malposture of the fetus but can be due to malposition or malpresentation.
- It can also result from abnormalities of the mare, (e.g., fracture of the pelvis, restrictions of the vaginal canal).

Essential Definitions

- *Presentation* is the relationship of the long axis of the fetus to the long axis of the dam, to include: anterior, posterior, or transverse presentation.
- *Position* is the relationship of the dorsum of the fetus to the quadrants of the mare's pelvis: dorso-sacral (normal), dorso-pubic (upside down), left or right dorso-ilial (dorsum of fetus is rotated to either the left or right).
- *Posture* is the relationship of the fetal extremities to its own torso (e.g., flexures of the carpus, shoulder, hips, hocks, lateral flexion of the head and neck).
- Postural defects (e.g., flexion of the extremities [limbs and head and neck]), are the most common cause of equine dystocia.
- Developmental or fetal congenital causes: ankylosis of joints, shistosomas reflexus, hydrocephalus, perosomus elumbis, wry neck, anasarca, and so on (Fig. 21.1).

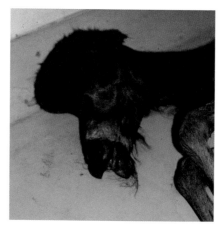

■ **Figure 21.1** Fetal hydrocephalus.
Image courtesy of C. L. Carleton.

ETIOLOGY/PATHOPHYSIOLOGY

Some dystocias are attributed to hereditary, nutritional, management, infectious, traumatic, or miscellaneous causes.

- Inherited abnormalities of the genital tract include twinning, size of the fetal head, ankylosis of joints, and hydrocephalus.
- Nutritional and managerial causes include a decrease in the mare's pelvic size (nutritional stunting), pelvic cavity fat (excess), failure to observe animals near term (management failure: an unattended, unresolved dystocia, can lead to uterine inertia/exhaustion), close confinement of mares during the entire gestation, and so on.
- Infectious conditions of the placenta or fetus can result in uterine inertia, incomplete cervical dilation, postural abnormalities due to fetal death, loss of placental attachment sites, and so on.
- Miscellaneous causes include traumatic damage of abdominal wall, which inhibits normal abdominal contractions; uterine torsion; pelvic fracture; fetal postural changes, which occur for no apparent reason; posterior presentation; and transverse presentation.

Systems Affected

- Reproductive
- Musculoskeletal
- Endocrine
- Others possibly affected as condition progresses, with development of systemic illness.

SIGNALMENT/HISTORY

Risk Factors

- Any breed and all ages of pregnant mares.
- All posterior presentations are potential dystocias.
- All deviations from normal position (dorsosacral), including dorsoilial and dorsopubic, are potential dystocias.
- Postural abnormalities such as flexion of the extremities (head and neck, limbs) account for the majority of dystocia. Included in these are carpal, shoulder, hip flexion; lateral flexion of the head and neck; and ankylosis of joints. It is impossible to determine why the fetus moves from a normal delivery presentation, position, and posture (anterior presentation, dorsosacral position, with extended head and neck and both forelimbs) to an abnormality of any order.
- Older mares and mares with insufficient exercise have an increased incidence for dystocia for unknown reasons.

Historical Findings

- Stage 2 of labor should not exceed 70 minutes or an abnormality of presentation, position, or posture should be suspected. The equine fetus survives for but a short interval once parturition begins. The reason for rapid fetal death is placental detachment while the fetus is yet *in utero*.
- A complete history includes: the mare's due date, any previous dystocia or abnormal gestations, recent systemic disease during the gestation, the length of active labor (Stages 1 and 2), timing of rupture of the allantoic membrane, when or if rupture of the amniotic membrane occurred, whether assistance was provided (potential for injury and contamination), and status of the mare's mobility.

 CLINICAL FEATURES

- An equine dystocia is always an emergency. Incidence of dystocia in the mare is less than 1%; miniature horses slightly higher. Always take a complete history and conduct a routine physical evaluation of the reproductive tract and a fetal examination *before* deciding how to handle a dystocia.
- Any mare in labor for longer than 70 minutes is at risk to deliver a dead fetus. Primary sign: failure of normal progression of fetal delivery during Stage 2 of labor.
- Client education: observe whether fetal soles are up or down during delivery as they emerge through the vulvar lips. They are visible through the intact amniotic membrane.
  - *Soles down*: the delivery may be either a normal anterior presentation or posterior presentation that is in dorso-pubic position.
  - *Soles up*: the delivery may be either posterior presentation in dorso-sacral position or anterior presentation in a dorso-pubic position.
- *Primary uterine inertia*: the uterus is overstretched (i.e., hydrops or twins); increased incidence in older or debilitated mares. Uterine infections may predispose mares to inertia. Failure of oxytocin release or failure of oxytocin to affect a uterine response may result in dystocia.
- *Secondary uterine inertia* is the result of uterine exhaustion. Active labor may fail due to the dam's pain during delivery. Prolonged dystocia with strong circular contractions may result in a fatigued uterus and become secondary uterine inertia.
  - When uterine inertia is maximal, the uterus is completely and tightly contracted around the fetus, the uterus may rupture if forced extraction is attempted.
- Immediate causes of dystocia can be relieved at the time of delivery; divided into maternal and fetal causes. Most immediate causes of equine dystocia are of fetal origin.
  - Maternal causes include stenosis of the birth canal (may be due to a small pelvis), a hypoplastic genital tract, lacerations and scars of the genital tract, pelvic tumors, persistent hymen, failure of cervical dilation, uterine inertia, abortions, twinning, etc.

- Fetal causes include an abnormal presentation, position, or posture; excessive fetal size, fetal anasarca, fetal ascites, fetal tumors, ankylosed joints, hydrocephalus, fetal monsters, posterior presentation, wryneck, and transverse presentation.

DIFFERENTIAL DIAGNOSIS

- The primary differential diagnosis for dystocia is prepartum colic.
- The signs of these two conditions can be similar, especially in early stages of dystocia.
- In the case of colic, signs of abdominal distress continue to worsen, whereas with dystocia it becomes obvious that the mare is not only uncomfortable, but is straining.
- In the case of true breech delivery (fetus is in dorso-sacral position, posterior presentation with bilateral hip flexion), the mare may not go into Stage 2 labor (due to the absence of point pressure on the cervix by fetal extremities) and straining is absent.
- Palpation of the reproductive tract, including transrectal and vaginal examinations, will be extremely rewarding to differentiate dystocia from colic. Certain inherited characteristics of a mare, (e.g., small pelvic size) may genetically influence the incidence of dystocia.

DIAGNOSTICS

If the history has confirmed breeding dates, the mare is known to be at or near term gestation, is demonstrating signs of labor, and/or there are indications the chorioallantoic membrane has ruptured.

Mare

- A thorough examination of the reproductive tract is indicated.
- If the mare is down and unable to rise, determine the cause. Return the mare to a standing position, if possible.
- An epidural may provide sufficient relief to allow a mare to stand that was previously unable. Reproductive manipulations are easier to perform with the mare standing, unless she is to be placed under general anesthesia.
- The mare's hydration status should be checked. Administer fluids if necessary before the manipulations begin, especially if the fetus is dead (a common outcome with the usual extended time from the onset of Stage 2 until the mare is presented for evaluation). Determine is she is sufficiently stable to administer local anesthetics, epidurals, general anesthesia or sedation, if necessary.
- Determine whether she is in shock or could go into shock before the procedures necessary to remove the fetus are complete. The presence of prolonged CRT and pale mucous membranes indicate the need for medications and fluids to be administered before proceeding.

- TRP of the genital tract should be performed before the vaginal examination: for possible lacerations, uterine tone, presentation, position, and posture of fetus; determine the degree of uterine contracture around the fetus.
- Vaginal examination of the genital tract: tail wrap and meticulous perineal washing to reduce further contamination of the birth canal. Use liberal amounts of lubricant to facilitate safe manipulation/mutation, fetal traction, or fetotomy. Determine if the birth canal size and degree of cervical relaxation are sufficient to permit fetal passage. Approximate the amount of space between the fetus and the maternal pelvis.
- At the outset of the vaginal examination, the vagina, cervix, and uterus should be examined for possible lacerations. Any lacerations should be brought to the client's attention, especially prior to palpation of the fetus or obstetrical manipulation.

Fetus

Methods to Determine Fetal Viability

- Gentle pressure over an eye to stimulate a blink reflex.
- Finger in fetus's mouth (for evidence of a suckling reflex).
- Pull on fetal limb to stimulate retraction by fetus.
- Maximally flex one of its limbs to stimulate pull away; or if one foot is presented through the vulvae, quick clamp with a Kelly forcep at the fetus' coronary band—very sensitive area—will stimulate a response if it is still alive.
- Finger in the anus to assess anal sphincter contraction if the fetus is in posterior presentation.
- U/S to determine presence of a heart beat or blood flow, may be difficult or too time-consuming—*time is of the essence.*
- Following viability assessment, note the fetal presentation, position, and posture.
- If the fetus is dead, attempt to determine how long (may not be possible until after delivery). Corneas can provide a rough estimate of the time of death; cloudiness indicates death *in utero* 6 to 12 hours prior to delivery. Emphysema and sloughing of fetus's hair indicates death occurred a minimum 18 hours prior to delivery.

Presurgical Option to Resolve Fetal Engagement in the Birth Canal

If C-section is not an option (not feasible, cost prohibitive) or the fetus is dead, an additional means to resolve the dystocia is with heavy sedation or light general anesthesia of the mare, followed by elevation of the mare's rear quarters by her hocks (Fig. 21.2). Even if the intent is to take a mare to surgery, a brief interval for elevation and attempted vaginal delivery may pay dividends and offer a reprieve from a C-section.

- Care must be taken to protect the hocks with padding or towels before attaching straps or ropes. Lifting may be accomplished by using a lift, front-end loader, overhead beam, etc., to elevate the rear end higher than the front. Once the mare is in lateral recumbency, *her hocks are elevated no more than 45 to 60 cm (18 to 24 inches)*. This is usually sufficient and avoids placing excessive pressure on the mare's diaphragm. Elevation allows the fetus to disengage from the pelvis (aided by gravity) and return (or be gently repulsed) to a more abdominal location.
- Permits mutation of the fetal extremities and increases the likelihood of vaginal extraction (live or dead fetus) or fetotomy (dead fetus). *See* Figure 21.3.

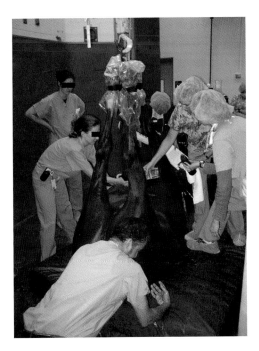

■ **Figure 21.2** Elevation of rear limbs of mare in dystocia to disengage the fetus from the birth canal and permit mutation and extraction.
Image courtesy of A. Tibary.

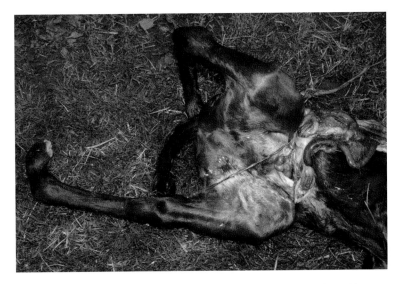

■ **Figure 21.3** Abnormal fetus (schistosomus reflexus with ankylosis) dead but delivered intact per vagina following elevation of the mare's rear quarters.
Image courtesy of C. L. Carleton.

CBC/Biochemistry/Urinalysis

- CBC and blood chemistries may be indicated if the animal is hospitalized and the results are rapidly available.

Pathologic Findings

Depends upon the cause of dystocia.

 THERAPEUTICS

- Essential to decide early in the intervention if a C-section is the best approach.
- If the fetus is alive and no other correction (mutation with extraction) is possible and if the surgical approach can be made in a short enough period of time to maintain fetal viability, that decision must be reached quickly and facilities must be available nearby.
- If the fetus cannot be delivered alive, consideration must be given to fetotomy, especially if this procedure can be accomplished on the farm with no more than one or two cuts.

Drug(s) of Choice

- Epidural anesthesia can assist in the delivery process by reducing contractions during an assisted delivery. The approximate dosage is 1 mL of 2% carbocaine per 40 kg of body weight. A portion of this is used to block the skin and tissue while inserting the needle into the appropriate place within the epidural space. Surgically shave and prep the area for the epidural injection. A 15-cm (6-inch) spinal needle is placed into the area of most movement near the sacral coccygeal junction and worked cranially into the canal. When it is in the proper place at least 10 to 12 cm (4 to 5 in) of the needle will be below skin depth to reach the spinal canal.
- Xylazine (0.5 to 1.0 mg/kg) can be used for sedation alone or combined with acepromazine (0.04 mg/kg).
- General anesthetic agents can be used to induce anesthesia for C-section or to accomplish further corrective procedures via elevation of the rear quarters of the anesthetized mare as described previously. If vaginal space is sufficient for delivery, a C-section may be avoided.
- Following delivery, the administration of oxytocin at a dosage of 10, but not more than 20, IU per 500 kg IM will hasten uterine contractions and involution of the postpartum uterus. Oxytocin should never be administered prepartum unless inducing parturition, due to its potential to cause further uterine contracture and further reducing the space for fetal manipulation. Exceeding recommended doses, especially early post-delivery, may result in uterine eversion (prolapse).

Alternative Drugs

- Other chemicals agents can be used including butorphenol (0.02–0.1 mg/kg IV), detomidine (0.02–0.04 mg/kg IV or IM), or morphine (0.6 mg/kg).

Appropriate Health Care

- Dystocia is generally best handled on the farm. Uterine size and space within which mutation and extraction can be accomplished, decrease with time and subsequent uterine contractions.
- Vaginal deliveries can best be accomplished shortly after a dystocia is diagnosed, whether mutation and forced extraction or fetotomy is to be performed.

Nursing Care

After delivery, follow-up care consists of thorough examination of the uterus, cervix, vagina, vestibule, and vulva.

- Broad-spectrum antibiotics should be placed into the uterus to reduce the number of organisms that were undoubtedly introduced during mutation and extraction of the fetus.
- Uterine stimulants such as oxytocin can be beneficial and enhance uterine involution, thus hastening its return to normal size postpartum.
- Systemic antibiotics may be necessary if indications of a systemic involvement develop.
- Uterine flushes or infusions may also be indicated to enhance uterine contractility.
- Other supportive therapy may be indicated for mares undergoing C-section.

Diet

- The diet of the mare requires no adjustments other than a possible reduction in the quantity fed, if indicated.
- The intent of maintaining the regular diet is to avoid intestinal upset due to dietary change. Changing the diet at the time of parturition further adds to the mare's stress and should be avoided.

Activity

- The mare's activity need not be restricted if a vaginal delivery was successful. However, mares undergoing C-section should be stall rested.

Surgical Considerations

- Important to decide early in the intervention if a C-section is the best approach.
- If the fetus is alive and no other correction (mutation, extraction) is possible, and if the surgical approach can be made in a short enough period of time to maintain fetal viability, then the decision must be reached quickly.
- If the fetus cannot be delivered alive, consideration must be given to fetotomy, especially if this procedure can be accomplished with one or two cuts on the farm.
- If a C-section is to be performed, timing is critical.

COMMENTS

Client Education

- It should be emphasized that mares should not languish in prolonged labor (exceeding 30 minutes without progress) because the probability of neonatal survival decreases rapidly.
- The position of fetal extremities should be examined closely during delivery; determine if the fetus is in an abnormal delivery presentation, position, or posture at the earliest possible time. If the soles of the fetus are pointed down, this indicates one of two possibilities: anterior presentation with dorso-sacral position or posterior presentation with dorso-pubic position. It is also essential to determine if the head of the fetus is resting on its metacarpi (normal presentation, position, and posture).
- The incidence of dystocia increases slightly in aged mares, possibly related to decreased uterine contractions.

Patient Monitoring

- TRP of the reproductive tract is indicated daily or every other day depending on the findings to determine the size and tone of the uterus.
- U/S examination can be combined with TRP to determine the presence or absence of fluid in the uterus.
- The owner should monitor the mare's mucous membranes and activity.
- Note should be made with regard to appetite and defecations, as well as lactation.
- Once a dystocia has been corrected, transrectal examinations should be performed to ascertain that uterine involution is occurring normally.

Prevention/Avoidance

- The only definite way to avoid dystocia is not to breed the mare. Close observation of near-term mares will aid in the early diagnosis of dystocia. There is no method to prevent dystocia without doing an elective C-section or not breeding a mare.

Possible Complications

- Oxytocin should never be administered prepartum due to its potential to induce further uterine contracture, reducing further the space for fetal manipulation.
- Exceeding recommended doses of oxytocin, especially early following delivery, may result in eversion (prolapse) of the uterus.
- Regardless of the approach selected, care must be taken when manipulating a fetus during delivery.
- After delivery, the uterus should be thoroughly examined for possible tears; tears may result in peritonitis.

- There may also be lacerations of the cervix, vagina, vestibule, or vulva.
- RFM and delayed uterine involution may occur following correction of a dystocia.
- Uterine inflammation or infection may result from dystocia or the corrective methods used.

Expected Course and Prognosis

- The best outcome occurs with the least amount of assistance necessary to deliver the fetus. For example, correction of one flexed limb would be less of a problem for the mare than a C-section. The latter also requires a longer period of recovery.
- Prognosis decreases with the duration of dystocia, inexperienced interference, the origin/cause of the dystocia, and other contributing factors. The prognosis for the mare is grave if it has been longer than 24 hours from onset of Stage 2.
- Fetuses have a guarded prognosis if it has been greater than 70 minutes from onset of Stage 2. After the initial examination of the mare, all factors should be discussed with the client, including prognosis, fees, and the best approach to resolve the dystocia.
- The choices of approach include the mare standing, in lateral recumbency, or with the rear-quarters elevated (*see* Fig. 21.2). Assisted forced extraction, manipulation (mutation) of the fetus, fetotomy, or C-section are the options to relieve dystocia.
- The last resort to handling a dystocia is euthanasia of the dam.
- Always give the client a realistic prognosis and permit him or her to make the decision.

Synonyms

- Difficult delivery/labor/parturition
- Parturition difficulties
- Difficult foaling
- Inability to foal

Abbreviations

CBC   complete blood count
CRT   capillary refill time
IM   intramuscular
IU   intrauterine
IV   intravenous
RFM   retained fetal membranes, retained placenta
TRP   transrectal palpation
U/S   ultrasound, ultrasonography

See Also

- Parturition
- Parturition induction

- Postpartum metritis
- Prolonged pregnancy
- Retained fetal membranes

Suggested Reading

Asbury AC. 1993. Care of the mare after foaling. In: *Equine Reproduction*. McKinnon AO and Voss JL (eds). Philadelphia, Lea & Febiger; 578–587.

Roberts SJ. 1986. *Veterinary Obstetrics and Genital Diseases (Theriogenology)*, 3rd ed, Woodstock, VT: Author; 326–351.

Author: Walter R. Threlfall

chapter 22

Early Embryonic Death

DEFINITION/OVERVIEW

Maternal structural or functional defects that prevent normal embryonic development from early pregnancy diagnosis at 14 to 15 days post-ovulation to the beginning of the fetal stage at approximately 40 days of gestation.

ETIOLOGY/PATHOPHYSIOLOGY

- The rate of EED has been estimated to be 5% to 10% in younger mares but much higher in older, subfertile mares
- Although rate of conception failure is generally approximately 30% in young mares, it approaches 50% to 70% in older, subfertile mares.
- The specific causes of EED are similar to those of conception failure, and some are listed:
  - Defective embryos associated with older mares and seasonal effects.
  - Unsuitable uterine environment associated with endometritis, endometrial periglandular fibrosis (Fig. 22.1), or endometrial cysts large enough to impede embryonic mobility during transuterine migration (Fig. 22.2) and interfere with *maternal recognition of pregnancy* (conception failure more likely).
  - Endometrial periglandular fibrosis associated with endometriosis can cause inadequate secretion of histotrophs necessary embryonic development.
  - Xenobiotics associated fescue toxicosis, ergotism, or phytoestrogens (anecdotal) can cause EED.
  - EED has also been associated with MRLS.
  - Endocrine disorders, such as hypothyroidism (anecdotal) and luteal insufficiency (anecdotal) have been proposed as causes of EED.
  - Maternal disease characterized by fever, stress, and pain (anecdotal) can be associated with EED.

Pathophysiology

Depending on the specific cause, the pathophysiological mechanisms for EED can involve one or more of the following:
- Embryonic defects or injury which prevent embryonic development and progression to the fetal stage.

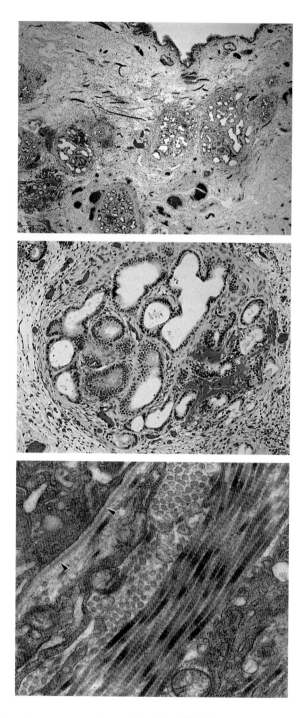

■ **Figure 22.1** In the top image, severe endometrial periglandular fibrosis and a relative lack of normal endometrial glandular architecture are shown in an endometrial biopsy sample collected from an older mare (bar = 200 μm). The severe fibrosis within and surrounding the fibrotic nests from this biopsy is shown in greater detail in the middle image (bar = 100 μm). The ultrastructural appearance of endometrial periglandular fibrosis is shown in the bottom image, where the cytoplasmic processes of fibroblasts alternate with bundles of collagen fibrils adjacent to glandular basal lamina *(arrowheads)* in a transmission electron micrograph. Image (bar = 350 nm).

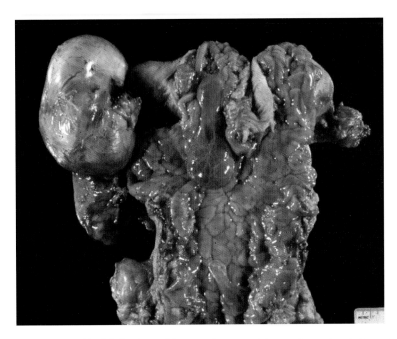

■ **Figure 22.2** Mare tract (died following colic) opened to reveal lumen. Large lymphatic cyst completely blocked the left uterine horn. Note: that was the mare's functional ovary and two large follicles were present. Image courtesy of C. L. Carleton.

- Unsuitable uterine environment which prevents normal embryonic or extraembryonic membrane development (might be associated with inadequate histotroph secretion) and progression to the fetal stage.
- Regression of CL associated with endometritis.
- Luteal insufficiency—anecdotal.
- Failure of *maternal recognition of pregnancy*

Systems Affected

Reproductive

 # SIGNALMENT/HISTORY

Risk Factors

- Older mares, more than 15 years of age, especially those with moderate/severe endometritis, endometrial periglandular fibrosis (*see* Fig. 22.1), or endometrial cysts.
- Anatomical defects predisposing the genital tract to endometritis.
- Seasonal effects
- Foal heat breeding: anecdotal and somewhat controversial.
- Inadequate nutrition
- Exposure to xenobiotics: fescue toxicosis and ergotism.
- Some heterospecific matings: stallion × jenny.
- Susceptibility to PMIE (more likely to cause conception failure).

Historical Findings

One or more of the following:

- Diagnosis of EED by transrectal U/S at least 14 or more days after ovulation, following previous confirmation of pregnancy.
- Diagnosis of failure of pregnancy by TRP at least 25 days after ovulation, following previous confirmation of pregnancy.
- History of PMIE
- History of abortion or dystocia.
- Return to estrus after diagnosis of pregnancy.
- Previous exposure to endophyte-infected fescue or ergotized grasses and grains.
- *Recent* systemic disease
- Geographical location, especially with relation to endophyte-infected fescue pastures/hay or ergotized grasses or grains.

 CLINICAL FEATURES

- Frequently, at least 40 days after ovulation, there is no evidence by transrectal U/S or TRP of a previously diagnosed pregnancy.
- Alternatively, at/up to 40 days after ovulation, there can be evidence by transrectal U/S of embryonic death in a mare previously diagnosed as pregnant.
- Transrectal U/S evidence of embryonic death includes decreasing embryonic vesicle size, change in appearance of the fluid within the embryonic vesicle, failure to visualize the embryo proper, the absence of a heartbeat after 25 days, or cessation of normal embryonic growth and development, with eventual disappearance of pregnancy-associated structures (Fig. 22.3).

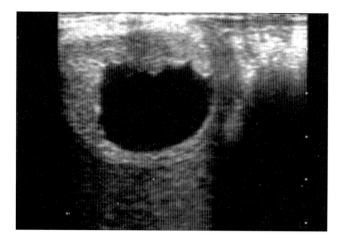

■ **Figure 22.3** Transrectal ultrasound evidence of early embryonic death: the embryo proper and the heart beat cannot be visualized in a 27-day pregnancy.
Image courtesy of D. Volkmann.

- Endometrial folds or intrauterine fluid might be visualized in the nonpregnant uterus.
- Luteal structures may or may not be present on the ovaries, and the mare's behavior may be cyclic or acyclic, depending on the circumstances.
- There may or may not be a mucoid or mucopurulent vaginal discharge

DIFFERENTIAL DIAGNOSIS

- Conception failure
- Previous misdiagnosis of pregnancy by transrectal U/S or TRP.
- Endometrial cysts, intrauterine fluid, paraovarian cystic structures, and small ovarian follicles can all be mistaken for pregnancies. They are distinguished from embryonic vesicles based on shape, size, location, and reexamination.
- Pregnancies move until 16 days post-ovulation (transuterine migration), increase in size, and develop/exhibit heartbeats.

DIAGNOSTICS

- CBC with differential, as well as serum biochemical data to determine inflammatory or stress leukocyte response, as well as other organ system involvement. Not usually indicated unless the mare has been ill recently.
- ELISA or RIA analyses for maternal progesterone may be useful up to 80 days of gestation (normal levels vary from greater than 1 to more than 4 ng/mL, depending on the reference laboratory). Maternal estrogen concentrations can reflect fetal estrogen production and viability, especially conjugated estrogens (e.g., estrone sulfate).
- Anecdotal reports of lower T_3/T_4 levels in mares with history of conception failure, EED, or abortion. The significance of low T_4 levels is unknown and somewhat controversial.
- Cytogenetic studies can be useful to detect chromosomal abnormalities.
- Endometrial cytology, culture, and biopsy procedures might be indicated to assess endometrial inflammation or fibrosis.
- Vaginal speculum examination and hysteroscopy might be indicated if structural abnormalities are suspected in the cervix or uterus.
- Feed or environmental analyses might be indicated for specific xenobiotics, ergopeptine alkaloids, phytoestrogens, heavy metals, or fescue endophyte (*Neotyphodium coenophialum*).
- Transrectal U/S is essential to confirm early pregnancy, as well as to detect intrauterine fluid and endometrial cysts.
- A thorough reproductive evaluation (i.e., transrectal U/S, vaginal speculum, endometrial cytology, culture, and biopsy) is indicated pre-breeding for individuals predisposed to EED (e.g., barren, older mares with history of conception failure, EED, or endometritis).

- In predisposed individuals (i.e., barren, older mares, or mares with history of EED, or conception failure, or endometritis), transrectal U/S should be performed at weekly intervals until at least 60 days of pregnancy.
- Transrectal U/S should be performed every 2 weeks until at least 60 days of pregnancy in normal mares to detect EED.
- It is necessary to follow embryonic growth and development and to distinguish the conceptus from cysts.

Pathological Findings

- An endometrial biopsy can demonstrate the presence of moderate to severe, chronic endometritis, endometrial periglandular fibrosis with decreased normal glandular architecture (*see* Fig. 22.1), or lymphatic lacunae (*see* Conception Failure in Mares).

 THERAPEUTICS

Drug(s) of Choice

Altrenogest

- Mares with a history of conception failure or moderate to severe endometritis (i.e., no active, infectious component) or fibrosis can be administered altrenogest (0.044–0.088 mg/kg PO, SID) beginning 2 to 3 days after ovulation or upon diagnosis of pregnancy, and continued until at least day 100 of gestation (taper daily dose over a 14-day period at the end of treatment).
- Altrenogest administration can be started later during gestation, continued longer, or used only for short periods of time, depending on serum progesterone levels during the first 80 days of gestation (greater than 1 to greater than 4 ng/mL, depending on the reference lab), clinical circumstances, risk factors, and clinician preference.
- If used near term, altrenogest frequently is discontinued 7 to 14 days before the expected foaling date, depending on the case, unless otherwise indicated by assessment of fetal maturity/viability or by questions regarding the accuracy of gestational length.

Precautions/Interactions

- Use altrenogest only to prevent conception failure of noninfectious endometritis.
- Use transrectal U/S to diagnose pregnancy at least 14 to 16 days after ovulation to identify intrauterine fluid or pyometra early in the disease course for appropriate treatment.
- If pregnancy is diagnosed, frequent monitoring (weekly initially) may be indicated to detect EED.
- Altrenogest is absorbed through the skin, so persons handling this preparation should wear gloves and wash their hands.

- Supplemental progestins are commonly and widely used to treat cases of conception failure, but their efficacy remains controversial.
- Primary, age-related, embryonic defects do not respond to supplemental progestins.

Alternative Drugs

- Injectable progesterone (150–500 mg/day, oil base) can be administered IM, SID instead of the oral formulation. Variations, contraindications, and precautions are similar to those associated with altrenogest.
- Other injectable and implantable progestin preparations are available commercially for use in other species. Any use in horses of these products is off-label, and little scientific data are available regarding their efficacy.
- Newer, repository forms of progesterone are occasionally introduced; however, some evidence of efficacy should be provided prior to use.
- T_4 supplementation has been successful (anecdotally) for treating mares with histories of subfertility. Its use remains controversial, however, and it is considered deleterious by some clinicians.

Appropriate Health Care

- Similar to that outlined in Conception Failure in Mares.
- Treat preexisting endometritis before insemination or breeding of mares during the physiologic breeding season.
- Mares being bred should have adequate body condition.
- Inseminate or breed foal heat mares if ovulation occurs at least 9 to 10 days (or more) postpartum and no intrauterine fluid is present.
- Prevention of PMIE (*see* Conception Failure in Mares)
- Depending on breed restrictions, various forms of advanced reproductive technologies manipulating/directly affecting the zygote or embryo are used in particular instances, (e.g., to retrieve embryos from the oviduct, approximately days 2 to 4 after ovulation) or uterus (days 6 to 8 after ovulation) for ET, and oocyte retrieval and successful IVF with subsequent ET.
- Primary, age-related embryonic defects are refractory to treatment.
- Most cases of EED can be handled in an ambulatory situation.
- Increased frequency of U/S monitoring of follicular development and ovulation, to permit insemination closer to ovulation, as well as more technical diagnostic procedures, may need to be performed in a hospital setting. Adequate restraint and optimal lighting might not be available in the field to permit quality U/S examination.

Nursing Care

- Generally requires none.
- Minimal nursing care might be necessary after more invasive diagnostic and therapeutic procedures.

Diet

- Generally no restriction, unless indicated by concurrent maternal disease or nutritional problems (e.g., under- or over-nourished).

Activity

- Generally no restriction of broodmare activity, unless contraindicated by concurrent maternal disease or diagnostic or therapeutic procedures.
- Preference may be to restrict activity of mares in competition because of the possible impact of stress on pregnancy maintenance, especially in mares with a history of EED.

Surgical Considerations

- Indicated for repair of anatomical defects predisposing mares to endometritis.
- Certain diagnostic and therapeutic procedures discussed above might also involve some surgical intervention.

 COMMENTS

Client Education

- Emphasize the *aged* mare's susceptibility to conception failure and her refractoriness to treatment.
- Inform clients regarding the cause, diagnosis, and treatment of endometritis.
- Inform clients regarding the seasonal aspects and nutritional requirements of conception.
- Inform clients regarding the role that endophyte-infected fescue and certain heterospecific breedings might play in conception failure.

Patient Monitoring

- Accurate teasing records.
- Reexamination of mares treated for endometritis before breeding.
- Early examination for pregnancy by transrectal U/S.
- Monitor embryonic and fetal development with transrectal or transabdominal U/S.

Prevention/Avoidance

- Recognition of at-risk mares.
- Management of endometritis before breeding.
- Removal of mares from fescue-infected pasture and ergotized grasses and grains after breeding and during early gestation.

- Use of ET procedures in at-risk mares.
- Prudent use of medications in bred mares.
- Avoid exposure to known toxicants.

Possible Complications

- High-risk pregnancy
- Abortion: infectious or noninfectious, depending on the circumstances.

Expected Course and Prognosis

- Young mares with resolved cases of endometritis or corrected anatomical abnormalities can have a fair to good prognosis to complete pregnancy.
- Older mares (more than 15 years of age) with a history of chronic, moderate to severe endometritis, endometrial periglandular fibrosis, or endometrial cysts, as well as conception failure or EED, have a guarded to poor prognosis for conception success, safe completion of pregnancy, and delivery of a healthy foal.

Synonyms/Closely Related Conditions

- Conception failure
- Infertility
- Pregnancy reabsorption
- Reabsorbed pregnancy
- Sterility
- Subfertility

Abbreviations

CBC	complete blood count
CL	corpus luteum
EED	early embryonic death
ELISA	enzyme-linked immunosorbent assay
ET	embryo transfer
IM	intramuscularly
IVF	in vitro fertilization
MRLS	mare reproductive loss syndrome
PMIE	post-mating induced endometritis
PO	per os (by mouth)
RIA	radioimmunoassay
SID	once a day
T_3	triiodothyronine
T_4	thyroxine
TRP	transrectal palpation
U/S	ultrasound, ultrasonography

See Also

- Abortion, spontaneous, infectious or noninfectious
- Conception failure in mares
- Conception failure in stallions
- Embryo transfer
- Endometrial biopsy
- Endometritis
- Metritis

Suggested Reading

Evans TJ, Rottinghaus GE, Casteel SW. 2003. Ergopeptine alkaloid toxicoses in horses. In: *Current Therapy in Equine Medicine 5*. Robinson NE (ed). Philadelphia: Saunders; 796–798.

Ginther OJ. 1992. *Reproductive Biology of the Mare: Basic and Applied Aspects*, 2nd ed. Cross Plains, WI: Equiservices; 499–562.

Paccamonti D. 2003. Endometrial cysts. In: *Current Therapy in Equine Medicine 5*. Robinson NE (ed). Philadelphia: Saunders; 231–234.

Vanderwall DK, Squires EL, Brinsko SP, et al. 2000. Diagnosis and management of abnormal embryonic development characterized by formation of an embryonic vesicle without an embryo in mares. *JAVMA* 217: 58–63.

Youngquist RS, Threlfall WR (eds). 2007. *Current Therapy in Large Animal Theriogenology*, 2nd ed. St. Louis: Elsevier-Saunders.

Author: Tim J. Evans

chapter 23

Eclampsia

DEFINITION/OVERVIEW

- Also known as puerperal tetany or lactation tetany.
- A rare metabolic condition resulting when serum calcium levels drop below 8 mg/dL in heavily lactating mares.
- Clinical signs are progressive and directly related to the level of serum calcium.
  - The mare develops muscle fasiculations beginning with the temporal, masseter, and triceps muscles.
  - She develops a stiff, stilted gait, and rear limb ataxia.
  - Becomes anxious.
  - Experiences tachycardia with dysrhythmias.
- It usually occurs within the 2 weeks after foaling and is associated with lactation and stress.

ETIOLOGY/PATHOPHYSIOLOGY

- The etiology is related to loss of calcium in the milk, particularly in those mares that milk heavily, especially when they are on lush pasture.
- It is seen most often in draft mares and heavy, well-muscled mares, Quarter Horse halter-type mares, that are working while lactating, or lactating mares that are transported over long distances.
- The condition is also recognized in the heavily milking mare 1 to 2 days post-weaning.

Systems Affected

- Mammary
- Musculoskeletal
- Cardiovascular
- Neurologic

SIGNALMENT/HISTORY

Based primarily on clinical signs in conjunction with the appropriate historical information:

- Lactating mare ten days postpartum and/or 1 to 2 days post-weaning.
- Prolonged exercise or transport.
- On lush pasture.
- Primarily due to hypocalcemia. Serum calcium values in the range of 5 to 8 mg/dL, coupled with associated clinical signs, confirm the diagnosis.
- Hypomagnesemia is an uncommon finding.
- Draft mares: Belgian, Percheron, Clydesdale.
- No age predisposition.
- Unlikely occurrence in primiparous mares.

Risk Factors

- Draft breeds, but not exclusively.
- Lactation, postpartum, heavier milking mares.
- Exercise or transport at the time of lactation
- Heavily lactating mare continuing after her foal has been weaned.

Historical Findings

- Incidence/Prevalence: Rare
- This condition occurs either late in gestation or the peripartal period.

 CLINICAL FEATURES

- Signs of eclampsia vary and include:
  - Muscle fasiculations involving the temporal, masseter and triceps.
  - Generalized increased muscle tone; stiff, stilted gait; rear limb ataxia; increased respiratory rate.
  - Some mares will demonstrate a delayed pupillary response (constriction) to a penlight.
  - Trismus (tonic contraction of the muscles of mastication); dysphagia; salivation.
  - May be mistaken for colic in the early stages: period of lying down, stretching out, rolling, looking at her flank, agitated, continuous walking.
  - Light to profuse sweating; elevated temperature; anxiety, tachycardia with dysrhythmia.
  - Synchronous diaphragmatic flutter, convulsions, coma, and death.
  - If untreated, the condition is progressive over a 24- to 48-hour period and some of these mares die.

- The clinical signs are directly related to the level of serum calcium.
  - Increased excitability: calcium levels are below normal (range 11–13 mg/dL), but more than 8 mg/dL.
  - Calcium levels of 5 to 8 mg/dL: usually produce signs of tetanic spasms and incoordination.
  - Serum calcium levels less than 5 mg/dL: often become stuporous and are recumbent.

DIFFERENTIAL DIAGNOSIS

- Colic
- Laminitis
- Myositis
- Tetanus
- Other neuromuscular disorders

DIAGNOSTICS

CBC/Biochemistry/Urinalysis

Parameters should be within normal limits, except for possibly elevated muscle enzymes.

Other Laboratory Tests

- Normal laboratory ranges reported for serum calcium vary (e.g., [1] from 8.5–10.5 and, [2] from 11–13 mg/dL). The majority of normal mares will be within the range of 11 to 13 mg/dL.
- It is best to know the normal range for serum calcium generated by *the laboratory that you regularly use.*
- In addition to abnormally low levels of serum calcium, many affected mares have been reported to have abnormalities in serum levels of magnesium and phosphorus.
- Hypocalcemia in the mare has been associated with hyper/hypophosphatemia and hyper/hypomagnesemia.
- Reports suggest that hypomagnesemia/hypocalcemia is most commonly associated with the transport of heavily lactating mares.

Other Diagnostic Procedures

- Evaluate serum calcium
- There may be excess protein in the mare's urine.

THERAPEUTICS

Drug(s) of Choice

- Intravenous calcium (slow infusion), in the form of 20% calcium borogluconate or 23% calcium gluconate.
- Rate: 250 to 500 mL per 500 kg body weight.
- Calcium solutions should be diluted 1:4 with saline or dextrose.

Precautions/Interactions

- Use caution when administering calcium solutions due to their potential cardiotoxic effects.
- It is imperative to monitor the heart for any alterations in rate or rhythm.
- If alterations occur, treatment should be stopped immediately.
- Dilution of the calcium with saline or dextrose reduces the potential for cardiotoxic effects.
- Safety measure: remove the foal from the mare until she is standing.

Appropriate Health Care

- Because of the progressive nature of this condition, therapy is recommended in nearly all cases.
- A few mildly affected cases will recover without treatment.

Nursing Care

- Occasional mare may require a second treatment, if a relapse occurs.

Diet

- Restrict access of heavily lactating mares to lush pasture if they have a history of eclampsia.
- Feed high-protein, high-calcium diets post-foaling to mares previously prone to eclampsia.

Activity

- Restrict transit of heavily lactating mares during the first 10 to 12 days postpartum, the most susceptible period.

COMMENTS

Client Education

- In addition to restricting access to lush pasture for mares with a history of eclampsia, reduce nutritional intake (quality) in heavily lactating mares for 1 to 2 weeks prior to weaning to reduce milk production.

Patient Monitoring

- A reduction in clinical signs and a positive inotropic effect, indicate treatment is effective.
- If no response is evident after the initial treatment, a second treatment may be necessary in 30 minutes.

Prevention/Avoidance

- Decreasing high-protein feeds in the mare's diet late in gestation may decrease the incidence in susceptible mares.
- In previously affected mares, decrease her intake of calcium 2 to 5 weeks pre-foaling.
- High-protein, high-calcium diets post-foaling for mares prone to eclampsia.
- See Client Education and Dietary Management for Susceptible Mares.

Possible Complications

Cardiovascular effects

Expected Course and Prognosis

- Most mares respond to treatment with a full recovery, however, relapses can occur necessitating additional therapy.
- Recurrence in the future if mares are foaling and maintained under the same management conditions.

Synonyms

- Hypocalcemia
- Lactation tetany
- Transport tetany

See Also

- Dystocia
- Parturition

Suggested Reading

Fenger CK. 1998. Disorders of calcium metabolism. In: *Equine Internal Medicine*. Reed SM and Bayly WM (eds). Toronto, WB Saunders; 930–931.

Freestone JF, Melrose PA. 1995. Endocrine diseases. In: *The Horse, Diseases and Clinical Management*. Kobluk CN, Ames TR and Geor RJ (eds). Philadelphia, WB Saunders; 1159.

Valberg SJ, Hodgson DR. 1996. Diseases of Muscle. In: *Large Animal Internal Medicine*, 2nd ed, Smith BP (ed). St. Louis, Mosby; 1498–1499.

Author: Carla L. Carleton

chapter 24

Embryo Transfer

DEFINITION/OVERVIEW

ET traditionally refers to the removal of an embryo from the uterus or oviduct of one mare (the donor) and placement into the uterus or oviduct of another (the recipient). Oocyte transfer and IVF are other, related assisted reproductive technologies also being further developed and used in horses.

Systems Affected

Reproductive

CLINICAL FEATURES

Indications/Potential Donors

- Mares that are older than 15 years with a history of conception failure, EED, or abortion.
- Mares with systemic disease or structural abnormalities that prevents them from carrying a fetus to term.
- Young mares with valuable genetics or those in competition.
- Certain extraspecific matings (e.g., zebra transferred into a horse recipient).

DIAGNOSTICS

Prebreeding/Embryo Collection Evaluations

- Indicated in individuals with a history of conception failure, EED, or abortion.
- Transrectal U/S, vaginal examination (both digital manual and speculum), endometrial cytology/culture, and endometrial biopsy to detect evidence of anatomic defects, endometritis, and fibrosis, which may predispose a mare to conception failure or EED.

- Similar procedures should be performed on mares being screened as potential ET recipients. These mares should have minimal reproductive abnormalities and be physically capable of carrying a foal to term.

Transrectal or Transvaginal U/S Examinations

- Transrectal U/S is used to evaluate follicular development and ovulation and to determine the appropriate timing for donor mare insemination or breeding. The ovulations of the donor and recipient mares should be synchronized with one another, with the recipient mare ovulating within 48 hours of the donor (may be clinician preference).
- Transrectal U/S examination is indicated for the donor and recipient mares at the time of flushing and transfer, respectively, to determine the absence of intrauterine fluid and the presence of a CL.
- Transvaginal U/S procedures have been used in the aspiration of oocytes.

Other Diagnostic Procedures

- Checking recipient's progesterone concentration may be indicated prior to transfer and at recipient's initial pregnancy examination to check for functional CL.
- ELISA or RIA for progesterone acceptable levels vary from greater than 1 to greater than 4 ng/mL, depending on the reference lab.

Pathological Findings

- An endometrial biopsy can demonstrate the presence of moderate to severe, chronic endometritis, endometrial periglandular fibrosis with decreased normal glandular architecture, and/or lymphatic lacunae (*see* Conception Failure in Mares and EED).

 THERAPEUTICS

Drug(s) of Choice

- Progestins, antibiotics, anti-inflammatory medications, or intrauterine therapy may or may not be used in the donor and, possibly, in recipient mares, depending on the circumstances, procedures involved, and clinician preference.
- eFSH has also been used with some success to superovulate mares for embryo collection.

Appropriate Health Care

Most ETs are best handled in a hospital setting with adequate facilities and personnel. It is important that all of the reusable and disposable equipment, as well as supplies, which will potentially come in contact with the embryo, be free of bacterial contamination and embryocidal residues.

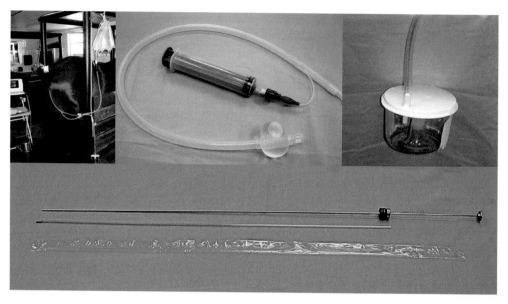

■ **Figure 24.1** The basic set-up for flushing a donor mare for an embryo *(top left)*, along with the type of intrauterine catheter used for flushing equine embryos *(top center)* and an embryo filtering device *(top right)*. The instrument below the other images can be used for nonsurgical intrauterine embryo transfer. Images courtesy of D. Volkmann.

Embryo Recovery Procedures

- For optimal success embryos are collected 6 to 8 days post-ovulation, depending on the circumstances, logistical considerations, and clinician preference.
- The flushing solution used for ET is commonly a modified PBS solution with added fetal or newborn calf serum, plus or minus antibiotics.
- Nonsurgical uterine flushing 6 to 8 days after ovulation (Fig. 24.1).
- Surgical oviductal flushing 2 to 4 days after ovulation.
- Laparoscopic and especially transvaginal U/S-guided recovery of oocytes.

Identification of Embryos

- After the flushing media is run into the donor mare, it is collected, usually in conjunction with some type of filtering device (*see* Fig. 24.1).
- Equine embryos can vary in size and appearance depending on their age (Fig. 24.2).
- Embryos are evaluated and graded using a standard grading scheme. Grade 1 denotes a high quality embryo, and Grade 4 denotes a very poor quality embryo.
- Multiple embryos can be collected if there are multiple ovulations, and, UFOs are also occasionally recovered (Fig. 24.3).
- Embryos are washed and can be transferred immediately.

ET Procedures

- Embryos can be transferred immediately, or they can be cooled and shipped to an embryo transfer center with multiple synchronized recipients, in containers devel-

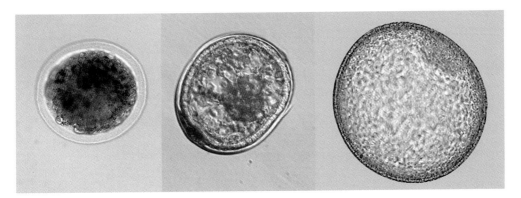

■ **Figure 24.2** An approximately 6- to 7-day-old morula and /-day-old early blastocyst (*left and center,* respectively). The early blastocyst has extruded blastomeres on its left; 8-day-old expanded blastocyst is shown on the right.
Images on left and center, courtesy of R. Foss; image on right, courtesy of D. Volkmann.

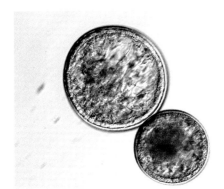
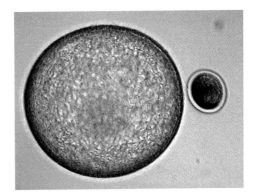

■ **Figure 24.3** Two slightly different aged blastocysts collected from the same mare *(left).* An expanded blastocyst and a much smaller, unfertilized oocyte (UFO) are shown on the right.
Image on left, courtesy of R. Foss; image on right, courtesy of D. Volkmann.

oped to transport cooled semen or specifically designed containers for embryos. The type of medium in which the cooled embryos are shipped might be different than the type of medium used to flush the donor mare (consult with the ET center prior to breeding the donor mare).

- Nonsurgical intrauterine transfer (the most commonly used technique; logistically simpler and less expensive than surgical transfer; instrument shown in Fig. 24.1).
- Surgical intrauterine transfer (initially more successful than nonsurgical transfer before improved nonsurgical equipment and methods became available).
- Oocyte collection and IVF to produce zygote, followed by laparoscopic or surgical oviductal transfer of zygotes (ZIFT).
- Oocyte collection with laparoscopic or surgical oviductal transfer of gametes (GIFT) into inseminated or bred recipient whose own follicles have been aspirated.

- Cryopreservation of embryos and unfertilized oocytes; cryopreservation schemes are still being developed and improved upon.

Nursing Care

Generally required after more invasive procedures in donor and recipient mares.

Diet

Normal diet, unless contraindicated by concurrent maternal disease or exercise restriction.

Activity

- Generally restricted after more invasive procedures in donor and recipient mares.
- Preference may be to restrict activity of donor mares in competition because of the possible impact of stress on pregnancy maintenance.

Surgical Considerations

- Surgical intervention might be indicated to repair anatomic defects predisposing to endometritis.
- Surgical oviductal recovery and implantation.

 COMMENTS

Client Education

- ET procedures are not approved by all breed registries.
- Success rates can be less than expected when donor mares are older, subfertile mares.
- Emphasize to the client that communication between the individuals breeding the donor mare and those performing the embryo collection and transfer is essential.
- Recipient mares generally need to be fairly closely synchronized with the donor mare, depending on the procedure (within 0 to 2 days).
- If the number of normal, synchronized recipients is limited, embryos can be transported to commercial facilities with large numbers of recipient mares.
- Embryo-freezing procedures are improving.

Patient Monitoring

- Accurate teasing records.
- Reexamination of donors diagnosed and treated for endometritis before ET.
- Early transrectal U/S of recipient mare for pregnancy.
- Transrectal U/S to monitor for embryonic and fetal development in the recipient mare.

Possible Complications

- Recipient EED or abortion.
- Endometritis in donor mares after the uterine flushing procedures.
- Pregnancy in donor mare following an *unsuccessful flush* (i.e., no embryo retrieved and follow-up prostaglandin injection not administered post-flush to the donor).

Expected Course and Prognosis

- Prognosis for successful pregnancy depends on the quality of the oocyte or embryo, and the reproductive health of the recipient mare.
- Prognosis for successful recovery of intrauterine embryo at 6 to 8 days after ovulation is approximately 70% in normal mares (less in subfertile mares).
- Prognosis for successful surgical intrauterine transfer of embryos is approximately 70% to 75% for embryos from normal mares (depends on facility and clinician; less from subfertile mares).
- Nonsurgical intrauterine transfer of embryos originally had potential to be less successful (large individual and facility variation) than surgical transfer but has become very widespread, with improved equipment and techniques.
- Other embryo, early zygote, and gamete procedures might have lower success rates than traditional ET, but they are still being improved.
- Embryo cryopreservation techniques have been developed and are being improved.
- Oocyte cryopreservation techniques are still being refined.

Synonyms/Closely Related Conditions

- GIFT
- IVF
- ZIFT

Abbreviations

CL	corpus luteum
EED	early embryonic death
eFSH	equine follicle stimulating hormone
ELISA	enzyme-linked immunosorbent assay
ET	embryo transfer
GIFT	gamete intrafallopian tube transfer
IVF	*in vitro* fertilization
PBS	phosphate-buffered saline
RIA	radioimmunoassay
UFOs	unfertilized oocytes
U/S	ultrasound, ultrasonography
ZIFT	zygote intrafallopian tube transfer

See Also

- Abortion, spontaneous, infectious or noninfectious
- Conception failure in mares
- Conception failure in stallions
- Embryo transfer
- Endometrial biopsy
- Endometritis
- Metritis

Suggested Reading

Carnevale EM. 2003. Oocyte transfer. In: *Current Therapy in Equine Medicine 5*. Robinson NE (ed). Philadelphia: Saunders; 285–287.

McCue PM, LeBlanc MM, Squires EL. 2007. eFSH in clinical equine practice. *Therio* 68(3): 429–433.

Moussa M, Duchamp G, Daels PF, et al. 2006. Effect of embryo age on the viability of equine embryos after cooled storage using two transport systems. *J Eq Vet Sci* 26(11): 529–534.

Squires EL. 2003. Management of the embryo donor and recipient mare. In: *Current Therapy in Equine Medicine 5*. Robinson NE (ed). Philadelphia: Saunders; 277–279.

Vanderwall DK. 2003. Embryo collection, storage, and transfer. In: *Current Therapy in Equine Medicine 5*. Robinson NE (ed). Philadelphia: Saunders; 280–285.

Youngquist RS, Threlfall WR (eds). 2007. *Current Therapy in Large Animal Theriogenology*, 2nd ed. St. Louis: Elsevier-Saunders.

Author: Tim J. Evans

chapter 25

Endometrial Biopsy

DEFINITION/OVERVIEW

Histopathological evaluation of the endometrium to help with the identification of infertility causes and to predict a mare's ability to carry a fetus to term.

ETIOLOGY/PATHOPHYSIOLOGY

Seasonal Variation

- Normal histological endometrial changes are driven by cyclic rise and fall of ovarian estrogen and progesterone. Variations reflect stage of estrous cycle and season.
- Winter anestrus: endometrial atrophy; luminal and glandular epithelium becomes cuboidal, glands straight, low in density, secretions accumulate from myometrial hypotonia.
- Vernal transition: increasing estrogen stimulates endometrial activity, reflected by luminal glandular epithelial activity and increasing gland density.
- Variations in luminal epithelium occur in the spring breeding season. Epithelial cells become tall columnar in estrus through early diestrus; low/moderately columnar and cuboidal through diestrus.
- Other springtime changes:
  - *Early estrus*: stromal edema develops, causing *physiologic nesting* of individual gland branches (Fig. 25.1).
  - *Estrus*: PMNs marginate on the sides of venules and capillaries, without migrating into the stroma. Glands are straight, some degree of edema (Fig. 25.2).
  - *Diestrus*: gland tortuosity increases (coiled glands described as *string of pearls*) and edema decreases.
- No seasonal effect on degree or distribution of histopathologic changes.

Assessment of Inflammation and Degenerative Changes

- Degree and extent of inflammation and degenerative changes of endometrium: alterations occur due to age, natural challenges (coitus, pregnancy), contamination by bacteria, pneumovagina, urovagina, DUC, and other unknown causes.

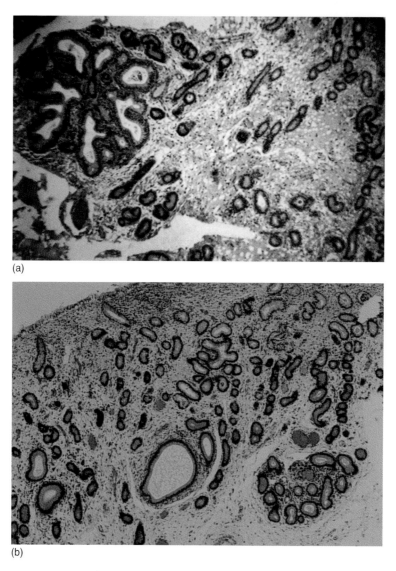

(a)

(b)

■ **Figure 25.1** Glandular nesting *(a, b)*.
Photos courtesy of A. Tibary.

- Nature of change: inflammatory cell infiltration, periglandular fibrosis, cystic glandular distention with/without periglandular fibrosis, and lymphangiectasia (Fig. 25.3).
- High correlation between degree of changes and ability of the endometrium to carry a fetus to term. As duration and degree of endometrial damage and insult increase, probability of term pregnancy decreases.

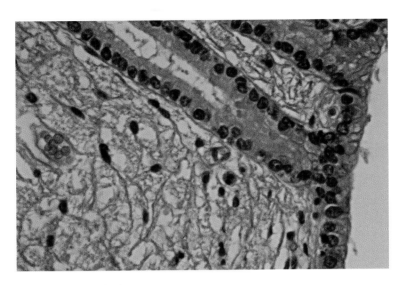

■ **Figure 25.2** Normal uterine gland.
Photo courtesy of A. Tibary.

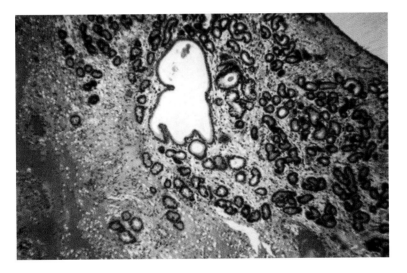

■ **Figure 25.3** Periglandular fibrosis, glandular cyst.
Photo courtesy of A. Tibary.

- Inflammation is associated with repeated natural challenges.
- Degenerative changes usually are progressive, associated with aging, clearly exacerbated by parity, chronic inflammation.

Systems Affected

Reproductive

SIGNALMENT/HISTORY

Risk Factors

- Age: Direct correlation of category to age.
  - Category I: primarily young, maiden mares.
  - Category II: old, pluriparous mares; high incidence of poor VC, pneumovagina, urovagina, DUC, periglandular fibrosis.
- Parity
- Anatomical abnormality: pneumovagina, urovagina, DUC.
- Repeated inflammation by/resulting from coitus, DUC, infectious endometritis.

Historical Findings

Infertility of variable degrees:
- Mare barren from previous/current breeding season, despite being bred within 48 hr pre-ovulation with proven semen.
- Anestrus mare during the breeding season.
- Mare with palpable reproductive tract abnormalities.
- History: EED, abortion, chronic inflammation.
- Mare with inconclusive cytologic/uterine culture findings to establish a diagnosis of clinical endometritis.
- Prior to urogenital surgery. If the biopsy category is found to be poor and future prospects for fertility are seriously compromised, surgical cost can be avoided.
- Essential for prepurchase examination of a broodmare prospect or ET recipient.

 CLINICAL FEATURES

Inflammation, the most common endometrial abnormality:
- Degree and cell type depend on severity of insult, length of exposure, and infection.
- Neutrophils predominate in acute endometritis; lymphocytes, plasma cells and macrophages in chronic endometritis. *See* Figure 25.4.
- Chronic/active is less common; PMNs, lymphocytes, and plasma cells may be present concurrently. Chronic changes are superimposed by acute changes, a result of persistent antigenic stimulation [contamination because of genital abnormalities (poor VC, RVF)]; semen placed in a DUC mare also results in fluid accumulation and inflammatory cell recruitment.
- Described by its distribution (focal, scattered, diffuse), frequency (slight, moderate, severe), and cell type present (acute, chronic, chronic/active).
- Inflammatory cells may be focal, scattered, or diffuse in their distribution in *stratum compactum* (including capillaries and venules) and luminal epithelium.
- Chronic inflammation also may affect the *stratum spongiosum*.

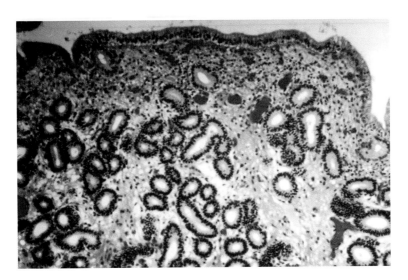

■ **Figure 25.4** Superficial inflammation.
Photo courtesy of Ahmed Tibary.

- Other types of cells occur less often: macrophages, siderophages, eosinophils.
- Macrophage presence is linked to irritating or poorly absorbed foreign matter in the lumen.
- Siderophages (macrophage that contains hemoglobin pigment from digestion of blood) indicate a previous foaling, abortion, hemorrhagic event that may have been as long as 2 to 3 years previously.
- Eosinophils often indicate acute irritation due to pneumovagina, urovagina, and, less often, fungal endometritis (Figs. 25.5a and 25.5b).
  Fibrosis is an irreversible change:
- Stromal cells deposit collagen in response to repeated acute/chronic inflammation, aging, other stimuli.
- Most collagen deposition is periglandular.
- *Nests* are clusters/branches of glands surrounded by collagen.

Periglandular Fibrosis exerts pressure within the gland and decreases blood flow to the gland, leads to cystic glandular distention, epithelial atrophy, and decreases uterine gland secretions (Fig. 25.6).

- Calculi, mineral/organic substances, may be in the lumen of endometrial glands.
- With periglandular fibrosis, a mare can usually conceive, but the pregnancy is lost prior to 90 days due to impaired secretion of glandular *uterine milk*, a critical secretion for conceptus' nutrition.
- Prognosis indirectly correlates with number of collagen layers and frequency of nests per LPF (i.e., more layers = poorer prognosis).
- Widespread distribution, any degree, correlates with low foaling rates.

Lymphatic Stasis is characterized by dilated, dysfunctional lymphatic vessels.

- Histology: dilated lymphatics are differentiated from widespread edema by endothelial cells lining a fluid-filled space.

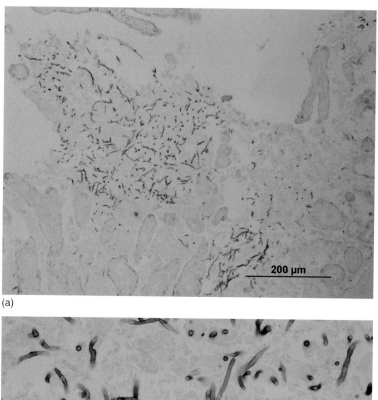

(a)

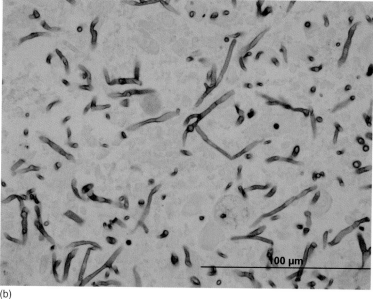

(b)

■ **Figure 25.5** Fungal hyphae, Gomori Methenamine Silver stain at 10× *(a)*. Fungal organisms identified by special staining, Gomori Methenamine Silver stain at 40× *(b)*.
Photos courtesy of D. Agnew.

- Common in mares with a pendulous uterus and DUC.
- TRP may reveal a thickened but soft uterus, poor tone in diestrus.
- When widespread, it is associated with low foaling rates.
- Coalescing lymphatic lacunae may become lymphatic cysts, 1 to 15 cm diameter.
- Lymphatic cysts identified by U/S, endoscopy, and, less frequently, TRP.

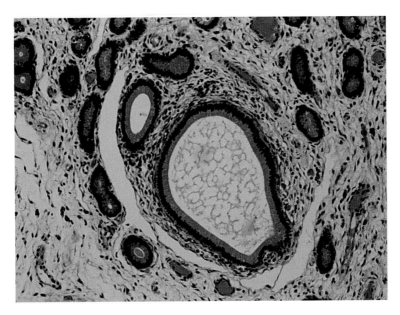

■ **Figure 25.6** Periglandular fibrosis.
Photo courtesy of A. Tibary.

Angiosis: Angiosclerotic changes of uterine vessels are associated primarily with parity, secondarily with aging.

■ Younger maiden mares have intact vessels. Older maiden mares develop mild sclerosis in the intima and adventitia. Pluriparous mares generally reveal all layers being affected; exhibit fraying and disruption of the intima, with medial and adventitial elastosis and fibrosis.

■ Severe angiosis with phlebectasia and lymphangiectasia decrease endometrial perfusion and drainage, resulting in edema formation.

Excessive Mucus production overlaying the epithelium or loss of epithelium may be associated with infectious/noninfectious chronic endometritis.

■ A consideration in prognosis for classification because it affects pregnancy outcome.

■ The degree and extension of angiosis or mucus production are not used in the traditional way of biopsy classification, but do have an impact on mare's fertility and ability to carry a pregnancy to term.

 DIFFERENTIAL DIAGNOSIS

Cystic Glandular Distention: If unassociated with fibrosis, may be due to uterine hypotonia and impaired flow of secretions:

■ Normal during anestrus and transition (seasonal variation).

■ During the breeding season: old, pluriparous mares with pendulous uteri; history of repeat breeding. Presents as clusters of cystic glands not surrounded by collagen (i.e., not fibrotic nests).

■ Cystic glands may have inspissated material and exhibit epithelial hypertrophy.

- Cystic glandular distention has been suggested to precede periglandular fibrosis.
- In normal mares, glands are uniformly dilated after a recent abortion or pregnancy.
- Gland *nest* associated with early estrus edema is a normal physiologic alteration; a gland *nest* secondary to irreversible, periglandular fibrosis is abnormal.
- Differentiate cystic glands (distention is up to 1 mm in diameter) from lymphatic cysts by origin and size.

Nonseasonal Glandular Atrophy or Hypoplasia:

- Decreased gland density during the breeding season is abnormal; associated with ovarian dysgenesis or secretory tumors (e.g., a granulosa cell tumor).
- Focal glandular atrophy can develop in old, pluriparous mares.

DIAGNOSTICS

- Component of a routine BSE. If pathology (e.g., endometritis) is suspected, culture and cytology must precede endometrial biopsy to avoid contaminating the uterine swab.
- Perform biopsy with a sterile endometrial biopsy forcep, preferably when the mare is cycling and, if convenient, during estrus (Fig. 25.7).
- Forcep is carried through the cervix into the uterine body. The sample(s) is taken from the caudal portion of the horn or at the junction of horn and body (i.e., approximate area for endometrial cup development during pregnancy). Unless a gross abnor-

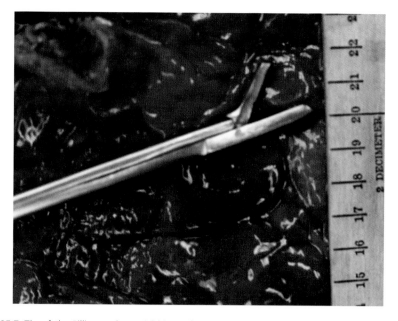

■ **Figure 25.7** Tip of the Pilling endometrial biopsy forcep positioned as it would be during collection of an endometrial biopsy.
Photo courtesy of A. Tibary.

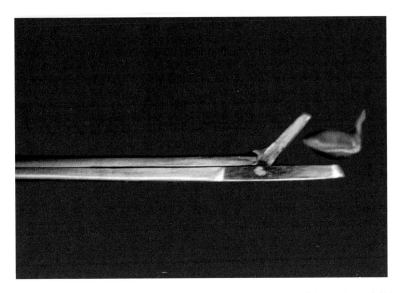

■ **Figure 25.8** Tip of the endometrial biopsy forcep; demonstrating the size of the endometrial biopsy sample as it has gently been teased from the biopsy basket. Care must be taken to minimize inducing any changes by spearing or otherwise rough handling of the sample as it is transferred into fixative.
Photo courtesy of A. Tibary.

mality is present, one sample is adequate to represent the entire endometrium; otherwise, take additional samples as needed (Fig. 25.8).

- Fix the biopsy sample in Bouin's for 4 to 24 hours, then transfer into 70% ethanol or 10% formalin until slides are prepared. Bouin exposure longer than 24 hours will make the sample brittle and difficult to section. Transferring directly into 10% buffered neutral formalin is satisfactory, but the fixed sample remains more *rubbery*; microtome cuts from the tissue block may lose a modicum of detail.
- H&E is the stain routinely used. Others may be requested to address specific concerns: van Geissen stain for angiosis, collagen and connective tissue; PAS for polysaccharides/mucus; GMS for fungi (*see* Figs. 25.5a and 25.5b).
- If a sample is to be sent to a lab for slide prep and interpretation, include complete history, stage of mare's cycle, and TRP findings on day of examination.
- Perform endoscopy to diagnose intraluminal adhesions, endometrial cysts.

Pathological Findings

Category I

- Endometrial health is optimal, expect at least 80% or more of Category I mares to conceive and carry to term.
- Histologic changes: slight, focal, and irregularly distributed (scattered).

Category IIA

- Fifty percent to 80% foaling rate with proper management.
- Conception and pregnancy maintenance slightly decreased.

- Histopathologic changes: slight to moderate, may improve with proper treatment, may include:
- Slight to moderate, diffuse cellular infiltration of superficial layers.
- Scattered, frequent inflammatory or fibrotic foci.
- Scattered, frequent periglandular fibrosis of individual branches, one to three collagen layers, or up to two fibrotic gland nests/LPF, examine at least five fields (*see* Fig. 25.3).
- Widespread lymphatic stasis without palpable changes.

Category IIB

- Ten percent to 50% foaling rate with proper management.
- Histopathologic changes: more extensive and severe than IIA, still may be reversible, may include:
    - Diffuse, widespread, moderately severe cellular infiltration of superficial layers.
    - Widespread periglandular fibrosis of individual branches, four or more collagen layers or two to four fibrotic gland nests/LPF in five fields.
    - Widespread lymphatic stasis, palpable changes in the uterus, usually noted as decreased uterine tone in diestrus.

Category III

- Foaling rate, even with optimal management and treatment, no more than 10%.
- Greatly decreased chances of conception and pregnancy maintenance; difficult-to-treat conditions or severe, irreversible changes in the endometrium.
- Histologic changes:
    - Widespread, severe cellular infiltration.
    - Glandular fibrosis (five or more fibrotic nests/LPF).
    - Severe lymphatic stasis.
- Endometrial hypoplasia with gonadal dysgenesis and pyometra with severe, widespread cellular infiltration and palpable endometrial atrophy.
- Electron microscopy
    - Reveals no major differences between categories I and II.
    - Category III, increased cells with degenerative structures, fewer organelles and cilia on surface.

 # THERAPEUTICS

Epicrisis

- Clinical evaluation of the biopsy requires interpretation in concert with patient history, physical examination findings, bacteriology results, and previous treatments.
- Include recommendations for treatment/management and prognosis.

Category I

A *normal* endometrium. If difficulties are encountered with conceiving or carrying to term and the mare is not infected; focus on semen quality, estrus detection, timing of breeding and insemination with respect to ovulation, anatomic or behavioral abnormalities.

Categories IIA and IIB

- Institute appropriate therapy to improve category.
- Inflammation decreases if the source of irritation is removed; contamination can be decreased before and at breeding.
- Pneumovagina and urovagina: surgical correction is required.
- Treat acute and chronic bacterial/fungal infections with appropriate local/systemic antibiotic/antifungal.
- Treat DUC: uterine lavage and oxytocin.
- Lymphatic circulation can be enhanced by cloprostenol (PGE2 analog) 12 to 24 hours before and after breeding.
- Fibrosis and angiosis are irreversible changes.
- Uterine edema: if due to impaired perfusion/drainage, may improve by increasing uterine tone with P + E. This is an empirical treatment and appears beneficial in some cases.

Category III

- Often become pregnant, but pregnancy is lost by 40 to 90 days gestation.
- Histopathologic changes are either difficult to affect or irreversible.
- Therapy is to decrease inflammation, diminish lymphangiectasia, couple with MCT at breeding.
- Extensive fibrosis decreases the likelihood that the category may improve with treatment.
- If allowed by the particular breed registry, consider the category III mare as an ET donor.
- If improvement is impossible, consider having a frank discussion with the owner regarding removing the mare from further breeding, or use her for nonbreeding purposes.

Drug(s) of Choice

- Antibiotic selection is based on culture and sensitivity.
- Endometritis treatment: refer to chapter and its recommendations.

Precautions/Interactions

- Do not treat with P + E if mare is infected because she may develop pyometra.
- Refer to Endometritis chapter.

Surgical Considerations

- Surgical correction of pneumo- and/or urovagina may improve biopsy category over time, especially if irritation is due to poor conformation.
- Always perform a biopsy to evaluate the extent of endometrial damage before committing to surgery to repair a cervical tear or other long-standing genital tract damage/contamination, e.g., recto-vaginal fistula, post-dystocia. If the biopsy category reveals extensive change and a poor prognosis for future fertility, surgery and its cost may not be justified.

 COMMENTS

Endometrial biopsy reveals structural changes but not etiology, unless also cultured positive and it is determined to be an infectious endometritis.

Patient Monitoring

- A repeat endometrial biopsy at approximately 2 weeks after treatment ends, to determine effectiveness of therapy and perhaps improvement in the biopsy category.

Prevention/Avoidance

- Do not collect a biopsy without first ruling out pregnancy (TRP and U/S).
- An absolute contraindication.

Possible Complications

- Biopsy is relatively safe.
- Possible complications: uterine perforation, excessive hemorrhage (rare).

Synonyms

Uterine Biopsy

Abbreviations

BSE   breeding soundness examination
DUC   delayed uterine clearance
EED   early embryonic death
ET   embryo transfer
GMS   Gomori Methenamine Silver
H & E   hematoxylin and eosin
LPF   low-power field
MCT   minimum contamination technique
P4   progesterone
PAS   Periodic Acid Schiff

P + E   progesterone and estradiol-17β in oil
PGF   natural prostaglandin
PMN   polymorphonuclear leukocyte
RVF   rectovaginal fistula
TRP   transrectal palpation
U/S   ultrasound, ultrasonography
VC   vulvar conformation

See Also

- Breeding soundness examination, mare
- Endometritis
- Metritis

Suggested Reading

Gruninger B, Schoon HA, Schoon D, et al. 1998. Incidence and morphology of endometrial angiopathies in relationship to age and parity. *J Comp Pathol* 119: 293–309.

Kenney RM, Doig PA. 1986. In: Equine endometrial biopsy. *Current Therapy in Theriogenology*. Morrow DA (ed). Philadelphia: WB Saunders; 723–729.

Nielsen JM. 2005. Endometritis in the mare. A diagnostic study comparing cultures from swab and biopsy. *Therio* 64: 510–518.

Schlafer DH. 2007. Equine endometrial biopsy: Enhancement of clinical value by more extensive histopathology and application of new diagnostic techniques? *Therio* 68: 413–423.

Author: Maria E. Cadario

chapter 26

Endometritis

DEFINITION/OVERVIEW

- Infectious/noninfectious endometrial inflammation.
- Major cause of mare infertility.
- Multifactorial disease classified in one of four groups:
  - Infectious (active/acute, active/chronic, or subclinical) endometritis
  - PMIE
  - Endometritis due to an STD
  - Degenerative endometritis due to aging (angiosis, periglandular fibrosis).
- May involve more than one group/origin.

ETIOLOGY/PATHOPHYSIOLOGY

Infectious Endometritis

- Uterus repeatedly exposed to contamination at breeding, parturition, and gynecological examinations.
- Uterine defense mechanisms to clear contamination, combination of:
  - Anatomic (physical) barriers
  - Cellular phagocytosis
  - Physical evacuation of uterine contents.
- Anatomic integrity: loss of the vulvar seal, vestibular sphincter and cervical integrity caused by aging, parity and associated perineal accidents, or breed predisposition.
  - Decreased function results in recurring aspiration of air (pneumovagina), urine (urine pooling), fecal material, or bacteria into the cranial vagina.
  - Contamination may increase during estrus, subsequent to vulvar and cervical relaxation.

PMIE

- Increased parity in aged mares and incomplete cervical dilation in maiden mares (old maiden mares, mares more than 12 years old) predisposes them to intrauterine fluid accumulation.

- Breeding (semen + bacterial contamination) induces a normal, transient, endometritis.
- Byproducts of inflammation normally are removed by uterine contractions through an open estrual cervix. Following ovulation, the cervix closes; fluids within the uterine lumen are cleared by the lymphatics.
- Intrauterine fluid is cleared (absent) by 12-hours post-mating in normal mares.
- The likelihood of fluid accumulation and lymphatic stasis increases if the uterine horns are suspended lower than the pelvic brim, uterine contractions are impaired, or normal contractions are coupled with negligible cervical dilation during estrus (i.e., as often occurs with maiden mares).
- Supportive structures of the genital tract stretch with each pregnancy.

Low Pregnancy Rate

- *Direct:* causes interference with embryo survival on its arrival into the uterus
- *Indirect:* by premature luteolysis; inflammation induces endometrial prostaglandin release.

Sexually Transmitted (Venereal) Endometritis

- Mode of transmission is coitus or AI with infected semen.
- Most common bacteria are *Pseudomonas aeruginosa*, *Klebsiella pneumonia*, and *Streptococcus zooepidemicus*.
  - All opportunistic organisms on the penile surface.
  - Can become overwhelming if the normal penile bacterial flora is disturbed/altered.
- *See* Venereal Diseases.

Systems Affected

Reproductive

 # SIGNALMENT/HISTORY

Infectious Endometritis

- Predisposition to contamination is caused by an inherent or acquired anatomical defect of the vulva, vestibular sphincter, or cervix.

PMIE

- *Pluriparous mares:* usually more than 12 to 14 years of age with a pendulous uterus.
- *Nulliparous mares:* young or old, having incomplete cervical dilation during estrus.

Risk Factors

- *Age:* more than 14 years old.
- Multiparous and nulliparous mares that are more than 12 to 14 years old.

- Abnormal VC.
- Excessive breeding (live covers or AI) during one or consecutive estrus periods.
- Pendulous uterine suspension.
- Cervix that fails to relax during estrus.

Historical Findings

- Infertility
- Accumulation of uterine fluid (luminal) before and/or after breeding
- Failure to conceive after repeated breeding to a stallion of known fertility
- Early embryonic loss
- Hyperemia of the cervix/vagina
- Vaginal discharge

 ## CLINICAL FEATURES

- Physical Examination can be inconclusive. Key diagnostic tools are patient history, cytology/culture, and U/S.
- Guarded swab (alone or combined with a cytology brush) to obtain samples for endometrial cytology and uterine culture (Fig. 26.1).
- Endometrial biopsy is indicated only in specific cases.

Infectious Endometritis

- Abnormal VC

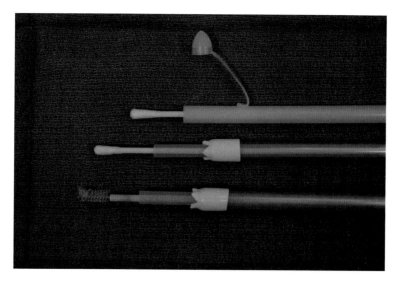

■ **Figure 26.1** Different type of swabs and brush for cytology: Kalayjian (top, single-guarded), double-guarded culture swab, cytology brush.

- TRP is not diagnostic.
- U/S usually reveals an accumulation of echogenic fluid in the uterine lumen.
- Hyperemia of vaginal and cervical mucosa; discharge may be observed at the cervix.
- Endometrial cytology and uterine culture reveal neutrophils (2 to more than 5 PMNs/hpf).
- Usually isolate a pure bacterial growth, single organism.

PMIE

- External genitalia not always abnormal.
- TRP, U/S, and cytology/culture results may be inconclusive in the spring, prior to onset of the breeding season.
- Signs of persistent inflammation usually appear post-breeding.
- May be hyperemia of the vaginal and cervical mucosa.
- Pendulous, edematous uterus in older mares.
- Presence of more than 2 cm (height, determined by U/S) of intrauterine fluid during estrus is diagnostic/predictive of PMIE.

U/S

- Normal mares retain small amounts of intrauterine fluid up to 12 hours post-breeding.
- Post-breeding U/S reveals luminal fluid that persists for 12 to more than 24 hours in the absence of treatment.
- Endometrial cytology reveals significant inflammation (more than 5 PMNs/hpf).
- Bacterial culture: usually negative.

 ## DIFFERENTIAL DIAGNOSIS

For Vaginal Discharge

- *Pneumovagina:* mucosal irritation by air, a foamy-appearing exudate accumulates on the vaginal floor.
- *Treatment-induced vaginitis or necrosis:* may result from antiseptics used for uterine lavage. Individual mares vary in their response to a similar treatment.
- *Bacterial vaginitis* secondary to pneumovagina.
- *Necrotizing vaginitis:* secondary to excessive manipulation and inadequate lubrication during dystocia or contamination during the delivery of a dead, necrotic fetus.
- *Urine pooling:* usually affects a population of mares with characteristics similar to those affected by endometritis.
  - Diagnosis (by vaginal speculum): presence of urine during estrus.
  - Transrectal U/S reveals nonechogenic intrauterine fluid present before and variably after ovulation.

- *Varicosities* in the region of the vaginovestibular sphincter.
  - May rupture and bleed during late pregnancy or during breeding.
  - Diagnosis by vaginal speculum.
- *Lochia:* a normal finding up to 6 days postpartum.
- *Postpartum metritis*
- *Pyometra*
- During pregnancy, a vaginal discharge may be a sign of placentitis.
- A serosanguinous cervical discharge with a negative bacterial swab: an indicator of premature placental separation.
- Premature mammary development may develop with placental insufficiency of any origin.

DIAGNOSTICS

Cytology

- Sample is of endometrial cells and intraluminal content.
- Scrape the endometrial surface with a swab tip, a cytology brush or a cap (if using a Kalayjian swab). Either cut off the cap (Kalayjian) and tap it on a slide or gently roll the swab onto a slide and stain with Diff-Quik.
- Evaluate a minimum of 10 fields of cytological specimens at 40× and under oil (100×).
  - Negative: epithelial cells and 0 to 2 PMN per 100×.
  - Moderate inflammation: epithelial cells and 2 to 5 PMN per 100×.
  - Severe inflammation: epithelial cells and more than 5 PMN per 100×.
- Neutrophils indicate active inflammation. Recent breeding or gynecologic examination results in a transient, positive cytology (Figs. 26.2 to 26.6).
- Persistent, positive cytology without bacterial growth, most often suggests a recurrent, noninfectious cause (e.g., pneumovagina, urine pooling, or early stages of DUC). If treatment or surgical correction fails to improve fertility, cannot rule out a previously missed infectious cause (e.g., a focal infection, an area not sampled because of a pendulous uterus, a subclinical endometritis).
- *Positive culture with positive cytology:* diagnostic for a uterine infection.
- *Positive culture with negative cytology:* indicates contamination during uterine sampling in 70% of the cases.
- May have a negative cytology result in 30% of subsequently confirmed endometrial infections, due to inability to reach the PMNs in the pendulous areas of the uterus (physically out of reach) or because of the type of microorganism isolated.
- There is less correlation between positive cytological findings and bacteria isolation when recovering *E. coli, P. aeruginosa,* and *Enterobacter cloaca* compared to *S. zooepidemicus, Staphylococcus* and *K. pneumoniae.*

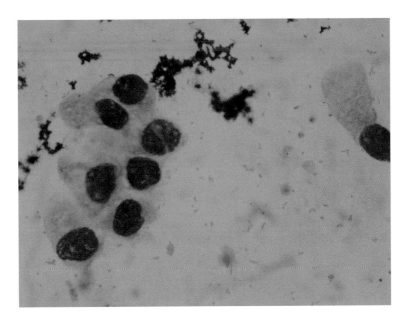

■ **Figure 26.2** Normal endometrial cytology. Modest degree of debris in evidence may sometimes be significant in chronic endometritis.

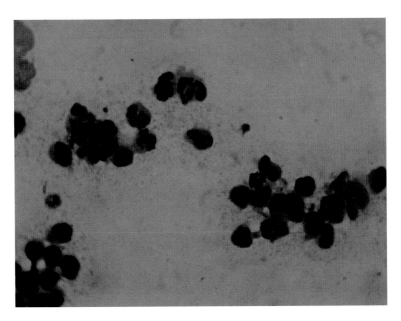

■ **Figure 26.3** Varying degrees of inflammation from mild to suppurative.

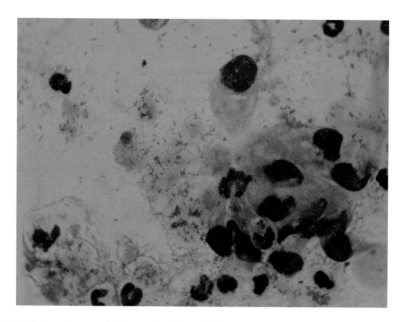

■ **Figure 26.4** Varying degrees of inflammation from mild to suppurative.

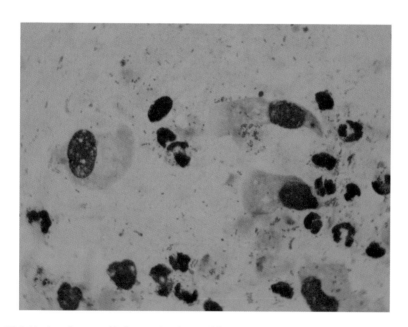

■ **Figure 26.5** Varying degrees of inflammation from mild to suppurative.

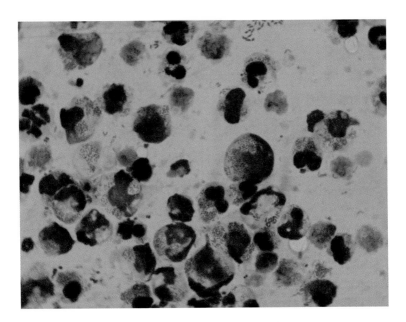

■ Figure 26.6 Varying degrees of inflammation from mild to suppurative.

Microbiology

Aerobes

- Most common isolates: *S. zooepidemicus* and *E. coli.*
- Use a guarded swab to sample the endometrial surface. Two different agar plates are used:
  - McConkey for gram-negative and blood agar for gram-positive and yeast.
  - Incubate plates at 37°C, examine at 24 and 48 hours.
- For subclinical endometrial infections, recommend culture be taken from endometrial biopsy sample or from the return solution of a small-volume uterine lavage.
- *E. coli,* a fecal contaminant, results from poor VC.
- *P. aeruginosa* and *K. pneumoniae* usually a venereal transmission.
- Overgrowth may occur secondary to excessive use of intrauterine antibiotics.
- Other bacteria: *Staphylococcus, Corynebacterium, Enterobacter, Proteus,* and *Pasteurella* spp.

Anaerobes

- *Bacteroides fragilis*
- May be recovered in some cases of postpartum metritis.

Yeasts

- Most common isolates: *Candida* and *Aspergillus* spp.
- Usually follow(s) excessive antibiotic uterine therapy.

- Use cytology slides and the blood agar plates for presence of *Candida* and *Aspergillus* spp.
- For a specific fungal culture, incubate in Sabouraud's agar for 4 days.

Small Volume Uterine Lavage

- For gross and bacteriologic evaluation of uterine content when chronic or subclinical endometritis is suspected, focalized fluid or hyperechoic lines are visualized in the uterus and/or mares are to be examined in diestrus.
- Flush uterus with 60 mL of sterile saline, evaluate cloudiness and pH of effluent; centrifuge and culture the pellet.
- Evaluate cytology smears for PMN, amount of debris, bacteria, and for the presence of urine crystals.

Endoscopy

- When other modalities fail to define the cause of infertility.
- Better method to visualize intrauterine adhesions affecting uterine drainage, luminal tumors, or uterine abscess (rare) that may not be palpable or visible by U/S.

Pathological Findings

Endometrial biopsy is useful to determine the presence or absence of endometritis when clinical and bacteriological findings are inconclusive.
- Culture and cytology taken from endometrial biopsy sample yield accurate results.
- Inflammatory cells (neutrophils) are diagnostic, if present, of active endometritis (*see* Figs. 26.2 to 26.6).
- Low numbers of lymphocytes and plasma cells (indicative of chronic endometritis) are not always associated with infertility.
- Lymphatic stasis is common in mares with a pendulous uterus and DUC.

Endometritis

- Cannot predict a mare's endometrial biopsy category, ranges from IIA to III (rarely).
- Category relates to the length of sexual rest, conformational abnormalities, and age.
- Histopathology associated with endometritis: mild, diffuse lymphocytic or neutrophilic infiltration; focally moderate fibrosis (one to four nests); lymphangiectasia.

PMIE

- Biopsy score at the beginning of the breeding season is not diagnostic.
- Category may be IIA or IIB, with mild inflammation and moderate fibrosis.
- After breeding, interstitial edema, lymphatic stasis, and diffuse, acute or subacute inflammation (PMN) usually develop.
- Serial sampling may be useful.

THERAPEUTICS

General Principles

- Administer treatments during estrus, when the cervix is open; however, this issue remains a topic of some controversy.
- Organism is eliminated chemically (antibiotics, antiseptics) or mechanically (uterine lavage, ecbolic drugs).
- Local placement of antibiotics is preferred to systemic treatment; higher concentrations achieved in the endometrium.
  - Cost of systemic treatment is more than local administration.
  - Most uterine infections in mares are luminal/endometrial.
  - Systemic treatment is optional when access to the mare is limited (e.g., unsafe or unsanitary conditions) or when attempting to avoid further uterine contamination.
- Uterine lavage is the treatment of choice for mares with DUC and to evacuate debris from the uterus before antibiotic instillation.
  - Also enhances local uterine defenses by local irritation and stimulates PMN migration to the lumen.
- Uterine lavage with LRS can be performed immediately prior to insemination when a mare has intrauterine fluid (e.g., rebreeding or multiple inseminations in a 24-hour period).
- If oxytocin is used during or after the lavage, wait for 45 to 60 minutes before inseminating the mare.

Endometritis

- *Active/acute endometritis:* <u>Morning</u>: Uterine lavage (daily or alternate days) followed by intrauterine infusion of chosen antibiotic/s. <u>Afternoon/Evening</u>: oxytocin administration.
- Antibiotics are chosen based on culture and sensitivity and should be diluted in 60 to 120 mL of sterile saline (maximum volume infused).
- *Chronic inflammation:* Do not breed mare until 45 to 60 days after treatment.
- *Chronic active endometritis:* surgical correction of defective anatomic barriers before intrauterine treatment of the bacterial isolate; uterine lavage and oxytocin if intrauterine fluid is present. Wait for a complete diestrus period before reevaluating.
- *Subclinical endometritis:* positive or negative cytology, no bacteria identified:
  - Uterine lavage with diluted antiseptics or antibiotics.
  - If history warrants; consider postbreeding treatment.
- *Yeast infection:* uterine lavage and oxytocin, followed by intrauterine infusion with antifungal drugs (Nystatin, Clotrimazole, etc.); alternatively, uterine lavage with diluted 0.01 to 0.05% povidone-iodine solution (to the approximate color of light iced tea, or better: 1.0 to 5 mL of 10% povidone iodine in 1 L saline), 2% acetic acid (vinegar) diluted with saline, or 20% DMSO.

- One or two treatments of intrauterine infusion with 540 mg of Lufenuron (Program, oral suspension for flea control in cats) diluted in 60 mL of saline has been effective in some few cases of fungal endometritis.
- Correct anatomic defects (poor perineal conformation, cervical incompetence) and culture and treat reservoirs of infection (e.g., vagina and clitoral fossa).

PMIE

- Manual cervical dilation (using sterile technique) pre- or post-breeding, followed by systemic or local antibiotics, may help intrauterine semen deposition and uterine clearance. Foaling, at least once, is highly recommended to improve cervical relaxation and drainage in old maiden mares.
- *Promote uterine clearance* by lavage and ecbolic drugs (oxytocin, carbetocin)

Mare with no history or characteristics of DUC:
- Begin her evaluation and treatment, if necessary, 12-hours post-breeding. Can then evaluate if her mechanisms of clearance are functioning normally.

If the mare has been diagnosed with PMIE: 4 to 8 hours post-AI or breeding (not ovulation), check for uterine fluid. The 4-hour interval ensures spermatozoa are in the oviduct, bacteria have not yet adhered or multiplied in the uterus.
- If fluid is present at a height of greater than 2 cm free fluid, lavage the uterus with 1 to 3 L of sterile saline or LRS. Administer oxytocin immediately before or after lavage.
- If only a small amount of free fluid is present, administer oxytocin only.
- Oxytocin immediately before or immediately after lavage stimulates strong uterine contractions; clears the remaining uterine contents and promotes lymphatic drainage.
- If possible, 12 hours after breeding, use cloprostenol if history has included dilated uterine lymphatics and poor drainage.
  - *$PGF_2\alpha$ and PGE2 analog (cloprostenol)* sustain smoother uterine contractions longer than oxytocin (4 to 5 hours versus 45 to 60 minutes).
  - *$PGF_2\alpha$ and PGE2 (cloprostenol)* are successful in reducing persistent uterine edema by stimulating lymphatic drainage.
- Twenty-four hours after breeding, if the mare has free intraluminal fluid, use lavage and oxytocin.
  - Small amounts of fluid require only the use of oxytocin.
  - If free fluid and persistent edema in the walls: lavage the uterus/oxytocin and add a regimen of IM oxytocin alternating with IM cloprostenol every 4 to 6 hr.
- If only edema is present, cloprostenol every 4 to 12 hours, up to 36 hours post-ovulation.
- Administer oxytocin every 2 to 4 hours in refractory cases, (e.g., older maiden mares).
- Forty-eight hours post-breeding: if the mare has not ovulated, rebreed, and oxytocin/cloprostenol sequence begins anew. Pre-breeding uterine lavage may be indicated.
- Treatment should continue, if necessary, no more than 3 to 4 days post-ovulation.
  - Embryo enters the uterus day 5 + 20 hours; allows treatment-induced uterine inflammatory response to subside.

Drug(s) of Choice

Antibiotics

- *Amikacin (1 to 2 g):* for gram-negative; *Pseudomonas* and *Klebsiella* spp. An intrauterine infusion of Tris-EDTA increases the permeability of the Pseudomonas capsule to the antibiotic.
- *Ampicillin (1 to 3 g):* for gram-positive; *Streptococci* and *E. coli.*
- *Carbenicillin (2 to 6 g):* broad spectrum; persistent *Pseudomonas* spp.
- *Gentamicin (1 to 2 g):* primarily for gram-negative; *Streptococci.*
- *Neomycin (2 to 4 g):* E. coli and *Klebsiella Streptococci* spp.
- *K-penicillin (5 × 10⁶ IU):* for gram-positive *Streptococci.*
- *Timentin (3 to 6 g):* broad spectrum; gram-positive and some *Pseudomonas spp.* Dilute with 60 to 150 mL of saline (proportional to uterine size).
- *Ticarcillin-clavulanic acid (3 to 6 g):* Enterobacter, S. aureus, B. fragilis. Dilute with 150 to 200 mL of saline
- *Ceftiofur (Naxel) (1 g):* broad spectrum; Do not use as first line of defense.
- Aminoglycosides must be buffered before infusion. Mix the antibiotic with an equal volume of sodium bicarbonate (e.g., 1 mL of $NaHCO_3$ (7.5%) for every 50 mg of gentamicin or amikacin), then dilute in LRS (neutral pH) or straight into a large volume (150 to 200 mL) of LRS, not saline (pH 5.5).

Systemic Antibiotics

- *K-penicillin:* 22,000 IU/kg IV, QID
- *Procaine penicillin G:* 22,000 IU/kg, IM, BID
- *Gentamicin:* 6.6 mg/kg IV, IM, SID
- *Amikacin:* 10 mg/kg IV, IM, SID
- *Ampicillin:* 20 mg/kg IV, IM; SID-BID
- *Trimethoprim-sulfamethoxazole:* 30 mg/kg PO BID

Local Antimycotics

- *Nystatin (0.5 to 2.5 × 10⁶ IU):* Candida spp.
- *Clotrimazole (500 to 700 mg):* Broad spectrum; *Candida* spp.
- *Amphotericin B (100 to 200 mg):* Broad spectrum; *Aspergillus, Candida,* and *Mucor* spp.; tablets must be crushed and well suspended in >100 mL of sterile saline.
- *Fluconazole (100 mg):* Candida spp.
- *Miconazole (500 to 700 mg):* Broad spectrum.
- Lufenuron (540 mg); Program (270 mg oral suspension for cats), may inhibit fungal growth by disrupting the cell walls. Limited success, rarely used anymore.

Others (Mucolytic agents)

- DMSO may remove excessive endometrial mucus to allow better access to the bacteria by the antibiotic.
  - At 5% to 10%: bacteriostatic.

- Greater than 10%: bacteriocidal.
- At 10% to 20%: decrease growth of *Candida albicans* in vitro.
- Intrauterine infusion with DMSO at more than a 25% concentration produces endometrial ulceration.

Uterotonic/Ecbolic Drugs

- *Oxytocin:* 10 IU IV or 20 IU IM.
- *Carbetocin:* long lasting oxytocin analogue; 014 to 0.17 mg IV or IM, once a day to BID. Not available in the United States.
- *Cloprostenol:* 250 to 500 microgram, IM. The prostaglandin of choice because of its effectiveness; fewer adverse effects.

Cervical Dilation

- Prostaglandins, Misoprostol ointment (*see* Cervical Lesions).

Immune System Modulators

- *Immunostimulants:* cell wall extracts from microoorganism (*Micobacterium phlei* or *Propionibacterium acnes*) appear to restore an impaired local immune response; chronic infectious endometritis
- *Immunodepressors:* Corticosteroids resulted in increased pregnancy rates in mares with a history of reproductive abnormalities (fluid accumulation after ovulation cervical incompetence) or infertility. Believed to decrease the post-mating inflammatory reaction (PMIE).
  - Dexametasone: 50 mg IV at breeding.
  - Prednisone: 0.1 mg/kg, BID for 4 days starting 48 hours before breeding.

Precautions/Interactions

- Do not administer prostaglandin or its analogs more than 36 hours post-ovulation; affects progesterone production by the CL; may result in EED.
- Adverse reactions may occur with natural or synthetic prostaglandin; transient sweating, ataxia, and increased GI motility.
- Do not administer corticosteroids if you suspect a uterine infection is present.
- Intrauterine infusion of enrofloxacin (Baytril) is contraindicated; not labeled for horses; highly irritating for endometrium.

Appropriate Health Care

Minimize contamination during breeding:
- Wash mare's perineum and stallion's penis with clean water; dry the stallion's penis prior to mating or semen collection for AI.
- Limit to one breeding (live cover or AI) per estrus.
- Breed as close to ovulation as possible.

- Immediately prior to natural breeding (live cover), infuse semen extender (60 to 120 mL) with nonspermicidal antibiotic (antibiotic concentration compatible with sperm viability); MCT.

Activity

Exercise: helps with uterine fluid evacuation.
- If exercise must be limited (e.g., because of laminitis or a sick foal at side), administer oxytocin every 3 to 6 hours to aid drainage.

Surgical Considerations

- Consider feasibility of surgical correction of predisposing causes before treating a uterine infection: Caslick's vulvoplasty (pneumovagina); vaginoplasty; urethral extension (urine pooling); repair of cervical tears.
- RVF and extensive cervical tears (foaling trauma): prudent to wait for results of an endometrial biopsy before the more extensive/expensive surgery, if the broodmare has been barren for more than a year. Chronic endometritis may have seriously diminished the mare's biopsy category in the interim.

 COMMENTS

Patient Monitoring

- Complete your gynecologic evaluation with special attention to uterine culture/cytology on day 1 or 2 of the estrus after treatment. Allow a complete diestrus for endometrial recuperation.
- If bacteria are isolated after treatment, contemplate local or systemic use of antiseptics/antibiotics.
- If no conception after several attempts, repeat the complete evaluation at 45 to 60 days after treatment.

Possible Complications

- Secondary bacterial/yeast overgrowth due to excessive use of antibiotics.
- Uterine adhesions
- Pyometra

Abbreviations

AI   artificial insemination
BID   twice a day
CL   corpus luteum
DMSO   dimethyl sulfoxide
DUC   delayed uterine clearance

EDTA   ethylenediaminetetraacetic acid
EED   early embryonic death
GI   gastrointestinal
hpf   high-powered field (microscopy)
IM   intramuscular
IV   intravenous
LRS   lactated Ringer's solution
MCT   minimum contamination technique
PGF   natural prostaglandin
PMIE   persistent mating-induced endometritis
PMN   polymorphonuclear (white) cell
QID   four times a day
RVF   rectovaginal fistula
SID   once a day
STD   sexually transmitted disease
TRP   transrectal palpation
U/S   ultrasound, ultrasonography
VC   vulvar conformation

See Also

- Cervical lesions
- Endometrial biopsy
- Parturition
- Postpartum metritis
- Pyometra
- Urine pooling/Urovagina
- Venereal diseases

Suggested Reading

Asbury AC, Lyle SK. 1993. Infectious causes of infertility. In: *Equine Reproduction*. McKinnon AO and Voss JL (eds). Philadelphia: Lea & Febiger; 381–391.

Brinsko S, Rigby SL, Varner DD, Blanchard TL. 2003. A practical method for recognizing mares susceptible to post-breeding endometritis. *Proc AAEP* 363–365.

LeBlanc MM. 2008. Treatment strategies for infertile mares. *Proc FAEP* 148–155.

Riddle WT, LeBlanc MM, Pierce SW, et al. 2005. Relationships between Pregnancy Rates, Uterine Cytology, and Culture Results in a Thoroughbred Practice in Central Kentucky. *Proc AAEP*. www.ivis.org; P2630.1205.

Vanderwall DK, Woods GL. 2003. Effect on fertility of uterine lavage performed immediately prior to insemination in mares. *JAVMA* 222: 1108–1110.

Author: Maria E. Cadario

Estrous Cycle, Manipulation, Synchronization

chapter 27

DEFINITION/OVERVIEW

- The estrous cycle of mares can be manipulated to maximize management's advantage by using hormone administration and artificial lighting programs.
- Some breeders rarely attempt to manipulate their mare's estrous cycles as an overall part of their breeding management.
- To effectively meet the demands of the equine industry relative to reproductive efficiency, it is necessary that the estrous cycle in the vast majority of mares be manipulated on a regular basis.

ETIOLOGY/PATHOPHYSIOLOGY

General Approaches or Goals of Manipulation

- Hasten the onset of ovulatory cycles in transitional mares.
- Induce ovulation in cycling mares.
- Synchronize estrus and ovulation in individual mares or groups of mares.
- Improve pregnancy rates in early postpartum mares.

Systems Affected

- Reproductive
- Endocrine

SIGNALMENT/HISTORY

- An intact mare must have reached an age consistent with puberty, but not be so old as no longer to be able to produce and ovulate follicles.
- Signs are variable depending on the reproductive status of the mare.
- Depending on the manipulative protocol applied, mares may be in:
  - Anestrus
  - Transition

- Diestrus
- Estrus

Risk Factors

- Industry norms
- Breed registry rules
- Management requirements
- Owner expectations

Historical Findings

- Desire or need to improve the efficiency of breeding management.
- Mares remaining barren at season's end because of the inability to match the mare's estrus activity and ovulations with the availability of semen from a particular stallion.

 CLINICAL FEATURES

- Periodic examination via TRP, U/S, or progesterone assay is indicated to monitor response to treatment.
- The interval for monitoring mares is dependent on the manipulation protocol being used and the expected response.

Clinical Findings/Justifications

Ovulation Induction

- The mare is checked for ovulation at intervals appropriate for the breeding management protocol being employed (e.g., for fresh, cool transported, or frozen AI).
- Typically mares are examined 1 to 2 days following administration of an OIA and at 24 to 48 hour intervals until ovulation is detected.
- One or more signs of impending ovulation may be detected with TRP or U/S.
  - Softening of the follicle wall.
  - Increased density of the follicle wall (preovulatory luteinization of the follicular wall) (Fig. 27.1).
  - Increase in the echogenic densities (i.e., ground glass speckles) in the follicle's antrum.
  - Decreased follicular width in at least one diameter.
  - Follicle develops a projection that extends to the ovulation fossa, site through which ovulation will take place (*see* Fig. 27.1)
  - Edema pattern decreases in the uterus pre-ovulation (Figs. 27.2 and 27.3a and b).
- Ovulation is most accurately confirmed with U/S (Figs. 27.4a and b).
- A CH/CL is generally detected between 24 and 48 hours after treating the mare with the OIA.

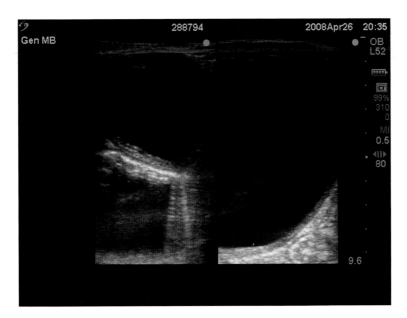

■ **Figure 27.1** Ultrasound images of two dominant follicles (same mare, same day). *Left*, demonstrates the luteinization of the follicular wall pre-ovulation and its point extending to the ovary's ovulation fossa; *right*, second, significantly bigger dominant follicle. Both ovulated and a twin crush was conducted on day 16 of gestation.

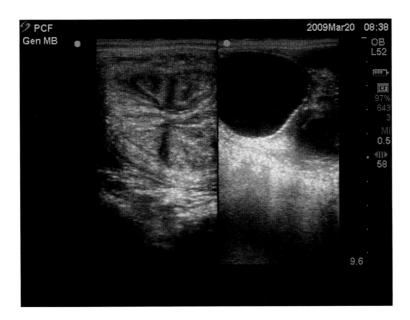

■ **Figure 27.2** Dominant follicle (*right*) coupled with typical preovulatory endometrial edema (*left*).

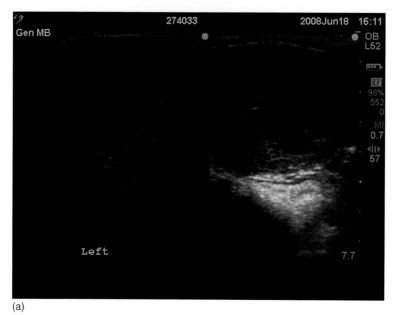

(a)

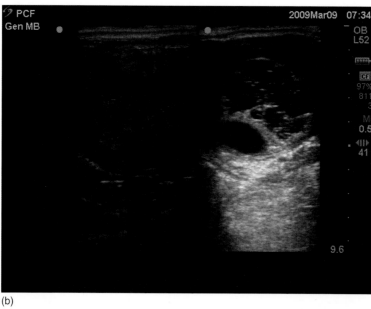

(b)

■ **Figure 27.3** In each ultrasound image, the uterus is on the left, the ovarian structure of interest on the right. They exhibit the decrease in uterine edema just prior to and following ovulation as the mare's cycle moves into diestrus. Note the increasing thickness of the corpus hemorrhagicum wall and filling by hemorrhage (clots, contracts, luteinizes) within the "former follicular space."

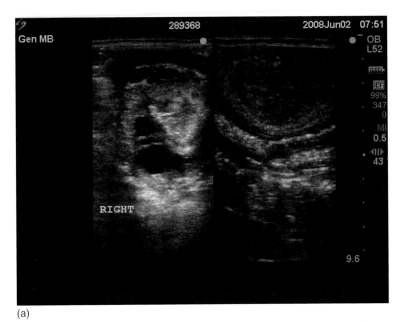

(a)

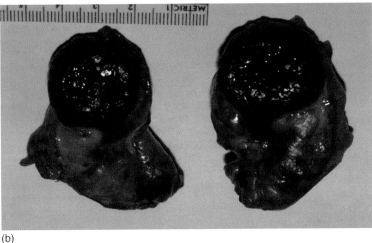

(b)

■ **Figure 27.4** *A*, The ultrasound demonstrates the sharp point of the developed corpus luteum (*left*) and lack of edema of the diestrus uterus (*right*). *B*, A cross-section of an ovary containing a mature corpus luteum. It demonstrates nicely the same track leading to the point at the ovulation fossa. The point of the prior ovulation can often be observed by U/S through to its regression to a corpus albicans.

Estrus and Ovulation Synchronization

■ Mares generally return to estrus within 3 to 5 days following the last day of treatment regardless of the protocol used.

■ Some mares ovulate during progestin treatment (the equivalent of a diestrual ovulation), hence the need to follow with prostaglandin on the last day of treatment.

   ■ Failure to return-to-estrus occurs most commonly because the mare ovulated during treatment and still has functional luteal tissue.

- P&E treatment is more reliable than progestins alone, because the estrogen suppresses follicular development, thus helping prevent ovulation during treatment. P&E still does not have FDA approval for use in the mare.
  - Because of this follicular suppression, return to estrus and subsequent ovulation is more delayed with P&E treatment than progestins alone.
  - P&E is the most effective protocol for synchronizing ovulation, with approximately 80% of mares ovulating on Days 19 to 22 following the last day of treatment.
- A two-dose prostaglandin protocol is more effective for synchronizing a return-to-estrus than a single treatment.
- Therefore, regardless of the protocol used, synchronizing ovulation within a useful window-of-time, further requires the use of an OIA.

Delaying "Foal Heat"

- The goal is to have a more suitable uterus in which to establish a pregnancy.
- Monitor the mare for uterine involution and luminal fluid following delivery and through her foal heat.
- Treating with P&E generally delays ovulation by approximately 1 day for every day of treatment.
- If the uterus involutes appropriately and does not contain any fluid at the foal heat, the mare can be bred on ovulations occurring Day 9 or later postpartum.
- If fluid remains during the foal heat, it is probably best to use the prostaglandin protocol and delay breeding until the second postpartum estrus.

Hastening Onset of the Ovulatory Season

- The principal method is exposing mares to an increased photoperiod (i.e., photostimulation, artificial lighting) during late fall and early winter. A transitional period (minimum of 60 days) still occurs, only its beginning is shifted to an earlier point in the calendar year.
- The most commonly used photostimulation protocols include:
  - *Traditional method*: 16 hours of light to 8 hours of dark (16L:8D) is most effective when the additional artificial light is added to the end of the day's natural photoperiod.
  - However, as little as 2 to 3 additional hours of artificial light may be sufficient to stimulate reproductive resurgence, known as *Night-Interruption* (aka Pulse or Flash lighting). The mare is exposed to 1 to 2 hours of artificial light during a photosensitive period 9.5 hours after the onset of darkness.
  - When artificial lights are started between November 1 and December 1, the majority of mares will have entered their ovulatory season by February 15.
  - Photostimulation must begin before the winter solstice to be of any advantage over the natural increase in photoperiod.
- When artificial lights are combined with dopamine antagonists, the time to the first ovulation can be as short as 15 days. Results are more reliable if the mare has entered vernal (spring) transition or is currently under photostimulation.
- It is essential to maintain mares under artificial lighting until at least May 1 or until they have been bred and are confirmed in foal (if prior to May 1). Earlier termination

of the lighting program may result in loss of the advantage/activity stimulated by the lighting program and the mare will often revert to a winter anestrus state. Her subsequent return to estrus activity during that season, may require an additional 60-days of increasing light ... a late breeding in the season.

- The response to native GnRH is highly variable. Many mares return to anestrus or a transitional state following a stimulated ovulation.
- hCG only works to induce ovulation in late transitional mares with steroidogenically competent follicles.
- P&E is most effective for synchronizing the first estrus and ovulation. It is only useful in mares that are in late vernal transition.
- Other methods used to hasten the onset of the ovulatory season include:
  - Dopamine antagonists used in conjunction with photostimulation and moderate ambient temperatures (a minimum of 50°F).
  - Administration of GnRH to stimulate follicular development and ovulation.
  - Administration of eFSH to stimulate follicular development and ovulation.
  - Administration of progestins or P&E to delay the first ovulation and synchronize the estrus.
  - Administration of hCG to induce ovulation in late vernal transitional mares.

Improving Pregnancy Rate on Foal Heat

- Prostaglandin or P&E are used at the same doses as for estrus and ovulation synchronization. See Drug(s) of Choice.

Protocols/Timing

Inducing Ovulation

- Ovulation can be induced by treating a mare with:
  - Releasing hormone to stimulate LH release from the anterior pituitary, or
  - Gonadotropin, with LH-like activity, that acts directly on the follicle and gonad.
- Conditions that help ensure a predictable response to treatment in the majority of mares.
  - An individual mare must be in her ovulatory season.
  - A follicle must have emerged as a dominant follicle.
  - A follicle must be steroidogenically competent (i.e., producing estradiol), as evidenced by uterine edema or the mare exhibiting signs of behavioral estrus.
- The most predictable response results when mares have a follicle that is at least 30 to 35 mm in diameter before being treated.
- Ovulation generally occurs 24 to 48 hours following treatment.

Synchronizing Estrus and Ovulation

- Synchronizing estrus in cycling mares generally involves modifying the luteal phase of the estrous cycle.
- The luteal phase can be shortened with prostaglandin or artificially prolonged with progestins.

- ▪ Prostaglandin is administered as a single dose, or two doses 14 days apart.
- ▪ Progestins are typically administered daily for 14 to 15 consecutive days.
- Combining estrogens with a progestin helps suppress follicular development and better synchronizes the cohort of follicles in the first follicular wave following treatment.
  - ▪ P&E is typically administered daily for 10 consecutive days.
- Prostaglandin is often used in conjunction with progestin, or progestin plus estrogen, therapy to ensure luteolysis in the event an unexpected ovulation occurred during treatment.
- Synchronizing ovulation to fall within a predictable window of time, additionally requires the use of an OIA.

Improving Pregnancy Rate on Foal Heat

- Manipulative therapy is designed to delay the onset of the foal heat or shorten the interval to the second postpartum estrus with the goal of improving the uterine environment for establishing a pregnancy.
- Once the placenta has been passed in the first 1 to 3 hours postpartum, progestin administration begins and is administered for 8 to 15 days postpartum to delay the onset of foal heat. Prostaglandin is administered on the last day of treatment.
- P&E can be administered for as little as 5 days to delay the onset of foal heat.
- P&E is started as soon as is practical on the day of foaling.
- Delaying foal heat results in the first postpartum ovulation occurring on or after the ninth postpartum day.
- Prostaglandin can be administered 5 to 7 days after the first postpartum ovulation to shorten the interval to the second postpartum estrus.
- Approximately 15 days are required postpartum for the endometrium to sufficiently repair to carry the next pregnancy. Transit time from the time of ovulation to entry into the uterus is approximately 6 days (ovary to uterus). Based on this, the recommendation to maximize conception at foal heat is to:
  - ▪ Breed a mare on foal heat if ovulation occurs on or after the ninth postpartum day and little or no fluid remains in the uterus.
  - ▪ If ovulation occurs before Day 9, then prostaglandin is administered ("short cycling") and the mare is bred in the subsequent estrus.

 # DIFFERENTIAL DIAGNOSIS

- To ensure a predictable response, it is important to establish the stage of cycle and the characteristics of the ovaries and tubular reproductive tract in a mare in deciding which manipulative procedures to apply.
- It is often important to determine:
  - ▪ Whether a mare has entered the ovulatory season.
  - ▪ Whether the mare is in diestrus and a CL is present on an ovary.
  - ▪ Follicular, uterine, and cervical characteristics.

DIAGNOSTICS

- Teasing
- TRP
- U/S
- Other laboratory tests: Progesterone assay can be helpful in establishing the stage of cycle and confirming the presence of a luteal structure.

Pathologic Findings

Conditions Causing Unpredictable Response to Some Forms of Manipulation

- Mares with hemorrhagic, anovulatory follicles.
- Anestrus mares
- Transitional mares

THERAPEUTICS

Drug(s) of Choice

Ovulation Induction

- Deslorelin, two forms have been used:
- An approved, implantable pellet (Ovuplant; Fort Dodge Laboratories).
  - Ovuplant is not currently available in the United States, although an injectable form can be imported from Canada with Food and Drug Administration permission.
  - Ovuplant (2.1-mg implantable pellet), 1 pellet is placed SC, preferably in a vulvar lip (to facilitate easier removal).
  - Placing the pellet in the vulva, lateral to the labia, facilitates removal following ovulation (see Precautions below).
- An unapproved, slow release injectable (Bio-Release Deslorelin injectable; BET Pharm).
  - Bio-Release Deslorelin injectable (1.5 mg/mL), 1 mL is injected IM.
- hCG (1,500 to 3,500 IU/dose), IM or IV. *Note*: 2500 IU is probably the most common dose administered. Exceeding 3000 IU IV may increase the likelihood of causing an anovulatory follicle (an anovulatory event).
- reLH, a recombinant reagent grade product, may be on the market in the near future and it has been evaluated thus far in clinical research projects.

Estrus and Ovulation Synchronization

- P&E
  - Progesterone (150 mg/day) and estradiol-17β (10 mg/day) in oil, IM.
- Progestins
  - Progesterone (150 mg/day), IM.
  - Altrenogest (Regumate; Intervet), 0.044 mg/kg/day, PO.

- Prostaglandin
  - Dinoprost tromethamine (Lutalyse; Pfizer), 1 mg/100 lbs BW, IM.
  - Cloprostenol (Estrumate; Schering-Plough), 250 µg/mL, IM.

Hastening Onset of the Ovulatory Season

- Sulpiride (0.5 mg/kg), BID, IM. *Note*: Available from veterinary compounding pharmacies.
- Domperidone (Equidone; Equitox, Inc.), 1.1 mg/kg, SID, PO.
- GnRH
  - Native GnRH (Cystorelin; Ceva), 50 to 100 µg, BID, IM or SC for 2 to 3 weeks.
  - Deslorelin can be administered in late vernal transition. Deslorelin injectable product is available from Canadian suppliers, but in the U.S. can only be purchased from a number of compounding pharmacies. The price is significantly less than it was in years past.
- eFSH (Bioniche) 6.25 mg, BID, IM for 5 to 7 days. *Note*: Treatment begins in transitional mares once follicles of 20 to 30 mm in diameter are present. Administer hCG when follicle reaches 35 mm in diameter.
- P&E (same dose as for estrus and ovulation synchronization, see Drug(s) of Choice) is administered for 10 days late in transition (or after approximately 60 days of artificial lighting) when the average diameter of the largest follicles is more than 30 mm.
- hCG (same dose as for ovulation induction in cycling mares, see Drug(s) of Choice) is administered once IM or IV once a follicle is at least 35 mm diameter in a mare that is displaying behavioral estrus for several days late in vernal transition.
  - May require multiple doses to hasten the first ovulation.

Precautions/Interactions

- Deslorelin implants have been associated with non-return to estrus in mares that fail to become pregnant at the first breeding and ovulation, due to an inhibitory feedback to the hypothalamus. Deslorelin can cause some mares to shut down for a variable period of time. This negative effect can be diminished by removal of the implant as soon as possible after ovulation has been confirmed.
- Progesterone administration may be contraindicated in mares with postpartum metritis.
- Age-Related Factors:
  - Protocols are not effective for prepubertal mares.
  - Protocols are not effective for geriatric mares that have stopped cycling.
  - Older mares tend to have a less predictable response to hCG.

Appropriate Health Care

- Apply routine preventative health care appropriate for the region, age, and reproductive status of the mare.

Diet

- A well-balanced diet, appropriate for the age and level of activity of the mare.
- Goal is to maintain good body condition. An overweight mare is undesirable.
  - A BCS of 6 to 8 is desirable.

Activity

- Routine activity is appropriate.
- Highly stressful activities may cause variable responses to some protocols designed to manipulate the estrous cycle.

 COMMENTS

Client Education

- Owner compliance and acceptance of programs designed to manipulate the estrous cycle in mares, is enhanced by taking time to thoroughly explain the rationale for and limitations of treatment, including the expected responses and potential benefits.

Prevention/Avoidance

- To avoid some mares shutting down following treatment with a deslorelin implant, it is advisable to remove the pellet following ovulation.

Possible Complications

- Some mares develop antibodies to hCG if treated with it 3–4+ times in a breeding season, which decreases its efficacy. The resistance (anti-hormone formation) abates by the next, subsequent breeding season.
- Hypersensitivity reactions to hCG are rare.

Expected Course and Prognosis

- Not every mare will respond with an expected outcome to a manipulative protocol described previously.
- Response is dependent on a number of factors, including mare age, body condition, general health, reproductive status, and the protocol used.
- Nevertheless, the majority of mares will respond with an expected outcome, when a protocol designed to manipulate the estrous cycle of a mare is properly applied to an appropriate candidate for treatment.

Abbreviations

AI   artificial insemination
BCS   body condition score

BID   twice a day
BW   body weight
CH   corpus hemorrhagicum
CL   corpus luteum
eFSH   equine follicle-stimulating hormone
GnRH   gonadotropin releasing hormone
hCG   human chorionic gonadotropin
IM   intramuscular
IV   intravenous
LH   luteinizing hormone
OIA   ovulation induction agent
P&E   progesterone and estradiol-17β in oil
PO   per os (by mouth)
SC   subcutaneous
SID   once a day
TRP   transrectal palpation
U/S   ultrasound, ultrasonography

See Also

- Abnormal estrus intervals
- Anestrus
- Delayed uterine involution
- Ovulation induction
- Ovulation synchronization
- Short-cycling

Suggested Reading

Blanchard TL, Varner DD, Schumacher J, et al. 2003. Manipulation of estrus in mares. In: *Manual of Equine Reproduction*. St. Louis: Mosby; 17–30.

Card C. 2009. Hormone therapy in the mare. In: *Equine Breeding Management and Artificial Insemination*, 2nd ed. Samper JC (ed). Philadelphia: Saunders/Elsevier; 89–97.

Duchamp G, Daels PF. 2002. Combined effects of sulpiride and light treatment on the onset of cyclicity in anestrous mares. *Therio* 58: 599–602.

Authors: Gary J. Nie and Carla L. Carleton

chapter 28

Estrus Detection, Fundamentals

DEFINTION/OVERVIEW

- Methods by which the stage of a mare's estrous cycle is determined.
- The intent is to breed a mare when she is either behaviorally receptive (with good records of teasing, cycle length, and estrus/diestrus responses) or characteristic signs are present based on the findings of TRP, U/S, and/or hormonal assays.

ETIOLOGY/PATHOPHYSIOLOGY

Systems Affected

- Reproductive
- Neuroendocrine

SIGNALMENT/HISTORY

Risk Factors

- Responds to the advances of a stallion (teasing response) appropriately through a 21-day cycle in diestrus or estrus.
- It's imperative to have facilities that allow safe exposure of the mare to the stallion (Figs. 28.1, 28.2, and 28.3).
- Safe palpation stocks or means of restraint in which a TRP can be conducted.

Historical Findings

- Assessment of the mare's responses to increasing day length, whether by teasing (mare to stallion, stallion to mare), TRP, U/S, hormonal assays.
- TRP findings in a normal mare during the ovulatory period will be synchronous (increasing/decreasing uterine tone and closed to relaxing cervix reflect specific ovarian activity during an estrous cycle).
- Asynchronous TRP, U/S, behavior: typical of mares in transition (vernal or autumnal), winter anestrus, or exhibition of a delayed return to estrus, a prolonged period of luteinization of an ovarian hematoma, an ovarian tumor (e.g., GTCT), and so on.

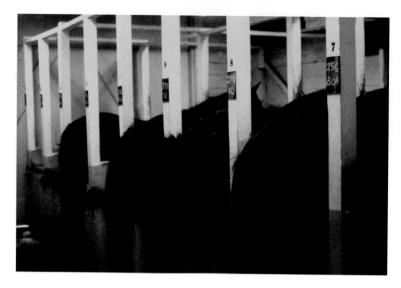

■ **Figure 28.1** Teasing stalls allowing safe, convenient teasing and palpation of mares in one barn.

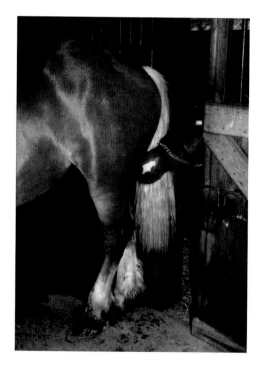

■ **Figure 28.2** Mare presented to stallion maintained in his stall with a handler.

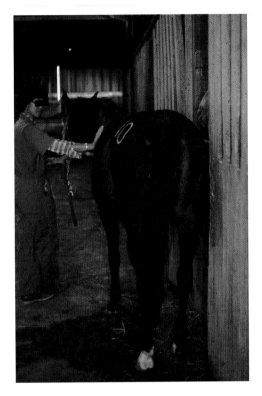

■ **Figure 28.3** Mare presented to stallion in his stall for teasing. Never get between the stallion and the mare; remain on the opposite side as demonstrated.

 CLINICAL FEATURES

Teasing

- Exposing the mare to a stallion to determine her interest, aggression, or passivity.
- Depending on a farm's routine, this may be done daily or every other day.
- Behavioral signs throughout an estrous cycle (degree varies, as waxing/waning):
  - A range of behavior from non-receptive to full, standing heat. The extremes are linked by periods of equivocal behavior as ovarian activity shifts from ovulatory follicle to CH to CL to CA and a return to estrus.
  - *Out of heat (nonreceptive, diestrus) behaviors* include: tail switching, moving around, squealing, ears back, kicking or attempting to kick (Figs. 28.4 and 28.5).
  - *Indifferent*: neither receptive nor non-receptive.
  - *In heat (receptive, estrus) behaviors* include: raises tail or deflects it to the side, stands still, winking (eversion) of the clitoris, urinates in squirts, lowers pelvis (posturing, breaking down), ears forward, leans toward stallion, refuses to move away from stallion, absence of nonreceptive behaviors (Fig. 28.6).

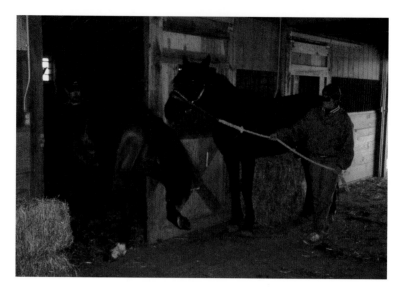

■ **Figure 28.4** Mare in diestrus, rejecting stallion's advances. Stall teasing; one of teasing team remains at the mare's head and presents her hind quarters to the stallion in the aisle.

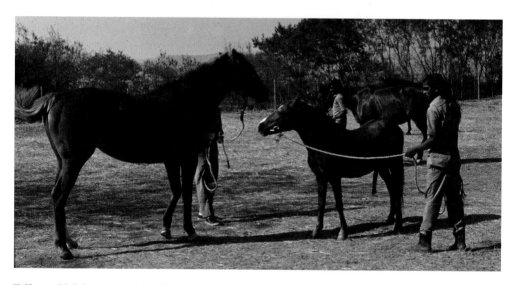

■ **Figure 28.5** Pasture teasing with a pony stallion; mare in diestrus: ears back, kicking.

- Multiple options for an acceptable teasing program, including:
  - Mares taken to the stallion that is held in a stall/paddock/pasture (Fig. 28.7).
  - Stallion brought to the mares that are held individually, or teased across a fence to the mares (in small pen, pasture, stall, or stock, or driven into a long tease chute).
  - Pony stallions are often used (smaller, lower purchase and maintenance costs, good libido, and unable to cover horse mares under normal circumstances (*see* Figs. 28.5 and 28.6).

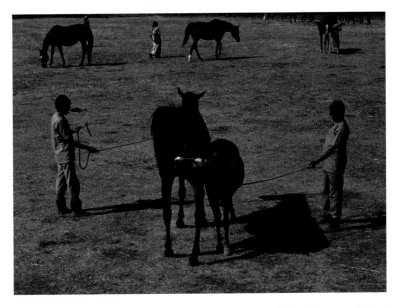

■ **Figure 28.6** Pasture teasing with a pony stallion; mare receptive to stallion's advances: tail elevated, deflected to one side, urinating.

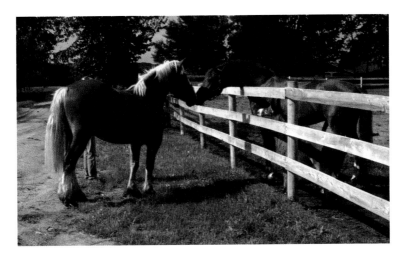

■ **Figure 28.7** Mare to stallion paddock teasing.

- Occasionally geldings serve as suitable teasers, less often mares treated with testosterone.
- Facilities to accomplish this also vary widely—dependent on experience of those handling the horses, numbers of individuals on the teasing crew, behavior/control of the horse; whether teasing a single mare versus a mare with a foal at side.
- Timing/frequency:
  - Early in the OBS when a high percentage of mares may yet be in vernal transition, TRP interval may be weekly while gauging the rate of follicular growth, uterine and cervical tone.

- Once signs that the ovulatory period is imminent are observed, the teasing interval should be decreased to every other day or daily.
- *Ovulation is close*: endometrial edema accompanies a large, late vernal transition follicle; an indicator of the steroidogenic competence of the follicle/s (estradiol).
- *Ovulation has occurred*: following a long period of irregular, transitional activity, the mare teases out for 2 weeks, an indicator of her first ovulation of the season (the first CL is present).
- Regular teasing should continue throughout the breeding season, including after breeding.
- The greatest loss of equine pregnancy occurs within the first 50 days of gestation.
- If loss can be identified (the mare teases in unexpectedly after early, positive pregnancy checks) prior to the formation of endometrial cups, the ability to detect the open mare and rebreed her within the same season is greatly enhanced.

TRP

- Diestrus TRP: increased uterine tone from that present during estrus; usually diestrual follicles present on the ovaries, the cervix is closed under the influence of progesterone (approximate proportion of 4:1, length to width; tubular and distinct).
- Estrus TRP: with regression of the prior CL, uterine tone decreases, edema of the endometrial folds can be felt by encircling a uterine horn with the palpation hand/fingers to its attached border; drawing the hand cranially, allowing the uterine horn to slip between one's fingers. The folds (5 to 10) will be felt; each providing a sensation similar to that detected with a cow's early pregnancy membrane slip. The mare's cervix becomes shorter and wider and less tubular as the prior CL regresses, as she enters estrus and progresses towards ovulation. Within 24 to 48 hours post-ovulation, as plasma progesterone level increase, the cervix closes again and uterine tone increases.

U/S

- Edema of the endometrial folds serves as an additional measure of the mare's hormonal milieu and whether she is responding appropriately.
- Edema is present during estrus in parallel with a dominant follicle and decreases in the hours prior to ovulation (Fig. 28.8).
- The presence/persistence of edema post-ovulation may be an indicator of endometritis and often accompanies postbreeding or postovulation uterine fluid accumulation.
- Endometrial fold edema present at early pregnancy checks often reflects the presence of a large follicle (greater than 25 mm at 16 days) or a pregnancy at risk (Fig. 28.9). In both instances, treatment with Regumate (0.44 mg/kg/day PO) at least through the formation of endometrial cups (and production of additional endogenous progesterone), may salvage the pregnancy. It would be essential to reassess the pregnancy at regular intervals. If it is not maintained, then Regumate treatment should immediately cease to permit the mare to return to estrus.

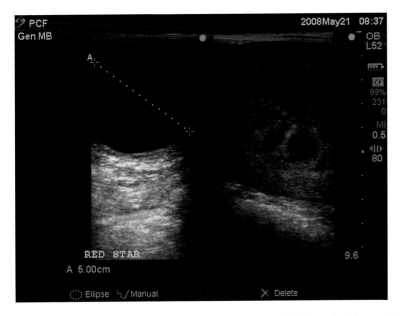

Figure 28.8 Ultrasound view of mare's tract during estrus: dominant follicle to the left, prominent edema of the endometrial folds to the right.

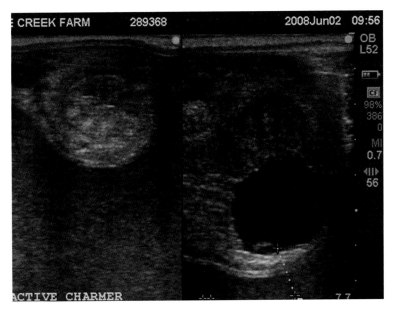

Figure 28.9 Ultrasound of a 23-day gestation showing edema in both nongravid and gravid (evident around the conceptus) horns.

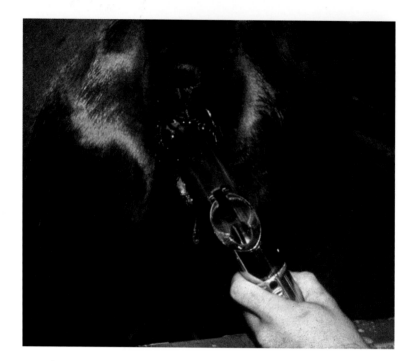

■ **Figure 28.10** Lighted vaginal speculum introduced through the mare's vulva.

- Edema may reflect endometritis due to poor VC and ascending infection/inflammation. If VC is less than ideal, a Caslick's vulvoplasty, as soon as possible after breeding and confirmation of ovulation, should be performed. Waiting to place the Caslick's until early pregnancy confirmation at 16 days, leaves the uterus vulnerable during 30% of the time most pregnancy loss occurs in the mare (within the first 50 days of gestation). Goal: minimize inflammation and maximize establishment of pregnancy.

Endocrine Evaluation

- Exhibition of estrus behavior is primarily due to the absence of progesterone. Mares begin to tease in when plasma progesterone is between 1–2 ng/mL and tease out within 24 to 48 hours post-ovulation when estrogens are low and progesterone is increasing.

Vaginal Speculum Examination

- A technique that is of least value and accuracy for close determination of a mare's estrus state is a vaginal speculum assessment of the relaxation of the external cervical os (Fig. 28.10). The external os of a closed cervix will appear as a rosette (note its dorsal phrenulum); closed, tight, off the vaginal floor (Fig. 28.11).
- As the mare comes into heat, the external os begins to relax toward the vaginal floor (Figs. 28.12 and 28.13).

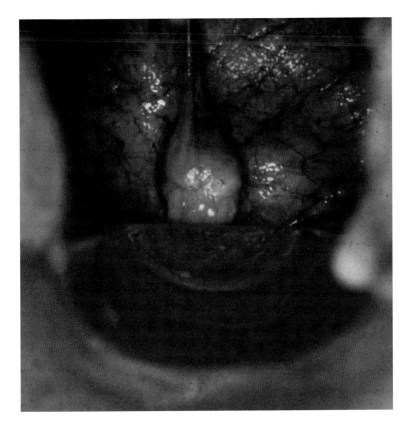

■ **Figure 28.11** Vaginal speculum of mare's external cervical os during diestrus (closed cervix).

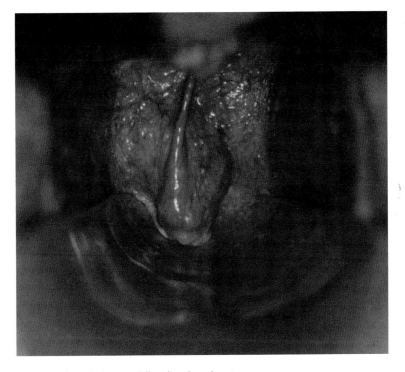

■ **Figure 28.12** External cervical os partially relaxed, early estrus.

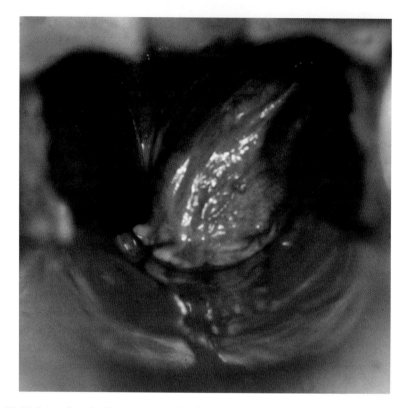

■ **Figure 28.13** External cervical is completely relaxed during estrus.

■ Results of TRP and U/S, assessment of endometrial edema, including TRP of the cervix' dimensions (length, width, tubularity), preclude the need to conduct a vaginal speculum exam to determine cervical relaxation. It is also inadvisable to contaminate the caudal genital tract when unnecessary. A vaginal speculum still has utility in diagnosing urine pooling in the mare's cranial vagina.

DIFFERENTIAL DIAGNOSIS

■ Normal estrus
■ Vernal or autumnal transition
■ Pregnant mare that continues to tease to the stallion

DIAGNOSTICS

Teasing, TRP, U/S as described.

COMMENTS

Client Education

- Economics: Teasing mares can be difficult, boring, and downright unpleasant early in the year in cold climates, but the time spent and the consistency of a regular teasing program can offset the need for many veterinary examinations and help identify the best days to breed a mare.
- Ovulation occurs 24 to 48 hours prior to the end of estrus. Knowing the length of each mare's prior period of receptivity helps determine when best to breed each one on the subsequent cycle.
- Continue teasing after breeding and confirmation of ovulation. Teasing is one of the best means for early identification of pregnancy loss and increases the likelihood the mare can be rebred within the same season.
- *Teasing, one person*: If either the mare or stallion is safely contained in a stall or small area with safe fencing, teasing can be done by one person, bringing the teasing stallion to the mares in stalls, or mares to the stallion's area. An adequate response by the mare may be missed, as the mare may fail to show signs of heat until the stallion moves away from her (e.g., mares with foals at side may be reticent to tease in); maiden mares may be fearful and only break down once the stallion is at a distance.
- *Teasing, two people*: The advantage of a team for teasing is that one observes the mare's specific responses (either behind the mare being led near a stallion) or following along (after the stallion is led by mares stalled in a barn) and observing mares for a minute or two after the stallion has departed from the immediate area.
- Most estrual mares respond to the stallion rather quickly and honestly. With good records and persistence a farm can identify individuals that require greater persistence, more time (e.g., 3 minutes versus 30 seconds), more contact or vocalization by the stallion, etc., to elicit a response when they are in estrus.

Synonyms

Heat, in Heat	in estrus
Out of heat	in diestrus
Teasing in	in estrus
Teasing out	going out of estrus or is in diestrus
Breaking down	mare exhibits signs of estrus during teasing, rotating pelvis
Standing heat	strong estrus, refusing to move away from the stallion

Abbreviations

BSE	breeding soundness examination
CA	corpus albicans
CH	corpus hemorrhagicum
CL	corpus luteum

GTCT   granulosa thecal cell tumor
OBS   operational breeding season
PO   per os (by mouth)
TRP   transrectal palpation
U/S   ultrasound, ultrasonography
VC   vulvar conformation

See Also

- Abnormal estrus intervals
- Anestrus
- BSE, components, mare
- Clitoral enlargement
- Conception failure
- Endometritis
- Estrous cycle, manipulation of
- Ovulation failure
- Ovulation induction
- Ovulation, synchronization of
- Transrectal palpation

Suggested Reading

Carleton CL. 2007. Clinical examination of the nonpregnant equine female reproductive tract. In: *Current Therapy in Large Animal Theriogenology*, 2nd ed. Youngquist RS, Threlfall WR (eds). Philadelphia: Saunders; 74–90.

Carnevale EM, Checura C, Coutinho da Silva MA, et al. 2002. Use of computer-assisted image analysis to determine the interval before and after ovulation. *Proc AAEP*, 48–50.

Górecka A, Jezierski TA, Słoniewski K. 2005. Relationships between sexual behaviour, dominant follicle area, uterus ultrasonic image and pregnancy rate in mares of two breeds differing in reproductive efficiency. *An Reprod Sci* 87: 283–293.

Pelehach LM, Greaves HE, Porter MB, et al. 2002. The role of estrogen and progesterone in the induction and dissipation of uterine edema in mares. *Therio* 58: 441–444.

Pryor P, Tibary A. 2005. Management of estrus in the performance mare. In: *Current Techniques in Equine Practice*. Philadelphia: Elsevier/Saunders; 197–209.

Samper JC. 1997. Ultrasonographic appearance and the pattern of uterine edema to time ovulation in mares. *Proc AAEP*, 189–191.

Author: Carla L. Carleton

chapter 29

Fescue Toxicosis

DEFINITION/OVERVIEW

- Tall fescue (*Lolium arundinaceum* [Schreb.]), a perennial grass, is infected with the endophyte *Neotyphodium coenophialum*. The endophyte produces toxins with severe adverse effects when ingested by late-term pregnant mares. [The standard author abbreviation, Schreb., is used to indicate Johann Christian Daniel von Schreber (1739–1810) as the author when citing a botanical name.]
- Reproductive abnormalities include:
  - Prolonged gestation
  - Late-term abortion
  - Premature placental separation
  - Dystocia
  - Traumatic injury to the reproductive tract
  - Thickened placentae
  - RFM
  - Agalactia
- A high incidence of foal mortality results from:
  - Prolonged gestation
  - Dystocia with anoxia/hypoxia
  - Dysmaturity
  - Weakness
  - Starvation
  - FPT
  - Septicemia

ETIOLOGY/PATHOPHYSIOLOGY

Toxins (Etiology)

- Multiple toxins are produced by the endophyte in fescue, including peramines, lolines, and ergopeptine alkaloids.
- *Peramines* do not affect animal health but do decrease insect herbivory.

- *Lolines* are pyrrolizidine alkaloids comprised of N-acetyl loline which causes vaso-constriction of the lateral saphenous vein and N-formyl loline. Characteristic hepa-totoxicity is not evident with tall fescue toxicosis.
- *Ergopeptine alkaloids* present include ergotamine, ergosine, ergovaline, ergonine, ergocristine, ergocryptine and ergocornine. However, ergovaline and ergosine are the most common isolates.

Ergot Alkaloids (Pathophysiology)

- Act as dopamine D_2 receptor agonists on prolactin secretory cells of the anterior pituitary (lactotrophs) causing decreased prolactin concentrations, resulting in aga-lactia and decreased priming of the mammary gland for development.
- Decrease tissue binding of estradiol, resulting in higher serum concentrations of estradiol-17β.
- Inhibit ACTH secretion, thus lowering fetal cortisol concentration which is needed for late gestation control of placental function.
- This compromise of placental function is reflected by decreased circulating P4 and relaxin.
- The decreased P4 is insufficient to stimulate lobuloalveolar growth of the mammary gland.
- The decreased P4 further compounds the agalactia initiated by decreased prolactin and increased estradiol-17β.
- May block CRH activity in the foal, which stimulates ACTH release.
- ACTH causes cortisol release from the adrenal.
- An increase of fetal cortisol signals parturition in the mare.
- Lack of fetal production of CRH, ACTH and cortisol could result in prolonged gestation.
- Ergovaline and N-acetyl loline have vasoconstrictive properties.
- These may produce hypoxia, resulting in further placental compromise.
- Interact with dopaminergic mechanisms capable of modifying gut motility with an effect on the feeding center of the hypothalamus.
- End result is decreased feed intake and decreased digestibility of endophyte-infected hay (weight loss).

Systems Affected

- Reproductive
- Mammary gland
- GI

 SIGNALMENT/HISTORY

- Pregnant mares who are more than 330 days of gestation grazing endophyte-infected fescue.
- Any horse grazing on endophyte-infected fescue.

Risk Factors

- *Mare*: uterine or cervical trauma during parturition.
- *Fetus/Neonate*: Hypoxemia of the foal during parturition. Failure of the fetus to rotate (abnormal presentation) just prior to parturition, larger fetal body size, and lack of *mare's readiness for parturition* increases the risk for dystocia.
- *Placenta*: Compromised placental function includes thickening and edema; increased difficulty rupturing placental membranes during parturition.
- *Endocrine*: Decreased prolactin and progesterone, increased estrogen: fails to prime and develop the mammary gland for colostrum and milk production.
- Fescue is one of the most abundant species of cool season perennial grasses. Fescue infected by endophyte results in a symbiotic relationship characterized by greater *stand survival* and increased yield.
- In addition, affected fescue has improved seedling performance, nitrogen assimilation, leaf water potential and turgor pressure. Shoot and root mass, and resistance to insect damage are increased. Drought tolerance is enhanced.

Historical Findings

- Approximately 75% of the 35 million acres of tall fescue grown in the United States is infected.
- Approximately 688,000 horses in the United States are pastured on tall fescue.
- Extends from Oklahoma to Texas and from Missouri to Virginia.

CLINICAL FEATURES

- Prolonged gestation by 20 to 27 days (360 ± 4 days).
- Lack of signs of imminent foaling (absence of classic signs: mammary gland development, hollowing of the paralumbar fossa, softening of the gluteal muscles or relaxation of the tail-head and vulvae).
- Dystocia
- Placental thickening at the cervical star and uterine body, premature placental separation.
- RFM
- Agalactia or hypogalactia.
- Decreased fertility.
- Weak or stillborn foals (50%–86%).
- Dysmature or hypothyroid foals.
- Reduced daily gains of yearlings, if not receiving supplementation.
- Increased sweating in pregnant mares.

DIFFERENTIAL DIAGNOSIS

- *Claviceps* sp. mycotoxicosis

DIAGNOSTICS

- Clinical signs
- Imaging: Prepartum transrectal U/S in the region of the cervical star. To evaluate placental thickening, edema, and separation from the endometrium.
- History of grazing endophyte-infected fescue within the last 30 days of gestation.
- Serum sampling with low progesterone, prolactin, relaxin; elevated estradiol-17β (results not available at all laboratories).
- Examination of placenta for increased thickening, edema, and weight.
- Sample pasture or hay: determine presence of endophyte by staining or analyze for ergovaline (analysis offered by a number of U.S. diagnostic laboratories).
- Foals: IgG, to rule out FPT
- Thyroid profile (hypothyroidism)

Pathological Findings

Placental Histopathology

- Inner, vascular portion, of the allantois: severe edema, accumulation of mucoid material.
- Congestion and mucoid degeneration of allantoic vessels, shortening of chorionic villi, prominent subepithelial collagen deposition of the chorion and allantois.

THERAPEUTICS

Drug(s) of Choice

Mare

Domperidone

- Dose at 1.1 mg/kg of body weight/day PO.
- A DA$_2$ dopamine receptor antagonist that does not cross the blood-brain barrier, therefore it has less potential to cause side-effects.
- If the mare is treated post-foaling, it can be given every 12 hours for several days to ensure optimum milk production.
- Effective in resolving pre- and postpartum agalactia and prolonged gestation.

Reserpine

- Dose at 0.01 mg/kg q. 24 hours PO.
- A Rauwolfian alkaloid that depletes serotonin, dopamine and norepinephrine depots in the brain and other tissues.
- Only effective in resolving postpartum agalactia.
- Crosses blood-brain barrier.
- Side effects include sedation and diarrhea, oral form has decreased side effects.

Sulperide

- Dose 3.3 mg/kg/day.
- Selective DA$_2$ dopamine receptor antagonist.
- Low prevalence of side effects even though it crosses the blood-brain barrier.
- Resolves prepartum agalactia, although not as effective as domperidone.

Fluphenizine decanoate

- Dose 25 mg IM one-time injection.
- Long-acting D$_2$-dopamine antagonist.
- Tranquilizes, may predispose animals to extrapyramidal or Parkinson-like side effects.
- Effective in maintaining systemic relaxin and improving pregnancy outcome.
- Additional research needed.

Foal

- Weak, dysmature foals may become septic due to FPT.
- Supplementation of IgGs (hyperimmune plasma), early IV treatment is better than PO due to potential for decreased absorption.
- Supportive care for dysmaturity or septicemia.

Appropriate Health Care

- Mare: (1) Start drug therapy 30-days prior to parturition or upon recognizing that a mare is/has been grazing endophyte-infected fescue. (2) Remove mare from endophyte-infected pasture or hay as soon as possible and treat for agalactia. (3) Attend parturition, the mare is at an increased risk of dystocia; close monitoring and assistance for mare during parturition.
- Neonate: supportive care for the dysmature, immunocompromised foal.

Diet

- Supplement yearlings or other horses with concentrate to alleviate decreased weight gain.
- Feed endophyte-free fescue or endophyte grass that contains peramine, not ergovaline (MaxQ).

Surgical Considerations

- C-section has not improved foal viability.

    COMMENTS

Client Education

- Mare: (1) Start drug therapy 30 days prior to parturition or upon recognizing that a mare is or has been grazing endophyte-infected fescue. (2) Remove mare from endophyte-infected pasture or hay as soon as possible and treat for agalactia. (3) Attend parturition, the mare is at an increased risk of dystocia; close monitoring and assistance for mare during parturition.

- Neonate: supportive care for the dysmature, immunocompromised foal.

Patient Monitoring

- Monitor mammary gland development in late gestation.
- Transrectal U/S for placental thickening and edema.

Prevention/Avoidance

Mare

- Remove mares from infected fescue pasture by 300-days gestation.
- If mares cannot be removed from pasture, treat mares with domperidone during the last 15 to 30 days of gestation.
- Monitor mammary gland development.
- Attend parturition to provide assistance, if needed.

Fetus

- Remove dam from infected pasture.
- Attend parturition to provide assistance, as needed.
- Prepare to provide neonatal emergency and critical care.
- Postpartum, supplement neonate with IgGs, IV plasma (Ig), and appropriate nutrients.

Pasture

- Test forage and seed samples to ascertain toxins, their extent in affected pastures.
- Burn fields and replant with uninfected fescue or other pasture grass.
- Dilution of infected pasture with legumes (red or white clover), or supplement mares with alfalfa hay.
- Minimize infection rate by frequent mowing, as the endophyte concentrates near the flowering seed head.

Expected Course and Prognosis

- Prognosis for mare and foal is excellent if mare is removed from infected fescue by 300-days gestation and/or treated appropriately.
- Gestational age of more than 330 days.
- Possible interference with nidation (controversial).

Synonyms

- Mycotoxicosis
- Agalactia

Abbreviations

ACTH   adrenocorticotropic hormone
CRH   corticotrophin-releasing hormone
FPT   failure of passive transfer
GI   gastrointestinal
IM   intramuscular
IV   intravenous
IgG   immunoglobulin G
P4   progesterone
PO   per os (by mouth)
RFM   retained fetal membranes
U/S   ultrasound, ultrasonography

See Also

- Toxinogenic fungi
- Tall fescue
- Pregnancy
- Dopamine
- Domperidone
- Agalactia

Suggested Reading

Blodgett DJ. 2001. Fescue toxicosis. *Vet Clin NA: Eq Pract*; 17(3): 567–577.

Cross DL, Redmond LM, Strickland JR. 1995. Equine fescue toxicosis: signs and solutions. *J An Sci* 73: 899–908.

Green EM, Loch WE, Messer NT. 1991. Maternal and fetal effects of endophyte fungus-infected fescue. *Proc AAEP* 37: 29–44.

Lane W. 2005. Endophytes in Common Forages. *Proc NAVC*, 319.

Author: Karen E. Wolfsdorf

chapter 30

Fetal Sexing, Early

DEFINITION/OVERVIEW

- Gender diagnosed by U/S examination of external genitalia, primarily GT location.
- Inaccurate before Day 60 of gestation.

ETIOLOGY/PATHOPHYISOLOGY

Systems Affected

Reproductive

SIGNALMENT/HISTORY

Risk Factors

- Fetal gender determination requires a deep transrectal examination, involving inherent risk (an extended examination increases the potential for a rectal tear).
- The U/S examination itself causes minimal risk to both mare and fetus.

CLINICAL FEATURES

- The GT is the embryonic precursor to the penis in the male and the clitoris in the female fetus.
- GT location is between the rear legs prior to Day 50 after ovulation.
- Its location is relative to surrounding fetal structures (i.e., UC, rear legs, tail) changes as the fetus grows rapidly.
- After Day 60, the GT is located immediately caudal to the UC in male fetuses and under the tail in female fetuses (Fig. 30.1).
- Ability to determine gender by U/S is dependent upon fetal accessibility, which becomes more difficult as the fetus ages and becomes located deeper within the abdomen. The transabdominal approach for U/S is useful after 100 days' gestation.

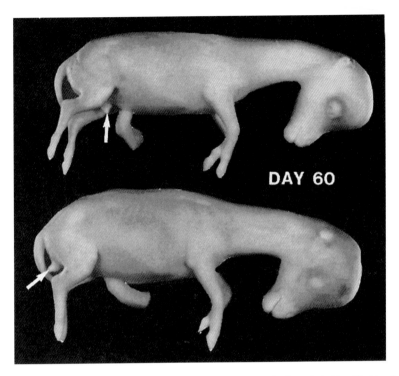

DAY 60

■ **Figure 30.1** Day 60 male (*top*) and female (*bottom*) fetuses. Genital tubercule is identified by the arrow. From Ginther OJ. 1995. *Ultrasonic Imaging and Animal Reproduction: Horses.* Cross Plains, WI: Equiservices Publishing; 236–246. Used with permission.

 DIAGNOSTICS

- In the younger fetus (less than approximately 80 days), the ultrasonic appearance of the GT is similar in male and female fetuses. It appears as a bilobed, hyperechogenic structure, protruding from the surface of the fetus.
- Gender determination is made by location of and not the ultrasonic appearance of the GT.
- Accuracy is high because each fetus has its own means of double checking/confirmation. The GT is always in one of two locations (caudal to the umbilical cord or under the tail near the anus) and its absence can be confirmed in the opposite position.
- As the fetus ages, the ultrasonic appearance of the penis changes, becoming trilobular and then circular with a hyperechogenic core. The penis may be pendulous or held close to the body wall.
- In the older female fetus, the ultrasonic appearance of the clitoris becomes trilobular, continues to protrude from the perineal region, and the labia can be demarcated.
- The anus may also protrude under the tail and must not be mistaken for the GT.
- The mammary gland can be seen as a hyperechogenic triangle between the rear limbs with identifiable teats in the older fetus.

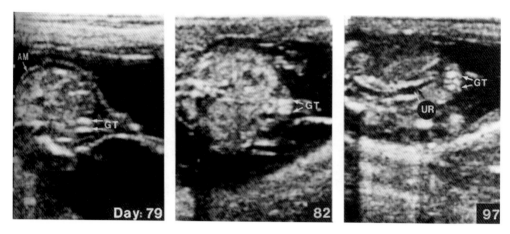

■ **Figure 30.2** Ultrasonic appearance of the genital tubercle in male fetuses on Days 79, 82, and 97. The genital tubercle is bilobed and hyperechogenic on Day 79. The appearance of the Day 82 genital tubercle is tri-lobed, as is the Day 97. AM, amnion; UR, urachus.
From Ginther OJ. 1995. *Ultrasonic Imaging and Animal Reproduction: Horses*. Cross Plains, WI: Equiservices Publishing; 236–246. Used with permission.

- The fetal ovaries appear homogeneous with a characteristic circular echo and may be identified from Day 100 to 134 of gestation.

Imaging

- Real time transrectal U/S is used earlier in gestation. A high quality machine is required.
- A 5.0-MHz transducer is useful for the transrectal examination. A 3.5-MHz transducer (probe) may be helpful for the transabdominal examination (Fig. 30.2).
- Transabdominal U/S can be used in later gestation when the fetus is no longer accessible transrectally, or after Day 60 in miniature horses.

Other Diagnostic Points

- Knowledge of normal ultrasonic fetal anatomy is essential.
- An understanding of ultrasound principles and artifacts is important.
- A thorough examination of the fetus is made, concentrating on the area between the umbilical cord and the tail.
- The GT is always located at one position (caudal to the umbilical cord or under the tail) and not in the other. It is essential to view both positions to determine gender with a high degree of accuracy.
- Cross-sectional views are useful to identify the GT. Frontal views help confirm location of the GT relative to surrounding structures and make mammary gland identification easier.

Pathological Findings

- Fetal abnormalities can be identified while determining fetal sex. This is easier early in gestation when the entire fetus can easily be examined.

COMMENTS

Client Education

- Accuracy is dependent upon the experience of the U/S operator, the demeanor of the mare, and the position of the fetus. An expected accuracy level can be determined for each examination.
- Knowledge of fetal gender may affect appraisal or insurance values, sale consignments, mating lists, sale of the mare or her offspring, or purchase decisions.

Patient Monitoring

Monitor the mare within the hours immediately after an examination for evidence of discomfort or colic; potential for a rectal tear is low, but nonetheless merits the client's observation.

Synonyms

- Fetal Sexing
- Fetal Gender Determination

Abbreviations

GT   genital tubercle
TRP   transrectal palpation
UC   umbilical cord
U/S   ultrasound, ultrasonography

See Also

- Equine Fetal Gender Determination (focus on mid to late gestation)
- Ultrasound assessment of feto-placental well-being, mid to late gestation

Suggested Reading

Curran S, Ginther OJ. 1989. Ultrasonic diagnosis of Equine fetal sex by location of the genital tubercle. *J Eq Vet Sci* 9(2): 77–83.
Equiservices Publishing Video: Fetal Gender Determination in Cattle & Horses.
Ginther OJ. 1995. *Ultrasonic Imaging and Animal Reproduction: Horses.* Cross Plains, WI: Equiservices Publishing; 236–246.
Renaudin CD, Gillis CL, Tarantal AF. 1999. Transabdominal ultrasonographic determination of fetal gender in the horse during mid-gestation. *Eq Vet J* 31(6): 483–487.

Author: Sandy Curran

chapter 31

Foal Heat/Postpartum Breeding

 ## DEFINITION/OVERVIEW

- Foal heat is the name given to the first estrus following parturition. It occurs anytime between 2 and 20 days postpartum.
- Postpartum or foal heat breeding is the breeding that occurs on the first estrus within the first 20 days postpartum.
- Uterine involution begins immediately following expulsion of the foal and continues for up to 45 days postpartum.
- Involution is demonstrated by a decrease in uterine size, elimination of fluid, maintenance of good tone, and regeneration of the endometrium.
- From existing information, the endometrium may be regenerated sufficiently to maintain a pregnancy by day 15 in most, but not all, mares. Therefore, the later postpartum the heat occurs, the better the probability of conception and subsequent pregnancy maintenance.
- Factors aiding in initiation of the first cycle postpartum:
  - With the end of placental function (discarding of fetal membranes soon postpartum), the mare experiences a rapid withdrawal of progestogens that dominated the hypothalamus and pituitary during gestation. Hypothalamic activity can resurge, and with that, the production of GnRH.
  - GnRH acts at the pituitary to cause production and release of FSH. FSH stimulates follicular development on the ovary and initiates the feedback of estradiol on the hypothalamus and pituitary.

 ## ETIOLOGY/PATHOPHYSIOLOGY

The mare exhibits normal signs of behavioral estrus or has detectable indicators of follicular development and changes characteristic of estrus occurring in the uterus and cervix.

Systems Affected

- Reproductive
- Endocrine

SIGNALMENT/HISTORY

- Mare is within 20 days postpartum and is demonstrating signs of estrus.
- It is uncommon for a mare not to have a postpartum heat, although she may not exhibit obvious signs of estrus.
- Typical foal heat mare behavior: her tail will be raised, clitoris exposed periodically (winking), frequent urinations, rear legs spread, ears forward when presented to a stallion, leans or moves toward a stallion, and resists moving away from a stallion when one is nearby.
- The mare also may not demonstrate any outward signs of estrus, but if examined (TRP and U/S) will have follicular development and other changes of the reproductive tract characteristic of estrus.

CLINICAL FEATURES

TRP and U/S

- Follicular size and appearance; may visualize the development of a "point" in the U/S image of the follicular fluid. The latter is the site through which ovulation will occur (the ovulation fossa), at the time of ovulation.
- U/S is an excellent tool to evaluate follicular development and the presence and degree of endometrial edema.
- The presence or absence of luminal fluid.
- TRP of the genital tract can help confirm postpartum estrus in mares that fail to exhibit external signs (e.g., often due to maternal instinct, protection of her foal, from things perceived as external threats).
- Similarly, a young, maiden mare (not postpartum) may not exhibit signs of estrus if she is intimidated by the stallion (his touch, vocalizations, aggression).

COMMENTS

Client Education

- Owners need to be aware that all mares do not exhibit signs of foal heat.
- Not all mares are good or suitable candidates for breeding 9 days postpartum.

Patient Monitoring

- Careful ovarian examination at the time of breeding. Presence of more than one dominant follicle increases the need for serial TRP and U/S evaluations to rule-out double ovulations; places the mare at an increased risk of twinning.
- If more than one ovulation has been detected, the early pregnancy check (at 15–16 days post-ovulation) is critical to monitor the uterus for the presence of twins and

to assist in early reduction (bicornual versus unicornual location of twin yolk sacs). Unicornual twins, if from synchronous ovulations, usually reduce without interference. Bicornual twins can be reduced early by pinch reduction.

- At an early postpartum check, a lymphatic cyst map can be drawn on a mare's palpation record (draw the shape of the uterine body and two horns and locate structures within it).
- Creation of a cyst map is highly recommended for all mare records at the first examination of the season or when presented for breeding (e.g., barren, foaling, maiden).
  - Record size and location of all cysts at the first TRP and U/S examination pre-breeding. Lymphatic cysts and the yolk sac of early pregnancy can be of similar size and shape and cannot be distinguished solely by U/S at a single, early pregnancy check.
  - Cysts are either slow growing or do not change their diameter at all within a breeding season. The normal, early conceptus, in contrast, increases its diameter significantly even within a 48-hour period between examinations.
  - Identify the location and relative size of lymphatic cysts that may be present within the uterine lumen.
  - The "map" serves as a guide of cystic structures present before breeding.
  - Makes it easier to rule-in or out what is a pregnancy and what is a cyst, at the earliest pregnancy check.
  - Avoid crushing the yolk sac of a pregnancy and leaving a cyst at a time of gestation prior to the embryo being evident within the yolk sac.
  - Determine pregnancy following breeding or insemination by TRP and U/S.

Possible Complications

- RFM (not passed/dropped for more than 3 hours postpartum).
- Poor or delayed uterine involution:
  - Determined by uterine horn size at TRP; remains too large at an 8-day postpartum check (the previously gravid horn is more than 15 cm diameter).
  - Uterine tone is insufficient, an indicator of delayed involution.
  - Lochia, or other fluid, remains in the uterine lumen (normal only to 6 days postpartum).
- Poor uterine tone, accumulation of large amounts of luminal fluid.
- Systemically ill mare in the peripartal period.
- Mares that suffered a dystocia or were assisted at parturition (increases likelihood of uterine contamination), increases likelihood of early conceptus loss.
- Dystocia, assistance rendered during delivery, RFM: all should preclude the mare being bred at her foal heat. Allow additional time for involution and clearance of contaminants that may have been introduced into the uterine lumen during procedures.
- Historical indicators that the uterine environment might have been compromised with the previous gestation and preclude breeding at foal heat:
  - Grossly abnormal placenta. Always examine the placenta once it has passed.

- A mare with compromised lactation. Another indicator that the hormonal milieu during late gestation may have been abnormal.
- Birth of a sick, weak foal (may reflect a previously hostile intrauterine environment).
- Natural service of mares, not exhibiting estrus (insufficient or negative, non-receptive behavior towards the stallion), can be dangerous to the stallion, mare, or bystanders.

Synonyms

Foal heat

Abbreviations

FSH	follicle stimulating hormone
GnRH	gonadotropin-releasing hormone
RFM	retained fetal membranes, retained placenta
TRP	transrectal palpation
U/S	ultrasound, ultrasonography

See Also

- Dystocia
- Mammary gland (normal, mastitis, lactation)
- Parturition
- Parturition induction
- Postpartum care, mare and foal
- Postpartum metritis
- Retained fetal membranes

Suggested Reading

Loy RG. 1980. Characteristics of postpartum reproduction in mares. *Vet Clin Sci N Amer Large Anim Prac* 2: 345–358.

Matthews P, Samper JC. 2009. Breeding the postpartum mare. In: *Equine Breeding Management and Artificial Insemination*, 2nd ed. Samper JC (ed). Philadelphia: Saunders Elsevier; 277–279.

Shideler RK, McChesney AE, Squires EL, et al. 1987. Effect of uterine lavage on clinical and laboratory parameters in postpartum mares. *Equine Pract* 9: 20–26.

Author: Walter R. Threlfall

chapter 32

High-Risk Pregnancy

DEFINITION/OVERVIEW

Pregnancy prone to early termination, delivery of a compromised foal, or prolongation by virtue of maternal, fetal, or placental abnormalities (structure or function).

ETIOLOGY/PATHOPHYSIOLOGY

- Those circumstances that raise concerns about premature initiation of labor, or prolonged gestation.
- The specific conditions associated with high-risk pregnancies are similar to those that raise concerns about fetal stress, distress, or viability and include the following:

Preexisting Maternal Disease

- Equine Cushing's-like disease
- Laminitis
- Chronic, moderate to severe endometrial inflammation, endometrial periglandular fibrosis, or endometrial cysts leading to impaired placental function.

Gestational Maternal Conditions

- Malnutrition
- Colic
- Endotoxemia
- Hyperlipidemia
- Prepubic tendon rupture
- Uterine torsion
- Dystocia
- Ovarian granulosa cell tumor
- Laminitis
- Musculoskeletal disease
- Exposure to ergopeptine alkaloids in endophyte-infected fescue or ergotized grasses or grains.
- Exposure to other xenobiotics.
- Exposure to abortigenic infections, especially EHV and bacterial contaminants on ETC setae.

Placental Conditions

- Placentitis
- Placental insufficiency
- Umbilical cord torsion or torsion of the amnion
- Placental separation
- Hydrops of fetal membranes
- MRLS

Fetal Conditions

- Twins (often resulting in placental insufficiency for one or both twins)
- Fetal abnormalities, such as hydrocephalus
- Delayed fetal development for gestational age; IUGR
- Fetal trauma

Pathophysiology

Depending on the specific circumstances, the pathophysiological mechanisms involved in high risk pregnancies are similar to those associated with fetal stress and distress and can involve one or more of the following:

- Maternal systemic disease; placental infection, insufficiency, torsion, or separation; and fetal abnormalities, all of which impede efficient fetal gas exchange and nutrient transfer.
- The fetus initially responds physiologically (i.e., stress) to these alterations in oxygenation and nutrient supply and might initiate the cascade of events leading to parturition at a time point in gestation when extrauterine survival is unlikely.
- In other instances of placental insufficiency, fetal growth and development are slowed, resulting in IUGR and, potentially, early termination of gestation.
- In equine fescue toxicosis, maternal prolactin concentrations are decreased and late-gestational 5α-pregnane secretion by the uterofetoplacental unit is impaired, resulting in prolonged gestation and fetal over-maturity at the time of parturition.

Systems Affected

- Maternal: Reproductive and other organ systems, depending on the nature of maternal systemic disease and complications (e.g., dystocia, RFM).
- Fetal: All organ systems.

 SIGNALMENT/HISTORY

Risk Factors

- May be nonspecific.
- Thoroughbreds, Standardbreds, draft mares, and related breeds are predisposed to twinning.

- Mares more than 15 years of age.
- American Miniature Horse mares.
- Other organ system involvement depends on the presence of placentitis, stage of gestation, presence of maternal disease, infection, or toxemia.
- Hyperlipemia is of special concern for over-nourished (highly conditioned, obese) American Miniature Horses, ponies, and donkeys.
- Same as those listed under Etiology/Pathophysiology.

Preexisting Maternal Disease

- Equine Cushing's-like disease.
- Laminitis
- Chronic, moderate to severe endometrial inflammation, endometrial periglandular fibrosis, or endometrial cysts, leading to impaired placental function.

Gestational Maternal Conditions

- Malnutrition
- Colic
- Endotoxemia
- Hyperlipemia
- Body wall tears/prepubic tendon rupture
- Uterine torsion
- Dystocia
- Ovarian granulosa cell tumor
- Laminitis
- Musculoskeletal disease
- Exposure to ergopeptine alkaloids in endophyte-infected fescue or ergotized grasses or grains.
- Exposure to other xenobiotics.
- Exposure to abortigenic infections, especially EHV and bacterial contaminants on ETC setae.

Placental Conditions

- Placentitis
- Placental insufficiency
- Umbilical cord torsion or torsion of the amnion.
- Placental separation
- Hydrops of fetal membranes.
- MRLS

Fetal Conditions

- Twins (often resulting in placental insufficiency for one or both twins).
- Fetal abnormalities, such as hydrocephalus.
- Delayed fetal development for gestational age; IUGR.
- Fetal trauma

Historical Findings

One or more of the following:

- Maternal disease during gestation, such as colic, hyperlipemia, body wall or prepubic tendon rupture, uterine torsion, etc.
- Mucoid, hemorrhagic, serosanguineous, or purulent vulvar discharge.
- Premature udder development and dripping of milk.
- Complete lack of late-gestational udder development.
- Previous examination indicating placentitis or fetal compromise.
- Previous abortion, high-risk pregnancy, or dystocia.
- History of delivering a small, dysmature, septicemic, or congenitally malformed foal.
- Preexisting maternal disease at conception, such as laminitis, equine Cushing's-like disease, endometrial inflammation, fibrosis or cysts.
- Previous exposure to endophyte-infected fescue or ergotized grasses or grains.
- Previous exposure to abortigenic xenobiotics or infections.

CLINICAL FEATURES

Maternal and Placental Signs

- Anorexia, fever, or other signs of concurrent, systemic disease.
- Abdominal discomfort.
- Mucoid, mucopurulent, hemorrhagic, serosanguineous, or purulent vulvar discharge.
- Premature udder development and dripping of milk (except in cases of fescue toxicosis where there is little or no udder development).
- Premature placental separation (red bag).
- Placentitis, placental separation, or hydrops of fetal membranes by transrectal or transabdominal U/S.
- Excessive abdominal distention.
- Excessive swelling along the ventral midline and evidence of body wall weakening or rupture by palpation or transabdominal U/S (Figs. 32.1a and b).
- Alterations in maternal circulating levels of progestins, estrogens, or relaxin reflecting changes in fetal well-being or placental function.

Fetal Signs

- The only clinical sign of fetal stress or distress might be the premature delivery of a live or dead foal or the late delivery of a severely compromised foal, unable to stand and suckle (Fig. 32.2).
- Fetal hyperactivity or inactivity (concurrent with maternal or placental abnormalities) may suggest a less-than-ideal fetal environment or fetal compromise.
- Can be assessed by visual inspection or by TRP of the mare.
- Alterations in the following parameters assessed using transrectal or transabdominal U/S (also see Diagnostics):

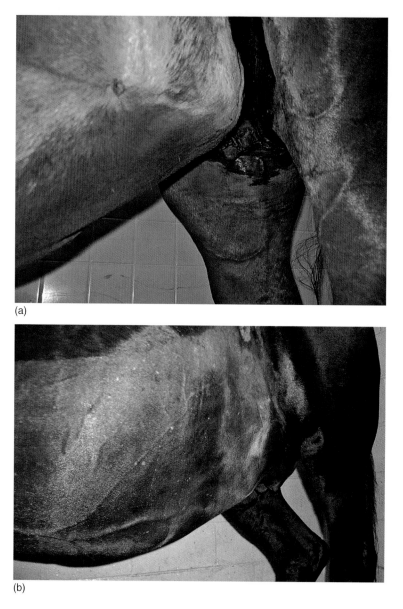

(a)

(b)

■ **Figure 32.1** *A, B,* These mares have body wall tears or ruptures that may affect management of their pregnancies and with potential adverse effects on fetal well-being.
Images courtesy of D. Volkmann.

- Fetal activity and normal muscle tone at less than 330 days of gestation: the normal FHR is less than or equal to 100 bpm after activity and at least 60 bpm at rest.
- Fetal activity and normal muscle tone at more than 330 days of gestation: the normal FHR is at least 50 bpm at rest and difference between resting and active rates is less than or equal to 40 bpm.

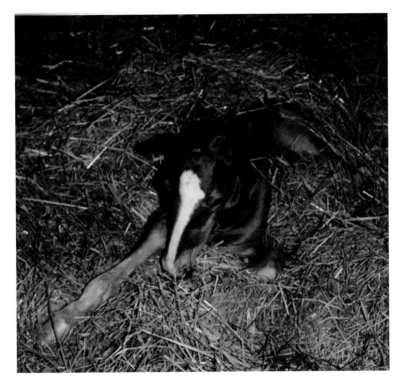

■ **Figure 32.2** Dysmature neonate with floppy ears (dysmature cartilage) delivered from a mare that had ruptured her prepubic tendon. It was weak, unable to rise unassisted.
Image courtesy of C. L. Carleton.

- Normal fetal heart rhythm, as assessed by U/S or ECG.
- Normal fetal breathing movements
- Increased amounts of amniotic fluid may reflect hydrops amnion (hydramnios); diminished amounts indicate fetal distress and longstanding, chronic hypoxia.
- Sudden changes in the echogenicity of the amniotic fluid in late gestation can indicate meconium expulsion and fetal distress.
- Appropriately sized fetus for gestational stage
- Fetal aortic diameter:
  - At 300 days of gestation approximately 2.1 cm.
  - At 330 days of gestation, 2.7 cm.
  - Record length and width of fetal orbit during the examination (relationship to stage of gestation).

Placental Health

- Normal uteroplacental thickness, by transabdominal U/S: 12.6 ± 3.3 mm.
  - Uteroplacental thickness greater than 19.2 mm is indicative of placentitis.
- Normal uteroplacental thickness by transrectal U/S:
  - Less than or equal to 8 mm at 271 to 300 days of gestation.

- Less than or equal to 10 mm at 300 to 330 days of gestation.
- Less than or equal to 12 mm at more than 330 days of gestation.
- Look for evidence of absence or very small areas of uteroplacental discontinuity.
- Increased echogenicity of the allantoic fluid more than 44 days prior to the mare's anticipated foaling date may reflect fetal distress; floating particulate matter normally gets gradually larger 10 to 36 days prior to foaling; sudden increases in the echogenicity of the allantoic fluid can be indicative of fetal or placental abnormalities.
- The mean vertical distance of the allantoic fluid in uncomplicated pregnancies from less than 300 days gestation to term is generally 19 ± 9 mm.

DIFFERENTIAL DIAGNOSIS

- Normal, uncomplicated, pregnancy with an active, normal fetus as assessed by TRP, transrectal or transabdominal U/S, or various laboratory tests.

DIAGNOSTICS

Maternal Assessment

- Complete physical examination
- CBC with differential, as well as serum biochemical data to determine inflammatory or stress leukocyte response, as well as other organ system involvement.
- ELISA or RIA analyses for maternal progesterone may be useful if fewer than 80 days of gestation (normal levels vary from greater than 1 to greater than 4 ng/mL, depending on the reference laboratory). At more than 100 days gestation, RIA detects both progesterone (very low if more than 150 days) and cross-reacting 5α-pregnanes of uterofetoplacental origin. Acceptable levels of progestins, including 5α-pregnanes, vary with stage of gestation and the laboratory used. Decreased maternal 5α-pregnane concentrations during late gestation are associated with fescue toxicosis and ergotism and are reflected in RIA analyses for progestins.
- Maternal estrogen concentrations can reflect fetal estrogen production and viability, especially conjugated estrogens (e.g., estrone sulfate).
- Decreased maternal relaxin concentration is thought to be associated with abnormal placental function.
- Decreased maternal prolactin secretion during late gestation is associated with fescue toxicosis and ergotism.
- There are anecdotal reports of lower T_3/T_4 levels in mares with a history of conception failure, EED, high-risk pregnancies, or abortion. The significance of low T_4 levels is unknown and somewhat controversial.
- Feed or environmental analyses might be indicated for specific xenobiotics, ergopeptine alkaloids, phytoestrogens, heavy metals, or fescue endophyte (*Neotyphodium coenophialum*).

Fetal Assessment

- Transrectal and transabdominal U/S can be useful in diagnosing twins; assessing fetal stress, distress, or viability; monitoring fetal development; evaluating placental health; and diagnosing other gestational abnormalities (e.g., hydrops of fetal membranes).
- In predisposed individuals (i.e., barren, older mares, or mares with history of high-risk pregnancy, placentitis, abortion, EED, conception failure, or endometritis), transrectal or transabdominal U/S should be performed on a routine basis during the entire pregnancy to assess fetal stress and viability.
- Confirmation of pregnancy and diagnosis of twins should be performed any time serious, maternal disease occurs or surgical intervention is considered for a mare bred within the last 11 months.
- Twin pregnancy can be confirmed by identifying two fetuses (easier by transrectal U/S when gestational age is less than 90 days) or ruled out by the presence of a nonpregnant uterine horn (transabdominal U/S during late gestation).
- Fetal stress, distress, or viability can be determined best by transabdominal U/S during late gestation. View the fetus in both active and resting states for at least 30 minutes. Note abnormal fetal presentation and position.
- Fetal ECG has been used to detect twins and to assess fetal viability and distress, but largely has been replaced by transabdominal U/S with ECG capabilities.
- Although it is a higher-risk technique in horses than in humans, U/S-guided amniocentesis or allantocentesis and analysis of the collected fluids might become a future means to assess fetal karyotype, pulmonary maturity, and to measure fetal proteins.
- Samples might reveal bacteria, meconium, or inflammatory cells.
- After the 2001 outbreak, MRLS research is underway to develop fetal catheterization techniques and other methods of prepartum evaluation.

Placental Assessment

- Evaluation of placental thickness, allantoic or amniotic fluid echogenicity and quantity.
- Alterations in fetal and placental parameters assessed using transrectal or transabdominal U/S (see Clinical Features).

Pathological Findings

- Evidence of villous atrophy or hypoplasia on the chorionic surface of the fetal membranes.
- Thickening and edema of the chorioallantois or allantochorion (Fig. 32.3).
- An endometrial biopsy can demonstrate the presence of moderate to severe, chronic endometritis, endometrial periglandular fibrosis with decreased normal glandular architecture, or lymphatic lacunae (see EED).

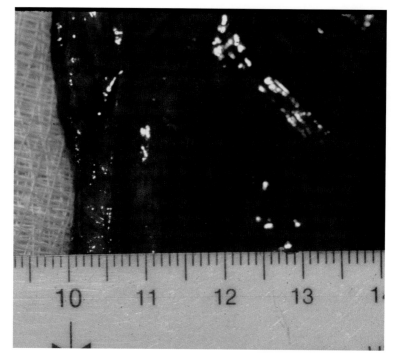

■ **Figure 32.3** Edematous and grossly thickened chorioallantois.
Image courtesy of C. L. Carleton.

 THERAPEUTICS

Drug(s) of Choice

- See recommendations for specific conditions associated with high-risk pregnancies, such as dystocia, fescue toxicosis, induction of parturition, prepubic tendon rupture, RFM, hydrops, and so on.

Altrenogest

- Depending on clinical circumstances, risk factors, and clinician preferences, altrenogest administration can start at various stages of pregnancy, continue until near term or at parturition, be used for only short periods (based on maternal progestin concentrations), or be decreased over time or discontinued abruptly.
- History of endometritis/previously aborted mare (without active infectious component) or mare with fibrosis: 0.044 to 0.088 mg/kg PO daily; commence 2 to 3 days after ovulation or upon diagnosis of pregnancy; continue to at least 100 days gestation; can decrease the dose over 14 days at the end of the treatment period (common practice: halve calculated dose for 1 week prior to stopping treatment or reassessment of cervical tone before treatment is stopped).

- Endotoxic/gram-negative septicemic mare less than 80 days of gestation: 0.088 mg/kg PO daily, initially, then 0.044 mg/kg daily until at least 100 days' gestation; can decrease dose over 14 days at the end of the treatment period.
- To prevent premature parturition by promoting uterine quiescence, following diagnosis of maternal disease, placentitis, or late-gestational twins: 0.088 mg/kg PO daily, initially, then 0.044 mg/kg daily.
- Near term, discontinue altrenogest 7 to 14 days before expected foaling date, unless otherwise indicated by assessment of fetal maturity/viability, question regarding accuracy of gestational age, or clinician preference.

Antibiotic or Antibacterial Therapy

- Indicated when there is a diagnosis of, or potential for diagnosis of, maternal, placental, or fetal infection.
- The specific antibiotics used depend on clinical circumstances, suspect organisms, therapeutic goals, clinician preferences and, potentially, financial considerations.

Domperidone

- Indicated for agalactia and late-gestational fetal maturation.
- When fescue toxicosis is diagnosed or when there is confirmation of prolonged gestation, based on breeding records: 1.1 mg/kg PO daily.
- Continue domperidone to parturition, with anticipated normal mammary development and lactation.

Flunixin meglumine

- Prophylaxis if endotoxin release is anticipated: 0.25 mg/kg IM (potential for injection reactions) or, preferably, IV or PO (once daily to QID).
- Dose can be doubled for analgesia and anti-inflammatory effect.
- May help decrease premature uterine contractions.

Pentoxifylline

- Anti-inflammatory and anti-cytokine effects, especially during endotoxemia.
- Dosing regimen varies from 4.4 mg/kg PO every 8 hours for laminitis, to 8.5 mg/kg PO twice daily to reduce cytokine effects in endotoxemia.

Precautions/Interactions

Altrenogest

- Only to prevent abortion or premature delivery in confirmed pregnancies, where a live fetus is present in utero.
- Not recommended to prevent spontaneous, infectious abortion other than those caused by placentitis and endotoxemia.
- Initially, weekly monitoring of fetal viability: retention of dead fetuses has been reported to result from continued treatment with supplemental progestins.

- Altrenogest is absorbed across skin: wear nitrile or rubber gloves and wash hands.
- Dependent on the etiology of the high-risk pregnancy, progestin supplementation might be unsuccessful.

Antibiotic or Antibacterial Therapy

- Depends on the specific drug.
- Some are potentially teratogenic (cause birth defects).

Domperidone

- Premature lactation; loss of colostrum: can generally be addressed by adjusting the treatment regimen.

Flunixin meglumine

- Can cause gastric ulcers and kidney problems.

Pentoxifylline

- Potentially, adverse GI, CNS and cardiovascular effects.

Alternative Drugs

- Injectable progesterone (150–500 mg/day, oil base) can be administered IM daily, instead of the oral formulation. Variations, contraindications, and precautions are similar to those associated with altrenogest.
- Other injectable and implantable progestin preparations are available commercially for use in other species. Any use in horses of these products is off-label, and little scientific data are available regarding their efficacy.
- Newer, repository forms of progesterone are occasionally introduced; however, some evidence of efficacy should be provided prior to use.
- See recommendations for specific conditions, such as dystocia, fescue toxicosis, high-risk pregnancy, induction of parturition, prepubic tendon rupture, RFM, hydrops, and so on.
- Phenybutazone can be used as an alternative to flunixin meglumine. Variations, contraindications, and precautions are similar to those associated with flunixin meglumine.
- T_4 supplementation has been successful (anecdotally) for treating mares with histories of subfertility and high-risk pregnancy. Its use remains controversial, however, and it is considered deleterious by some clinicians.
- Medications for other maternal diseases: potential risks are dependent on the specific drug.

Appropriate Health Care

Depending on the circumstances, monitoring/managing high-risk pregnancies (especially close to anticipated foaling date), including the prolonged examination times required for complete serial transabdominal fetal assessments, is best performed at a facility prepared to manage these types of pregnancies, especially if distress is severe and parturition (induction or C-section) is imminent.

- Early diagnosis of at-risk pregnancies is essential for successful treatment. The impact of maternal disease on fetal and placental health cannot be underestimated.
- With a maternal body wall tear, fetal/foal survival is improved when circumstances allow conservative management without induction of parturition or an elective C-section.
- With prolonged fetal stress or distress, maintenance of pregnancy (while attempting to treat the cause of fetal compromise) must be balanced with the need to induce parturition (with or without C-section), if that becomes necessary to stabilize the mare's health.
- Parturition requires close supervision in cases of fetal stress and distress. The neonatal foal will likely require intensive treatment.
- Individual circumstances and their sequelae will require consideration to determine nature and timing of treatment:
  - Physical examination findings.
  - CBC and biochemistry profile results.
  - Stage of gestation
  - Nature of maternal disease.
  - Hydrops of fetal membranes.
  - Evidence of fetal stress, distress, or impending demise.
  - Maternal mammary development.
  - Maternal health risks or impending maternal demise.
  - Occurrence of complications such as dystocia, RFM, FPT, or fetal dysmaturity, with or without septicemia.
  - Financial considerations; relative value of mare and foal.
  - Refer to individual topics for treatment recommendations.

Nursing Care

- Depending on the nature of the maternal disease, the occurrence of fetal stress or distress, and the necessity for surgical intervention, intensive nursing care might very well be required for the neonatal foal and the mare.
- Special attention should be given to the possibility of FPT in the neonate, which would require that the foal receive a plasma transfusion.

Diet

- Feed the mare an adequate, late-gestational diet with proper levels of energy, protein, vitamins, and minerals, unless contraindicated by concurrent maternal disease.

Activity

- For most cases, exercise will be somewhat limited and supervised.
- Body wall tears, prepubic tendon rupture, laminitis, or fetal hydrops may necessitate severe restrictions on or complete elimination of exercise.

Surgical Considerations

- C-section may be indicated when vaginal delivery is not possible or in dystocias not amenable to resolution by manipulation alone.
- Surgical intervention might be indicated for future repair of anatomical defects predisposing mares to endometritis and placentitis.
- Depending on the specific circumstances, certain future diagnostic and therapeutic procedures might also involve some surgical interventions in the mare or the foal.

 COMMENTS

Client Education

- Clients should be aware that early diagnosis is essential for fetal survival.
- Predisposing conditions compromising fetal well-being must be corrected or managed for a successful outcome.
- Induction of parturition and C-section are not without risk to the mare and foal.

Patient Monitoring

- Mare and fetus need frequent monitoring until termination of pregnancy.
- Specific monitoring depends on the therapy undertaken, nature of the maternal or fetal disease, and complications that might develop.
- Mares should be carefully monitored for premature or inadequate udder development.
- Within 24 hours of delivery, the foal should be assessed and, if necessary, appropriately treated for FPT.
- Vaginal speculum examination and uterine cytology and culture (as indicated) can be performed 7 to 10 days postpartum or sooner, depending on the circumstances.
- Endometrial biopsy may be indicated as part of the postpartum examination as a prognostic tool for future reproduction.
- Appropriate therapeutic steps should be taken based on these findings.

Prevention/Avoidance

- Early recognition of at-risk mares and potential high-risk pregnancies.
- Correction of perineal conformation to prevent placentitis.
- Management of preexisting endometritis before breeding.
- Early monitoring of mares with a history of fetal stress, distress, or viability concerns.
- Complete breeding records, especially for recognition of double ovulations, early diagnosis of twins (at less than 25 days; ideally, days 14 to 15) and selective embryonic or fetal reduction.
- Careful monitoring of pregnant mares for vaginal discharge and premature mammary secretion.

- Removal of pregnant mares from fescue pasture or ergotized grasses or grains during last trimester (minimum of 30 days prepartum).
- Use ET procedures with mares predisposed to EED or high-risk pregnancies.
- Avoid breeding or using ET procedures in mares that have produced multiple stressed, distressed, or dead foals due to congenital and potentially inheritable conditions.
- Prudent use of medications in pregnant mares.
- Avoid exposure to known toxicants.
- Management of ETCs for prevention of MRLS.
- If history of abortion, evidence of moderate to severe endometritis or fibrosis, evaluate and treat the mare prebreeding.

Possible Complications

- Abortion, dystocia, RFM, endometritis, metritis, laminitis, septicemia, reproductive tract trauma, or impaired fertility, which will all affect the mare's well-being and reproductive value.
- Fetal stress or distress
- Fetal death
- Stillbirth
- Neonatal death
- Neonatal foals from high-risk pregnancies have potentially been compromised during gestation and are more likely to be dysmature, septicemic, and subject to FPT or angular limb deformities than foals from normal pregnancies.

Expected Course and Prognosis

- The ability to prevent and treat the conditions associated with high risk pregnancies has improved dramatically over the last 20 years. However, the successful management of these pregnancies requires rigorous monitoring of the mare, fetus, and neonatal foal. The goal is to address treatable health concerns as soon as possible during the pregnancy and to avoid or minimize challenges to maternal, fetal, and placental health.
- If the predisposing conditions can be treated or managed, pregnancies in which fetal stress has been diagnosed have a guarded prognosis for successful completion.
- If there is evidence of fetal stress progressing to distress, and the distress continues in the face of treatment for the predisposing conditions, fetal viability and maternal health become major concerns. The prognosis for successful completion of gestation under these circumstances is guarded to poor.

Synonyms/Closely Related Conditions

- Abortions, spontaneous infectious and noninfectious
- Fetal stress, distress and viability
- Placental insufficiency
- Twins

Abbreviations

BPM	beats per minute
CBC	complete blood count
CNS	central nervous system
ECG	electrocardiogram
EED	early embryonic death
EHV	equine herpesvirus
ELISA	enzyme-linked immunosorbent assay
ET	embryo transfer
ETC	Eastern tent caterpillar
FHR	fetal heart rate
FPT	failure of passive transfer
GI	gastrointestinal
IM	intramuscularly
IUGR	intrauterine growth retardation
IV	intravenously
MRLS	mare reproductive loss syndrome
PO	per os (by mouth)
QID	four times a day
RIA	radioimmunoassay
RFM	retained fetal membranes, retained placenta
T_3	triiodothyronine
T_4	thyroxine
TRP	transrectal palpation
U/S	ultrasound, ultrasonography

See Also

- Abortion, spontaneous, infectious or noninfectious
- Dystocia
- EED
- Endometrial biopsy
- Endometritis
- ET
- Fetal stress, distress and viability
- Hydrops amnion/allantois
- Induction of parturition
- Placental insufficiency
- Placentitis
- Twins

Suggested Reading

Christensen BW, Troedsson MH, Murchie TA, et al. 2006. Management of a hydrops amnion in a mare resulting in birth of a live foal. *JAVMA* 228(8): 1228–1233.

Evans TJ. 2002. High risk pregnancy. In: *The Five Minute Veterinary Consult—Equine*. Brown CM, Bertone JJ (eds). Philadelphia: Lippincott Williams & Wilkins; 518–519.

Koterba AM, Drummond WH, Kosch PC. 1990. *Equine Clinical Neonatology*. Philadelphia: Lea & Febiger.

Madigan JE. 2003. *Manual of Equine Neonatal Medicine*, 3rd ed. Woodland, CA: Live Oak.

Robinson NE, ed. *Current Therapy in Equine Medicine 5*. Philadelphia: Saunders.

Ross J, Palmer JE, Wilkins PA. 2008. Body wall tears during late pregnancy in mares: 13 cases (1995–2006). *JAVMA* 232(2): 257–261.

Sertich PL. 1999. Fetal ultrasonography. In: *Equine Diagnostic Ultrasound*. Reef VB (ed). Philadelphia: WB Saunders; 425–445.

Youngquist RS, Threlfall WR (eds). 2007. *Current Therapy in Large Animal Theriogenology*, 2nd ed. St. Louis: Elsevier-Saunders.

Author: Tim J. Evans

chapter 33

History Form, Mare

DEFINITION/OVERVIEW

- In order to understand the multitude of aspects that may affect a mare's fertility, it is essential to review the impact of management decisions (vaccinations, anthelmintics, housing, level of performance), breadth of the mare's activities/training, nutrition, exposure to pathogens, transportation, etc., that impact her performance (positively or otherwise).
- All factors should be taken into account when reviewing a mare's reproductive history, including endometrial biopsy category and its interpretation (stage of cycle and season when collected), relationship of uterine culture to cytology and endometrial biopsy findings.

ETIOLOGY/PATHOPHYSIOLOGY

Systems Affected

Reproductive

SIGNALMENT/HISTORY

A comprehensive review of aspects affecting mare health: management (vaccinations, anthelmintic administration), training, nutrition, and so on, as well as a detailed reproductive history in its many aspects, should accompany any routine mare BSE (Fig. 33.1).

Risk Factors

- Age (pubertal, mature, aging, when first bred, age at first foaling)
- Season when evaluated (BSE)
- Breeding status: maiden, foaling, barren, barren by choice.
- Methods of breeding: live cover versus AI (fresh, chilled, frozen semen).
- Foaling history: dystocia, RFM, health of her foals.
- Vulvar conformation
- Aged mares experience fewer ovulations during the ovulatory period. They are also more likely to present with delayed uterine clearance, to have compromised endometrial health (biopsy), and experience a higher rate of EED. They are best bred during the PBS to increase their likelihood of conceiving.

Historical Findings

- Breeding injuries (lacerations, fistula, cervical tears; surgical repairs).
- Prior infections, reports of fluid accumulation before or after breeding.
- Placentitis, high-risk pregnancies.
- Assessment of her lactation, colostrum production, mammary gland evaluation.
- Prior treatments that may impact uterine health (by whom, with what, duration, frequency).
- Prior reports: uterine cultures, cytology, endometrial biopsies.
- Nonreproductive factors that influence reproductive health (lameness, vision, neurologic, etc.).

 CLINICAL FEATURES

- Primary breeding season in the northern hemisphere falls between Feb. 15 (onset of the OBS) through the PBS (June/July).
- The February start of the OBS results from the use of the Universal Birth Date of January 1 that is recorded for equine births occurring within a calendar year. It is primarily employed by particular breeds (usually racing stock). The influence it has on equine breeding practices is not positive, in that breeding activity commences at a time of year when estrous cyclic activity is poorly established (mares still in anestrus or vernal transition).
- Management programs such as artificial lighting, treatment with altrenogest, or progesterone and estradiol combinations coupled with prostaglandin at the end of the progesterone regimen, are meant to assist in establishing estrous cycle activity earlier in the calendar year.

 COMMENTS

- The will to exert influence on the larger horse breeding industry is lacking and practices such as the universal birth date will continue. The OBS terminates by mid to late June, and breeding of all but the oldest and subfertile mares ceases, while the PBS is just getting into full swing.
- Mare fertility, estrous cycles, and body condition are all enhanced by breeding during long days (the PBS), when good pasture is available, and foals are less stressed by winter foaling conditions.
- The point of early breeding is to have mares foaling as early as possible in the following calendar year.
  - Offspring of racing breeds are usually marketed at yearling sales the year after their birth.
  - Earlier born foals are larger, stronger, better developed and able to train and compete in the 2- and 3-year-old races, than foals born in May, June, and so on, against which they will compete.

- Failing to enter the early breeding, early foaling, early training and racing schedule, would result in later born offspring. Because of the potential 5- to 6-month-age differential, late foals (born in May, June and later) are less developed at 2- and 3-year-old competitions.
- That industry practice has a negative impact on management and production practices. Normal horse physiology and husbandry would better be served by breeding during the physiologic breeding season.

Abbreviations

AI   artificial insemination
BSE   breeding soundness examination
EED   early embryonic death
OBS   operational breeding season
PBS   physiologic breeding season
RFM   retained fetal membranes

See Also

- BSE, mare
- Cervical lesions
- Endometrial biopsy
- Endometritis
- Estrus detection, fundamentals
- High-risk pregnancy
- Nutrition, broodmare
- Perineal lacerations/Recto-vaginal fistulas
- Pneumovagina/Pneumouterus
- Retained fetal membranes
- Vaccination program, broodmare
- Vulvar conformation

Suggested Reading

Carleton CL. 2007. Clinical examination of the nonpregnant equine female reproductive tract. In: *Current Therapy in Large Animal Theriogenology*, 2nd ed. Youngquist RS, Threlfall WR (eds). Philadelphia: Saunders; 74–90.

Hinrichs K. 1997. Irregularities of the estrous cycle and ovulation in mares (including seasonal transition). In: *Current Therapy in Large Animal Theriogenology*, 2nd ed. Youngquist RS, Threlfall WR (eds). Philadelphia: Saunders; 144–152.

Jeffcott LB, Rossdale PD, Freestone J, et al. 1982. An assessment of wastage in thoroughbred racing from conception to 4 years of age. *Eq Vet J* 14(3): 185–198.

Jeffcott LB, Whitwell KE. 1973. Twinning as a cause of foetal and neonatal loss in the thoroughbred mare. *J Comp Pathol* 83(1): 91–106.

Author: Carla L. Carleton

Michigan State University
Veterinary Teaching Hospital

MARE HISTORY FORM

Date: Age: Weight, current: kg / lbs

Date purchased: Losing weight

Presenting Complaint: Gaining weight

PART ONE—NONREPRODUCTIVE INFO:

1. GENERAL INFO: *Use Medical Record PE/HX form for recording this info.

2. IDENTIFICATION/INSURANCE INFO:

Note type of identification:

Lip tattoo   Insurance company:

Freeze brand   Neck tattoo   Name of Breed Association:

Microchip (AVID or other?) and #   Registration Number   Cross registration (QH & Paint; Hanoverian & Dutch, etc.)?:

3. MEDICAL MANAGEMENT INFO:

A. Note Vaccine/s

                            Type given & route of administration (5-way [specify], rhino, PHF, WNV, Rabies, etc.) (MLV, killed, attenuated - if known)

                            Date given
                            Date of most recent Coggins

B. Note Anthelmintic/s

                            Type given (Panacur, Ivermectin, etc.)
                            Date given/Frequency of Administration
                            EPM Status (evaluated/treated):

C. Management of Cyclicity (Artificial lighting?)   Maintained under lights to induce earlier estrus?

                            Date lighting therapy began?

Hormonal regimen for transition mgt (Details)?

                            Wattage, stall/paddock size, ft candles of exposure?

                            Length of time mare is under supplemental light/day?

                            Added to AM, PM, or Flash lighting?

■ **Figure 33.1** Mare History Form.

Please check box or fill in blank which best describes patient's current environment:

_____ Pasture
_____ Racetrack
_____ Boarding facility

Stall time: _____

Hrs turned out/day:

Hrs turned out/night: _____

_____ Paddock/Pasture

List any current or previous disease conditions present at barn/stable:

Current feeding regimen (include amounts, cutting (1st, 2nd, 3rd) of hay, type of hay; concentrate (plain oats, sweet feed, custom mix, % protein; beet pulp, etc.):

Number of feedings per day (once, twice, etc.):

List any current medications/supplements:

List any previous injuries (non-repro & repro related)

List previous medications given, i.e. steroids, antibiotics, etc.

List any previous surgeries, dates, outcomes:

Check current performance level that best describes the mare's use::

_____ **High Level Performance**: (racing, endurance training, dressage, polo)
Low Level Performance: (broodmare, pleasure, trail riding)

PART TWO—REPRODUCTIVE INFORMATION:

Please check any of the following areas related to breeding that have been problematic:

_____ Early embryonic death _____ Chronic uterine infections _____ Other (Describe):
_____ Mid-late term abortions _____ Irregular cycles

■ **Figure 33.1** continued

Please check box which best describes patient's status and fill in the blanks accordingly:

_____ Maiden

_____ Barren; last foaling date:

_____ Lactating; last foaling date:

_____ Pregnant; last breeding date: is date of ovulation known?

_____ Unknown?

_____ >Aggression (to ☐ mares, ☐ people, ☐ stallions)

_____ >Intensity/duration of estrus

_____ Behavioral anestrus (during phys. breeding season)

Onset of behavior change:

_____

month/yr (season)

2. ESTRUS DETECTION METHODS

_____ Teasing

_____ TRP (transrectal palpation)

_____ U/S

_____ Teasing & TRP (describe TRP program; how often, +/- U/S, check for ovulation?)

_____ None of the above

Describe teasing methods used:

_____ Stallion to mare

_____ Mare to stallion

_____ Teaser pony

_____ Gelding

_____ Other (ex. behavior change w/paddock mates)

_____ Frequency of checks:

3. CYCLING INFO:

_____ Number of cycles in previous season

_____ Number of cycles bred in previous season

_____ Currently in foal heat?

_____ Onset of foal heat, date

_____ Age when first estrus occurred

_____ Length of estrous cycle

_____ Length of heat (estrus) period

_____ Duration of each standing estrus

_____ Size of follicle at ovulation (if known)

4. BREEDING INFO: (current season)

_____ Live cover

_____ AI

_____ Raw

_____ Extended

_____ Fresh, cooled

_____ Frozen

_____ Age when first bred

_____ Age when last bred (or) last breeding date

_____ # of covers/conception

_____ Total book of stallion used, for current season

_____ # of covers/cycle

Describe breeding methods used (how are breedings timed to ovulation +/- post-ovulation checks, when do breedings begin and stop, how long to breed)

Provide detail re: relevant points:

Covers	Year	Total Covers	Dates and Outcomes

■ Figure 33.1 continued

5. FOALING INFO:

_____ Date of last foaling

FOALINGS: Date (Yr)	Outcome: live foal, abortion, stillborn, retained fetal membranes	Assisted delivery/normal delivery C-section/Fetotomy	Gestation length

	History of Retained Fetal Membranes (RFM): Year(s) Occurred:
	Prescribed treatment
	Oxytocin
	Antibiotics
	Dose
	Frequency of treatment
	Route (IM, IV, IU):
	Duration:
	History of abortion (describe): History of early embryonic loss (EED):
	Repeated abortions?	How many years?
	Within the season?	At what gestational age?

6. PRIOR BREEDING SOUNDNESS EVALUATIONS:

History of genital/uterine infections

_____ Exposure to infected stallion

_____ Exposure to CEM

_____ Exposure to other VD: (EHV3, EVA, etc.)

_____ Frequency

Isolate? (bacterial, viral)

_____

_____ Date of most recent uterine culture

Notes re: last uterine treatments

_____ Antibiotics

_____ Dose

_____ Frequency of treatment

Route of administration

Prior endometrial biopsy?

_____ Year

_____ Category (I,IIA,IIB,III)

Reported changes:

Inflammation

Acute

Chronic

Periglandular fibrosis

_____ Cystic glandular degeneration

History of uterine cultures

Uterine culture taken by

_____ DVM

Other (Technician, Manager, Owner) _____

Results: _____

_____ Duration of treatment

_____ Follow-up culture?

_____ Date of follow-up culture

Time elapsed between last

treatment date and reculture

Therapy to improve Bx findings?

_____
_____
_____
_____
_____
_____
_____

7. OTHER REPRO TRACT INFO:

Vagina

_____ RVF

_____ other abnormality

Cervix

_____ Competent

_____ Incompetent

■ **Figure 33.1** continued

Vulva/Perineum

_____ VC

_____ Caslicks

_____ other Sx

_____ Lacerations

_____ Laceration repair?

PART THREE—CLINICAL EVALUATION, MSU

Date: _____

WNL = within normal limits

8. PROCEDURES USED:

TRP

LO	RO	Uterus	Cervix	VC

Vaginal, abnormalities?

(Note location of cervical abnormalities/tears/adhesions on the "cervical circle" to the left. Identify site/s and depth of involvement).

Cervical evaluation

_____ Intact

_____ Thinning

_____ Tears

Ultrasonography -
location/presence of:

a) Cysts: _____

b) Fluid: _____

c) Other: endometrial
folds, apparent
sacculations of
horns, etc.? _____

_____ Uterine culture (pending)

Uterine cytology

Results: _____

_____ Endometrial biopsy (pending)

Uterine lavage

_____ Volume used (cc)

_____ % Return

_____ Saline or
LRS?

_____ Uterine   Before: After:
tone

Antibiotic instillation? Which?

_____ Treatment days   Frequency   Dose

_____ Reculture,
when?   _____

Additional comments from today's examination:

■ **Figure 33.1** continued

297

Hydrops Allantois/Amnion in the Mare

chapter 34

DEFINITION/OVERVIEW

- Excessive fluid accumulation in either the allantoic or amniotic cavity of the pregnant uterus.
- Hydrops allantois is related primarily to placental dysfunction or insufficiency.
- Hydrops amnion is attributable to abnormalities of the fetus, contributing directly to fluid accumulation by virtue of or secondary to congenital anomalies. Segmental aplasias (primarily GI in origin) preclude swallowing and processing or recycling of amniotic fluid. The fetus may be delivered alive, but is nonviable.

ETIOLOGY/PATHOPHYSIOLOGY

- Dysfunction of either the placenta or the fetus results in accumulation of excessive amounts of allantoic or amniotic fluid, undermining the dam's health by the accumulation of excessive weight (modest to rapid rate of increase), contributing to her dehydration, compromised GI function, and labored respiration.
- Clinical management for both conditions is the same, induction of parturition to save the dam's life, and to prevent rupture of the ventral abdominal wall or the uterus.
- There may be a hereditary role in development of hydropic conditions.
- Incidence/Prevalence: Rare.

Systems Affected

Reproductive, dam and fetus

SIGNALMENT/HISTORY

- No breed or age predisposition, although more cases have been reported in draft mares.
- Abnormal accumulation of fluid (up to 100 L) in the allantoic cavity; abdominal size is abnormally large for stage of gestation.
  - Time-frame for accumulation of fluid in the uterus, can be moderate to rapid (allantoic or amniotic).
  - Frequently a rapid onset, a few days to a few weeks.

- Commonly occurs from 6 to 10 months gestation.
- Most mares develop a tremendous amount of ventral abdominal edema.
- Abdominal or uterine rupture can result due to excessive weight of the accumulated allantoic or amniotic fluid.
- With a rapid increase in abdominal size or shape, accompanying signs may include: abdominal pain (moderate to severe), severe ventral edema, elevated pulse, labored respiration due to pressure on the diaphragm, difficulty walking, and recumbency as the condition progresses.
- TRP reveals an abnormal accumulation of fluid.
- The fetus is difficult or impossible to detect (TRP or U/S).

Risk Factors

- Draft mares
- Older, multiparous mares but has been reported in all ages.

DIAGNOSTICS

CBC/Biochemistry/Urinalysis

- Possible increase or decrease of the PCV (secondary to hypovolemia or dehydration, respectively).
- Possible increase in BUN and creatinine secondary to dehydration.

Imaging: U/S

- Fluid compartments are grossly enlarged, either allantoic or amniotic.
- Torso/abdomen of the hydramnios fetus may have a grossly widened diameter as a result of ascites.

Other Diagnostic Procedures

- U/S and TRP
- Abdominocentesis, U/S guided, may be of use to detect abnormal free fluid in abdomen, in cases of uterine rupture.

Pathologic Findings

- Placental insufficiency secondary to placentitis.
- Hydrops amnion: fetal swallowing defects (segmental aplasia(s) prevent swallowing and processing of amniotic fluid; leading to fluid accumulation in excessive amounts.
- Fetal defects such as growth retardation and hydrocephalus have been reported, as well as brachygnathia.
- Torsions of the umbilical cord and amnion have been reported.

DIFFERENTIAL DIAGNOSIS

- Twin pregnancy: mid-to-late gestation.
- Prepubic tendon rupture.
- Herniation or rupture of ventral abdominal wall.
- Possibly, uterine torsion.

 ## THERAPEUTICS

Drug(s) of Choice

- Since most hydrops mares spontaneously abort, treatment should be directed at terminating the pregnancy. (See Abortion, Inductive of/Elective Termination).
- The use of oxytocin usually is not effective because most of these mares will have uterine inertia (atony) due to the stretching of the uterine musculature.

Appropriate Health Care

- Manual dilation of the cervix, completed gradually over a 10- to 20-minute period.
- Measured, controlled drainage of allantoic/amniotic fluid via aseptic insertion of a sterile drain tube through the cervix and fetal membranes.
- Slow removal of fluid is important to prevent hypovolemic shock in the mare.
    - A sudden loss of pressure on the abdominal vessels may result as the uterus is drained, and lead to vascular pooling. Monitor PCV and TP throughout.
    - If removal can be well-managed, achieving a gradual decrease of her uterine volume over a 12- to 24-hour period is best for the mare.
    - One method: manually dilate the mare's cervix, administer serial cloprostenol injections (250 μg at 12-hour intervals for two to four doses). Place NG tube through the cervix or the membranes (will be at the approximate region of the placental cervical star). Achieve rate outflow restriction (control of outflow) by tying off (a simple loop either around the external cervical os or the membranes extending through the cervix). Remove no more than 5 to 10 L at a time, clamping off in between increments to keep the mare stabilized.
    - Continue with IV fluid delivery and care, as follows.
- For the dam:
    - IV fluids: balanced electrolyte solutions, LRS, or hypertonic saline solution.
    - Corticosteroids: Solu-Delta-Cortef® (prednisolone sodium succinate). Initial dose is 50 to 100 mg; IV or IM. Initial IV should be given slowly (30 sec to 1 minute).
    - Dexamethasone: 0.1 to 0.5 mg/kg; used at the higher end of the dose range to decrease the likelihood of hypovolemic shock.
    - Oxytocin is often ineffective due to chronic uterine stretching (atony/inertia).
- Once sufficient fluid has been removed by a slow, controlled rate removal, the CA membrane should be further ruptured/opened and the fetus removed by forced extraction.

- *Note*: In some cases the CA membrane may be thickened and difficult to rupture, in which case, the membrane should be pulled caudally, into the anterior vagina, to facilitate easier opening of the membrane and extraction of the fetus.
- Continuing monitoring the mare, fluids and antibiotic administration, as indicated.

Nursing Care

Close monitoring of the mare for signs of shock or infection after removal of fluids and fetus.

Activity

Limited by inability of dam to move.

Surgical Considerations

- Induction of parturition.
- C-section but keep in mind that fetal survival is unlikely.

 COMMENTS

Client Education

Mares that appear excessively large for stage of gestation should be evaluated, particularly if signs of systemic disease or disability develop.

Patient Monitoring

- Once a diagnosis is made, termination of pregnancy is the appropriate follow-up.
- Monitor for respiratory distress, stability of dam's vital signs.

Prevention/Avoidance

- Hydrops amnion:
  - The fetus is abnormal; the dam is normal.
  - Breed to a different sire once the mare has recovered from either controlled vaginal delivery or C-section.
- Hydrops allantois:
  - The dam's uterus is abnormal resulting in abnormal placentation incapable of sustaining the pregnancy to term; the fetus is usually normal (but can't be saved at the late stage of gestation).
  - As the abnormal placentation may reflect ineffective placental attachment because of an abnormal endometrium, placentitits, or primary placental failure, rebreeding may result in a similar outcome.
  - The dam could still be a suitable embryo donor.

- Adventitious placentation has been reported in cattle and is an effort by the placenta to generate additional, however ineffective, sites for placental transfer. Normal placentation is essential to sustain the fetus to term (O_2 in, CO_2 out, removal of fetal waste).
- Placentitis may compound pregnancy and exacerbate difficulties linked with an abnormal endometrium.

Possible Complications

- Loss of pregnancy
- Prepubic tendon rupture
- Rupture of ventral belly wall
- Maternal death

Expected Course and Prognosis

- Prognosis for fetal survival is poor.
- Prognosis for survival of the dam is guarded, if parturition is induced before more serious damage occurs.
- Prognosis for future reproduction:
  - Guarded for the dam if the diagnosis is hydrops allantois, the endometrium is the problem.
  - Guarded for the fetus of the hydrops amnion mare; recommend she be bred to a different stallion.

Abbreviations

BUN   blood urea nitrogen
CA   chorioallantoic
CBC   complete blood count
GI   gastrointestinal
IM   intramuscular
IV   intravenous
LRS   lactated Ringer's solution
NG   nasogastric
PCV   packed cell volume
TP   total protein
TRP   transrectal palpation
U/S   ultrasound, ultrasonography

See Also

- Dystocia
- Placentitis
- Placental basics
- Placental insufficiency, mare
- Premature placental separation

Suggested Reading

Frazer GR. 1998. The Pregnant Mare. In: *Equine Internal Medicine*. Reed SM, Bayly WM (eds). Philadelphia: WB Saunders; 1079–1130 [hydrops: 1096–1097].

Honnas CH, Spensley MS, Laverty S, et al. 1988. Hydramnios causing uterine rupture in a mare. *JAVMA* 193: 332–336.

Löfstedt RM. 1993. Miscellaneous diseases of pregnancy and parturition. In: *Equine Reproduction*. McKinnon AO, Voss JL (eds). Philadelphia: Lea & Febiger; 596–597.

Palmer JE. 2005. The high risk mare. Presented to *Belgian Eq Pract*. Ithaca: IVIS, P2001.1105

Reimer JM. 1997. Use of transcutaneous ultrasonography in complicated latter-middle to late gestation pregnancies in the mare: 122 cases. *Proc AAEP*, 259–261.

Vandeplassche M, Bouters R, Spincemaille J, et al. 1976. Dropsy of the fetal sacs in the mare: Induced and spontaneous abortion. *Vet Rec* 99: 67–69.

Author: Carla L. Carleton

chapter 35

Large Ovary Syndrome

 DEFINITION/OVERVIEW

- Includes a number of conditions, both normal and abnormal, that result in one or both ovaries achieving a size that is significantly larger than considered normal, as detected by TRP or U/S.
- Definition of the cause is reached by a systematic process which considers:
  - History
  - Season/time of year
  - Behavior
  - Physical examination findings (TRP and U/S)
  - Hormone analysis
  - Response to some routine treatments to elicit alterations in either size of the enlarged gonad or a change in behavior.

Most common causes of LOS:

- Persistent follicles
- Hematoma
- Pregnancy

Rare causes:

- GCT/GTCT (the most common ovarian tumor, but still a rare occurrence)
- Teratoma
- Dysgerminoma
- Cystadenoma
- Abscess
- and multiple single reports of additional tumor types.

 ETIOLOGY/PATHOPHYSIOLOGY

Physiology

- Equids are long-day breeders (i.e., estrous cycles and the ovulatory period normally occur during spring and summer months).
- Light is the predominant influence on ovarian activity and estrous cycles.
- Outside the optimal season for breeding activity, the gonads are waxing or waning relative to follicular activity and the occurrence of ovulation.

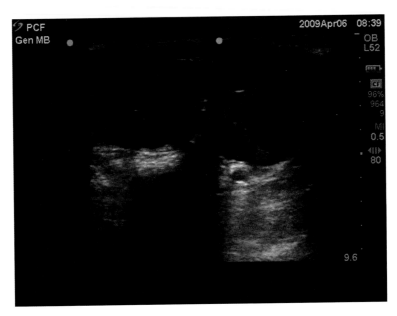

■ **Figure 35.1** Typical ultrasound appearance of normal mare ovaries during the physiologic breeding season, multiple follicles of varying sizes.

- Light is perceived by the pineal gland, a neuroendocrine transducer, and relays its perception of available light by increasing or decreasing the production of GnRH from the hypothalamus.
- Suppression of hypothalamic activity by the pineal gland diminishes as day length increases. Increased amounts of melatonin-like substance suppress hypothalamic activity during the winter months.
- As GnRH increases (springtime, increasing day length), FSH and LH increase, and result in increased ovarian activity.
- There is a lag time of 60 to 90 days following the winter equinox (late December, shortest day of year in the northern hemisphere) for the increasing light to be reflected in consistent/regular estrous cycles and ovulation.
- It is normal for mares to have multiple follicles present on both ovaries through her ovulatory period (Fig. 35.1).
- After the summer solstice (late June, longest day of the year), day length begins to decrease, GnRH production tapers, followed by a decrease in LH and FSH to a point that their available levels are insufficient to complete maturation and/or induce ovulation of follicles.
- *Persistent follicles in vernal (spring) transition:*
  - Variable sizes throughout transition. Those late in vernal transition, may regress after persisting for a month or more, or,
  - Eventually ovulation will occur (of its own accord, if time is not a management issue) with sufficient light, FSH, and LH.
  - Ovulation, late in spring transition, may be stimulated by the administration of hCG.

- *Persistent follicles in autumnal (fall) transition:*
  - Early in fall transition it is possible to stimulate additional ovulations, especially those identified in the first half of autumnal transition and if follicles are at least 35 mm.
  - All follicles will eventually regress (decrease in size) as daylight wanes and endogenous GnRH, LH, and FSH decrease, and the mare slips into winter anestrus (when bilaterally the ovaries are small and inactive).

Normal Ovary, Persistent Follicles

- The most common cause cited for LOS.
- May be single or multiple, present on one or both ovaries.
- Presence/characteristics are primarily due to season (late spring/early fall) and increasing or decreasing duration of light.
- Their presence does not indicate ovarian disease (i.e., normal structures that will resolve if left alone).

Normal Ovary, Hematoma

- Second most common cause of LOS.
- Enlargement resolves without assistance over time unless treated with prostaglandin to stimulate earlier initiation of estrous cyclic activity.
- Only considered pathologic if the hematoma causes sufficient destruction of ovarian tissue that future normal activity is precluded.

Abnormal Ovary, Tumors and Other Causes

- Hormone treatments fail to elicit a desirable response (PGF, hCG, deslorelin).
- TRP, U/S, radiography: reveal appearance inconsistent with normal ovarian structures.
- Systemic illness of the mare is rare.
- Type of cell identified on histopath examination of ovarian tissue following OVX.

Systems Affected

Reproductive

 ## CLINICAL FEATURES

- Females of breeding age (postpubertal and preovarian senescence).
- All breeds
- Incidence/Prevalence

Persistent Follicles

- Potentially more than 80% of reproductively normal mares.

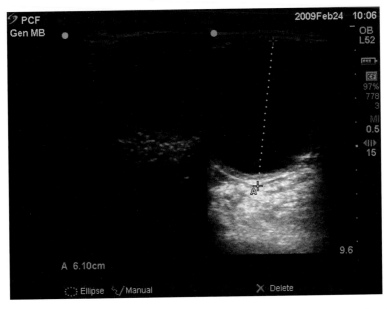

■ **Figure 35.2** A persistent follicle present late in vernal transition (Feb. 24) of a mare housed under lights the previous 90 days. Note the endometrial edema just beginning to be evident. Follicles late in transition are finally steroidogenic.

- Approximately 20% of northern hemisphere mares continue to experience estrous cycle activity year-round, albeit with some variation in length from the "normal" of a 21-day estrous cycle.
- Signs, Behavior and TRP associated with persistent follicles
  - Seasonal component: typically during one of the two transition periods.
  - Usually tease in, demonstrate a positive response to a stallion, for extended periods of time (1+ month).
  - Estrus behavior persists longer than during a normal estrous cycle (longer than 12 to 14 days in the spring).
  - TRP and U/S reveal the presence of follicles, may be multiple of varying size (Fig. 35.2); their appearance is still as follicles (i.e., they don't take on the irregular appearance of the multilocular/fenestrated spaces typical of a granulosa cell tumor).
  - May increase in size/diameter with time, but the increase is slower than observed with dominant follicles (dominant follicle increases approximately 5 to 6 mm/day during estrus) during the ovulatory period.
- Causes associated/linked with persistent follicles
  - Vernal transition: increasing day length between winter anestrus and the ovulatory period.
  - Autumnal transition: decreasing day length between the ovulatory period and winter anestrus.

Hematoma

- Uncommon, but a few cases a year will be recognized within a normal population of mares during the breeding season.

Tumors

- GCT/GTCT is the most common ovarian tumor, but its occurrence is rare.
- All other tumors occur even less frequently (but, all are rare).

 DIFFERENTIAL DIAGNOSIS

Ovaries during pregnancy (more than 37 to 40 days gestation):
- With formation of endometrial cups and subsequent production of eCG, secondary follicles luteinize to become secondary CL. The ovaries of the pregnant mare become bilaterally enlarged.
- Mare's behavior may mimic the aggression of some mares with a GCT/GTCT.
  - Most likely related to increased circulating testosterone stemming from fetal gonads.
  - May be in excess of 100 pg/mL by 60 to 90 days gestation.
  - Peaks at approximately 200 days gestation; declines to basal levels by time of foaling.

Ovarian Hematoma

- Behavior and TRP: This event occurs following estrus and ovulation (key history: the mare was recently in estrus). Serial palpations will confirm that (as with a normal postovulatory CH to CL) uterine tone will increase and the cervix will close (the influence of progesterone) and mare teases out.
- The CH increases to a size substantially larger than the follicle that preceded it.
- Usually by the time of diagnosis, the acute pain associated with the rapid stretch of the ovarian tunic has subsided, and the mare's behavior is that of a diestrus mare (i.e., normal; teases out; rejects the stallion's advances).
- Although the initial rise of progesterone may be delayed slightly compared with a normal CH, blood progesterone will rise (greater than 1 ng/mL) by 5 to 6 days post-ovulation, confirmation that ovulation occurred.
- Contralateral ovary is normal.
- U/S of hematoma is eventually similar to a CH, albeit a large one (Fig. 35.3a).
- The rapid size increase of the hematoma, stretches the tunic surrounding the ovary, and the mare may exhibit pain or colic in the short term.
- Resolution: time or prostaglandin. Complete luteinization may be delayed and thus delay responsiveness to PGF (will require longer than 6 days post-ovulation to respond as would an otherwise normal, mature CL; may be as long as 2 weeks, occasionally longer) (Figs. 35.3b and c).

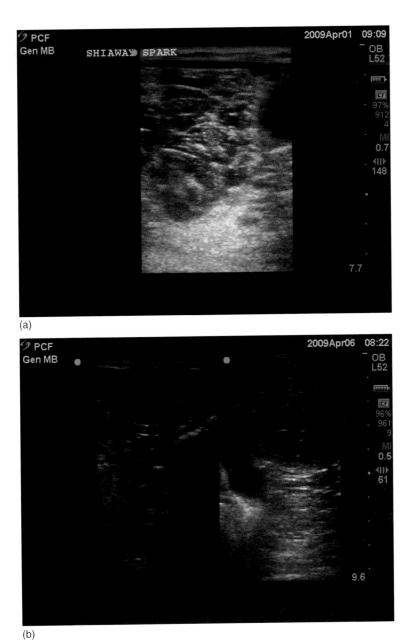

(a)

(b)

■ **Figure 35.3** Ovarian hematoma: Follicle prior to its formation was only 40 mm diameter *(a)*; luteinization of corpus luteum is delayed *(b)*; beginning to decrease in size. Uterine tone finally began to increase and the cervix to close with the rise in progesterone *(c)*.

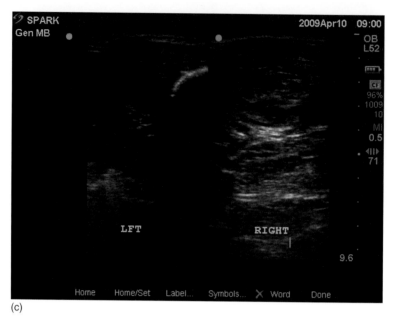

■ **Figure 35.3** continued

GCT/GTCT

- TRP: characterized by a unilateral gonad enlargement (rate of tumor growth varies significantly by case).
  - Surface of tumor remains smooth, but may have gentle lobulations (Fig. 35.4).
  - Ovulation fossa disappears (indentation, central area of germinal epithelium fills in) early in development of the tumor.
  - Over time, contralateral ovary shows evidence of suppression. Early on the number/size of follicles decreases, then the total volume/size of parenchyma decreases.
  - Chronic GCT/GTCTs will be coupled with a contralateral ovary that may become so small it is difficult for the novice to detect.
  - Rare/uncommon, the contralateral ovary may continue to exhibit follicular activity and ovulations.
- Circulating levels of inhibin (produced by the granulosa cells) are elevated in 90% of GCT/GTCT.

Behavior

- Mares typically exhibit one of three primary behaviors: chronic anestrus (80%), stallion-like (increased aggression, 15%), persistent estrus (nymphomaniac, 5%).
- Because of the slower increase of size that stretches the ovarian tunic, mares rarely exhibit pain (contrast this with the rapid formation of a hematoma).
- Mare may exhibit discomfort at the trot or refuse to go over jumps. Weight of the enlarging ovary coupled with impact, bounces ovary; felt as a sharp, painful stretch-

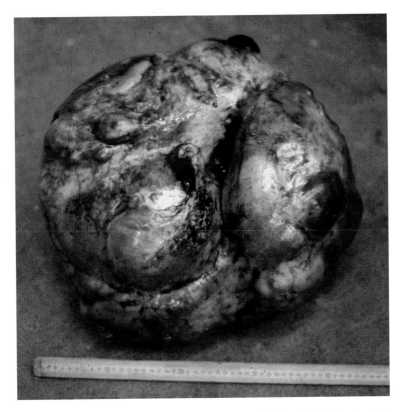

■ **Figure 35.4** A granulosa thecal cell tumor removed via a ventral abdominal incision (note the meter stick lying alongside it). The mare had a year-long history of having been anestrus in her behavior.

ing of the mesovarium and may elicit behavioral changes (pain, anger, reticence to perform).

Teratoma

- Rare, not hormonally active (no distinctive behavior change).
- TRP: contralateral ovary is normal. Surface of teratoma may exhibit some sharper protuberances reflecting its potentially eclectic content.
- No effect on behavior or estrous cycle activity.
- Teratoma is benign.

Dysgerminoma

- Rare
- Initial presentation for intermittent chronic colic, weight loss, stiff extremities.
- Presence of tumor may only be discovered once mare's health deteriorates due to metastases.
- Potentially/can be highly malignant.

Cystadenoma

- Unilateral, no effect on contralateral ovary.
- No effect on behavior.
- Appearance: large, cystic structures, may be confused early on with persistent follicles, remains nonresponsive to hCG.
- Rare hormonal impact. If it does occur, it's usually as elevated testosterone.

Ovarian Abscess

- Rare
- Early reports may have been associated with attempts to reduce the size and number of persistent follicles via a flank approach aspiration. As knowledge grew regarding the normalcy of persistent, transitional follicles, such aggressive, ill-conceived procedures are no longer accepted/practiced (Figs. 35.5a and b)
- Contralateral ovary is normal.
- No affect on behavior or estrous cycle activity.

Other Laboratory Tests

GCT/GTCT

- Elevation of circulating inhibin levels (in excess of 0.7 ng/mL) in 90% of GCT/GTCT.
- Elevation of testosterone (more than 50 to 100 pg/mL) in 50 to 60% of affected mares.
- Progesterone levels are usually less than 1 ng/mL.

Ovarian Hematoma

- Blood progesterone will increase by 5 to 7 days of start of hematoma formation (the day of ovulation, when rapid stretch began).

Dysgerminoma

- Reports of hypertrophic pulmonary osteoarthropathy developing secondary to metastatic dysgerminoma.
- Initial presentation is for intermittent chronic colic, weight loss, stiff extremities.
- Radiography, biopsies for metastasis.

Imaging: U/S

One of the most important adjunct tools to evaluate/differentiate cases of LOS.
Persistent follicle: except for larger size, appearance is similar to normal follicles.

Hematoma:

- Recent event: fluid-filled space (black, similar to follicular fluid on U/S exam).
- Within 2 to 10 days hyperechoic "speckles" began to appear; ongoing clotting of blood, contraction of the clot within the CH, and invasion of luteal cells (becoming an over-sized CL).
- Eventually takes on the uniform hyperechoic appearance of a CH (a large one), and over time, a CL. U/S appearance of luteinization is delayed (*see* Figs. 35.3a, b, and c) and it will not respond to prostaglandin by 5 to 6 days post-ovulation.

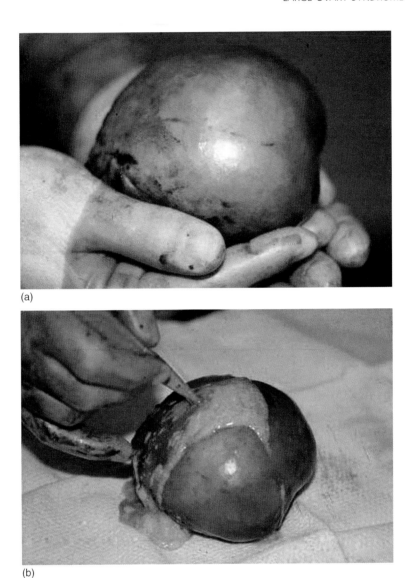

(a)

(b)

■ **Figure 35.5** Postoperative appearance of ovarian abscess *(a)*. When the ovarian tumor was excised, it revealed a total loss of normal internal stroma from long-standing pressure necrosis *(b)*.

- Unlike a normal CH that is usually smaller than the size (diameter) of the follicle that preceded it, a hematoma is larger in diameter than the preceding follicle, ranging from slightly larger to extremely larger ("grapefruit" and bigger).

GCT/GTCT

- Multicystic, the spaces of which can appear quite irregular, sizes of fluid pockets range from a few mm to multiple centimeters (Figs. 35.6a and 35.6b).
- Size/location of the tumor during an U/S scan may range from readily accessible off the tip of uterine horn at the lateral end of the proper ligament to very pendulous

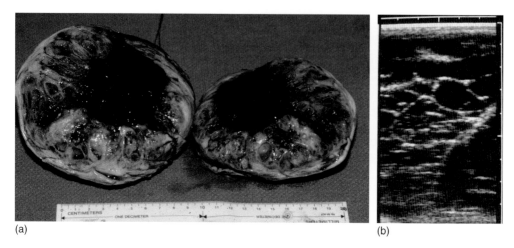

(a)   (b)

■ **Figure 35.6** A cross-section of a granulosa cell tumor showing the irregular, fluid-filled pockets so typical of this type of tumor *(a)*. Ultrasound view revealing the typical *Swiss cheese* fenestrations of a granulosa cell tumor *(b)*.

(dependent on weight & stretch of the mesovarium/broad ligament) within the caudal abdomen.

- Recorded weights have ranged from less than 1 to more than 45 kg (MSU veterinary teaching hospital, over a 20-year period).
- At the time of detection, the majority will be less than 30 cm diameter.

Teratoma

- Variable echogenicity, reflecting the nature of its contents (i.e., soft tissue, fluid, hair, bone, and teeth).

Other Diagnostic Procedures

In addition to serial TRP and U/S, blood hormone evaluations are valuable:

Hormone	Normal range	GCT/GTCT
Progesterone, estrus	Less than 1 ng/mL	
Progesterone, diestrus	More than 1 ng/mL	
Progesterone, GCT/GTCT		Less than 1 ng/mL
Testosterone		More than 50 to 100 pg/mL
Inhibin	0.1 to 0.7 ng/mL	More than 0.7 ng/mL

Pathologic Findings

- Persistent follicles: N/A
- Hematoma: N/A
- Neoplasms can potentially arise from any of the tissue types present in the ovary.

- Classification is based on their origin in surface epithelium: sex cord-stromal tissue, germ cell, or mesenchymal tissue.
  - GCT/GTCT: sex cord-stromal tumor, endocrine effects, specific in mare: inhibin production by thecal cells (GTCT).
  - Teratoma: many tissue types, including germ cells, within the mass; can include hair, skin, respiratory epithelium, tooth, and bone. High metastatic potential in mice and humans, not a routine concern in the mare. Immature teratomas: tissue resembles embryonic origins; mature teratomas are also known as dermoid cysts.
  - Cystadenoma: from epithelium; forms cystic neoplastic masses.
  - Dysgerminoma: from germ cells, analogous to seminoma of the testis; cells are arranged in sheets and cords with a dense population of large pleomorphic cells; all malignant.

 # THERAPEUTICS

Drug(s) of Choice

Hematoma

- No treatment, wait for the ovary to regress in size and other follicular activity to develop.
- PGF$_2\alpha$, 5 to 10 mg IM, no fewer than 7 to 10 days post-ovulation and formation of the hematoma.
- May be unresponsive to treatment within first 2 weeks.
- Successful treatment is noted by the mare returning to estrus within 2 to 5 days.

Persistent Follicles

- Can elect "no treatment, but for time": wait for estrous activity to begin (vernal transition) or cease (autumnal transition) on its own.
- To shorten the duration of vernal transition:
  - Regu-mate®, but do not institute treatment before significant follicular activity is present (multiple 15–20 mm follicles present on both ovaries). During transition a mare is experiencing behavioral, not physiologic estrus. See Estrus, abnormal intervals. Wear protective gloves. Dose PO at 0.044 mg/kg (1 mL per 110 lbs BW), SID, 15 days. Can be delivered by dose syringe PO or placed on grain at feeding time.
  - hCG: 2,500 to 3,000 IU, IV; may induce ovulation late in vernal transition. See Estrus, abnormal intervals. Wait until a follicle of at least 35 mm is present. Anticipate ovulation within 36 to 44 hours.
  - Deslorelin, GnRH analogue, is available as an injectable product. Results in ovulation within 38 to 60 hours. Little difference (deslorelin cost has decreased significantly in recent years) in percent of mares responding (approx. 80%), time to ovulation, and conception rate, compared to hCG. As a decapeptide, it doesn't stimulate antibody production as can hCG. A subset of mares will experience persistent anestrus if PGF is administered 1 week after deslorelin administration.

- Progesterone plus estradiol 17β: 10 days: Results in more effective ovulation and follicular suppression than progesterone alone. Administered IM, SID, 150 mg/day progesterone and 10 mg/day estradiol-17β; PGF on the last day of treatment. hCG may be used once a follicle of at least 35 mm has been detected for ovulation induction.
- Other progesterone products are available: P4 in oil (100 mL vial for IM injection); Bio Release P+LA (long-acting) also in a 100-mL vial (150 mg progesterone + E17β, IM); and P+ in oil (50 mg/mL progesterone + 3.3 mg/mL E17β, IM).
- Future products to come on the market with a 2-week interval of administration: P+ microspheres and SABER progesterone for injection.

Precautions/Interactions

Some behavior changes can be dramatic. Use caution around mares that are showing aggressive behavior; may need individual paddock, distance from other mares in estrus, separation from foals, stallions.
- Large ovarian tumors can develop extensive blood supplies.
- Intraoperative time can be significantly lengthened due to time required to properly ligate vessels supplying the tumor; increases surgical risks.
- Intraoperative intravenous fluid replacement to overcome vascular pooling (compartmentalization) at the time the largest tumors are removed from the abdomen.

Appropriate Health Care

Only as specified for particular conditions as discussed previously.

Nursing Care

- None specific to conditions.
- General postoperative medical care recommended following an OVX.

Surgical Considerations

Recommendation for OVX

- GCT/GTCT : removal of affected gonad for reproductive function to return, prognosis fair to good depending on size of tumor, surgical route, duration of suppression of contralateral ovary.
- Cystadenoma: rare, reported testosterone production.
- Abscess, Teratoma: dysfunctional ovary.

 COMMENTS

Client Education

- Importance of conducting serial examinations to reach an accurate diagnosis of LOS and thus avoid an unnecessary ovariectomy.

- Vast majority of LOS cases are due to persistent follicle(s) and hematoma.
- GCT/GTCTs are the most common tumor causing ovarian enlargement, but they are still an uncommon or rare occurrence.

History

- Season: during transitional periods, persistent follicle(s) is first rule-out.
- Estrous activity: a mare recently showing estrus, is now out of estrus, may be painful, and an enlarged ovary is detected. Hematoma is the first rule-out.
- Response to treatment: progesterone supplementation, prostaglandin, hCG.
- Behavior changes: prolonged anestrus, increased aggression, nymphomania?

Serial TRP

- At an interval of 7 to 10 days, may require 3 to 5 examinations.
- Avoid too frequent examinations (at intervals too short to expect or detect a significant decrease or increase in the size of an affected ovary); avoids unnecessary cost or surgery. Allow for at least two examinations within the span of a potential estrous period: (1) for comparison of affected and contralateral ovary, (2) rate of size increase, and (3) activity of opposite gonad.

U/S

- It is a most effective tool to evaluate the internal characteristics of the enlarging gonad. See Imaging.

Circulating Hormone Levels

- Inhibin, testosterone, progesterone.
- Inhibin assay developed at UC Davis Endocrinology Lab, Davis, CA, offers an ovarian tumor panel to evaluate for most likely rule-outs.

Patient Monitoring

Routine postoperative care for OVX.

Possible Complications

- Any operative procedure or anesthesia holds potential risk for death.
- GCT/GTCT: time from OVX to resumption of estrous cycle activity is influenced by the months or years of suppression.
  - Most have usually been present for more than 1 to 3 years at the time of diagnosis.
  - Rare cases of permanent suppression (usually a tumor has been present for many years, opposite ovary is ultimately incapable of recovering).
  - Rare case of remaining ovary also developing into a GCT/GTCT.
  - A few mares with this tumor will continue to develop follicles and ovulate on the contralateral ovary.

Expected Course and Prognosis

Prognosis, Poor

- *Dysgerminoma*: potential for metastasis.
  - Usually in a advanced state of metastatic disease by the time of diagnosis.

Prognosis for Future Reproduction, Good

- *Hematoma:* large size returns nearly to normal over 1 to 6 months.
  - Rarely will a hematoma destroy remaining ovarian tissue (pressure effect within the tunic).
  - Some mares will develop a hematoma on subsequent cycles within a season.
- *Persistent follicles*: 100% resolution with time and season.

Prognosis for Life, Good:

- *GCT/GTCT*
- *Abscess*
- *Cystadenoma*
- *Teratoma*

Associated Conditions

- *Dysgerminoma:* hypertrophic pulmonary osteoarthropathy developing secondary to metastatic dysgerminoma; initial presentation was for intermittent chronic colic, weight loss, stiff extremities.
- Behavior modification with GCT/GTCT.

Age-Related Factors

- Of breeding age (capable of estrous activity):
  - Hematoma
  - Persistent follicles
- Tumors
  - No age limitation

Synonyms

- Ovarian tumors
- Transitional ovaries

Abbreviations

BW   body weight
CH   corpus hemorrhagicum
CL   corpus luteum
eCG   equine chorionic gonadotropin
FSH   follicle stimulating hormone

GCT   granulosa cell tumor
GTCT   granulosa thecal cell tumor
GnRH   gonadotropin releasing hormone
hCG   human chorionic gonadotropin
IM   intramuscular
IV   intravenous
LH   luteinizing hormone
LOS   large ovary syndrome
OVX   ovariectomy
P4   progesterone
PGF   prostaglandin F (natural prostaglandin)
PO   per os (by mouth)
SID   once a day
TRP   transrectal palpation
U/S   ultrasound, ultrasonography

See Also

- Abnormal estrus intervals
- Anestrus
- Estrus cycle, Mare, manipulation of
- Ovulation failure
- Ovulation, induction of
- Pregnancy
- Prolonged diestrus

Suggested Reading

Carleton CL. 1996. Atypical, asymmetrical, but abnormal? Large ovary syndrome. *Proc Mare Reprod Symp, Soc for Therio,* 27–39.

Foley GL. 1997. Ovarian neoplasms of domestic animals. *Proc Reprod Pathology Symp, Soc for Therio* 60–65.

Hinrichs K. 2007. Irregularities of the estrous cycle and ovulation in mares (including seasonal transition). In: *Current Therapy in Large Animal Theriogenology,* 2nd ed. Younguist RS, Threlfall WR (eds). Philadelphia: Saunders Elsevier; 144–152.

McCue PM. 1998. Review of ovarian abnormalities in the mare. *Proc AAEP,* 125–133.

Schlafer DH. 1997. Non-neoplastic lesions of the ovaries of the mare. *Proc Reprod Pathology Symp. Soc for Therio,* 69–72.

Stangroom JE, Weevers R de G. 1962. Anticoagulant activity of equine follicular fluid. *J Reprod Fert* 3: 269–282.

Author: Carla L. Carleton

Leptospirosis

chapter **36**

DEFINITION/OVERVIEW

- Leptospirosis is a worldwide disease caused by pathogenic serovars of the spirochete *Leptospira interrogans*.
- It affects wildlife and domestic animals and has a zoonotic potential. Serologic surveys show that equine exposure to leptospires is common but clinical disease is uncommon.
- Clinical leptospirosis in horses is primarily associated with recurrent uveitis, abortions, stillbirths, and neonatal disease.
- Hepatic and renal disease in adults is uncommon.

ETIOLOGY/PATHOPHYSIOLOGY

- Leptospires are spirochetes that are both host and non-host adapted. Infection by host adapted serovars results in an increase in endemic disease or clinical disease in immunologically naïve animals. Infection by non-host-adapted serovars results in sporadic infections or disease outbreaks.
- If the serovar is host adapted, then infection is often for life; if the serovar is non-host adapted, then infection and shedding are usually brief.
- *L. interrogans* serovar bratislava is the presumed host-adapted serovar of horses. Leptospires penetrate mucosal and skin surfaces and result in a bacteremia and an invasion of internal organs 4 to 10 days later. Outcome of infection depends on the horse's humoral response and the pathogenicity of the serovar. Organisms multiply in organs and release metabolites that combined with immune-mediated damage cause the clinical signs associated with the disease.
- Pathogenic serovars of *L. interrogans*:
    - In North America, most abortions have resulted from infections by leptospires in the serovar kennewicki and less frequently serovars grippotyphosa and hardjo.
    - Leptospiral abortions previously reported as *Leptospira pomona* have been reclassified as *L. interrogans* serovar kennewicki.
    - In northern Ireland, the serovar bratislava is identified most frequently.
- Leptospires evade the immune system in the proximal renal tubules, genital tract, CNS, and eyes. Leptospira are shed into the environment in high concentrations in the urine, although all body secretions may contain leptospires during the bacteremic phase.

Systems Affected

- Ophthalmic: recurrent uveitis
- Reproductive: abortion, stillbirth
- Renal/urologic: renal disease and pyuria
- Neonatal disease: hepatic and renal disease, weakness, pulmonary hemorrhage.
- Hepatobiliary: liver disease and jaundice.

 SIGNALMENT/HISTORY

- Serologic surveys have identified worldwide exposure to leptospires. Predominant serovars vary with geographic area and leptospire antigens used in the surveys.
- Signs associated with:
  - Bacteremia: includes pyrexia, depression, lethargy, and anorexia.
  - Organ invasion: indicative of the specific organ involved.
- Are usually no premonitory signs observed prior to abortion.
- Chronic disease is associated with recurrent uveitis.
- Subclinical infections and carrier states are asymptomatic.

Risk Factors

- Direct transmission with host-to-host contact via infected urine, exposure to posta-bortion discharge, and aborted fetuses.
- Indirect transmission via contaminated environment from exposure to shedding maintenance hosts. Skunk and raccoons are maintenance hosts for serovars kenne-wicki and grippotyphosa, and cattle for serovar hardjo.
- Warm, moist environment; neutral to slightly alkaline soil pH; and a high density of carrier and susceptible animals.

 CLINICAL FEATURES

- Ophthalmic: initially, blepharospasm, excessive tearing, photophobia, chemosis, miosis, aqueous flare, hypopyon, and corneal edema. Chronic sequelae include syn-echia formation, retinal detachment, chorioretinitis, cataracts, atrophy of corpora nigra, and phthisis bulbi.
- Reproductive: abortion (usually late gestation), stillbirth, or premature birth or neo-natal disease depending on stage of gestation and infection.
- Renal/urologic: azotemia, polyuria/polydipsia, pyuria, hematuria, and pyrexia.
- Neonatal disease: weakness, icterus, renal failure, hematuria. One outbreak also reported respiratory distress, pyrexia, and depression.
- Hepatobiliary: jaundice, pyrexia, and lethargy.

DIFFERENTIAL DIAGNOSIS

Recurrent Uveitis

- *Toxoplasma* spp., *Onchocerca cervicalis*, *Streptococcus* spp., viral agents, ocular trauma.
- Onchocerca microfilariae and viral inclusion bodies are found in conjunctival scrapings and biopsy.
- Rising serum titers are associated with Toxoplasma spp.

Abortion

- *Infectious causes*: EHV-1 is differentiated by characteristic histologic lesion of intranuclear eosinophilic inclusion bodies and indirect immunofluorescent tests. Placentitis (bacterial and fungal) is differentiated by gross evidence of placentitis, isolation of organisms from the placenta and fetal organs, especially the stomach. EVA is differentiated by viral isolation from placental and fetal tissues. Ehrlichia risticii is differentiated by histopathology of the fetus and isolation of the organism from the fetus.
- *Noninfectious causes*: placental abnormalities, twinning, twisted umbilical cord, and maternal systemic disease.

Renal/Urologic

- Bacterial pyelonephritis is identified by pyuria and the presence of bacteria in the urine.
- Hemodynamic renal dysfunction is differentiated by other physical examination findings.
- Nephrotoxicity is identified by exposure to a source.

Neonatal Disease

- Neonatal isoerythrolysis is associated with hemolytic anemia.
- Tyzzer's disease is seen in older foals; organisms are seen in the liver with Warthin-Starry stain.
- EHV-1 is differentiated on a severe leukopenia and pneumonia.
- Septicemia is differentiated by other physical examination findings, blood culture and postmortem specimens.

Hepatobiliary

- Hemolytic anemia, fasting, cholelithiasis, neoplasia, hepatic abscess, acute and chronic hepatitis.
- Differentiated on U/S findings, hematology, and serum biochemistry.

DIAGNOSTICS

CBC/Biochemistry/Urinalysis

- Serum biochemistry profile reflects specific organ involvement; leukocytosis, hyperfibrinogenemia.
- Urinalysis (if renal involvement) shows RBC, WBC, and casts.

Other Laboratory Tests

- Culture of *Leptospira* is difficult due to fastidious growth requirements and length of time required for culture. Dark-phase microscopy and FAT are also used.
- Antemortem body fluids (i.e., urine, blood, and aqueous humor) or postmortem tissues (i.e., kidney, liver, fetus, and placenta) must be placed in transport media recommended by the diagnostic laboratory. The collection of midstream urine samples from second urination after furosemide administration enhances isolation, and repeat sampling increases the chances of isolation.
- MAT results need to be interpreted with caution as normal adults can have titers of greater than 1:100. Paired samples taken 2 to 4 weeks apart showing a fourfold increase also need cautious interpretation as the duration and strength of the response is variable. Comparison with other farm individuals may assist with interpretation. Mares with MAT titers greater than 1:6400 that are in contact with a mare that has aborted should be isolated and treated accordingly.
- MAT and culture can be performed on vitreous humor samples.
- No PCR is available, at this stage, for routine use.

Imaging

U/S may assist in the evaluation of hepatic and renal disease.

Pathologic Findings

Fetus and neonates: Most common findings are icterus, generalized petechial and ecchymotic hemorrhages, and microabscesses of kidneys. Placenta is edematous with a necrotic chorion covered with mucous exudates. Allantoic membrane may contain cystic nodular masses.

THERAPEUTICS

Drug(s) of Choice

- Effectiveness of treatment for leptospirosis in horses in unknown.
- Combination of penicillin (200,000 IU/mL) and dihydrostreptomycin (250 mg/mL) 20 mL IM BID for 7 days resulted in no urine shedding. Potassium penicillin (20,000 IU/kg IV every 6 hours) has been recommended in infected pregnant mares to prevent infection of the fetus.

Ophthalmic

Therapy is aimed at reducing immune-mediated inflammation and providing mydriasis and analgesia.

Reproductive

Antimicrobial therapy is indicated to prevent and decrease shedding of spirochetes in urine or prophylactic treatment of pregnant in-contact mares with high titers.

Precautions/Interactions

Avoid use of potentially nephrotoxic drugs if renal disease is suspected.

Alternative Drugs

Oxytetracycline (5–10 mg/kg) for 7 days has been used.

Appropriate Health and Nursing Care

Reproductive

Aborting mares should be isolated and the area they inhabited be disinfected. Contaminated bedding, fetal and placental tissues should be rapidly removed and disposed. Mares can shed leptospires in urine for up to 4 months post-abortion.

Renal/Urologic

Appropriate antimicrobials and supportive care to ensure adequate renal function.

Neonatal Disease

Appropriate antimicrobials and supportive care should be administered. Foals should be isolated, as high numbers of leptospires are shed in urine.

Hepatobiliary

Appropriate antimicrobials and supportive care should be administered.

Activity

Activity should be restricted to decrease environmental contamination.

 COMMENTS

Client Education

The client should be informed as to the zoonotic potential. Infection can occur through contact of mucous membranes or skin lesions with urine or tissue from an infected animal.

Patient Monitoring

Ophthalmic

Recurrent episodes of uveitis.

Reproductive

Therapy should be instituted if fetal membranes are retained or if signs of systemic illness become evident. Monitor in-contact mares' serum titer levels and consider antibiotic therapy of in-contact pregnant mares.

Renal/Urologic/Neonatal Disease/Hepatobiliary

Monitor hepatic and renal function.

Prevention/Avoidance

- Approved vaccinations are not available for use in horses in North America.
- Extra-label uses of vaccines are being investigated as prevention for recurrent uveitis.
- Isolate affected animals, and consider antibiotic therapy for in-contact pregnant mares.
- Limit access to wet environments, and avoid contamination with other domestic animals and wildlife.

Possible Complications

- Ophthalmic: blindness associated with recurrent uveitis.
- Reproductive: abortion outbreak.
- Neonatal disease: Foals from infected dams may be born with clinical disease.
- Zoonotic potential: Clinical signs are variable from asymptomatic infection to sepsis and death. Most common complaints are flu-like symptoms and vomiting; however, neurologic, respiratory, cardiac, ocular, and gastrointestinal manifestations can occur.
- Pregnancy: Abortion, stillbirths, and neonatal disease can be sequelae, depending on the stages of infection and gestation.

Expected Course and Prognosis

- Ophthalmic: alternating periods of acute and quiescent disease.
- Reproductive: uneventful recovery of mare.
- Neonatal disease, renal/urologic, and hepatobiliary: Prognosis is guarded in severe acute disease and depends on the extent of organ invasion and the severity of tissue injury.

Abbreviations

BID   twice a day
CBC   complete blood count

CNS central nervous system
EHV equine herpes virus
EVA equine viral arteritis
FAT fluorescent antibody test
IM intramuscular
IV intravenous
MAT mixed agglutination test
PCR polymerase chain reaction
RBC red blood cells
U/S ultrasound, ultrasonography
WBC white blood cells

See Also

- Agalactia/Hypogalactia
- Mammary gland: mastitis, lactation
- Prolonged pregnancy

Suggested Reading

Bernard WV. 1993. Leptospirosis. *Vet Clin North Am Equine Pract* 9: 435–444.
Donahue JM, Williams NM. 2000. Emergent causes of placentitis and abortion. *Vet Clin North Am Equine Pract* 16: 443–456.

Author: Jane E. Axon

chapter 37

Mammary Gland, Normal

DEFINITION/OVERVIEW

- The equine mammary gland or udder is situated in the inguinal region. It is not easily visible in maiden or nonpregnant, nonlactating mares.
- In the term pregnancy and lactating mare, the gland becomes easily visible from a distance both laterally and caudally. Mammary gland function is fundamental for protection of the newborn foal (colostrum), and for its growth and development (lactation).
- Examination of the mammary gland and its secretion during pregnancy is an important part of pregnancy health and prediction of time of foaling.
- The mammary gland should be examined:
  - In the immediate postpartum period.
  - When normal growth of the foal is in question or appears to be compromised.
- Examination of the mammary gland is an important part of the prepurchase examination of broodmares as well as mares to be used as ET recipients.

ETIOLOGY/PATHOPHYSIOLOGY

Anatomy

Mammae

The equine mammary gland is composed of two halves (mammae) divided by a septum along the longitudinal intermammary groove. The gland is supported medially by an elastic medial suspensory ligament and laterally by the fibrous lateral suspensory ligaments (Fig. 37.1).

- The mammae are divided into loosely distinct lobes by the suspensory ligament trabeculae. Each gland is made of two (sometimes three) lobes (lactiferous duct systems) with the cranial system being the largest. The glands (generally four) are completely independent.
- In the nonlactating mare, the gland is very small and lies caudal to two folds of abdominal skin. The teats are small and laterally flattened (Figs. 37.2a, b, and c).

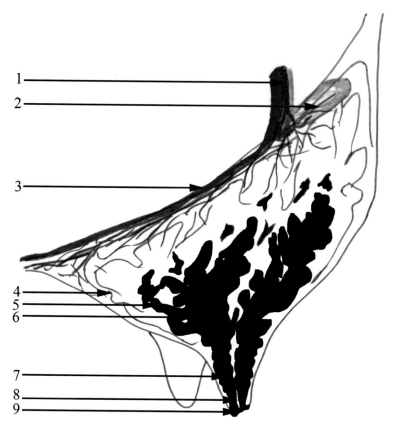

■ **Figure 37.1** Schematic drawing of the cross section of the equine mammary gland: (1) mammary (external pudendal) artery and vein; (2) supramammary lymph node; (3) subcutaneous abdominal (milk) vein; (4) parenchyma (lobule and alveoli) tissue (glandular tissue); (5) lactiferous duct; (6) gland cistern (lactiferous sinus of the glandular part); (7) teat cistern (lactiferous sinus of the papillary part); (8) papillary duct; and (9) rosette of Furstenberg.

Teats

In the term pregnancy and lactating mare, the teats and mammae enlarge and extend cranially and caudally. The gland becomes easily visible from a distance both laterally and caudally (Figs. 37.3a and b).

■ Each teat presents two and sometimes three orifices (Fig. 37.2c). Each corresponds to a separate papillary duct (streak canal) leading to a separate papillary part (teat cistern) and a glandular part (gland cistern of the lactiferous sinus). The teats do not have an organized sphincter (*see* Fig. 37.1).

Duct System

The lactiferous duct system is lined by bistratified columnar epithelium. Smaller ducts leading to the alveoli are lined by simple columnar epithelium. The alveoli are composed of specialized epithelial cells (lacteal cells) surrounding a lumen which collects

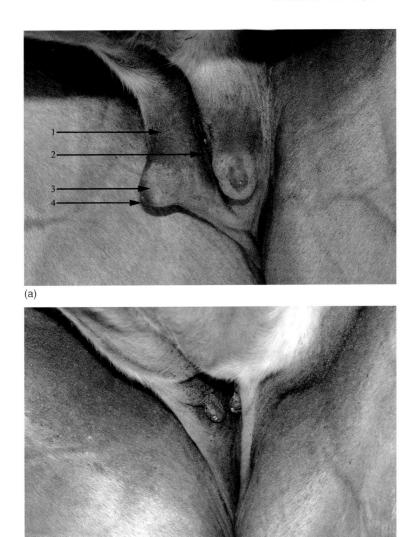

(a)

(b)

■ **Figure 37.2** *A,* Nonlactating parous mare: (1) mammae; (2) longitudinal intermammary groove; (3) teat (papilla); and (4) rosette of Furstenberg. *B,* Nonlactating maiden mare. *C,* Lactating mare showing two teat milk streaks.

milk and channels it via a small duct into a common lobular duct. The alveoli are grouped in lobules surrounded by myoepithelial cells which contract under the effect of oxytocin and cause milk ejection.

Blood and Lymphatic System and Nervous Innervation

■ Arterial supply is provided by the external pudendal artery which branches into a cranial and a caudal mammary artery as it emerges from the inguinal canal and enters the caudal part of the gland.

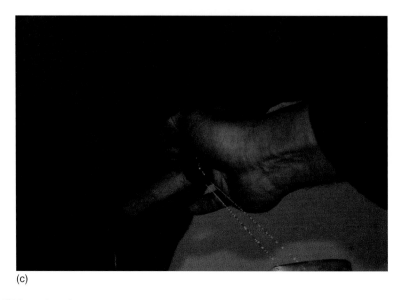

(c)

■ **Figure 37.2** continued

- Venous drainage is provided primarily by the venous plexus collecting laterally into external pudendal veins on each side and cranially into the caudal superficial epigastric vein which connects with the superficial vein of the thoracic wall (obvious during lactation). Supplemental venous drainage is provided by connection with the obturator veins and branches of the internal pudendal vein.
- Lymphatic drainage leads to superficial inguinal (mammary) LN at the base of the udder. Accessory LN drain from the subcutis.
- Innervation is provided mainly by the genitofemoral nerves via the inguinal canals. The mammary skin is innervated by branches from the pudendal nerve and nerves of the flank.

Mammary Development

- Mammogenesis is evident during early fetal life as differentiated cells proliferate and form mammary buds.
- Teats are present at births in colts and fillies.
- Allometric growth of the mammary gland is noticed in fillies after puberty.
- The gland is very small and not visible from a distance in nonpregnant maiden females. The exceptional neonate fillies may show some development and lactation (see "witch's milk").
- The most important development of the mare's mammary gland occurs in the last third of pregnancy and predominantly in the last 4 weeks of gestation.
- Both estrogens and progestagens are required for mammary gland development. The rise of prolactin during the last week of pregnancy, combined with the decrease in progestagens, is thought to be the primary mechanism for initiation of lactation.
- Lactation can be initiated in progesterone/dopamine antagonist-treated mares.

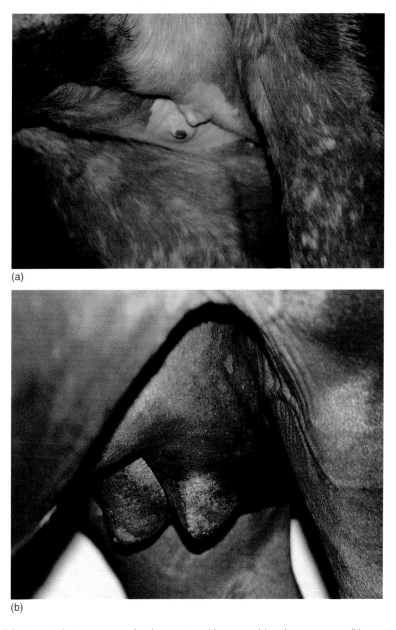

Figure 37.3 Preparturient mammary development: maiden mare *(a)* and parous mare *(b)*.

- Prolactin increases post-foaling, but lactation can be maintained without prolactin after it peaks.
- Milk ejection is caused by oxytocin release in response to mammary stimulation or psychological factors.
- Electrolytes in mammary gland secretions change as foaling time approaches, evidenced by a decrease in Na+ and increases in potassium and calcium.

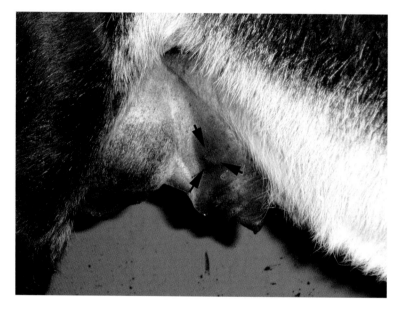

■ **Figure 37.4** Rudimentary teats in male donkey *(arrows)*.

- Colostrogenesis (concentration of IgG from serum into the mammary gland) takes place during the last 4 weeks of pregnancy. Leakage of colostrums during this period can result in a significant reduction of IgG content post-foaling.

Genetics

- Some breeds of mares and donkeys are selected for mammary conformation and milk production.
- Mules have rudimentary mammae that can develop into a normal producing gland with appropriate hormonal stimulation or pregnancy and birth (ET).
- Male donkeys have more obvious rudimentary teats on each side of the prepuce (Fig. 37.4).

Systems Affected

Mammary gland

 ## SIGNALMENT/HISTORY

- Normal female equines
- Pregnancy
- Lactation: postpartum, post-abortion, or subsequent to hormonal treatments.

Risk Factors

Pregnancy

Historical Findings

- Advanced pregnancy (third trimester), physical examination findings: The normal mammary gland should present a smooth surface. In late pregnancy the mammary gland is enlarged. Edema of the cranial region of the mammary gland frequently occurs the last few days pre-foaling. In late pregnant and lactating mares, veins are visible on the surface of the mammary gland. The gland and teats should be symmetrical and non-painful.
- Postpartum or aborting mares.

 ## CLINICAL FEATURES

General Appearance of Milk

- Milk secretions may be serous to thick, flocculent, purulent or hemorrhagic.

Cytology

- Cytological evaluation is important to diagnose mastitis because bacterial culture results are frequently negative.

 ## DIAGNOSTICS

Imaging

- U/S of the mammary gland may be helpful in identifying deep lesions.
- U/S evaluation of the mammary gland can be accomplished with 7.5-, 5.0-, or 3.5-MHz linear or sector transducers, depending on the size and depth of a lesion.
- Normal U/S appearance of the mammary gland reveals heterogeneous mammary tissue, as well as the anechoic gland cistern of the lactiferous sinus (Fig. 37.5).
- U/S evaluation of the retromammary and inguinal lymph nodes should be included in the evaluation.
- Doppler U/S may help identify vascular problems.

Pathological Findings

See Mastitis.

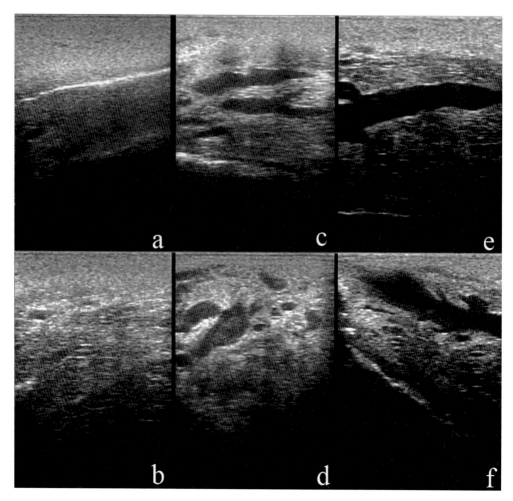

■ **Figure 37.5** Ultrasound of the normal equine mammary gland: (a) maiden non-lactating; (b) parous non-lactating; (c) lactating glandular cistern and parenchyma, longitudinal view; (d) lactating glandular cistern and parenchyma, cross-sectional view; and (e) and (f) of a teat cistern.

THERAPEUTICS

Drug(s) of Choice

See Mammary Gland, Lactation, Induction of.

COMMENTS

Abbreviations

ET embryo transfer
IgG immunoglobulin G
LN lymph nodes
U/S ultrasound, ultrasonography

See Also

- Lactation
- Mastitis

Suggested Reading

Chavatte-Pamer P. 2002. Lactation in the mare. *Eq Vet Educ Manual* 5: 88–93.
Knottenbelt D. The mammary gland. 2003. In: *Equine Stud Farm Medicine and Surgery*. Knottenbelt DC, Pascoe RP, Leblanc M, et al (eds). Philadelphia: Saunders; 343–352.

Author: Ahmed Tibary

chapter 38

Mammary Gland, Mastitis

DEFINITION/OVERVIEW

- An inflammatory process of the mammary gland that can be infectious, primarily due to bacteria.
- Other causative agents include fungi, nematode migration, or subsequent to complication of trauma or neoplasia.
- Mastitis may be clinical or subclinical.

ETIOLOGY/PATHOPHYSIOLOGY

- Infectious organisms can colonize the mammary gland tissue by routes that are:
  - Hematogenous
  - Percutaneous
  - Ascending
- Establishment of the infection and production of a disease state depend on:
  - Virulence of the organism.
  - Ability/effectiveness of local defense mechanisms.
  - Local defense mechanisms in the mammary gland rely primarily on prevention of entry at the teat level, physical elimination by ejection of milk, and local immunity.
- *Hematogenous* infection is generally a sequel of septicemia or a specific localization of a pathological process (e.g., as with *Corynebacterium pseudotuberculosis* abscesses).
- *Ascending* infection can occur via the teat canal or via a breach in the mammary gland integument (e.g., cutaneous neoplasia, cutaneous *Habronema*, lacerations, insect bites).
  - Accumulation of milk in the gland predisposes it to ascending infection.
  - Mastitis is generally seen in heavy-milking mares at the time of weaning.
  - Mastitis can occur in nonlactating mares and immature fillies, with similar routes to develop an infectious mastitis (hematogenous, percutaneous or ascending).
- Abscesses: can be caused by complications of mastitis or penetrating wounds. Abscesses due to hematogenous spread of *Corynebacterium pseudotuberculosis* have been reported.

Systems Affected

- Mammary gland
- Other systems may be affected as a complication of septicemia, endotoxemia.

 SIGNALMENT/HISTORY

- Mastitis is often seen in mares just after weaning. Accumulation of milk in the gland predisposes it to ascending infections.
- Mastitis can develop any time lactation occurs, even in dry mares and immature fillies.

Risk Factors

- Draft breeds, some breeds of donkeys, and dairy mares are predisposed to mastitis.
- Incidence of mastitis and mammary gland neoplasia is low.
- Incidence of mammary gland neoplasia is reported to be 0.11% to 0.19% of all equine tumors.
- Unsanitary conditions
- Other causes of local edema and swelling, or trauma that create an opportunity for an infection to become established.
    - Weaning
    - Excessive manipulation of the mammary gland (milking).

Historical Findings

- Foal's failure to thrive or it is losing weight.
- Mare's refusal to let the foal suckle.
- Depression, fever, sudden enlargement of the mammary gland, or increased sensitivity in the region.

 CLINICAL FEATURES

Physical Examination Findings

- Mammary gland enlargement (Fig. 38.1).
- The gland may be asymmetrical if only half of the gland is affected.
    - The affected gland may show edema (swelling), increased firmness, or increased heat.
    - Acute mastitis is associated with a painful mammary gland and, in some cases, hind limb lameness.
    - Mammary secretions may be serous, serosanguinous, bloody or purulent (Fig. 38.2).
- Puerperal edema or mastitis may be observed during the neonatal period and are usually associated with the foal's failure to nurse or possibly septicemia in the mare.

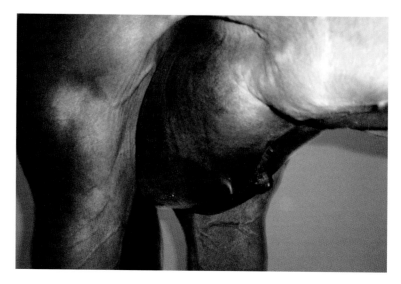

■ **Figure 38.1** Mammary gland enlargement due to acute mastitis.

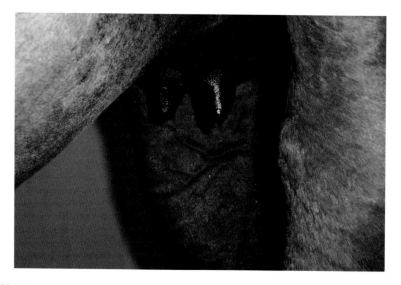

■ **Figure 38.2** Serosanguinous secretion in a term gestation mare.

- Fever and signs of endotoxemia are associated with peracute mastitis.
- Reactive mammary LN are observed in acute mastitis.
- Subclinical mastitis may not be asymptomatic.
- Chronic mastitis may be revealed by the presence of fibrosis or loss of function of all or part of the gland.

Causes

- Bacterial infections are the most common.
  - Most common isolates are *Streptococcus equi* subspecies *zooepidemicus*.
  - Other isolates include *Staphylococcus aureus*, *S. epidermis*, *Klebsiella* sp., *Pseudomonas* sp., *Corynebacterium* sp. and *Escherichia coli*.
  - Staphylococcus infections are associated with a recurrent granulomatous mastitis (botryomycosis).
  - *Corynebacterium pseudotuberculosis* may be isolated from mammary gland abscesses.
- Fungal infections are rare.
  - *Aspergillus* spp.
  - *Coccidioides immitis*
- Parasitic lesions include strongyle larva migrans and cutaneous habronemiasis.
- Noninfectious cause of local inflammation of the mammary gland may be due to neoplasia (mammary adenocarcinoma).

 DIFFERENTIAL DIAGNOSIS

- Enlargement of the mammary gland may be due to neoplastic changes (adenocarcinoma, melanoma, mastocytoma, lymphosarcoma, cutaneous lymphosarcoma). Adenocarcinomas are aggressive, malignant, and can metastasize through lymphatic and hematogenous routes.
- Differential diagnosis of mammary gland enlargement or asymmetrical development:
  - Diffuse mastitis
  - Mammary abscess
  - Neoplasia
  - Edema
  - Normal prepartum enlargement
  - Placentitis
  - Impending abortion
- Visible or palpable multifocal nodules on the mammary skin:
  - Cutaneous lymphosarcoma
  - Melanoma
- Visible or palpable multifocal nodules in deeper tissue:
  - Adenocarcinoma
  - Ulcerative lesions may be seen involving the skin and deeper tissue.
- Increased size of the regional LN may be observed with adenocarcinoma.
- Weight loss and other systemic signs may be present if tumors are aggressive and have metastasized.

DIAGNOSTICS

- Normal in chronic and subclinical mastitis.
- Leucocytosis with neutrophilia and hyperfibrinogenemia may be seen in acute mastitis.
- If systemic endotoxemia is present, may see leucopenia, azotemia, increased nonsegmented WBC, and toxic changes in neutrophils.

Other Laboratory Tests

General Appearance of Milk

- Milk secretions may be serous to thick, flocculent, purulent, or hemorrhagic.

Cytology

- Cytological evaluation is important particularly for mastitis because bacterial cultures are not always positive (false-negative). Cytology of milk samples can be done on sediment or direct smears stained with Trichrome or Diff Quick® stain. Gram staining is helpful in determining the type of bacteria involved in mastitis to enable earlier onset of antimicrobial treatment.
- Cytological evaluation of nodular lesions may be done by fine needle aspiration. Biopsy of some lesions may be required for definitive diagnosis of neoplastic and parasitic lesions.
- Expected appearance of cytology samples:
  - Colostrum(s): normal or homogenous protein background with karyorrhectic debris and red-to purple spheres (Fig. 38.3).
  - Milk from lactating mares will reveal protein background; sometimes some neutrophils may be present.
  - Dry mare mammary secretions will be characterized by the presence of foam cells (uniformly vacuolated macrophages), a few neutrophils, and a few inspissated casts (Fig. 38.4).
  - Supporous lactation secretion may present a variety of secretory cells and neutrophils (Fig. 38.5).
- With mastitis, there is an increase in degenerated and non-degenerated neutrophils and necrotic debris. Infectious agents (bacteria or fungi) may be visualized on cytology (Figs. 38.6 and 38.7).
- With neoplasia, various cytological changes may be observed depending on the type of tumor.

Culture

- Samples should be submitted for aerobic bacterial as well as for fungal culture.
- Anaerobes are not a common cause of mastitis in the mare.
- Cultures may be positive as a result of:
  - Secondary infectious condition

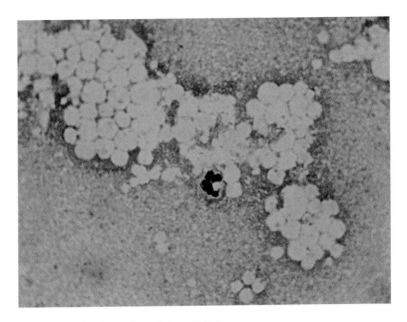

■ **Figure 38.3** Mammary gland secretion cytology: Colostrum.

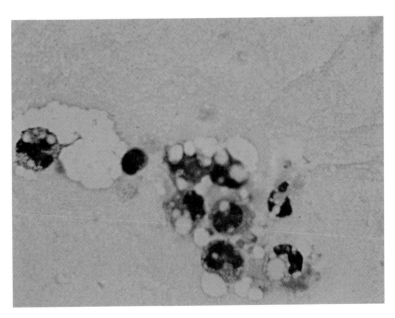

■ **Figure 38.4** Mammary gland secretion cytology: Normal milk mid-lactation. Note the presence of some foam cells and leucocytes.

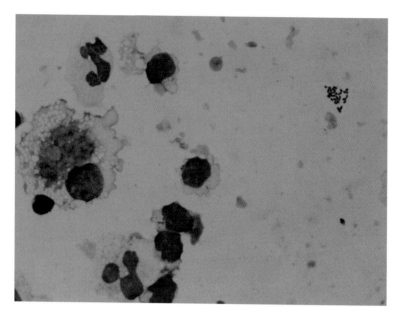

■ **Figure 38.5** Mammary gland secretion cytology: Supporous lactation secretions (bacteria on the right are surface contaminants).

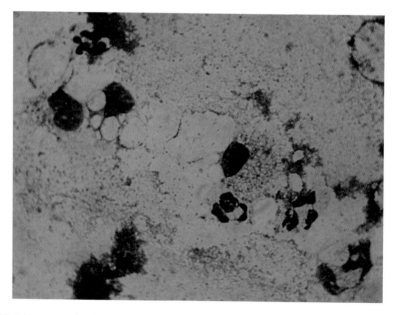

■ **Figure 38.6** Mammary gland secretion cytology: Milk from subclinical mastitis.

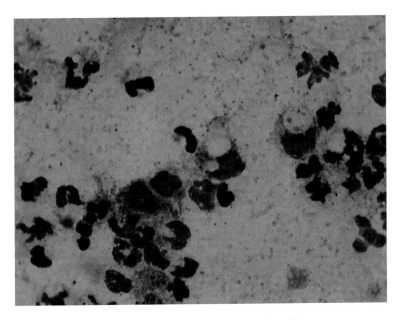

■ **Figure 38.7** Mammary gland secretion cytology: Milk from clinical mastitis.

- ■ Ulcerative neoplastic lesion
- ■ Parasitic lesions
- ■ Cultures are negative in up to 30% of mastitis cases.

Histopathology

- ■ Mammary gland biopsy may be helpful to identify the cause of inflammation or determine the type or nature of neoplasia.

Imaging

- ■ U/S of the mammary gland may be helpful in identifying deep lesions (abscesses or neoplasia).

 THERAPEUTICS

Drug(s) of Choice

- ■ Cattle mastitis preparations (intramammary) are available and contain various antimicrobials: cefquinone, amoxicillin, cephapirin benzathine, cephapirin sodium, cloxacillin, cloxacillin benzathine, erythromycin, ampicillin, pirlimycin hydrochloride, penicillin dihydrostreptomycin and ceftiofur hydrochloride.
  - ■ Caution should be exercised when inserting these bovine preparations.
  - ■ The nozzle of the syringe is too long for the mare's short teat canal.

- Introduction of intramammary antimicrobials should be preceded by thorough disinfection of the teat with iodine or chlorhexidine solution.
- Solutions of gentamicin (100 mg in 100 mL of sterile saline) or ceftiofur sodium (1 to 2 g in 100 mL of sterile water) may be administered directly into the mammary gland.
- Systemic antimicrobial therapy consists primarily of trimethoprim sulfadiazine (15 mg/kg q 12 h) or a combination therapy, such as procaine penicillin (20,000 units/kg IM, every 12 hours) and gentamycin (8 mg/kg IM, every 24 hours).
- Anti-inflammatory treatment is frequently necessary. Either flunixin meglumine (1.1 mg/kg IV or PO every 24 hours) or phenylbutazone (2 to 4 mg/kg IV or PO every 12 or 24 hours).

Precautions/Interactions

- Effects of treatment on the foal (mare's milk will contain antibiotics).
- Foal should be given supplemental feed.

Appropriate Health Care

- Frequent stripping of the mammary gland to eliminate infectious organisms, inflammatory cells and products.
- Hot packing or hydrotherapy.
- Intramammary infusion may be sufficient/appropriate in some cases.
  - The use of lactating cow intramammary preparations has been reported.
  - This is more difficult due to the peculiar anatomy of the mare's mammae.
  - Intramammary therapy often requires sedation.
  - The teat should be thoroughly cleansed pre-treatment to avoid introduction of bacteria.
- Systemic broad-spectrum antibiotics for two weeks (e.g., trimethoprim sulfonamide, penicillin in combination with gentamicin).
- NSAIDs
- Abscesses require drainage.
- Chronic recurrent mastitis, non-responsive to therapy, may require amputation.

Traumatic and Parasitic Lesions

- Deep lacerations should carefully be evaluated for integrity of the teat canal. Corrective surgery may be attempted if tissue integrity is not overly compromised.
- Habronemiasis lesions require total excision.

Nursing Care

- Mastitis: Slight exercise may help to decrease edema in the mammae.
- Postsurgical care is dependent on the extent of surgery.

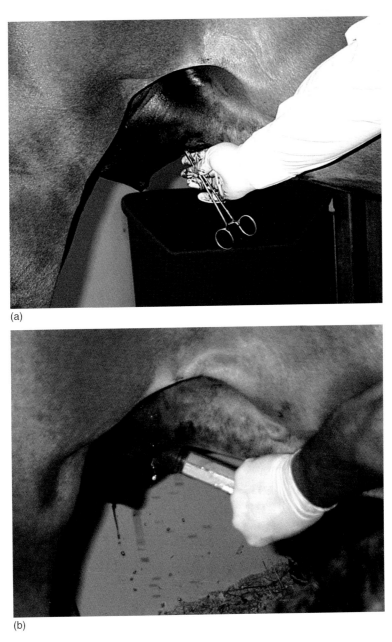

(a)

(b)

■ **Figure 38.8** Drainage *(a)* and flushing *(b)* of a mammary abscess.

Surgical Considerations

- Surgical drainage is the best approach for walled-off abscesses (Fig. 38.8).
- Surgical ablation of the gland and LN is the treatment of choice for malignant tumors.
  - Ablation is usually performed under general anesthesia, with the mare in dorsal recumbency.

- After scrubbing and drainage of the LN and cystic nodules, the skin is incised in an elliptical shape.
- The incision extends from the anterior edge to the posterior edge of the udder centered on the teat.
- The skin flap is elevated by sharp dissection to isolate the deeper mammary tissue.
- Blunt finger dissection allows separation of the gland from the raphé and abdominal wall.
- The blood vessels within the inguinal area are exposed and dissection is continued using electrocautery.
- All major vessels (external pudendal artery, obturator vein, branches of the internal pudendal and contralateral external pudendal vein, caudal superficial epigastric vein) are double ligated before total ablation.
- A drain tube or roll of gauze soaked with povidone iodine is inserted in the surgical cavity and the skin is closed.
- Transudate may be evident for up to 10 days.
- Drain is removed after 14 days.
- Nonmalignant tumors may be treated by surgical excision or cryotherapy. Mastocytoma and equine sarcoid may require total excision.
- Local cryotherapy has been performed using liquid nitrogen.
  - Direct contact of cooled brass cryoprobe (−20°C) on the lesion.
  - Slow thaw and refreeze technique.
- Melanomas are best left undisturbed unless they become aggressive.

 COMMENTS

Client Education

- Regular monitoring of foal growth/weight gain provides a good gauge of the mare's satisfactory lactation.
- Regular monitoring of mammary gland appearance and the mare's reaction to the gland being palpated.

Patient Monitoring

- The mare should be evaluated daily during treatment.
- Response to treatment should be noticeable after 3 days, with complete resolution of signs within a week. Preferably the treatment should be continued for an additional week.
- CBC and biochemistry should be performed on mares that exhibited severe clinical signs or toxic changes before treatment, or for those necessitating long-term administration of aminoglycoside or NSAIDs.
- Mares that underwent surgical ablation of tumors or the mammary gland should be monitored daily until the surgical site is healed.

- Mares with aggressive tumors should be monitored periodically with CBC and biochemistry.

Possible Complications

- Loss of function or decreased milk production, decreased protein and calcium concentration in future lactations may affect quality of colostrums, foal health, growth and development.
- Recurrent bouts of mastitis may develop in cases resistant to treatment.
- Metastasis to other organs and systemic involvement may be seen, particularly in the case of adenocarcinoma.
- Complications from surgery are always a possibility when mammary gland ablation is attempted.
- Abortion if systemic signs are severe.

See Also

- Mammary gland, normal
- Lactation

Abbreviations

CBC	complete blood count
IM	intramuscular
IV	intravenous
LN	lymph node(s)
NSAIDs	nonsteroidal antiinflammatory drugs
PO	per os (by mouth)
U/S	ultrasound, ultrasonography
WBC	white blood cells

Suggested Reading

Freeman KP. 2002. Cytological evaluation of the equine mammary gland. *Eq Vet Educ Manual* 5: 97–98.

McGladdery AJ. 2002. Differential diagnosis and treatment of diseases of the equine mammary gland. *Eq Vet Educ Manual* 5: 94–96.

Perkins NR, Threlfall WR. 2002. Mastitis in the mare. *Eq Vet Educ Manual* 5: 99–102.

Author: Ahmed Tibary

chapter 39

Mammary Gland, Lactation

DEFINITION/OVERVIEW

- Lactation is the normal secretory (lactogenesis) and excretory function (milk let-down) of the lactiferous duct system of the mammary gland resulting in the production and ejection of colostrum or milk.
- Lactation is induced by the hormonal changes occurring during pregnancy.
- Lactation can be induced by exogenous hormone treatments in nonpregnant, non-lactating mares.
- In the normal parturient mare without human intervention, lactation lasts up to 12 months. In modern horse breeding lactation lasts 4 to 6 months, dependent on the timing of weaning.

ETIOLOGY/PATHOPHYSIOLOGY

Initiation of Lactation

- The mammary gland develops in the last third of pregnancy and predominantly in the last 4 weeks of gestation.
- Both estrogens and progestagen are required for initial development of the lobulo-alveolar system of the mammary gland.
- In the late pregnant mare, the main active progestogens are 5α-pregnanes which have an affinity for progesterone receptors.
- The estrogens involved in the late pregnant mare are composed of estradiol-17α which rises just before foaling as well as other estrogens (equilin and equilenin).
- Progesterone inhibits milk production.
- The rise of prolactin during the last week of pregnancy combined with the decrease in progestagen is thought to be the primary mechanism for initiation of lactation.
- Prolactin plays the major role for lactogenesis and initiation of lactation, but not for its maintenance. Plasma prolactin levels peak 2 to 3 days post-foaling and remain higher in lactating than in nonlactating mares for 10 weeks post-foaling.
- Lactation can be initiated in progesterone/dopamine antagonist-treated mares.
- Milk ejection is caused by oxytocin release in response to mammary stimulation or psychological factors.

- However, oxytocin discharge prior to milk let-down does not seem to be critical to initiate lactation for mares.
- In the mare, the mammary gland has two distinct secretions: (1) prefoaling secretions and colostrogenesis, and (2) milk.

Prefoaling Mammary Secretion

- Electrolytes in mammary gland secretions change as the time of foaling approaches. This is demonstrated by a decrease in sodium and increase in potassium and calcium.
- Colostrogenesis (concentration of IgG from serum into the mammary gland) takes place during the last 4 weeks of pregnancy. Leakage of colostrums during this period can result in a significant reduction of the IgG content that is available post-foaling.
- Final mammary development occurs in the last 2 weeks of pregnancy. Mammary secretions change from straw-colored to gray and become sticky just prior to parturition.
- Colostrum is "produced" only for the first 24 hours. Total protein in colostrum is around 150 g/L. IgG concentration is 60 to 150 g/L in the first 24 hours and declines rapidly thereafter.

Lactation

- Lactation in the free-ranging mare may last as long as 11 months.
- Current horse breeding practices generally limit lactation to the first 20 weeks following delivery. Lactation stops with early weaning.
- Total milk production in an average lactation for most light-breed horses is 2,500 kg.
  - An average horse mare produces a volume equal to 3% of her BW in the first 3 months, and 2% BW in the last 3 months of lactation.
  - Ponies: 4 to 5% of BW in the first 3 months and 2 to 3% in the last 3 months.
- Peak lactation occurs at about 6 to 8 weeks postpartum; approximately 2.5 to 3 kg milk per 100 kg BW.
- Daily milk yield in average riding-type mares (approximately 454 kg) varies between 15 and 20 kg.
- Draft horses and some breeds of donkeys produce more milk and the duration of lactation persists longer.

Milk Composition

- Mare's milk is low in total protein, fat, and energy and high in lactose. Lactose concentration increases during lactation (Table 39.1).

Systems Affected

Mammary gland

TABLE 39.1 Composition of Equine Milk.

Species and Weeks of lactation	Energy (Kcal/100 G)	Protein (%)	Fat (%)	Lactose (%)	Total Solids (%)
Mare 1–4	58	2.7	1.8	6.2	10.7
Mare 5–8	53	2.2	1.7	6.4	10.5
Mare 9–21	50	1.8	1.4	6.5	10.0
Donkey	52	1.84	1.47	6.25	10

(National Research Council: *Nutrient Requirements for Horses*. 5th ed. Wash, DC. National Academic Press, 1989 and Lu, et al, 2006).

 # SIGNALMENT/HISTORY

- Postpartum nursing mares
- Nurse mares prepared with hormonal treatment.
- Draft breeds, some breeds of donkeys, and dairy mares are selected for higher milk yield.

Historical Findings

- Normal pregnancy and foaling
- Exogenous hormonal induction of lactation
- Mammary gland enlargement and secretion
- Result of hormonal changes during pregnancy
- Hormonal treatments/induction of lactation

 # CLINICAL FEATURES

Associated Conditions

- Agalactia is the failure of lactogenesis. This is a syndrome often associated with tall fescue toxicosis or oats infected with the fungus *Claviceps purpurea* (Brazil). The syndrome is the result of decreased prolactin concentration by dopamine agonist and serotonin antagonist activity of the alkaloids.
- Premature lactation: mammary gland development and premature lactation signal a disorder in the endocrinologic activity of the uteroplacental unit and of impending abortion (see twinning, placentitis, abortion).
- Inappropriate lactation
  - Mammary gland development and production of a serous secretion (soporous lactation) is seen in nonpregnant mares or fillies in spring and early summer and is believed to be due to seasonal hormonal (prolactin) changes and the presence of phytoestrogens.
  - Lactation in newborn fillies, known as "witch's milk," is a common phenomenon. It may be associated with high lactogenic hormone concentration.

- Eclampsia/hypocalcemia: observed primarily in the immediate postpartum period in draft horses, miniature mares, and some breeds of donkeys.
- Mastitis
- Poor reproductive performance may result from loss of condition during lactation.

Age-Related Factors

- Poor lactation may be observed in primiparous mares and older mares with chronic changes in mammary tissue.

Pregnancy

Condition for development of mammary glands and initiation of lactation.

 # DIFFERENTIAL DIAGNOSIS

Mammary gland enlargement can be the result of:
- Diffuse mastitis
- Mammary abscess
- Neoplasia
- Edema
- Normal prepartum enlargement.
- Impending abortion

Differentials for poor mammary development should include:
- Agalactia due to fescue toxicosis.
- Agalactia due to poor nutrition (body condition).
- Chronic fibrotic changes of the mammary tissue.

 # DIAGNOSTICS

General Appearance of Milk

- Milk secretions may be serous to thick, flocculent, purulent or hemorrhagic.

Cytology

- Cytological evaluation is important particularly for diagnosing mastitis as bacteriologic culture is not always positive.
  - Cytological evaluation can be made of smears stained with Gram stain, Diff Quick®, Pollack trichrome, or Papanicolaou stain.
  - Diff Quick® is relatively easy for use in a practice situation.
  - Pollack Trichrome and Papanicolaou staining produce the best cytological differentiation, but are time-consuming.
- First milk (colostrums) will have a normal or homogenous protein background with karyorrhectic debris, and red-to-purple spheres.

- Milk from lactating (wet) mares has a green-to-rust protein background; sometimes neutrophils will be present.
- Mammary secretions of non-lactating (dry) mares are characterized by the presence of foam cells (uniformly vacuolated macrophages), a few neutrophils, and a few inspissated casts.

Pathologic Findings

See Mammary gland and Mastitis

 THERAPEUTICS

- Lactation may be induced in nonparturient mares.
- Induction of lactation is a combination treatment: Progesterone and estradiol to induce mammary development, and a dopamine D2-antagonist (Sulpiride) to increase plasma prolactin concentration and promote lactogenesis.

Drug(s) of Choice

For induction of lactation

- Progesterone-in-oil, 150 mg IM daily
- Estradiol-in-oil, 50 mg IM daily
- Altrenogest (500 mg) vaginal sponge
- Estradiol (50 mg), vaginal sponge
- $PGF_2\alpha$ (dinoprost, 5 mg IM)
- Sulpiride (50 mg IM BID, or 1 mg/kg BW, IM, BID)

Treatment Protocol 1

Week 1: Altrenogest (500 mg) and estradiol benzoate (50 mg) delivered by intravaginal sponge.
Week 2:
- Day 8, $PGF_2\alpha$ (5 mg dinoprost, IM).
- Place a new vaginal sponge (a repeat of week 1), and administer daily Sulpiride (1 mg/kg IM, BID).
- Day 9: start milking the mare. Five milkings (important for stimulation) per day, beginning 2 minutes after administration of oxytocin (5 IU IM).

Treatment Protocol 2

Week 1: Daily IM administration of progesterone (150 mg) and estradiol 17β (50 mg).
  Day 7: $PGF_2\alpha$ (5 mg dinoprost, IM).
  Days 1 to 10: Sulpiride (500 mg, IM, BID).
  Place foal with mare on day 1 of treatment.

To Stop Lactation

- Bromocryptine (0.08 mg/kg[75] BW BID to 0.8 mg/kg[75] BW daily) to effect.
- Note: this treatment will have a negative effect on follicular activity.

Appropriate Health Care

- Regular observation of mare's body condition.
- Regular observation of foal growth.

Nursing Care

- Special attention should be given to the concentration of amino acids in the lactating mare diet.
- Lysine and methionine are critical for the foal.

Diet

- In its first 3 months of life, the foal receives its nutrition for growth and development predominantly from milk.
- Average daily energy expenditure for lactation is approximately 12 Mcal.
- Mares may develop a negative energy balance if not fed properly.
- Energy should be provided at maintenance requirement, plus (BW × 0.792)% for production.
- Protein requirement is 0.5 g/Mcal of DE for the first 3 months.
- If a diet has an energy density of 2.6 Mcal/kg (1.2 Mcal/lb), it should contain 13% protein.
- A diet of an energy density of 2.45 Mcal/kg, should contain 11% crude protein.
- Particular attention should be given to the amino acids lysine and methionine.
- Feeding a high fat diet (22%–25%) is indicated in mares experiencing weight loss during lactation.
- Supplementation of a foal's diet with copper and iron may be indicated, as these elements may not be provided in sufficient quantities by milk.

 # COMMENTS

Client Education

- BCS or weigh the nursing mare
- Regular monitoring of foal growth
- Early identification of agalactia and factors that may induce agalactia or poor milk production.
- Milk production is negatively affected by tall fescue toxicosis, dystocia, pain, uterine infection, or photoperiod.
- If lactation has been negatively affected, proper supplementation of the foal is critical.

- Supplementation of the neonate is dependent on the stage of lactation.
  - In the first 5 weeks of life: specially formulated equine milk replacer provided at about 20 to 25% of the foal's BW per day.
  - Between 5 to 8 weeks: decrease milk replacer to 17% to 20% of the foal's BW per day and encourage creep feeding (mostly grain).
  - After 2 months, foals can be weaned and fed as a weanling.
- ADG of foals:
  - ADG in kg/day = 0.95 − 0.05(Mcal DE/day).
  - This formula can be adjusted based on the foal's daily gain to determine how much creep (supplemental) feeding is needed to achieve the desired gain for a particular breed.

Possible Complications

- Agalactia
- Mastitis

Abbreviations

ADG	average daily gain
BCS	body condition score
BID	twice a day
BW	body weight
DE	digestible energy
IM	intramuscular
IgG	immunoglobulin G
PGF	natural prostaglandin

Suggested Reading

Chavatte-Palmer P. 2002. Lactation in the mare. *Eq Vet Educ Manual* 5: 88–93.

Deals PF, Duchamp G, Massoni S, et al. 2002. Induction of lactation in non-foaling mares and foal growth of foals raised by mares with induced lactation. *Therio* 58: 859–861.

Deichsel K, Aurich J. 2005. Lactation and lactational effects on metabolism and reproduction in the horse mare. *Livestock Prod Sci* 98: 25–30.

Lu DL, Zhang DF, Liu PL, et al. 2006. Chemical composition and nutritive value in donkey milk. *Xinjiang Agri Sci* 43: 335–340.

Steiner JV. 2006. How to induce lactation in non-pregnant mares. *Proc AAEP* 52: 259–269.

Vivrette SL, Kindahl H, Munro CJ, et al. 2000. Oxytocin release and its relationship to dihydro-15-keto PGF$_2\alpha$ and arginine vasopressin release during parturition and to suckling in postpartum mares. *J Reprod Fert* 119: 347–357.

Author: Ahmed Tibary

chapter 40

Miniature Horse Reproduction

DEFINITION/OVERVIEW

- The AMHA standards define two types according to height.
  - Type A must be less than 34 inches at the withers.
  - Type B must measure 34 to 38 inches at the withers.

ETIOLOGY/PATHOPHYSIOLOGY

Female Reproduction

- Their general reproductive physiology is similar to full-sized mares, but miniatures present some peculiarities relative to infertility and pregnancy complications.
- Type A mares should not be bred before 3 years of age.
- The estrous cycle is slightly longer than that of full-sized mares, ranging from 21 to 24 days.
  - Estrus lasts 3 to 7 days.
- Gestation length in Type A mares averages 319 days (range 300–350 days).
- Parturition events are similar to those of full-sized mares.
  - Premonitory signs are discrete.
  - Mammary gland development is minimal prior to parturition; waxing is rarely exhibited.
  - Mammary gland softening may be a good indicator of impending parturition.
- Placental delivery after foaling is relatively faster than in full-sized mares (less than 30 minutes).
- Miniature mares have a high incidence of premature placental separation.
- Uterine involution is completed by 2 weeks postpartum.

Reproductive Loss

- Reproductive performance is largely unstudied.
- Miniature mares have a higher incidence of early pregnancy loss (as high as 40% in the first 90 days of gestation) and mid-to-late term abortions.
  - Most pregnancy losses are due to congenital disorders.
  - Dwarfism has been associated with these late pregnancy losses.

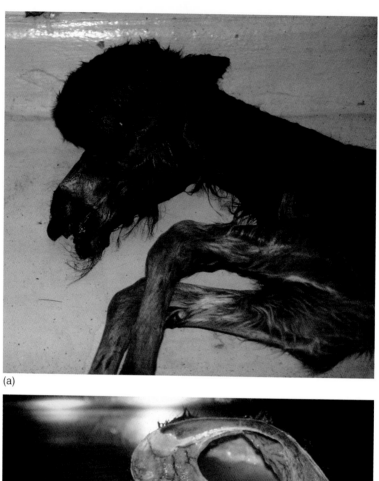
(a)

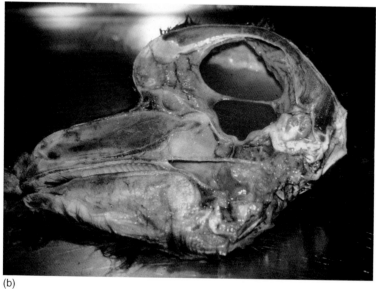
(b)

■ **Figure 40.1** *A*, Hydrocephalus and domed head shape are a common cause of abortion or dystocia in miniature mares. *B*, Postmortem of hydrocephalic foal; its skull, halved.
Images courtesy of C. L. Carleton.

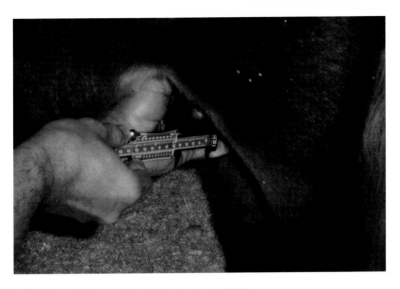

■ **Figure 40.2** Miniature stallion genitalia: Testicular measurement.

- Dystocia is more common than in full-sized mares, especially those that terminate in abortion.
  - Hydrocephalus and dome-headed foals are often the cause of dystocia (Figs. 40.1a and b).

Male Reproduction

- Testicular descent in the miniature seems to be slower that in full-sized horses (Fig. 40.2).
  - Breeders often wait until 3 years of age before declaring a colt a cryptorchid.
- Average testicular length and width:
  - Type A stallion: 6.3 by 3.9 cm.
  - Type B stallion: 7.2 by 4.5 cm.
- Total spermatozoa in the ejaculate is lower in Type A (4.3 billion) than Type B (5.4 billion).
- The bulbourethral glands each measure 21 mm length (range 16–27 mm) by 14 mm height (range 10–11 mm).
- The prostate is approximately 18 mm (range 11–29 mm) wide.
- The seminal vesicles measure 9 mm in diameter (range 5–15 mm); luminal measurement of 4 mm (range 2–11 mm).
- The ampullar diameter is 10 mm (range 5–20 mm); luminal measure of 1 mm (range of 0–3 mm).

Artificial Breeding

- The AMHA allows registration of foals conceived by AI, *if*:
  - Cooled semen is used in mares on the same premises as the stallion or
  - Within 72 hours of collection and with an appropriate permit.

- Use of frozen semen is not allowed.
- Stallions should not breed more than a total of 20 mares by AI per season.
- ET techniques are similar to those used in the horse, but this technology is not allowed by the AMHA (foals resulting from ET may not be registered).

Systems Affected

Reproductive

 SIGNALMENT/HISTORY

Physical Examination Findings

Examination of the Open Female

- The perineal area and vulva are small and tight.
- TRP may be possible in some individuals. Sedation and infusion of lubricant mixed with lidocaine into the rectum is recommended.
- Vaginal examination is best performed with a small Polanski speculum (Figs. 40.3a and b).

Examination of the Pregnant and Parturient Female

- Diagnosis of pregnancy by TRP is similar to horses. However, it may not be possible in small mares.

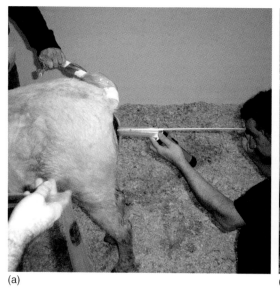
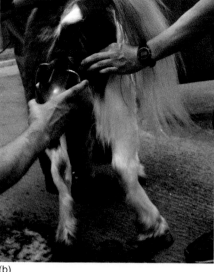

(a)   (b)

■ **Figure 40.3** Vaginal examination with the tube speculum is easy and allows collection of endometrial cytology and bacteriology samples if the mare in heat *(a, b)*. A small Polanski speculum is the best method for postpartum evaluation.

- Sick pregnant females should always be checked for hyperlipidemia.
- Dystocia is more common in miniature horses. Imaging techniques are often required to determine fetal position and fetal viability.
- Obstetrical management is similar to that used in the full-sized mare.

Examination of the Male

- The protocol for examination of miniature stallions is similar to that used for evaluation of full-sized stallions. Total scrotal width varies from 7 to 8 cm.
- Semen can be collected by a small Missouri AV (best choice), by manual stimulation, or by using a nonspermicidal human condom.
  - A standard-sized Missouri model can also be used. Preparation is similar, but when filled, lubricated, and its leather cover in place, add additional water (at the appropriate fill temperature. If the filling device ends with a tire valve connect, it will be easier to overfill/inflate it further) to increase the internal pressure for the smaller, miniature stallion's penis.
  - If using the standard length Missouri AV to collect a miniature stallion (corollary of using the Colorado-type AV in a 1,000-lb horse): as soon as possible after pulsations have been detected (ejaculation): (1) the AV is removed from the stallion as he dismounts, (2) the valve on the side of the AV is unscrewed, while the length of the AV is held almost parallel to the floor with only the AV's proximal (large end) slightly elevated to prevent back flow [loss] of semen; (3) water escapes from the double walled AV, creating a rapid decrease in the internal pressure, and semen within the AV quickly flows to the collection bag/bottle. (4) This quick deflation of the water jacket prevents semen from remaining in contact with the warmer AV temperature for more than a minute, thus preserving its quality.
- Semen volume varies from 15 to 30 mL depending on Type A or B.
- Average ejaculate parameters:
  - Motility: 65%
  - Morphology: 55%
  - Total number of spermatozoa in the ejaculate ranges from 2 to 5 billion.
  - Total number of *motile* sperm about 1.5 billion.

Risk Factors

Genetics

- Congenital abnormalities are common and some are hereditary:
  - Dwarfism
  - Parrot (Brachygnathia)
  - Sow mouth (Prognathia)

○ CLINICAL FEATURES

- In the female, specific causes of infertility and abortion are assumed to be similar to those found in horses. Miniatures are susceptible to all infectious organisms that are

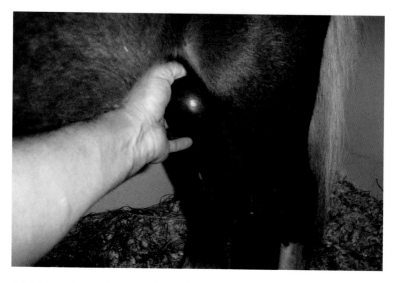

■ **Figure 40.4** Miniature stallion after correction of bilateral testicular torsion (180 degrees).

causative agents in full-sized horses. It is estimated that 8% to 9% of miniature stallions are positive for EVA.
■ Type A mares have a higher incidence of reproductive problems.
■ Reported causes of anestrus include:
  ■ Hypothyroidism
  ■ Equine Cushing's disease
  ■ Ovarian dysgenesis (63XO karyotype) has been described in a miniature mare.
■ Infertility in the male is often due to severe testicular degeneration.
■ Testicular torsion has been reported in miniature stallions (Fig. 40.4).

 # DIAGNOSTICS

■ Approaches to diagnosing and resolving common reproductive problems, are similar to those used in full-sized horses.
■ Miniature mares are more prone to:
  ■ Hyperlipidemia
  ■ Pre- and postpartum hypocalcemia.
■ Indications similar to horses for specific conditions.
■ Blood lipids should be determined in sick pregnant females.
■ Hypocalcemia is common in females with:
  ■ RFM (Figs. 40.5a and b).
  ■ Pre- or postpartum depression.
  ■ Muscle fasciculations (*Thumps*) or synchronous diaphragmatic flutter.

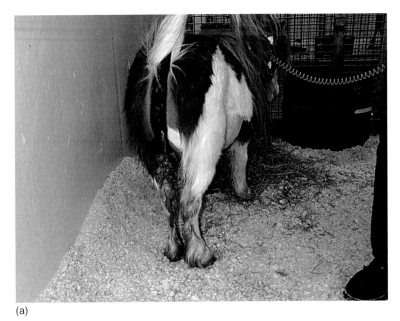

(a)

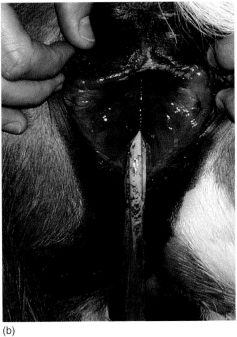

(b)

■ **Figure 40.5** A dystocia with subsequent retained fetal membranes in a miniature mare with *thumps* and hypocalcemia *(a)*. Retained fetal membranes and the vulva showing slight bruising *(b)*.

Microbiology

■ Similar to horses

Cytology

■ Similar to horses

Imaging

U/S of the female reproductive tract

■ U/S characteristics of the uterus at different phases of the estrous cycle are similar to those described in the mare. Transrectal U/S in miniature mares is best accomplished using an U/S probe mounted on a rigid extension plastic rod (Fig. 40.6).
■ The rectum can completely be emptied of feces by administration of an enema.
■ Preovulatory follicle size ranges from 28 to 35 mm.
■ Transrectal U/S diagnosis of pregnancy is possible at 12 days post-ovulation and becomes easier after 18 days.
  ■ The appearance and growth of the conceptus is comparable to that of full-sized horses in the first 30 days.
  ■ Fetal heart beat is detected at 26 days.
■ Transabdominal U/S diagnosis of pregnancy is possible at 30 days but easier after 45 days (Fig. 40.7).
  ■ The U/S transducer should be placed deep into the inguinal area (near the mammary gland).

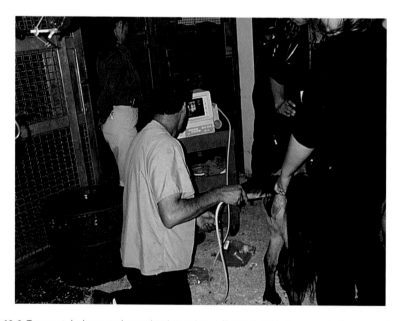

■ **Figure 40.6** Transrectal ultrasound examination using a linear transducer mounted on an extension pipe. This technique is helpful if transrectal palpitation is not possible. It can be difficult to master.

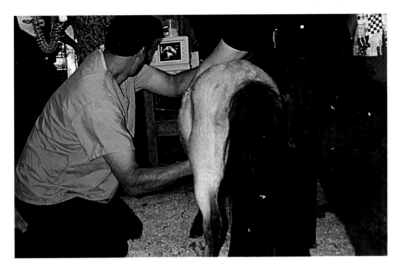

■ **Figure 40.7** Transabdominal ultrasound for pregnancy and fetal evaluation. Pregnancy diagnosis by trans-abdominal ultrasound can be done reliably starting at 45 days of pregnancy.

- The bladder is the main landmark to identify the uterus.
- Fetal well-being and utero-placental thickness are evaluated in the same manner as in the mare.
- CTUP values are 2 mm less than those reported for full-sized mares.

U/S of the Male Genital Organs

- Examination technique is similar to that for full-sized stallions.

Other Diagnostic Procedures

- Endometrial biopsy technique is similar to that used in full-sized mares.
  - Sedation of the mare is highly recommended.
- Endocrinological evaluation is helpful for pregnancy diagnosis.
  - eCG can be used from 40 to 100 days but may yield a high rate of false-positives due to the high rate of pregnancy loss after the endometrial cups have formed.
  - A blood estrone sulfate value greater than 30 ng/mL indicates pregnancy; accurate after 100 days gestation.
  - Fecal estrone sulfate greater than 100 ng/gm after 150 days, is indicative of pregnancy.
  - Combining two tests, eCG and estrone sulfate, improves diagnostic accuracy.

THERAPEUTICS

Drug(s) of Choice

Hormone Therapy

- Treatment of RFM: Oxytocin at 30 IU in LRS, with an IV drip-rate of 1 IU every 2 minutes.
- Induction of ovulation: hCG (1,000 to 1,500 IU, IV), when the follicle is larger than 32 mm in diameter and the female is in estrus.
- Induction of luteolysis (short-cycling): cloprostenol (125 µg IM).

Appropriate Health Care

- Similar to horses
- Pregnant miniature mares should be carefully monitored for hyperlipemia if off-feed.

Surgical Considerations

Similar to full-sized mare

See Also

See specific conditions in mares.

Abbreviations

AI	artificial insemination
AMHA	American Miniature Horse Association
AV	artificial vagina
CTUP	combined thickness of the uterus and placenta
eCG	equine chorionic gonadotropin
ET	embryo transfer
EVA	equine viral arteritis
hCG	human chorionic gonadotropin
IM	intramuscular
IV	intravenous
LRS	lactated Ringer's solution
RFM	retained fetal membranes
TRP	transrectal palpation
U/S	ultrasound, ultrasonography

Suggested Reading

Campbell ME. 1992. Selected aspects of miniature horse reproduction: Serologic and ultrasonographic characteristics during pregnancy and clinical observations. *Proc Soc Therio*, 89–96.

Paccamonti DL, Buiten AV, Parlevliet JM, et al. 1999. Reproductive parameters of miniature stallions. *Therio* 51: 1343–1349.

Pozor MA, McDonnell SM. 2002. Ultrasonographic measurements of accessory sex glands, ampullae, and urethra of normal stallions of various size types. *Therio* 58: 1425–1433.

Tibary A. 2004. Reproductive patterns in donkeys and miniature horses. *Proc NAVC*, 17–21, 231–233.

Tibary A, Sghiri A, Bakkoury A. 2008. Chapter 17: Reproduction. In: *The Professional Handbook of the Donkey*, 4th ed, Svenden ED, Duncan J and Hardill D (eds). The Donkey Sanctuary, Whittet Books; 314–342.

Author: Ahmed Tibary

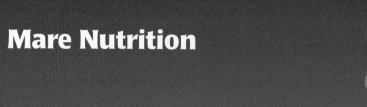
Mare Nutrition

 DEFINITION/OVERVIEW

Phases of nutrient concerns and requirements for broodmares follow.

Pre-breeding

- Before breeding, mares need to be gaining or at least maintaining BW to optimize conception rates, which can be a challenge if the mare is lactating.
- Ensure adequate calorie and protein intake to accomplish these goals.

Early Pregnancy (First 6–7 Months)

- The first two trimesters of pregnancy do not impose great nutritional strain on the mare, but are the time when potential teratogens (i.e., Vitamin A) can cause the most damage to the fetus.
- Feed to maintain body condition.
- Avoid over-supplementing, especially Vitamin A.

Late Pregnancy

- In the last trimester, when the fetus is growing most rapidly, there is an increased need for protein, energy and minerals, especially calcium, phosphorus, copper, and perhaps zinc. This coincides with late winter/early spring conditions, when only dry hay is available. Additional vitamin A and E might be beneficial.
- Gradually increase protein, calcium, and phosphorus intakes, assuming the mare was previously on maintenance intake.

Early Lactation

- Lactation increases demands for water and energy in addition to the still elevated need for protein and minerals.
- Feed to maintain good body condition.
- Energy, protein, and mineral intakes are the highest at this time.
- Coincides with weather-induced stresses and rebreeding.
- Antioxidant vitamin supplementation may be beneficial if not on good pasture.

Late Lactation

- Reduce energy intake if mare is overweight.

SIGNALMENT/HISTORY

- Female to be bred or one that is pregnant or lactating.
- Some mares are "hard keepers;" others are remarkably efficient.
- The challenge is to keep the weight on the former and to provide adequate minerals while avoiding obesity in the latter.
- Improper nutrition will result in:
  - Weight loss, emaciation.
  - Poor body and hair coat condition of mare.
  - Poor conception rates.
  - Weak, small, or deformed foals.

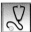

DIFFERENTIAL DIAGNOSIS

- Weight loss, emaciation: Clinical infection/illness, organ failure, toxicity.
- Poor hair coat/hoof condition: poor grooming/hygiene.
- Poor conception rates: management errors.
- Weak, small, or deformed foals: teratogens, fescue toxicity, genetics.

DIAGNOSTICS

Precautions/Interactions

Avoid
- Obesity
- Excessive weight loss.
- Inadequate calcium, phosphorus, copper, and selenium intake.
- Excessive grain, especially sweet feeds.
- Over-supplementation of fat-soluble vitamins, herbal nutraceuticals.

Possible Interactions

- Excess Selenium will interfere with copper absorption or utilization and vice versa.
- Excessive Vitamin E will interfere with Vitamin A absorption and possibly vice versa.
- Excessive grain will predispose to obesity and colic.
- Obesity will predispose mare to laminitis, colic, dystocia.

CBC/Biochemistry/Urinalysis

- Use to rule out clinical infection and illness, organ failure, or toxicity.
- Blood concentrations of most nutrients do *not* reflect intake or dietary adequacy, especially with respect to calcium, phosphorus and vitamins such as A and E.

Other Laboratory Tests

▪ If a nutrient imbalance is suspected, get the feed (i.e., hay, pasture, concentrates) analyzed to determine actual intake.

Diet

Pre-breeding

▪ Free choice (2%–3% BW) good quality forage (hay or pasture), high fat (7%–10%) concentrates at less than 0.5% BW per feeding, if weight gain is needed.
▪ Possibly vitamin A (60 IU vitamin A/kg BW) and E (2 IU vitamin E/kg BW) supplements for 2 weeks before breeding.

Early Pregnancy (Non-Lactating, First 6–7 Months)

▪ Feed to maintain good body condition (5–7 on the Henneke scale of 1–10) but avoid letting the mare get obese.
▪ Do *not* supplement minerals and vitamins if their concentrations are adequate in the ration for maintenance.
▪ Especially avoid over-supplementing the active form of vitamin A (Retinyl/retinol compounds).
    ▪ Potentially teratogenic if given in excess (more than 600 IU/kg BW).

Late Pregnancy (Last Trimester)

▪ Gradually increase mineral and protein intake by feeding concentrates designed specifically for broodmares and foals.
▪ Type and amount really depends on the condition of the mare and hay/forage being fed.
▪ Key is to feed as little high starch concentrate as possible while maintaining increased intakes of protein and minerals.

Early Lactation (First 3 months)

▪ Feed to maintain good body condition.
▪ Energy, protein, and mineral intakes are the highest at this time, plus it often coincides with weather-induced stresses and rebreeding.
▪ Concentrates formulated specifically for broodmares and foals should be used, especially because the foals will often "steal" their dam's concentrates.
▪ Straight grains such as oats, corn, or barley do not have adequate mineral content. The mare's ration will affect her milk mineral content but not the volume produced to any great extent. Avoid excesses or imbalances in the mineral intake by using feeds formulated specifically for lactating mares and that are appropriate for the type of hay used (i.e., calcium/protein content can be lower if fed with alfalfa versus grass hay).
▪ Antioxidant supplementation (vitamins A and E: see preceding recommendations) may be beneficial if not on good pasture.

Late Lactation

- Reduce energy (concentrates) intake if mare is overweight.

Activity

- No restrictions
- Best if on 24/7 turnout or regular exercise program, especially pre-breeding.

 COMMENTS

Client Education

- Horse owners should disregard most of what they see on the Internet and most of what appears in lay magazines.

Patient Monitoring

Body condition assessed weekly or biweekly.

Possible Complications

Old mares may need special senior type feeds.

Abbreviations

BW   body weight
CBC   complete blood count

See Also

- Nutrition of the foal
- Nutrition of the stallion

Suggested Reading

National Research Council. 2007. *Nutrient Requirements for Horses*, 8th ed. Washington, D.C.: National Academy Press.
Body Condition scoring techniques www.equineprotectionnetwork.com/cruelty/henneke.htm.
Ralston SL. 1993. Analysis of Feeds and Forages for Horses. www.rcre.rutgers.edu/pubs/publication.asp?pid=FS714.
Ralston SL. 1997. Diagnosis of Nutritional problems in horses. www.rcre.rutgers.edu/pubs/publication.asp?pid=FS894.
Ralston SL. 2001. Feeding the "easy Keeper" horse. www.rcre.rutgers.edu/pubs/publication.asp?pid=FS799.

Author: Sarah L. Ralston

chapter 42

Ovulation Failure

DEFINITION/OVERVIEW

The ovulatory follicle in a mare is generally 35 mm or larger in diameter. Follicles that obtain that size, but fail to ovulate, are addressed.

ETIOLOGY/PATHOPHYSIOLOGY

- Waves or "clutches" of oocytes are recruited for development into antral follicles during diestrus.
- Ultimately, one or two follicles become dominant and progress to ovulation, while the remaining follicles undergo atresia. The mechanism for this selection is not well understood.
- Estradiol (follicular origin) stimulates an increase in LH secretion (pituitary origin) that ultimately induces ovulation. The LH rise in mares is prolonged compared to other species.
- Deficiencies of either follicular estradiol or pituitary LH secretion can contribute to ovulation failure.

Systems Affected

Reproductive

SIGNALMENT/HISTORY

- Mares of any breed and age may be affected.
- Multiple dominant follicle formation is more common in thoroughbred, standard-bred, warmblood, and draft mares.
- Multiple dominant follicles are most frequently observed from March through May in the northern hemisphere.

Historical Findings

- Mares may exhibit prolonged estrus behavior.
- Discomfort from ovarian enlargement (especially if its increase in size is rapid) can mimic pain associated with colic or a sore back.

CLINICAL FEATURES

- TRP: At least one large (more than 35 mm) fluid-filled structure or simply an enlarged ovary.
- Ovarian U/S: Single or multiple follicle(s), polycystic structures typical of neoplasia, a fluid-filled cavity filled with echogenic particles or fibrin-like strands that are indicative of a hematoma, or, rarely, an ovarian abscess.

 DIFFERENTIAL DIAGNOSIS

- If TRP is the sole means used to determine follicular growth and ovulation, the presence of two or more adjacent follicles may wrongly be interpreted to be one follicle that fails to ovulate. Transrectal U/S is recommended to avoid this dilemma.
- Ovarian neoplasia can mimic persistent follicular development due to similarities of behavior, cycling/teasing, and the presence of fluid-filled cavities on TRP and U/S (see LOS).
- Ovarian abscesses have been reported to develop secondary to invasive ovarian procedures or as a result of hematogenous infection. Abscesses may be confused with persistent follicles on palpation, but the contents most often appear very echogenic on U/S examination. The mare may be systemically ill, but equally if the abscess is walled off, her health may not be compromised at all.
- Paraovarian cysts can be confused with ovarian follicles if they are in close proximity to the ovary. Distinguish from ovarian structures by careful and thorough TRP and U/S.
- Large antral follicles can form during the luteal phase of the estrous cycle (diestrus). Diestrual follicles frequently undergo atresia rather than proceeding to ovulation.
- Hemorrhagic Anovulatory Follicles
  - Normal follicular development occurs, but ovulation does not. These follicles can become quite large (60–110 mm diameter), are filled with blood, and may or may not exhibit luteinization of the follicular wall.
  - Such follicles may be estrogen-deficient or result from insufficient hypothalamic GnRH release. Decreased pituitary LH secretion/synthesis may be involved in their pathogenesis.
  - The occurrence of hemorrhagic anovulatory follicles is most common during autumn transition, but can occur during the breeding season.
- Persistent Follicles
  - These are not ovarian cysts, which rarely occur in the mare, but are follicles that fail to undergo final maturation and ovulation.
  - Most common during late vernal or early autumnal transition.
- Luteinized Follicles
  - Described in humans, luteinized follicles may also occur in mares. An association with reproductive senility has been proposed.

- This form of ovulation failure may occur in the normal mare when secondary CLs form during pregnancy.

DIAGNOSTICS

- Historical review: Rule out problems related to season, sexual behavior, and teasing methods.
- TRP: Ovarian size, shape, and activity; uterine size and tone; and cervical relaxation should be evaluated three times per week over the course of several weeks to characterize the mare's reproductive status.
- U/S: Essential to fully evaluate the abnormal ovary.
    - The follicular fluid of normal follicles may exhibit increasing echogenicity and its shape may change from spherical to pear/triangular shape as ovulation approaches.
    - Hematomas may have a distinctly echogenic fluid content with large, criss-crossing fibrin-like strands (see LOS).
    - Persistent follicles appear normal on U/S examination (see LOS).
    - The U/S appearance of ovarian neoplasia varies depending on the tumor type. Although all ovarian tumors in the mare are rare, the most common is the GCT/GTCT. Its most common U/S image is of an irregularly polycystic/multilocular structure (see LOS).
- Serum progesterone concentration: basal levels of less than 1 ng/mL indicate no active/mature CL is present. Mature CL function is associated with levels of greater than 4 ng/mL. Follicles can develop during diestrus when progesterone concentrations are greater than 1 ng/mL.
- Serum testosterone and inhibin concentrations: Mares typically have testosterone values less than 50 to 60 pg/mL and inhibin values less than 0.7 ng/mL. Hormone levels suggestive of a GCT/GTCT (in a nonpregnant mare) are: testosterone levels greater than 50 to 100 pg/mL, inhibin greater than 0.7 ng/mL, and progesterone less than 1 ng/mL.
- Transrectal U/S is routinely used to evaluate the equine reproductive tract. The reader is referred to other texts for a comprehensive discussion on this technique.

THERAPEUTICS

- If ovulation failure is related to season (transition, anestrus), no treatment is necessary. Transitional follicles eventually regress, though it may take 30 to 45 days.
- Luteinized follicles and some hematomas may respond to prostaglandin treatment. Hematomas may be unresponsive to treatment for 2 weeks or longer after they first develop.
- Ovulation of persistent follicles may be induced using either hCG or deslorelin implants, if they occur late in vernal transition (hCG receptors are present by that time).
- Ovariectomy is the recommended procedure to eliminate ovarian tumors or abscesses.

Drug(s) of Choice

- $PGF_2\alpha$ (Lutalyse® [Pfizer], 10 mg, IM) or its analogs to lyse persistent CL tissue.
- Ovulation can be stimulated if a follicle is at least 30 mm by deslorelin, or if at least 35 mm by hCG (2500 IU, IV).
- Altrenogest (Regu-Mate® [Intervet], 0.044 mg/kg, PO, SID, minimum 15 days) can be used to shorten the duration of vernal transition, providing follicles at least 20 mm diameter are present and the mare is demonstrating behavioral estrus. $PGF_2\alpha$ (Lutalyse® [Pfizer], 10 mg, IM) on day 15 of the altrenogest treatment increases the reliability of this transition management regimen.

Precautions/Interactions

Horses

- $PGF_2\alpha$ and its analogs are contraindicated in mares with asthma, COPD, or other bronchoconstrictive disease.
- Prostaglandin administration to pregnant mares can cause CL lysis and abortion. Carefully rule out pregnancy before administering this drug or its analogs.
- $PGF_2\alpha$ causes sweating and colic-like symptoms due to its stimulatory effect on smooth muscle cells. If cramping has not subsided within 1 to 2 hours, symptomatic treatment should be instituted.
- Antibodies to hCG can develop after its use in the mare. It is desirable to limit its use to no more than two or three times during one breeding season. The half-life of these antibodies ranges from 30 days to several months; they typically do not persist from one breeding season to the next.
- Deslorelin implants have been associated with suppressed FSH secretion and decreased follicular development in the diestrus period immediately following use. This causes a prolonged interovulatory period in non-pregnant mares. Implant removal within 1 to 2 days post-ovulation decreases this possibility.
- Altrenogest, deslorelin and $PGF_2\alpha$ should not be used in horses intended for food purposes.

Humans

- $PGF_2\alpha$ or its analogs should not be handled by pregnant women, or people with asthma or bronchial disease. Any accidental exposure to skin should immediately be washed off.
- Altrenogest should not be handled by pregnant women or people with thrombophlebitis and/or thromboembolic disorders, cerebrovascular disease, coronary artery disease, breast cancer, estrogen-dependent neoplasia, undiagnosed vaginal bleeding or tumors that developed during the use of oral contraceptives or estrogen-containing products. Any accidental exposure to skin should immediately be washed off.

Alternative Drugs

Cloprostenol sodium (Estrumate® [Schering-Plough Animal Health], 250 μg, IM), is a prostaglandin analog. This product is used in similar fashion as the natural prostaglandin, but it has been associated with fewer side effects. It is not currently approved but is widely used in horses.

 COMMENTS

Patient Monitoring

Until normal cyclicity has been established, regular reproductive examinations are recommended.

Possible Complications

Individual mares may be prone to develop more than one hemorrhagic or anovulatory follicle in a season.

Synonyms

Hemorrhagic anovulatory follicle = autumn follicle

Abbreviations

CL	corpus luteum
COPD	chronic obstructive pulmonary disease
FSH	follicle stimulating hormone
GCT/GTCT	granulosa cell tumor/granulosa theca cell tumor
GnRH	gonadotropin releasing hormone
hCG	human chorionic gonadotropin
IM	intramuscular
IV	intravenous
LH	luteinizing hormone
LOS	large ovary syndrome
$PGF_2\alpha$	natural prostaglandin
PO	per os (by mouth)
SID	once a day
TRP	transrectal palpation
U/S	ultrasound, ultrasonography

See Also

- Abnormal estrus intervals
- Anestrus
- Large ovary syndrome

Suggested Reading

Carleton CL. 1996. Atypical, asymmetrical, but abnormal? Large ovary syndrome. In: *Proc Mare Reproduction Symp, ACT/SFT* 27–39.

Ginther OJ. 1995. Ovaries. In: *Ultrasonic Imaging and Animal Reproduction: Horses.* Cross Plains, WI: Equiservices; 23–42.

Hinrichs K. 2007. Irregularities of the estrous cycle and ovulation in mares (including seasonal transition). In: *Current Therapy in Large Animal Theriogenology.* Youngquist RS, Threlfall WR (eds). St. Louis: Saunders Elsevier; 144–152.

Pierson RA. 1993. Folliculogenesis and ovulation. In: *Equine Reproduction.* McKinnon AO, Voss JL (eds). Philadelphia: Lea & Febiger; 161–171.

Sharp DC, Davis SD. 1993. Vernal transition. In: *Equine Reproduction.* McKinnon AO, Voss JL (eds). Philadelphia: Lea & Febiger; 133–143.

Author: Carole C. Miller

chapter 43

Ovulation, Induction of

DEFINITION/OVERVIEW

Mares remain in estrus for 5 to 7 days and ovulate 24 to 48 hours before going out of heat. A routine management strategy is to breed mares every other day while in heat. As a consequence, a mare may be bred two to three times per cycle, if no OIA is used. The goals of administration of an OIA are to advance (hasten) the time of ovulation in the cycle so that ovulation will occur within a predictable time period.

ETIOLOGY/PATHOPHYSIOLOGY

- hCG binds to the equine LH receptor in gonadal tissue.
- The "LH-like bioactivity" of hCG causes maturation and ovulation of the dominant follicle.
- Recombinant equine LH has similar biologic activity as that of native LH and will induce ovulation when administered to mares in estrus.
- Agonists of GnRH, such as deslorelin, stimulate release of endogenous LH from the anterior pituitary, which subsequently advances follicle maturation and ovulation.

Systems Affected

Reproductive

SIGNALMENT/HISTORY

The guidelines for administration of an OIA are:
- The mare is in estrus.
- Diameter of the largest follicle is at least 35 mm; it may be much larger (or a size appropriate for the breed).
- Edema of the endometrial folds is present (at least or more than Grade 1 on a scale of 0–3).

Risk Factors

- Failure of ovulation after drug administration.
- Adverse reactions to OIAs are rare.

CLINICAL FEATURES

- Breed differences exist as to the minimum follicular size at which an OIA should be administered with the expectation of a predictable ovulation.
- The normal size ranges of preovulatory follicles in mares of various breeds are:
  - Quarter Horses and Arabians: 35 to 45 mm
  - Thoroughbreds and Standardbreds: 40 to 50 mm
  - Warmbloods: 45 to 55 mm
  - Draft breeds: 50 to 60 mm
- Administration of an OIA before the dominant follicle is capable of responding will result in failure to ovulate.
- Quarter Horse, Arabian, Thoroughbred, and Standardbred mares will usually respond if an OIA is administered when a growing follicle is at least 35 to 40 mm in diameter.
- It is recommended that an OIA not be administered to warmblood and draft mares until the dominant follicle is 40 to 45 mm and 45 to 50 mm, respectively.
- Indications for use of an OIA include breeding to a stallion with limited availability, breeding with cooled-transported semen or frozen semen, or if a single mating or insemination is desired (i.e., for a mare with a history of PMIE).

DIFFERENTIAL DIAGNOSIS

- Diestrus dominant follicles (i.e., detection of a large follicle in the presence of a CL). Such mares will not be in estrus and will not have endometrial edema present. Expect uterine tone to be increased and the cervix closed (findings also characteristic of diestrus).
- Parovarian cysts (i.e., fluid-filled structures adjacent to the ovary that have the appearance of a large ovarian follicle on U/S).

DIAGNOSTICS

- Detection of a large preovulatory follicle in a mare in behavioral estrus or in a mare with endometrial edema by TRP and U/S.

Pathological Findings

- Mares may develop anovulatory or hemorrhagic follicles with or without administration of an OIA.

- Detection of echogenic particles or strands within the lumen of the dominant follicle is the first sign of impending ovulation failure and formation of a hemorrhagic follicle.
- Currently there are no management practices or medications to prevent the occurrence of anovulatory follicles in predisposed mares.
- A single dose of prostaglandin, natural or an analogue (e.g., cloprostenol, 250 μg cloprostenol sodium, IM) is effective in causing regression of a luteinized anovulatory follicle.
  - The structure will regress and a new wave of follicular development will commence.
  - Wait approximately 7 days after the structure has started to form, or until it is fully luteinized, before administering prostaglandin.

 ## THERAPEUTICS

To advance (hasten) the time of ovulation in the cycle so that ovulation will occur within a predictable time period.

Drug(s) of Choice

- hCG: Chorulon® (Intervet, Millsboro, DE) is effective at dosages ranging from 1,500 IU to 2,500 IU. May be administered IV or IM. The dose used by the author is 2,500 IU, IV.
- reLH (EquiPure LH™, AspenBio Pharma Inc., Castle Rock, CO) is administered at a dose of 750 μg, IV.
- The GnRH agonist, deslorelin (available through several compounding pharmaceutical companies), is administered at a dose of 1.5 mg, IM.
- Approximately 85% to 90% of mares will ovulate in response to any of the three OIAs.
- The percentage of mares ovulating after treatment is not significantly different between the OIAs.
- The average time interval from treatment to ovulation for hCG and reLH is approximately 36 to 40 hours and 40 to 44 hours for deslorelin.

Precautions/Interactions

- OIAs should not be administered before the dominant follicle is mature (see Clinical Features) or the follicle may fail to respond (i.e., does not ovulate).

Alternative Drugs

- Currently, only hCG, reLH, and deslorelin are routinely used to induce ovulation in mares.
- A recent study reported the hormone kisspeptin may be effective in ovulation induction.
  - Kisspeptin is not commercially available at present.

- Additional studies are needed to verify its potential as an OIA for routine clinical use.

COMMENTS

Patient Monitoring

- Palpation or U/S daily or every other day.
- Ovulation should occur within 36 to 48 hours following administration of an OIA.

Possible Complications

- A SC implant form of deslorelin containing 2.1 mg of the GnRH agonist (Ovuplant™, Ft. Dodge Animal Health, Inc., Ft. Dodge, IA) was reported occasionally to result in prolonged interovulatory intervals in treated mares.
- The implant is no longer commercially available in the United States.

Expected Course and Prognosis

- Ovulation should occur within 36 to 48 hours following administration of an OIA.
- Efficacy at inducing a timed ovulation may be reduced in mares that are older than 20 years of age.

Synonyms

Estrus   heat

Abbreviations

CL	corpus luteum
GnRH	gonadotropin releasing hormone
hCG	human chorionic gonadotropin
IM	intramuscular
IV	intravenous
LH	luteinizing hormone
OIA	ovulation inducing agent
PMIE	persistent mating-induced endometritis
reLH	recombinant equine luteinizing hormone
SC	subcutaneous
TRP	transrectal palpation
U/S	ultrasound or ultrasonography

See Also

- Abnormal estrus intervals
- Anestrus
- Ovulation failure

- Prolonged diestrus
- Mare's estrous cycle, manipulation of

Suggested Reading

Briant C, Schneider J, Guillaume D, et al. 2006. Kisspeptin induces ovulation in cycling Welsh pony mares. *Animal Reprod Sci* 94: 217–219.

Farquhar VJ, McCue PM, Nett TM, et al. 2001. Effect of deslorelin acetate on gonadotropin secretion and ovarian follicle development in cycling mares. *JAVMA* 218: 749–752.

McCue PM. 2003. Induction of ovulation. In: *Current Therapy in Equine Medicine 5*. Robinson NE (ed). Philadelphia: Saunders; 240–242.

Meinert C, Silva JFS, Kroetz I, et al. 1993. Advancing the time of ovulation in the mare with a short-term implant releasing the GnRH analogue deslorelin. *Eq Vet J* 25: 65–68.

Author: Patrick M. McCue

chapter 44

Ovulation, Synchronization

DEFINITION/OVERVIEW

- Estrus length is variable in the mare.
- Timing of ovulation is a prerequisite for breeding management and use of assisted reproductive techniques such as:
  - AI with frozen-thawed semen using the minimal dose of semen, or when a low number of sperm from subfertile, valuable stallions is used.
  - Limited availability of a stallion.
  - Natural service of mares and the stallion has a full book of mares.
  - Timing of embryo collection and synchronization with recipients.
  - Timing of oocyte collection.
  - Timing for oocyte transfer.
- Individual and seasonal conditions may produce variable results.

ETIOLOGY/PATHOPHYSIOLOGY

- Synchronization of ovulation in mares requires two steps:
  - Synchronization of follicular waves.
  - Induction of ovulation.
- Synchronization of follicular waves in the cyclic mare is primarily achieved by combined administration of estrogen and progesterone.
- Treatment with progesterone alone does not inhibit follicular development.
- Estradiol 17-β causes follicular regression.
- Ovulation is induced by either GnRH, hCG, or reLH when the size of the follicle and uterine edema are appropriate.
- Synchronization of ovulation in transitional mares may be achieved by eFSH combined with an ovulation induction agent

Systems Affected

Reproductive

DIAGNOSTICS

Imaging

- Transrectal U/S to determine ovarian activity.
- Transrectal U/S to monitor follicular growth and endometrial edema.

THERAPEUTICS

Drug(s) of Choice

P & E

- Progesterone (50 mg/mL) and estradiol 17-β (3.3 mg/mL) (P&E, a compounded drug). Daily IM injection of 3 mL of P & E for 10 days followed by $PGF_2\alpha$ or a prostaglandin analogue administered at the time of the last dose of P & E.
- Follicular growth is monitored starting 3 to 5 days after the end of treatment.
- Ovulation is induced when endometrial edema is present and follicular diameter is at least (or greater than) 30 mm (for deslorelin) or at least (or greater than) 35 mm (hCG)
- Eighty percent of treated mares are ready for ovulation induction by day 7 to 9 following the last injection.

Progesterone and Progestagen Therapy

- All of this progesterone and progestagen therapies are combined with an ovulation induction treatment such hCG or GnRH analog (deslorelin).

Altrenogest (Regu-Mate®)

- Dose is 0.044 mg/kg PO, every 24 hours for 8 to 14 days.
- Mares should be administered one dose of $PGF_2\alpha$ at the end of the treatment.
- Most of the mares come into heat in about 3 days following the final day of treatment.
- Ovulation synchronization is obtained with a GnRH analogue or hCG.

Progesterone in Oil

- Dose is 150 mg IM, once a day for 10 days.
  - Similar results as with altrenogest, but ovulation needs to be synchronized with hCG or a GnRH analogue.
- Long-acting progesterone or altrenogest
  - New compounded slow release formulation allows effective delivery of progesterone or altrenogest for 8 to 12 days following a single IM injection.

CIDR

- CIDR, containing 1.9 g of progesterone, is inserted into the vagina for 10 to 12 days.

PGF$_2\alpha$ and an Analogue

- Effective in inducing luteolysis starting no sooner than 5 days post-ovulation if a single dose is given.
- The two most common in use are dinoprost tromethamine (5–10 mg per 450 kg, IM) and cloprostenol (250 µg per 450 kg, IM).
- Mares return to estrus 2 to 7 days after treatment, with ovulation occurring 9 to 14 days after administration.
- Onset of estrus and ovulation can be variable depending on the size and status of the follicles at the time of treatment.
- It is not the best option to synchronize estrus and ovulation.

U/S-Guided Transvaginal Follicular Aspiration

- Follicular aspiration, day 0, may be performed on all follicles greater than 10 mm diameter.
- Administration of 2 doses of PGF$_2\alpha$ (or an analogue) 12 hours apart, 4 to 5 days after aspiration is recommended when follicles are mature because some mares may develop luteal tissue.
- More than 90% of the mares will ovulate within 48 hours of hCG treatment.

hCG

- hCG has LH activity for several hours and produces a predictable time to ovulation when mares are selected based on follicular diameter (a follicle of at least 35 mm) and signs of estrus (endometrial folds evidencing edema) are present
- hCG is given IV at a dose of 2500 to 3000 IU.
- More than 80% of treated mares will ovulate within 36 to 48 hours post-treatment.
- Efficacy of hCG to induce ovulation is less predictable early and late in the breeding season.

reLH (Ovi-Stim™)

- A single chain of reLH was shown to have biological activity similar to LH and has been used in mares as an alternative to hCG.
- A dose of 0.75 mg reLH, IV, induces ovulation 48 hours post-treatment in 90% of estrus mares.
- Mares should be treated when a dominant follicle of at least 35 to 39 mm diameter is present.
- reLH does not affect interovulatory intervals.

GnRH (Deslorelin)

- A dose of 2.2-mg implants of deslorelin SC in the neck or submucosal placement in the vulva. The latter site allows for easier removal.

- Slow release injection (compounded deslorelin, 1.5 mg IM).
- Ovulation is induced 36 to 48 hours after treatment when the follicle is at least 30 mm in diameter and endometrial edema is present.

Precautions/Interactions

- Pregnancy
- Abnormal cyclicity
- Endometitis or uterine infection

Appropriate Health Care

- Monitor mare for injection site reaction (usually not very severe).

 COMMENTS

Client Education

- Client should be warned that there is individual variation in the response to these treatments.
- Some of the drugs are compounded and their use is extra-label.

Patient Monitoring

Mares should be monitored for reactions.

Possible Complications

- Injection site reaction is a problem with some of compounded progesterone/estrogen drugs:
  - Administration of progesterone/estrogen may result in fluid accumulation in the uterus especially in mares with endometritis.
  - CIDR treatment is associated with mild vaginitis or mucopurulent vaginal discharge that usually resolves spontaneously 48 hours after the CIDRs removal.
  - PGF$_2\alpha$ is associated with variable signs of GI upset, sweating, and colicky signs.
  - GnRH implants are associated with delayed return to the next natural estrus. This may be avoided by removing the implant shortly after ovulation.

Expected Course and Prognosis

- Good

Age-Related Factors

Geriatric mares may have changes in ovarian function that prevent them from responding to any treatment.

Abbreviations

AI	artificial insemination
CIDR	Controlled Internal Drug Release
eFSH	equine follicle stimulating hormone
GI	gastrointestinal
GnRH	gonadotropin releasing hormone
hCG	human chorionic gonadotropin
IM	intramuscular
IV	intravenous
P&E	progesterone and estradiol
PGF	prostaglandin F
PO	per os (by mouth)
reLH	recombinant equine luteinizing hormone
SC	subcutaneous
U/S	ultrasound, ultrasonography

See Also

- Manipulation of estrus

Suggested Reading

Card C. 2009. Hormone therapy in the mare. In *Equine Breeding Management and Artificial Insemination,* 2nd ed. Samper JC (ed). Philadelphia: Saunders-Elsevier; 89–97.

Authors: Jacobo Rodriguez and Ahmed Tibary

chapter 45

Parturition

DEFINITION/OVERVIEW

- Normal delivery of the fetus and fetal membranes after a normal pregnancy length (345 ± 12 days).
- Parturition is the result of endocrinologic, anatomic, and physiologic changes occurring both in the mare and the fetus during the last few days to weeks of pregnancy.
- Most foaling occurs during the night or early morning when barn activity is at a minimum.
- Usually divided into three stages:
  - Stage 1: fetal positioning and preparation for delivery.
  - Stage 2: fetal expulsion.
  - Stage 3: fetal membrane delivery (and passing of the placenta).
- Full-term, healthy pregnancies: 95% to 98% result in a normal parturition (uncomplicated, no dystocia).

ETIOLOGY/PATHOPHYSIOLOGY

Gestation Length and Its Variation

- Pregnancy length is extremely variable; affected by genetics (i.e., breed and individual animal), sex of the fetus, season, and nutrition.
- Birth of normal foals has been reported after pregnancies ranging from 315 to 406 days.
  - American Miniature Horse pregnancies are short, ranging from 296 to 340 days.
  - Donkey pregnancies are longer than in mares, ranging from 340 to 395 days.
- Foals delivered before day 300 are generally not viable.
- Foals delivered between 300 and 320 days of pregnancy are considered premature and have low viability.
- Maturity of the foal is not directly correlated to pregnancy length.
- Full-term pregnancy length of mares foaling in winter and spring is 10 to 15 days longer than of mares foaling in late spring and summer.
- Additional artificial photoperiod (supplemental light program) during the winter tends to reduce the seasonal variation of pregnancy length.

- Mares bred to a jackass (mule fetus) have a longer gestation by 2 to 3 weeks.
- Mares carrying a male fetus have a 2- to 3-day longer gestation than if carrying a female fetus.

Premonitory Signs of Parturition

- Mammary development begins 4 to 6 weeks prepartum in response to decreasing concentration of estrogens and increasing concentrations of progesterone.
- Notable increase in mammary gland size is seen in the last 2 weeks of pregnancy.
- Maximum distension of the mammary gland and teats and waxing (dried colostrum) at the ends of the teats occurs 24 to 48 hours before parturition (Fig. 45.1).
- Mammary gland secretion changes include increased viscosity.
- Mammary secretion electrolytes are a good indicator of impending parturition:
  - Calcium concentration greater than 10 nmol/L (or greater than 40 mg/dL) and inversion of the sodium (decreasing) and potassium (increasing) concentration indicate fetal readiness for birth.
- Relaxation of the sacrosciatic ligament may be seen several days before parturition.
- Relaxation and enlargement of the vulva is most noticeable a few hours before foaling.

Endocrinology of Parturition

- Maternal progestagen rises during the last weeks of pregnancy:
  - ACTH stimulates the fetal adrenal cortex, which leads to production of pregnolone.
  - Pregnolone is produced by placental metabolism to 5α-pregnanes.

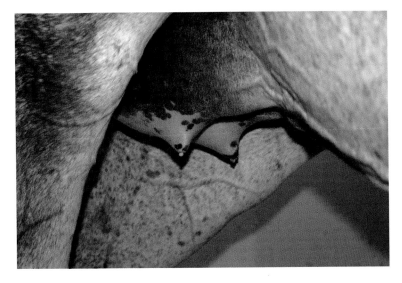

■ **Figure 45.1** Waxing, 48 hours prepartum.

- During the final maturation of the equine fetus (last 48 hours of pregnancy):
  - The fetal adrenal switches from production of pregnolone to cortisol.
  - This causes a decrease in progestagen.
- Increased fetal cortisol and a sharp increase in placental release of relaxin, initiate release of oxytocin and $PGF_2\alpha$, which mediate cervical relaxation and myometrial contractions.
  - Relaxin, oxytocin, and $PGF_2\alpha$ activity peak during the second stage of labor.

Stage 1

- Lasts 1 to 4 hours. However, mares seem to have some control on the timing of parturition and may delay parturition if disturbed during this stage.
- Myometrial contractions, in response to their increased sensitivity to oxytocin, cause a colicky syndrome in the periparturient mare (Fig. 45.2a).
- Myometrial activity is probably exacerbated by fetal movement and pressure against the cervix. These pressures induce increased oxytocin release (Ferguson's reflex).
  - During this stage the fetus shifts from a dorso-pubic or dorso-ilial position to a dorso-sacral position with its head and legs extended.
  - This repositioning stimulates further dilation of the cervix as a result of fetal feet and head pressure (also called point pressure) with each contraction.
- Mares on pasture may seek isolation from the herd and appear depressed.
- Abdominal pain and discomfort causes a colicky syndrome:
  - Increased sweating along the neck, shoulders, and flank (Fig. 45.2b).
  - Restlessness
  - Frequently stands up and lies back down (Fig. 45.2c).
  - Tail switching
  - Squatting
  - Self mutilation (biting her side)
  - Frequent micturition
  - Defecation and yawing
  - The parturient mare may be seen exhibiting the Flehman response.
- Milk ejection (dripping or full-stream) may be seen during this phase.
- During this stage, myometrial contractions assist in fetal orientation, forcing the fetus against the cervix, causing further cervical dilation with each contraction.
- The cervical star of the CA ruptures (Fig. 45.3a):
  - The cervical star is the avillous, thin area of the CA immediately apposed to the internal cervical os.
  - Its breaking allows the fetus to engage/move into the cervix and birth canal.
  - Rupture of the CA is commonly referred to as breaking water, the first "water compartment" of the placental membranes is released (usually amber colored) (Figs. 45.3b, c, d, and e).

Stage 2

- Lasts 15 to 30 minutes, encompasses delivery of the fetus, its passage through the birth canal.

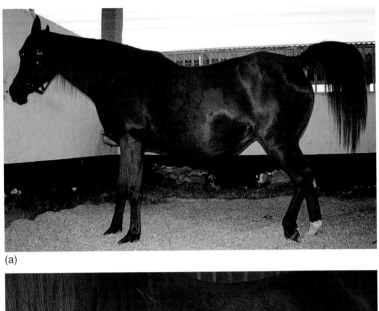
(a)

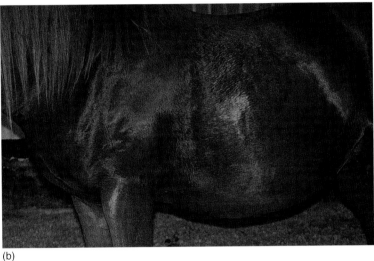
(b)

■ **Figure 45.2** Stage 1 of parturition in the mare: Stretching and abdominal discomfort *(a)*, sweating *(b)*, and rolling *(c)*.

- Intensity and frequency of abdominal and uterine contractions increase.
- Abdominal muscle contractions are likely initiated by stretching of the soft tissue of the birth canal.
- Expulsion of the fetus results from forceful, synchronized contractions of the abdominal muscles and diaphragm, combined with the increased intra-abdominal pressure due to closure of the mare's glottis.
- Abdominal muscle contractions occur in clusters of three to four every 2 to 3 minutes.
- The amniotic sac (a whitish-blue membrane) appears at the vulva within 5 to 10 minutes of the end of stage I (*see* Figs. 45.3a and c).

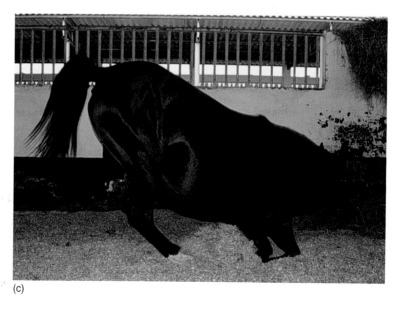

(c)

■ **Figure 45.2** continued

- One hoof, or a hoof and the nose, may be seen within the normally transparent amnion (*see* Fig. 45.3d).
- The amniotic sac is ruptured by movement of the fetal legs and head.
- The fetus may be delivered with the amnion intact. It should immediately be torn and moved off of the fetus' nares/face to avoid asphyxiation.
- This is the rupture of the placenta's second water compartment.
- The mare may alternate between standing and lateral recumbency.
- Anterior (head first) is the most common presentation for normal foalings.
  - Fetus's head is aligned with the forelimbs and lies between the two carpal joints.
  - One of its forelimbs is slightly ahead of the other (extended), which narrows its shoulder diameter for easier passage through the birth canal.
- The areas of maximum fetal diameter are its head and shoulders, which require expulsive efforts by the mare.
  - Once the fetus's head and shoulders are out, the rest of its body follows with minimal abdominal contractions.
  - Abdominal contractions cease once the fetus's pelvis has been delivered.
- The majority of foals are delivered with the mare in lateral recumbency.
- Mares will often lie for a few minutes with the rear legs of the foal still resting in the vaginal canal (*see* Fig. 45.3e).
- The umbilical cord ruptures when the foal attempts to move or the mare stands (Fig. 45.4a).
- *Immediate* vaginal examination and obstetrical evaluation is indicated if:
  - Failure to progress from Stage 1 to Stage 2 within 10 minutes.
  - Failure to make progress within 10 minutes of the appearance of the amnion at the vulvae.

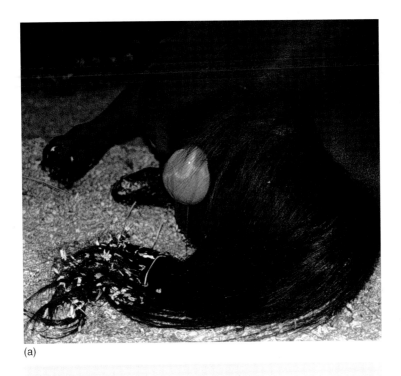

(a)

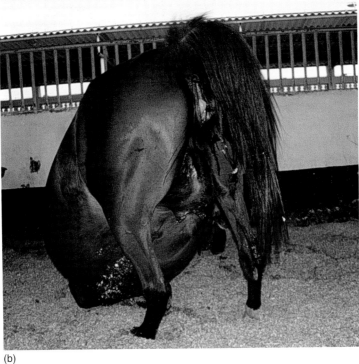

(b)

■ **Figure 45.3** Stage 2: Rupture of the chorioallantoic sac and appearance of the amniotic sac *(a)*, mare alternating between standing and lateral recumbency *(b)*, increased expulsive efforts *(c)*, rupture of the allantoic sac with amnion still intact *(d)*, and expulsion of the foal with the mare in lateral recumbency *(e)*.

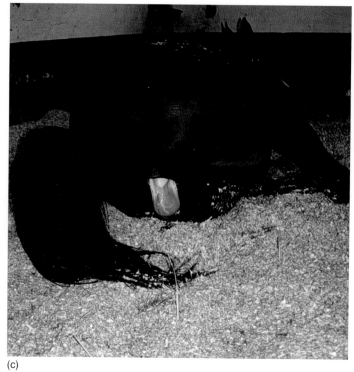

(c)

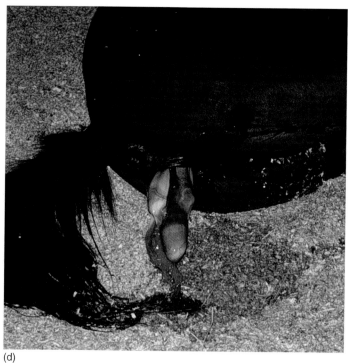

(d)

■ **Figure 45.3** continued

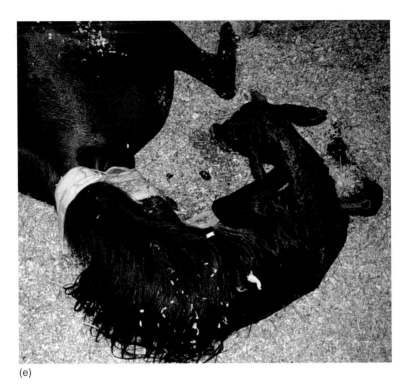

(e)

■ **Figure 45.3** continued

■ Stage 2 longer than 60 minutes is associated with poor outcome, fetal viability is compromised.

Stage 3

■ Placental detachment and expulsion:
  ■ Result of the combined effect of loss of blood tension following rupture of the umbilical cord and,
  ■ Rhythmic myometrial contractions originating at the tip of the uterine horns.
■ Mares may exhibit abdominal discomfort (e.g., restlessness, pawing, increased heart rate, rolling or lateral recumbency) during this stage.
■ The chorionic villi progressively detach:
  ■ From the endometrial crypts at the tip of the horn, the fetal membranes invaginate within themselves as their release progresses along the uterine horn (Figs. 45.4b and c).
  ■ They are expelled inside-out (amniotic or fetal side visible).
■ Delivery of the placenta takes less than 1 hour in most mares.
  ■ Should be completed by 3 hours postpartum in nearly all mares.
■ The placenta is considered retained and intervention is required if it fails to pass in its entirety by 3 (time frame most often used in United States) to 6 hours (common time frame accepted in the United Kingdom) postpartum.

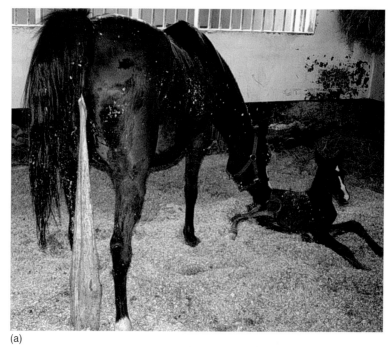

(a)

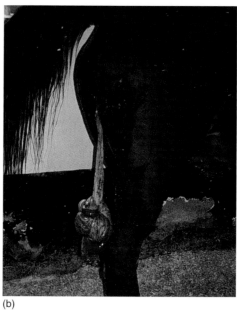

(b)

■ **Figure 45.4** Stage 3: Ruptured umbilical cord *(a)*, tying the placenta *(b)*, and placenta delivered with the amniotic surface (fetal side) visible *(c)*.

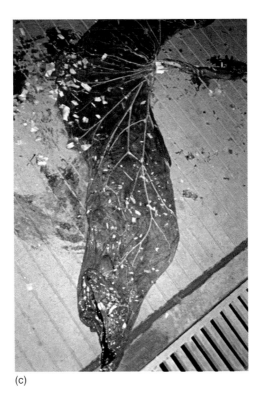

(c)

■ **Figure 45.4** continued

- Treat to address risk of developing metritis and toxemia.
- Placenta should *always* be examined for completeness, size (i.e., weight, edema), and evidence of lesions or abnormalities.
- Normal placental weight is 10% to 11% of the foal's birth weight.

Systems Affected

- Reproductive
- Fetus/neonate

SIGNALMENT/HISTORY

Historical Findings

- Normal pregnancy after mating, AI, or ET.
- Fetal readiness for birth.
- Breeding date is compatible with term pregnancy.
- Duration of pregnancy falls within normal range.

Physical Examination Findings

- Signs of impending parturition
- Relaxation of sacrosciatic ligaments
- Mammary development and waxing
- Vulvar relaxation and edema

 DIFFERENTIAL DIAGNOSIS

Abortion

- History: breeding date, abnormal pregnancy
- Twinning
- Fetal hydrops (hydrops amnion, hydrops allantois)
- Uterine torsion
- Prolonged pregnancy

 DIAGNOSTICS

CBC/Biochemistry/Urinalysis

Required only if there is an OB emergency.

Other Laboratory Tests

- Determination of calcium, sodium, and potassium concentration in mammary secretion.
  - Predictive timing of parturition.
- Use of stall-test kits for determination of electrolytes changes:
  - Titrets®, Softcheck®, Predict-A-Foal®
  - May be helpful in predicting readiness for birth.
  - Not always accurate because they test all divalent cations.
  - Titret® seems to be the most reliable for prediction of foaling within 24 hours, but it is time consuming.
- $CaCO_3$ concentration:
  - Equal or greater than 200 ppm equates the likelihood of foaling within 24, 48, or 72 hours, to be 54%, 84% and 95%, respectively.
  - Mares with $CaCO_3$ concentration of 300 to 500 ppm will foal within 12 to 18 hours.
- These preexisting conditions (e.g., placentitis, and premature lactation).
  - Should be interpreted on an individual basis after clinical assessment of the mare.
  - Primarous mares often have insufficient prepartum mammary gland secretions to permit testing.

Diagnostic Procedures

Required if an OB problem arises.

THERAPEUTICS

Nursing Care

Preparation for foaling:
- Large clean foaling stall or pasture.
- Tail wrap
- Use of electronic foaling monitor.
- Cleanse the perineal area and udder.

Diet

- Broodmare nutrition is increased by 20% to 25% of maintenance requirement during the last trimester.
- Contrarily to common belief, obesity does not increase risk for dystocia.
- Calcium-to-phosphorus ratio should be maintained at 1.2 to 1.5:1 during last trimester.
- Maintain good body condition to promote lactation.

Activity

- Depends on outcome of foaling. With normal foaling and healthy foal, paddock exercise is beneficial for uterine involution.
- Limited activity imposed by foal factors:
  - Angular limb deformities
  - Maladjustment syndrome
  - Failure to nurse (high risk for FPT)
- Limited activity imposed by mare factors:
  - Broad ligament hemorrhage
  - RFM

Surgical Considerations

- C-section may be considered if vaginal delivery is not possible.

COMMENTS

Client Education

- Maintain good breeding records.
- Familiarize client with signs of impending parturition and all stages of parturition.

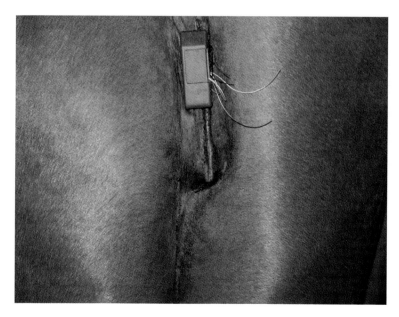

■ **Figure 45.5** Foal-Alert® system for monitoring parturition in the mare. The alarm sounds at the time the magnet is separated from the transmitter box when the vulvar lips are pulled apart during foaling.

- Increase the frequency of observation once waxing is observed.
- Encourage use of surveillance or monitoring systems such as closed-circuit TV, video-Internet.
  - Electronic detection devices to monitor mare position (Birthalarm®, EquiPage®, or Breeder Alert®), or vulvar stretching (Foal-alert®) are helpful when used properly (Fig. 45.5).
  - Monitoring devices are *not* an excuse to forego frequent observation of mares.
- Encourage use of kits monitoring electrolytes changes in mammary secretions.
- Have client assemble a foaling and neonatal foal kit and have it ready and available on farm (e.g., towels, buckets, tail wrap, lubricant, and oxygen).
- Have a clear plan of action and educate clients:
  - When to call the veterinarian.
  - What to do while waiting for the veterinarian to arrive.

Patient Monitoring

- Immediately postpartum:
  - Monitor the mare for any signs of weakness, muscle fasciculation, ataxia, colic, or excessive blood loss.
- First 2 days postpartum:
  - Monitor the mare for agalactia or mammary gland disorders, foal rejection.
- Examine the vulva, vagina, and cervix after the placenta has passed.
- If foaling has been relatively uneventful, allow time for the mare and foal to bond. Constant, continuing interruptions can interfere with bonding (Fig. 45.6).

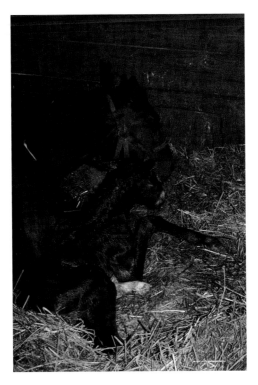

■ **Figure 45.6** Once foaling is complete, allow mare and foal bonding, and avoid unnecessary interference. Image courtesy of C. L. Carleton.

■ Tease and perform a complete reproductive examination at the beginning of foal heat or by a week to 10 days after foaling.

Prevention/Avoidance

■ Avoid breeding mares with chronic health problem (COPD, liver, or kidney failure), recent abdominal surgery, recurrent colic, severe orthopedic problems, previous birth canal injury.
■ Use ET or associated ART if a mare is at high risk for complications from pregnancy or parturition.
■ Young fillies (2 year olds) suffer an increased incidence for dystocia.
■ Older mares are at risk for increased complications.
■ High-risk pregnancies or abnormal pregnancies may increase the likelihood of dystocia.

Possible Complications

■ Premature placental separation (red bag)
■ Failure of amnion to rupture
■ Dystocia of fetal or maternal origin

- Lactation failure
- Behavioral problem (foal rejection)
- Cervical or vaginal trauma
- Rectovaginal tears/RVF
- Postpartum metritis
- RFM
- Broad ligament hemorrhage
- Colon torsion

Expected Course and Prognosis

- Normal course and duration of each stage is associated with an excellent prognosis.
- Incidence of dystocia is low (less than 10%) in the equine.
- Excess prolongation of any stage of parturition is associated with a reduction in neonatal survival.
- Prognosis for the life of the mare and survival of the foal is increased by rapid and adequate intervention.
- Prognosis for reproductive life is excellent following an uncomplicated birth.

Synonyms

- Birthing
- Foaling
- Labor
- Delivery

Abbreviations

ACTH	adrenocorticotropic hormone
AI	artificial insemination
ART	advanced reproductive technologies
CA	chorioallantoic
$CaCO_3$	calcium carbonate
CBC	complete blood count
COPD	chronic obstructive pulmonary disease
ET	embryo transfer
FPT	failure of passive transfer
OB	obstetrical
$PGF_2\alpha$	natural prostaglandin
ppm	parts per million
RFM	retained fetal membranes, retained placenta
RVF	rectovaginal fistula

See Also

- Abortion
- Dystocia
- Prolonged pregnancy
- Fetotomy
- C-section
- Induction of parturition
- Induction of abortion
- Placentation
- Placentitis
- Pregnancy
- Postpartum complication
- RFM

Suggested Reading

Dolente BA, Sullivan EK, Boston R, et al. 2005. Mares admitted to a referral hospital for postpartum emergencies: 163 cases (1992–2002). *J Vet Med Emer Crit Care* 15: 193–200.

Frazer GS, Perkins NR, Embertson RM. 2002. Normal parturition and evaluation of the mare in dystocia. *Eq Vet Educ Manual* 5: 22–26.

Morel MCGD, Newcombe JR, Holland SJ. 2002. Factors affecting gestation length in the thoroughbred mare. *Anim Reprod Sci* 74: 175–185.

Ousey JC. 2004. Peripartal endocrinology in the mare and foetus. *Reprod in Domes Anim* 39: 222–231.

Wessel M. 2005. Staging and prediction of parturition in the mare. *Clinical Tech Eq Pract* 4: 228–238.

Author: Ahmed Tibary

chapter 46

Parturition Induction

DEFINITION/OVERVIEW

- Elective pharmacological initiation of labor in a mare under specific conditions and at a selected time prior to initiation of Stage 1 parturition.
- An elective procedure meant to guarantee presence of qualified personnel for a supervised foaling.
- Should only be attempted if there is sufficient historical and clinical data to support the fetus's readiness for birth.

ETIOLOGY/PATHOPHYSIOLOGY

- Relies primarily on stimulation of myometrial contractions in response to a bolus dose or continuous rate infusion of oxytocin.
  - To mimic the hormonal pattern of normal Stage 1 parturition.
  - The length of Stage 1 is shortened.
  - Once Stage 1 is completed, Stage 2 and Stage 3 will follow as per a normal foaling (durations normal, as per an uninduced parturition).
- Delivery occurs within 15 to 90 minutes of administration of oxytocin.

Systems Affected

Reproductive

SIGNALMENT/HISTORY

- Procedure is most considered for:
  - Valuable mares
  - Mares with a previous history of complications from birthing.
  - Mares that previously have delivered compromised foals.
- Justifications for induction may include:
  - Delayed parturition due to uterine atony.
  - Older mare

- Mare with weak abdominal musculature.
- Prolonged gestation
- Mare with previous injuries to the pelvic canal.
- Mare with fetal hydrops.
- Rupture (partial or full) of the prepubic tendon.
- History of premature placental separation.
- Mare known to have produced a NI foal.
- Imminent death of the mare due to an injury or disease.

CLINICAL FEATURES

An abbreviated Stage 1 labor, evidenced by rapid onset of restlessness, sweating, pawing, circling, and milk ejection; clinically more intense than in naturally foaling mares.
- Induction results in a shortening of the timeline to the onset of Stage 2 labor.
- Stage 1 usually begins within 10 to 90 minutes of oxytocin administration (dependent on the dose, method, and route of administration).
    - Relatively short duration compared with Stage 1 of a natural parturition.
- Stage 2 (begins with the rupture of the CA sac) occurs within 10 to 30 minutes of onset of Stage 1.
    - Progression and monitoring of Stage 2, as well as Stage 3, should be similar to that provided for a normal foaling (see Parturition).

Mare Evaluation

- Gestation length minimum 330 days.
    - Gestation length alone is not a good indicator of fetal maturity or readiness for birth.
    - The closer a mare is to her previously recorded term gestation length, the better.
- Mammary gland should be well-developed and colostrum present.
    - Mammary gland secretions and electrolyte concentrations are the most reliable indicators of fetal maturity.
    - Mammary gland secretions should be monitored during the last weeks of gestation.
    - Secretions generally change from straw-colored and watery to more viscous and smoky grey or opaque-white at term.
- Relaxation of the perineum and sacrosciatic ligaments should clearly be evident.
- Cervical relaxation is considered by some to be the most important criteria to reach a decision of whether or not to induce.
    - The expectation is that the cervix should be soft and allow insertion of least 3 fingers (4–8 cm in width) before proceeding with an induction.
    - Some mares will have a completely dilated cervix for days, and some as long as 2 weeks, before parturition occurs.

- Mares can respond to an induction regimen even with a closed cervix, but the fetus may experience increased risk for intrapartum asphyxia, post-delivery delayed adjustment, and prolonged times to stand and nurse.
- Cervical dilation may be enhanced by local application of prostaglandin E_2 prior to administering oxytocin.

Mammary Gland Secretions

- Mammary secretion concentrations of calcium, sodium, and potassium are evaluated.
- Commercial kits to predict time of foaling:
  - Measure only changes in calcium and therefore are not 100% accurate.
  - Precise biochemical laboratory testing (flame spectrophotometer or laboratory chemistry analyzer) of mammary secretions is more accurate and useful.
- Electrolyte concentrations in mammary secretions may not be well-correlated with readiness for delivery if the mare has been leaking colostrums or milk at the end of pregnancy (prepartum).
- Values indicating parturition is imminent:
  - Calcium concentration should be greater than 40 mg/dL (more than 10 mmol/L).
  - Sodium concentration should decrease to less than 30 mEq/L.
  - Potassium concentration should increase and surpass sodium concentration (more than 35 mEq/L).
  - If water hardness test are used, $CaCO_3$ concentration should be more than or above 300 ppm.

DIAGNOSTICS

- Outcome depends on several criteria to ensure the dam is ready for delivery and that fetus is ready for extra-uterine life.
- No single criterion can guarantee success of an induced parturition.

CBC/Biochemistry/Urinalysis

Not necessary, unless indicated by the mare's health status.

Other Laboratory Tests

Evaluation of concentrations of calcium, sodium, potassium, and magnesium in mammary secretions.

Imaging

Transabdominal U/S is useful to assess fetal membranes, fetal orientation and well-being.

THERAPEUTICS

Drug(s) of Choice

- Oxytocin is the drug of choice for induction of parturition in the mare.
- Oxytocin dose and route of administration:
  - Range 2.5 IU to 120 IU
  - IV, IM, SC
  - Variable time intervals
- Large bolus oxytocin doses (40–60 IU, IV) result in an explosive Stage 1.
- Low dose or multiple small doses (2.5–20 IU; IV, IM, or SC every 15 minutes) produce a smoother, more physiologic, foaling.
- Administration via intravenous catheter (2.5–10 IU in 30–60 mL of saline, every 20 minutes) or continuous rate infusion at 1 IU/minute (60–120 IU in 1 L of saline) may better mimic normal release of oxytocin, but this may be more difficult to administer in field conditions.
- Small doses (2.5 IU, IV) are effective if the mare is ready to foal.
  - Treatment is initiated when the mammary secretion calcium concentration reaches 8 nmol/L.
  - A mare ready to foal will do so within 2 hours of treatment.
  - If she does *not* foal, treatment is repeated 24 hours later.
  - Most mares will require only one treatment; a small number may require two, and sometimes three, treatments.
  - This technique appears to be safer; however it may not be practical in field conditions.
  - Also, administration of small doses of oxytocin still can produce a premature foal even with mammary secretion calcium concentration greater than 8 nmol/L.

Precautions/Interactions

- Mare with an abnormal vaginal discharge.
- Insufficient information available with regard to gestation length or fetal health.

Alternative Drugs

- The natural prostaglandin, PGF$_2\alpha$, dinoprost tromethamine, at a dose of 5 to 12 mg, IM, is ineffective unless a mare is close to foaling.
- PGF$_2\alpha$ and its analogues have several adverse effects on the mare and fetus:
  - Premature placental separation.
  - Prematurity
  - Stillbirths and maladjusted foals.
  - Thus, they are *not* a good choice for induction of parturition in the mare.
- Synthetic analogues of PGF$_2\alpha$ (e.g., Protalene [4 mg SC] and fenprostalene [0.5 mg SC] have been used successfully. Foals are delivered within 4 hours of treatment.

- Prostaglandin E_2 (2–2.5 mg) applied intracervically enhances cervical dilation and improves delivery times when given in combination with oxytocin.

Appropriate Health Care

- The mare should be prepared as for parturition.
- The tail should be wrapped and the perineal area and udder cleaned.
- Induction should be performed in a clean, large foaling stall.

Nursing Care

- The foaling should be closely supervised; avoid hasty intervention.
- Intervention to verify position and posture of the fetus should be attempted only when indicated, as per a normal foaling.
- Mare and foal postpartum evaluation and care should be performed, as per a normal routine.

 COMMENTS

Client Education

- Clients should be warned that induction of parturition is not without risks particularly for the fetus or foal.
- Induction should not be used as a routine, elective procedure.
- An on-site, mare-side veterinarian is required during an induction.

Possible Complications

- Delivery of premature or weak foals.
- Premature placental separation and fetal hypoxia or anoxia.
- Dystocia
- RFM
- FPT (insufficient colostral IgG absorption) in foals

Expected Course and Prognosis

In carefully selected cases, the prognosis for the mare and foal is good.

Synonyms

- Induction of foaling
- Elective attended parturition

Abbreviations

CA   chorioallantoic, chorioallantois
CBC   complete blood count

CaCO₃   calcium carbonate
FPT   failure of passive transfer
IgG   immunoglobulin G
IM   intramuscular
IV   intravenous
NI   neonatal isoerythrolysis
PFG   prostaglandin (natural)
PPM   parts per million
RFM   retained fetal membranes
SC   subcutaneous
U/S   ultrasound, ultrasonography

See Also

- Induction of abortion
- Parturition
- Pregnancy

Suggested Reading

Camillo F, Marmorini P, Romagnoli S, et al. 2000. Clinical studies on daily low dose oxytocin in mares at term. *Equine Vet J* 32: 307–310.

Macpherson ML, Chaffin MK, Carroll GL, et al. 1997. Three methods of oxytocin-induced parturition and their effects on foals. *JAVMA* 210: 799–803.

Ousey J. 2003. Induction of parturition in the healthy mare. *Equine Vet Ed* 15: 164–168.

Rigby S, Love C, Carpenter K, et al. 1998. Use of prostaglandin E-2 to ripen the cervix of the mare prior to induction of parturition. *Therio* 50: 897–904.

Author: Ahmed Tibary

chapter 47

Perineal Lacerations, Recto-Vaginal Vestibular Fistulas

DEFINITION/OVERVIEW

Perineal lacerations: perineal body damage is defined by the degree of damage present:

- A first-degree laceration involves the skin and the mucous membrane of the vulva (Fig. 47.1).
- A second-degree laceration involves the next deeper layer of the vestibule or the vaginal wall, extending into the perineal body and deeper layers of the vulva.
- A third-degree laceration involves full-thickness tears through the perineal body, extending through the rectal wall and anal sphincter, and full-thickness through the vulva (Figs. 47.2 and 47.3).

Recto-vaginal lacerations and fistulas are defined as follows:

- Recto-vaginal lacerations are full-thickness tears through the rectal wall and, possibly, involve the perineal body, but do not involve the anal sphincter or vulva
- Recto-vestibular fistulas are much more common than recto-vaginal fistulas (Fig. 47.4).

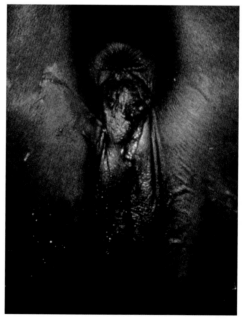

■ **Figure 47.1** Perineal laceration, first degree.
Image courtesy of C. L. Carleton.

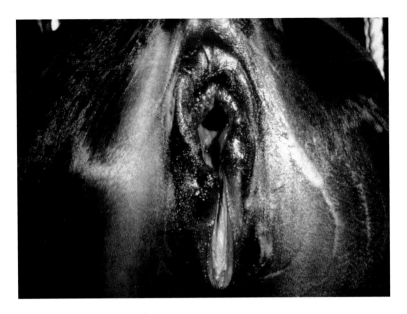

■ **Figure 47.2** Perineal laceration, third degree.

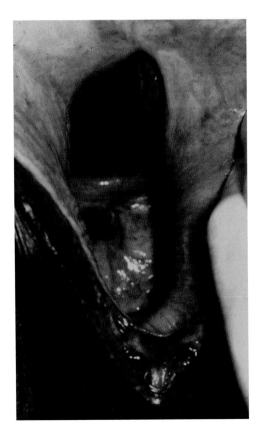

■ **Figure 47.3** Perineal laceration with vulvae held laterally. The cranial, intact portion of the perineal body can be seen dividing the rectum from the vagina.

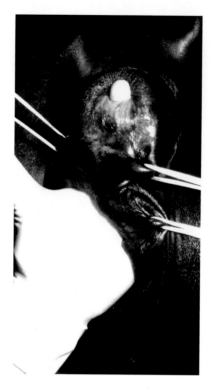

■ **Figure 47.4** A rectovaginal fistula.

 ETIOLOGY/PATHOPHYSIOLOGY

Perineal lacerations occur at parturition because of abnormal posture or position of the fetus, which causes fetal extremities to be pushed further dorsal than normal, forcing the fetus's feet into or through the wall of the vagina or vestibule.

- Lacerations of the rectum or vagina can occur at breeding, but perineal lacerations are rare at breeding.
- Genetics plays a role only if, for some reason, the mare has an inherited narrowing of the vagina.
- Partial- to full-thickness lacerations of the vestibule, vagina, anal sphincter, or rectum can occur.
- Air can be aspirated into the vagina or uterus secondary to the damaged normal barrier tissues that protect the genital tract (i.e., vulvar lips, vestibular sphincter).
- Fecal contamination of the vagina and vestibule, followed by inflammation of the vestibule, vagina, cervix, and possibly the endometrium, can occur following laceration.

Systems Affected

- Reproductive
- Muscular (in the perineal area)

SIGNALMENT/HISTORY

All breeds and all ages of breeding stock can be involved.

Risk Factors

- There are no statistics available regarding incidence. It is infrequent, but not rare.
- Lacerations can occur at term and parturition. Abnormal fetal position or posture is associated with this condition. Because fetal posture and position can change within minutes before parturition, examinations conducted much before parturition, are of little value except for determining fetal presentation.

Historical Findings

- The mare may have a history of assisted delivery, but this is not essential. Because of the extreme forces generated by the mare's abdominal musculature during the Stage 2 of labor, it is possible for the mare to deliver a live foal unassisted, while creating a perineal laceration within the same time frame.

CLINICAL FEATURES

- This condition is not an emergency. Because of the tearing, bruising, and edema that occur at and after injury, surgical correction is delayed until the initial inflammation and bruising has subsided; generally at least at 30 days (Figs. 47.5 and 47.6). Careful

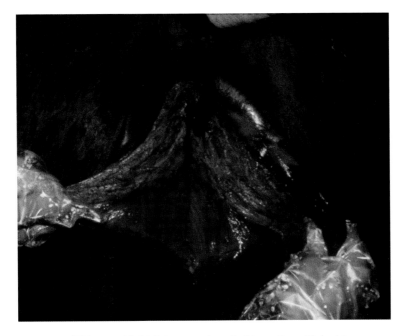

■ **Figure 47.5** A recent (30-hours-old) third-degree rectovaginal laceration with bruising.

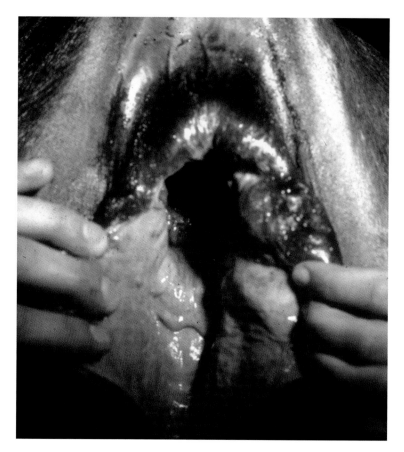

■ **Figure 47.6** The benefit of the passage of time. Thirty days after the tear occurred, bruising has subsided, inflammation has resolved, and the likelihood of surgical success has been enhanced.

physical examination should be made of the perineum, perineal body, vagina, and rectum, including TRP and vaginal examination.

 # DIAGNOSTICS

Differentiate perineal lacerations from rectovaginal fistulas.

 # THERAPEUTICS

Activity

- It is essential to determine if the laceration extends into the peritoneal cavity. Although rare, it is a possibility with a perineal laceration or recto-vaginal fistula. It is important to emphasize to the client that systemic antibiotics seldom are indicated or necessary to control infection with these injuries. Local medication is rarely indicated. Lacerations should be repaired before attempting to rebreed. Boosting the tetanus vaccination, if not recent, should be mandatory.

Surgical Considerations

- Surgical repair can be attempted once inflammation and bruising have subsided, a minimum 30 days. Postoperatively, it is imperative that feces remain soft until healing is complete.
- If surgery will be done early in the spring, place the mare on pasture, and return her to pasture immediately after surgery. Green grass has a high-moisture content, which should soften her stool. Other methods of stool softening include bran and mineral oil, but these are less effective in the author's opinion.

Two-Stage Repair

Stage 1

- Epidural anesthesia is administered using a 15-cm (6-in) spinal needle; the mare is sedated, her tail is wrapped and elevated over her back and attached to a support directly above the animal. The rectum and vagina/vestibule are emptied of feces and thoroughly, but gently, cleaned. Use of irritating scrubs is contraindicated because they may stimulate postoperative straining. Reconstruction of the perineal body is accomplished by an incision made into the remaining shelf 2 to 3 cm anterior to the cranial limit of the laceration. The incision is continued posteriorly along the sides of the existing laceration in a plane approximately equal to the original location of the perineal body. The vestibular and vaginal mucosa is reflected ventrally 2 cm.
- Simple interrupted sutures are placed through the area of the perineal body so that the perineal body is reapposed and the submucosal vaginal or vestibular tissue is brought together in the same suture pattern.
- After placement of one or two of these sutures, a continuous suture pattern is begun in the reflected mucosal membrane to appose the submucosal surfaces. This suture pattern continues cranial to caudal, as additional simple interrupted sutures are placed.

Stage 2

- This step is completed after complete healing of Stage 1. Debride the anal sphincter and dorsal vulvar commissure, and place sutures in these tissues to reestablish the sphincters, if possible. Optimal success is achieved if sphincter tone is regained after repair.

One-Stage Repair

- Similar to two-stage repair, except that repairs of the anal sphincter and dorsal vulvar commissure are completed at the time of the initial surgery.

COMMENTS

Client Education

- Advise the owner regarding the importance of close/frequent observation of foaling mares. Many lacerations occur before a problem is detected, even in the presence of trained foaling attendants. Observation is critical.

Patient Monitoring

- An immediate examination is indicated if there is a possibility or concern that a laceration has occurred. If a laceration has occurred, but it doesn't extend into the peritoneal cavity, reexamine the area in 2 weeks to assess the degree of inflammation and formation of granulation tissue at the laceration site.

Prevention/Avoidance

- Occurrence is difficult to predict. It cannot be prevented by any method other than not breeding the mare.

Possible Complications

- Abscesses may develop in the laceration area, but this is uncommon, aided in part by the abundant surface area that facilitates drainage and formation of granulation tissue from the deeper layers outward. If the laceration is sutured immediately after the occurrence, the potential for abscessation may actually increase.

Expected Course and Prognosis

- Without surgical correction, mares with third-degree lacerations and recto-vaginal fistulas have a very low probability of conceiving and maintaining a pregnancy to term. Therefore, surgical correction is strongly recommended before attempting breeding.

Abbreviations

TRP   transrectal palpation

See Also

- Delayed uterine involution
- Dystocia
- Prolonged pregnancy
- Urine pooling/urovagina

Suggested Reading

Aanes WA. 1964. Surgical repair of third degree perineal lacerations and recto-vaginal fistulas in the mare. *JAVMA* 144: 485–491.

Belknap JK, Nickels FA. 1992. A one-stage repair of third-degree perineal lacerations and rectovestibular fistula in 17 mares. *Vet Surg* 21: 378–381.

Colbern GT, Aanes WA, Stashak TS. 1985. Surgical management of perineal lacerations and recto-vestibular fistulae in the mare: a retrospective study of 47 cases. *JAVMA* 186: 265–269.

Heinze CD, Allen AR. 1966. Repair of third-degree perineal lacerations in the mare. *Vet Scope* 11: 12–15.

Stickle RL, Fessler JF, Adams SB, et al. 1979. A single stage technique for repair of recto-vestibular lacerations in the mare. *J Vet Surg* 8: 25–27.

Author: Walter R. Threlfall

chapter 48

Placental Basics

DEFINITION/OVERVIEW

The equine placenta begins its development by the migration of fetal trophoblasts from the developing conceptus into the adjacent endometrium with which it is in contact. As with other species, placental classification is based on five attributes:

- Shape: diffuse with the normal placenta being covered by villi allowing attachment to the entire endometrial surface.
- Origin of placental tissues: the placenta is allantochorionic, formed by fusion of fetally derived allantoic sac and chorion.
- Degree of invasion: equine placentation is epitheliochorial. Fetally derived chorionic tissue directly apposes maternal endometrial epithelium.
- Vascular structure: microcotyledonary/villous. The unit of exchange is a villous-like maternal and placental vascular apposition found all over the chorionic surface. Normal sites that are avillous are present (see exceptions).
- Degree of attachment: equine placentation is adeciduate, that is, no loss of maternal tissue occurs with placental formation or upon its expulsion.

ETIOLOGY/PATHOPHYSIOLOGY

Formation of the equine placenta is a complex multistage process.

- The equine conceptus is mobile up to day 16 following conception, allowing trans-uterine migration and signaling for pregnancy recognition and maintenance. The conceptus remains spherical until approximately day 35, becoming ellipsoid thereafter.
- The first physical connection between the conceptus and the endometrium is formed beginning day 34 to 37 by fetal trophoblastic cell invasion of the maternal endometrium forming the endometrial cups. Pregnancy maintenance by allantochorionic placentation begins at approximately day 40.
- The placenta has expanded to contact the entire endometrial surface by approximately day 77. The placenta can be considered fully developed by day 150.
- The endometrial cups produce eCG and are responsible for the formation and function of accessory CL. Peak function occurs around day 70, with necrosis occurring

by day 120 to 150. Cups are eventually sloughed (by immunological rejection). The residual cup material is trapped in invaginations of the overlying allantois. These areas may be seen during a placental evaluation and are called the allantochorionic pouches.

 # CLINICAL FEATURES

Appropriate placental development is vitally dependent on the reproductive competency of the mare.

- Chorionic surface: considered to be a reflection of the endometrial health of the mare. If significant pathology develops (e.g., with uterine infection or degenerative fibrotic changes), it results in diminished diffusion between the maternal and fetal circulations, thus nutrient, gas, and fetal waste transfer are decreased.
- Microcotyledons: structural development and surface density over the chorion is influenced by mare age and parity. This has been found lowest in aged multiparous mares, with primiparous mares also having decreased density compared to young multiparous mares. A "priming" effect on microcotyledonary surface density is hypothesized to occur with the first pregnancy, increasing microcotyledonary surface density and foal birthweight in subsequent gestations.
- Maternal size and genetics: maternal weight is positively correlated to mass and gross surface area of the allantochorion, with maternal size interacting with both maternal and fetal genotypes to control fetal growth. Foal birth weight is positively correlated with the mass, gross surface area, and tissue volume of the allantochorion.

 # DIFFERENTIAL DIAGNOSIS

Avillous Areas

- There are five normal avillous areas of the equine placenta:
  - Location of the endometrial cups
  - The cervical star
  - Ostia (each UTJ, an ostium) near the tip of each uterine horn.
  - Site of the umbilical attachment
  - Invaginated/redundant folds of the allantochorion (appear longitudinal and symmetric). (See Figure 48.1)
- Pathologic avillous areas: apposition of placentae in a twin pregnancy, placentitis, and endometrial fibrosis can lead to abnormal avillous areas.

Placental Thickening

- See Placentitis.

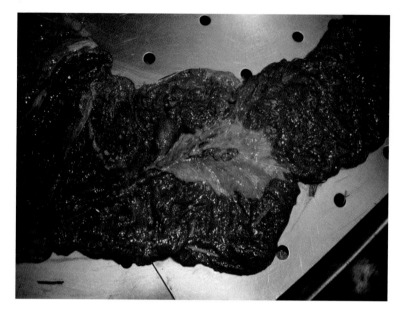

■ **Figure 48.1** Redundancy of the placental folds that creates a symmetrical avillous "lesion" when separated, pulled apart. One hypothesis is that it results from chronic umbilical cord traction on the adjacent allantochorion. This should not be confused with a pathologic process.

 # DIAGNOSTICS

Placental evaluation: the allantochorion is usually expelled inside out, with the fetal surface (i.e., allantois) exteriorized. During a normal delivery, the fetus ruptures the placenta at the cervical star leaving only remnants of it around the periphery of the fetus's point of exit. To examine the placenta, expose the chorionic surface and lay it out on a level surface in the shape of an "F." To ensure none has been retained, confirm that the tips of both horns are present. If areas of the placental surface are torn, match blood vessels on the exposed allantoic surface to ascertain the size or limits of the defect; this method is the easiest means to rule out that any portions are missing/retained.

- Allantochorion: Normally appears as a "red velvet" surface because of the diffuse microvilli over the entire surface. The tip of the pregnant horn is of greater diameter. It is usually thicker and more edematous when compared to the nonpregnant horn. It is abnormal if the allantochorion is edematous or grossly thickened because this may indicate vascular disturbances or fescue toxicosis.
- Amnion: The equine amnion is completely separate from allantochorion. It normally appears white, translucent, and is a thin membrane. Abnormal findings include: discoloration and edema (fetal distress leading to *in utero* [prior to fetal expulsion] meconium passage also known as fetal diarrhea) or thickening (amnionitis), which may also indicate the extension of an allantochorionitis.
- Umbilical cord: There are normally distinct allantoic and amniotic portions, with approximately four longitudinal twists along its entire length. Abnormal length is

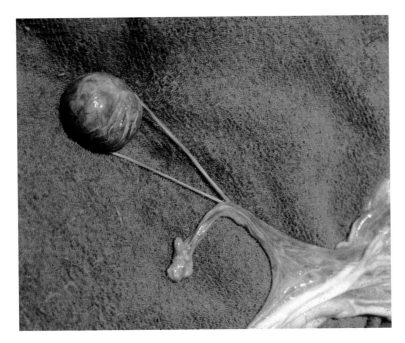

■ **Figure 48.2** Yolk sac remnant attached to the umbilicus; a relatively common finding during a placental evaluation.
Image courtesy of C. L. Carleton.

the most common finding. If the umbilical cord is longer than 100 cm, the risk of fetal strangulation and umbilical cord torsion is increased. This may be manifested as fetal autolysis, vascular damage, thrombi formation (from abnormal, excessive twisting leading to vascular stasis), and urachal tearing. Occasionally will observe remnants of the yolk sac from earlier stage of development; often mistaken for a twin because of its appearance: typically a hollow, bony sphere on a pedicle (Figs. 48.2 and 48.3)

- Allantoic fluid: usually clear to amber in color. This fluid is essentially hypotonic urine and fetal excretory products.
- Hippomane (allantoic calculus): found within the allantoic fluid and composed of concentric layers of cellular debris. Of rubbery consistency and a dark brown, green, or tan coloration.
- Amniotic fluid: translucent white viscous fluid, formed from respiratory and buccal secretions of the fetus.

Pathological Findings

- Placentitis
- Placental insufficiency

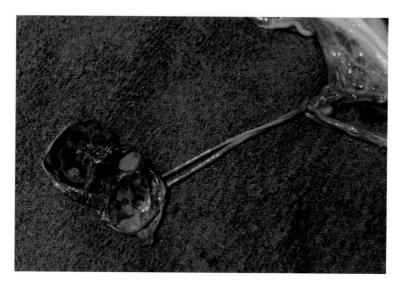

■ **Figure 48.3** Yolk sac remnant transected. Routinely misidentified as a twin within the placenta. Image courtesy of C. L. Carleton.

 COMMENTS

Client Education

Keep placenta in water-tight container for evaluation to prevent fluid loss making assessment of edema difficult.

Abbreviations

CL   corpus luteum
eCG   equine chorionic gonadotropin
UTJ   uterotubal junction

See Also

- Placentitis
- Placental insufficiency
- Twin (Multiple) Pregnancy
- Endometrial Biopsy

Suggested Reading

Asbury AC, LeBlanc MM. 1993. *The placenta.* In: *Equine Reproduction.* McKinnon AO, Voss JL (eds). Philadelphia: Lea & Febiger; 509–516.

Author: Peter R. Morresey

chapter 49

Placental Insufficiency

DEFINITION/OVERVIEW

In cases of placental insufficiency, the feto-placental exchange unit cannot adequately meet fetal demands. The resulting fetal malnutrition may lead to IUGR, prolonged gestation, or pregnancy loss.

ETIOLOGY/PATHOPHYSIOLOGY

A number of factors can contribute to this condition.

- Physical constrictions to placental development: body pregnancy and intraluminal adhesions from previous endometritis.
- Area available for placental villus exchange between the endometrium and fetus is decreased. This may result from both non-formation and separation of the micro-cotyledonary attachments between the chorion and endometrium (Fig. 49.1).

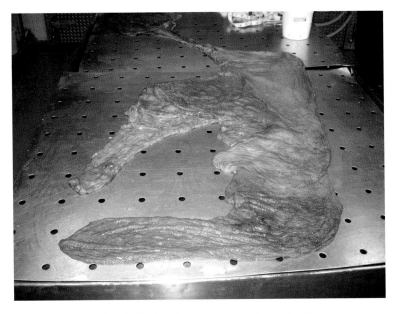

■ Figure 49.1 Pale chorionic surface indicative of sparse microcotyledon development.

- Diminished histiotrophe (uterine milk) production. Histiotrophe production, secretion, and absorption occurs between the microcotyledonary attachments of the placenta and endometrium. Histiotrophe production increases during pregnancy, however, this is dependent on the health and number of endometrial glands.

Systems Affected

Multiple organ systems of the fetus can be affected:
- Cardiovascular: decreased development.
- Musculoskeletal: decreased development.
- Nervous: chronic deprivation leads to hypoxic insult.
- Endocrine/Metabolic: insulin abnormalities are detected throughout life.
- Gastrointestinal: decreased development.

SIGNALMENT/HISTORY

- Pregnant female, usually aged or multiparous, that may have a previous history of endometritis.
- Mares bearing twins: the occurrence of placental insufficiency in these mares highlights the inability to sustain two placentas and two fetuses.

Risk Factors

- Placentitis: inflammation and separation compromise the microcotyledonary attachments.
- Degenerative endometrial changes: evidence of inflammation and fibrosis lead to a low Kenney grade endometrial biopsy score.
- Age and parity: occurrence of problems increases with age or repeated pregnancy. However, maiden mares have decreased endometrial gland formation compared to parous mares and have comparatively decreased placental growth and development.
- Chronic endometritis: leads to degenerative endometrial change.
- Poor vulvar conformation: loss of vulvar or vestibular seal permits aspiration of irritants/contaminants into the cranial vagina.

Historical Findings

- Repeated early pregnancy loss.
- History of birthing underweight foals of abnormal gestational lengths.
- Pale, small placenta with evidence of avillous areas.
- Endometrial changes that are irreversible: endometrial biopsy previous to current pregnancy commonly shows evidence of fibrosis, glandular nesting, or decreased numbers of endometrial glands.

CLINICAL FEATURES

- Placental insufficiency is highly correlated with the delivery of pre-term, or the abortion of, a small, emaciated fetus (or fetuses) in the absence of infectious disease.
- Alternatively, an appropriate ("normal") or prolonged gestation length may result in the delivery of a small-for-gestational-age, dysmature fetus that is underweight with a silky haircoat and with behavioral abnormalities.

 ## DIFFERENTIAL DIAGNOSIS

- Infectious causes of abortion: bacterial, viral, and fungal.
- Noninfectious causes of abortion: endotoxemia caused by systemic illness.
- Other causes of prolonged gestation: fescue toxicosis and fetal endocrine abnormalities.
- Other causes of fetal malnutrition: twinning, maternal disease leading to catabolism.

 ## DIAGNOSTICS

- Hematology: abnormalities reflect systemic pathologic processes, if any, in the mare. Will not show evidence of placental dysfunction.
- Transabdominal U/S: small-for-gestational-age fetus: fetal crown-rump length and fetal orbit diameter are decreased compared to cohorts of similar gestational age.
- Transrectal U/S: can visualize thickness or detachment of the placenta cranial to the cervix. It is most readily apparent late in gestation.
- Neonatal examination: IUGR effects are more pronounced when limitation of growth occurs later in gestation. Asymmetrically affected fetal and neonatal development can be seen, with a fetus/neonate having a long head, thin body, and relatively little body fat.

Pathological Findings

- Gross Findings: Placental examination may reveal thickened, edematous, or discolored areas on the chorionic surface. In addition, avillous areas other than those previously described as normal may be present (see Placental Basics). With twin pregnancies, the classic placental lesion is at the site of apposition of the two placentas, which prevents it from completely attaching to the endometrium. This is grossly visible as an avillous (pale) area at which no exchange can occur. The usual outcome is abortion of both fetuses or one dead or mummified. If the mare reaches term, the remaining twin is small for gestational age.
- Histopathologic Findings: endometrial biopsy reveals pronounced fibrosis, glandular nesting and lymphatic stasis of the endometrium. Varying degrees of inflammation may be present.

THERAPEUTICS

Goals of treatment are to improve maternal health (if it is compromised) and attempt to increase fetal nutrition via improving mare nutrition and boosting histiotrophe production. If other placental disease is present (placentitis), treat it concurrently.

Drug(s) of Choice

Progestin supplementation may be helpful to boost endometrial histiotrophe production.

- Altrenogest: 0.044 mg/kg PO every 24 hours. Dosage may be safely doubled in severe cases.
- Progesterone-in-oil (150 mg to 300 mg IM) has also been recommended.

Alternative Drugs

See placentitis treatment (if present).

Appropriate Health Care

Before beginning treatment, establish the viability of the fetus by transabdominal fetal U/S. Note fetal heart rate and placental dimensions/thickness.

Nursing Care

Minimize environmental and social stressors.

Diet

Correct any nutritional inadequacies or deficiencies in the mare's ration.

Activity

Maternal confinement and rest from forced exercise is appropriate.

Surgical Considerations

Avoid surgical procedures and excessive pain to the mare if possible because decreased uterine blood flow from anesthesia may increase fetal compromise.

 COMMENTS

Client Education

Endometrial health declines with age and increasing parity of mares.

Patient Monitoring

- U/S: *Fetus*: monitor regularly for signs of viability. Note fluctuations and values of the heart rate. *Placenta*: thickness, presence of detachment from the endometrium.

- Maternal hormonal levels: progesterone and estrogen levels are considered measures or indicators of uteroplacental function.

Prevention/Avoidance

Evaluation of a mare when she is not pregnant (i.e., a breeding soundness evaluation [BSE]). The endometrial biopsy is useful to evaluate the density of endometrial glands, the presence of inflammation (acute, neutrophilia; chronic, plasmacytic, lymphocytic), presence of pneumovagina (eosinophilia), and scar tissue (diffuse periglandular fibrosis; lymphatic dilation and stasis).

Possible Complications

- Abortion
- Placentitis: premature placental separation *in utero* and at parturition.
- Birth of an undersized, weak neonate: neonatal hypoxic insult, sepsis (e.g., bacterial, fungal).

Expected Course and Prognosis

- Abortion: placenta is inadequate to meet the needs of pregnancy.
- Fetal compromise: underweight, physiologically stressed fetus.
- Neonatal compromise: hypoxic insult due to premature placental separation.

Abbreviations

BSE   breeding soundness evaluation/examination
IUGR   intrauterine growth retardation
U/S   ultrasound, ultrasonography

See Also

- Endometrial biopsy
- Endometritis
- Placental basics
- Placentitis
- Twin (Multiple) Pregnancy

Suggested Reading

Adams R. 1993. Identification of the mare and foal at high risk for perinatal problems. In: *Equine Reproduction.* McKinnon AO, Voss JL (eds). Philadelphia: Lea & Febiger; 988–989.

Giles RC, Donahue JM, Hong CB, et al. 1993. Causes of abortion, stillbirth, and perinatal death in horses: 3,527 cases (1986–1991). *J Am Vet Med Assoc* 203: 1170–1175.

Author: Peter R. Morresey

chapter 50

Placentitis

 ## DEFINITION/OVERVIEW

Placentitis results from inflammation of the placenta by infection with a bacterial, viral, or fungal agent.

 ## ETIOLOGY/PATHOPHYSIOLOGY

- An infectious agent (e.g., bacterial, viral, and fungal) invades the placenta and multiplies leading to an inflammatory response. Placental thickening and detachment may follow decreasing functional exchange with the fetus.
- Modes of entry to the placenta include ascending infection via the cervix (most common), hematogenous spread as part of a systemic illness, or direct spread and inoculation from a pre-existing focus (Figs. 50.1 and 50.2).

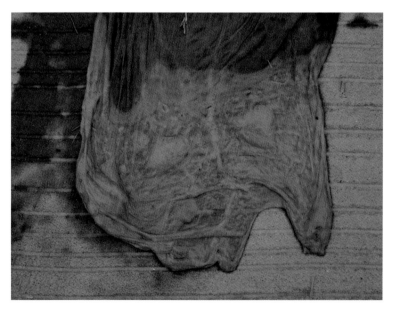

■ **Figure 50.1** Ascending placentitis with significant involvement at the cervical star and caudal uterine body of the fetal membranes.

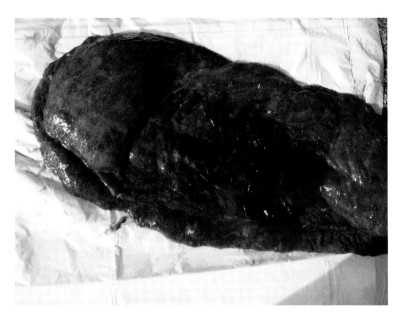

■ **Figure 50.2** Focal placentitis on the pregnant uterine horn of the fetal membranes.

Systems Affected

Reproductive: infectious agent and associated inflammation may spread to the fetus from the placental tissue.

 # SIGNALMENT/HISTORY

Placentitis is a condition of the pregnant mare chiefly during late gestation.

Risk Factors

Bacterial placentitis may occur at any time throughout gestation with two presentations reported.
- Acute: focal or diffuse, with neutrophilic infiltration, necrosis of chorionic villi. Primarily occurs in early to mid gestation.
- Chronic: focal or extensive, centered around the area of the cervical star. Characterized by eosinophilic chorionic material, necrosis of villi, adenomatous hyperplasia, mononuclear cell infiltration. Primarily seen in mid to late gestation.
- Common pathogens include *Streptococcus equi var zooepidemicus*, *Streptococcus equisimilis*, *Pseudomonas aeruginosa*, *Klebsiella pneumoniae*, and *Escherichia coli* (the latter being a fecal contaminant).
- *Leptospira* sp.: diffuse placentitis inoculated by hematogenous spread only.
- Nocardioform: *Crossiella* sp., a Gram-positive filamentous bacillus. Lesions tend to be situated at the horn base and it is chronic in nature.

Viral

- EVA: thickening of the chorioallantois is attributable to the longer incubation time before abortion occurs compared with EHV-1 (and either none or nonspecific placental changes).

Fungal

- Mycotic placentitis usually occurs at 300 days or later of gestation.
- *Aspergillus* sp.: chronic lesions appear as a focal placentitis at the cervical star; similar in nature to chronic bacterial cases.
- *Candida* sp.: a diffuse, necrotizing and proliferative placentitis.
- *Histoplasma* sp.: multifocal granulomatous changes present.

Anatomic

- Cervical incompetence: laceration, age-induced degeneration.
- Production of $PGF_2\alpha$ by endotoxin release, leading to cervical relaxation.

Historical Findings

- Vulvar discharge
- Precocious mammary development
- Previous history of placentitis or late-term abortion

 CLINICAL FEATURES

- Vulvar discharge: mucoid, progressing to purulent, sometimes hemorrhagic
- Cervical incompetence: inflammation and discharge visible via speculum examination
- Mammary: swelling and discharge suggests prepartum lactation
- Relaxation of pelvic musculature: vulvar tissue and sacrosciatic ligament
- Restlessness and premonitory foaling behavior with impending abortion
- Placental: thickening; edema; and discoloration with plaque formation often centered on the cervical star

 DIFFERENTIAL DIAGNOSIS

- Impending parturition: liquefaction of cervical mucus plug may be mistaken for vulvar discharge.
- Fescue toxicosis: placental edema present. Parturition date delayed, often accompanied by decreased colostrum production and depressed subsequent lactation.
- Other infectious causes of vulvar discharge: vaginitis, endometritis, pyometra, and metritis.
- Uterine trauma or intraluminal hemorrhage.
- Urinary tract infection: may observe mucopurulent to hemorrhagic urine being voided.

- Urine pooling: poor vaginal and vulvar conformation are likely complicit. Assess patency of the urethral orifice and its sphincter.
- Uterine or vaginal neoplasia: evaluate by speculum and manual examination per vaginum.
- Other causes of spurious lactation: may be linked with season or an endocrine abnormality.
- Other cause of pelvic relaxation: impending normal parturition.

 # DIAGNOSTICS

Clinical examination findings:
- Hematology: leukocytosis with neutrophilia is variably present because infection is not usually systemically important.
- Hyperfibrinogenemia: possible in advanced cases.
- Biochemistry: usually normal, major organ function unaffected.
- Urinalysis: normal.
- U/S: both transrectal and transabdominal are indicated. Increased uteroplacental thickness, especially in the cervical region, is highly suggestive of a problem. Areas of folding or detachment may be seen with transabdominal examination. Allantoic fluid debris may be present.
- Speculum examination: avoid excessive air aspiration when possible because this can compound vaginal inflammation. Allows visual assessment of cervical integrity and the presence and nature of discharge. It is non-invasive and therefore preferable to manual cervical palpation because the latter may stimulate PG release and initiate uterine contractions.
- Microbiology: Swab cervical discharge and submit for culture and sensitivity. Cytology of the discharge will provide preliminary information and may observe degenerate PMNs with or without bacteria or fungal elements.

Pathological Findings

- Gross examination of the allantochorion: findings include a thickened, discolored chorioallantois, with the normal areas of bright red chorion having been replaced by grayish/brown chorion. Raised plaques with exudate and avillous areas may be present.
- Histopathology: it is necessary to differentiate bacterial from mycotic agents. Findings include an inflammatory infiltrate, with fibrosis, thrombosis, and edema of affected tissues. The causative agent may be directly visualized.
- Microbiology: isolation of bacterial, fungal, or viral agent.

 # THERAPEUTICS

- Eliminate inciting cause: control infectious agent (bacterial, fungal).
- Maintain fetoplacental function.

- Prevent fetal expulsion: if the mare carries her pregnancy to 300 days, the chance of fetal survival, even with the mare's placentitis, increases as the stress of intrauterine environment accelerates maturity.

Drug(s) of Choice

Antimicrobials

- Penicillin G: 22,000 units/kg IM every 12 hours.
- Gentamicin: 6.6 mg/kg IV every 24 hours.
- Trimethoprim-sulfamethoxazole: 25 mg/kg PO every 12 hours.
- Selection of antimicrobial is based on sensitivities of the most likely culpable pathogen, however broad-spectrum therapy initially is warranted; not all drugs penetrate the placenta.

Anti-Inflammatories

- Phenylbutazone: 2.2 mg/kg PO every 12 to 24 hours.
- Flunixin meglumine: 1 mg/kg PO every 12 to 24 hours.
- Decrease endotoxin production and thereby reduce luteolytic potential and myometrial contractility. Anti-inflammatories are also useful to decrease the incidence of laminitis from the absorption of any systemic inflammatory mediator.

Progestogen Supplementation

Altrenogest 0.044 mg/kg PO every 24 hours. This dose rate may safely be doubled.
- Maintain production of histiotrophe: fetal nutrition.
- Quiets myometrium
- Aids cervical competency

Precautions/Interactions

If fetal death occurs:
- Discontinue progestagens and NSAIDs
- Allow abortion to occur
- Avoid *in utero* fetal decomposition

Alternative Drugs

Pentoxifylline 8.5 mg/kg PO every 8 hours has been used adjunctively for purported diminishment of cytokine production.

Appropriate Health Care

Mare

- Vaginal speculum examination to monitor the cervix: make note whether the cervix is closed and has the appropriate pale coloration, or alternatively, if it appears to be relaxing and is inflamed with overt discharge.

- Transrectal U/S of the cervix and caudal uterine body: to evaluate the thickness of the placenta and uterine wall and to detect the presence of placental detachment and folding.
- Attend the parturition: Cases of placentitis have an increased incidence of premature placental separation or a failure of the thickened chorioallantois to tear readily at the cervical star as the fetus is born (Stage 2 parturition). There is a higher risk of neonatal asphyxiation.
- Preterm mammary development (especially if it occurs more than 30 days before parturition) leads to premature lactation and loss of colostrum. Provide supplemental colostrum for foal after birth (test for absence of alloantibodies).
- Placental examination: ensure the placenta has been passed in its entirety and no fetal membranes have been retained within the uterus.

Neonate

- With placentitis, there is an increased potential for sepsis due to possible *in utero* challenge.
- Prepartum lactation may have depleted the mare's colostral antibodies. Ensure adequate intake.

Nursing Care

Minimize maternal and fetal stress.

Activity

Stall rest the mare.

 COMMENTS

Client Education

Endometrial health and cervical competence decline with age and increasing parity of mares. Placentitis is likely to be repeated in subsequent pregnancies.

Patient Monitoring

Regular monitoring of known affected mares or those with a history of placentitis.

Prevention/Avoidance

- BSE of the mare before pregnancy. Important to include examination of cervical competency, this is best performed in diestrus when maximal closure (greatest cervical tone) should be present.
- Prebreeding preparation of the mare and stallion: hygiene before collection and of equipment, during semen collection, and artificial breeding.
- Keep environment and housing of pregnant mares as clean as possible.

Possible Complications

- Abortion
- Sick, weak neonate
- Premature placental separation.
- Laminitis
- Fetal sepsis: bacterial; fungal

Expected Course and Prognosis

Successful management of a pregnancy to term is dependent on the chronicity of placentitis and the severity of disease at the time it is discovered. A long-term, comprehensive treatment course will be required. Abortion may still occur despite aggressive treatment.

Abbreviations

BSE	breeding soundness examination
EHV	equine herpes virus
EVA	equine viral arteritis
IM	intramuscular
IV	intravenous
NSAID	nonsteroidal anti-inflammatory drug
PG	prostaglandin
PGF	natural prostaglandin
PMN	polymorphonuclear
PO	per os (by mouth)
U/S	ultrasound, ultrasonography

See Also

- BSE
- Placental Basics
- Placental insufficiency

Suggested Reading

Adams R. 1993. Identification of the mare and foal at high risk for perinatal problems. In: *Equine Reproduction*. McKinnon AO, Voss JL (eds). Philadelphia: Lea & Febiger; 988–989.

Asbury AC, Leblanc MM. 1993. Placental abnormalities. In: *Equine Reproduction*. McKinnon AO, Voss JL (eds). Philadelphia: Lea & Febiger; 514–515.

Hong CB, Donahue JM, Giles RC, et al. 1993. Etiology and pathology of equine placentitis. *J Vet Diagn Invest* 5: 56–63.

Author: Peter R. Morresey

chapter 51

Pneumovagina/Pneumouterus

DEFINITION/OVERVIEW

- Air in the vagina or uterus.
- Usually results from vulvar conformational defect.

ETIOLOGY/PATHOPHYSIOLOGY

- Air accumulates subsequent to poor VC and relaxation of the vestibular sphincter.
- The negative pressure within the lumen of the genital tract aids in movement of air into the vestibule, vagina, and uterus; elicits a *wind sucking* sound.
- With motion (e.g., running, rolling), air is forced back out, resulting in a characteristic expulsive sound.

Systems Affected

Reproductive

SIGNALMENT/HISTORY

General Comments

- Described as potential reproductive problem as early as 1937.
- Condition remains a major cause of subfertility/infertility.

Physical Examination Findings

- Determine if VC is normal:
    - Assess relationship of dorsal vulvar commissure to the pubis; it should lie at or below the floor of the pubis (Figs. 51.1, 51.2, and 51.3).
- Effect of poor VC on fertility is confirmed by the presence of vaginitis, pneumovagina, or pneumouterus.

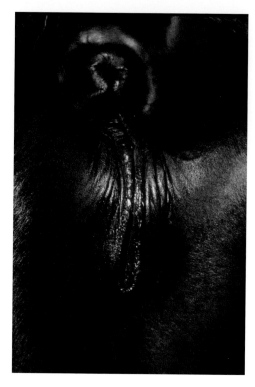

■ **Figure 51.1** Example of poor vulvar conformation. There appears to be a good seal between the vulvar lips, but the cranial slant is unmistakable and undesirable.
Image courtesy of C. L. Carleton.

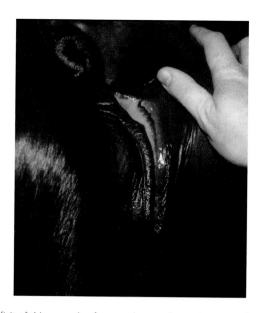

■ **Figure 51.2** The full deficit of this example of poor vulvar conformation, extending well over the caudal brim of the pubis, places this mare at severe risk of pneumovagina and ascending uterine contamination.
Image courtesy of C. L. Carleton.

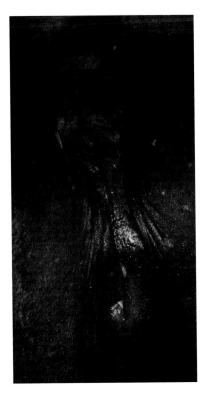

■ **Figure 51.3** Poor vulvar conformation. Anterior slant compounded by deficits in the seal between the vulvae. Image courtesy of C. L. Carleton.

- As age/parity increase:
  - Anus is pulled cranially and thus attached soft-tissue structures move forward with it.
  - The vulva is pulled in a cranial slant, up over the posterior brim of the pubis.
- Predisposing Factors:
  - Changes in general conformation (e.g., sway back).
  - Loss of body condition or vaginal fat.
  - Age, genetics, trauma-related changes of VC.
  - Weakness or stretching of the supporting soft-tissue structures in the perineal area.

Risk Factors

- All breeds, but breeds/individuals with less perineal muscle (Thoroughbreds, in particular) are more severely affected.
- All of breeding age.
- Older pluripara mares most commonly affected.
- Diminishes protective barrier of a normal vulva by age, parity, and genetic predisposition.

- VC also influenced by pregnancy as a result of the additional stretching of the perineal soft tissues.
- Poor body condition may contribute to decreased VC.
- Normal estrual tissue relaxation may slightly affect VC.

Historical Findings

- May exhibit signs of chronic pneumovagina, including vaginal flatus, abnormal redness of the vaginal mucosa and accumulation of air in the uterus, coupled with abnormal VC.
- Subfertility/infertility linked with uterine infections or inflammation is also common.

 ## CLINICAL FEATURES

- Possible genetic influence for less-than-ideal VC.
- No statistics available regarding incidence. Condition is common and one of the major causes of equine infertility.

 ## DIAGNOSTICS

Imaging

U/S: not necessary, unless to confirm pneumouterus.

Pathologic Findings

- Evidence of vaginitis and endometritis:
  - Indicators of pneumovagina or pneumouterus.
  - Other possible causes exist, but with poor VC, the diagnosis is conclusive.
- This condition may result not only in subfertility and infertility but also a cause of abortion in pregnant mares after vaginitis and cervicitis develops.

 ## THERAPEUTICS

Drug(s) of Choice

- No antibiotics are indicated.
- Selection of local anesthetic is at the discretion of the surgeon.

Appropriate Health Care

- Little justification to treat a mare for uterine infection or inflammation if poor VC is not corrected.

Surgical Considerations

- Surgical correction for poor VC (vulvoplasty or episioplasty) was first described by Dr. Caslick in 1937.
- First, wrap and tie the mare's tail away from the field of surgery and thoroughly clean the perineal area with cotton and soap.
- Carbocaine or other local anesthetic is infiltrated into the mucocutaneous junction of the vulva; about 10 to 12 mL typically used to infiltrate both sides of the vulva.
- The tissue edges are freshened before suturing, either by:
  - *Strip removal*: very narrow strip of tissue is cut away from the edge of the each vulvar lip, or by
  - *Split-thickness technique*: incising (no. 10 scalpel blade) at the mucocutaneous junction along the line dilated with local anesthetic (i.e., no tissue is removed). The incised line on the mucocutaneous junction, dilated with anesthetic, separates approximately 1 cm wide. The horseshoe shaped incision reaches from right vulvar lip, dorsally in an arch over the top of the vulvar commissure, continuing to the left vulvar lip. The lateral aspects (skin to middle of the cut line) of the right and left vulvar lip incision are closed. Creates an appropriately thin and protective barrier to prevent further fecal and air contamination.
  - The latter is tissue-sparing and preferred for the long-term reproductive welfare of the mare.
  - Over the reproductive life of a mare, the split-thickness technique helps to retain the normal elasticity of vulvae during labor by minimizing prior, annual damage (scar formation).
  - Both described techniques are in common use and considered acceptable.
  - Suture patterns may vary: Ford interlocking (allows adjustment of preplaced sutures to minimize likelihood of gaps in suture line), simple interrupted (increased likelihood to form gaps in my experience), simple continuous, etc.
- Use nonabsorbable suture material or staples, with removal in about 10 to 12 days.
  - At the time of suture/staple removal, evaluate surgical site for presence of small fistulae through which contamination may continue.
- The *Pouret technique* is another surgical option only considered for cases of very poor VC. In cases of severe/extremely poor VC, it may be necessary to dissect the perineal body in a caudal (widest) to cranial (complete the dissection in a narrower point) flat plane, creating a pie-shaped wedge. It permits the genital tract, ventral to the rectum, to slide caudally and slightly ventral; out of the line of fecal contamination as well as aspiration of air; only the skin is closed (i.e., no deep reconstruction of dissected tissue) between the anal sphincter and dorsal vulvar commissure. The degree/depth of dissection determines the degree of correction that is attained.
  - Restraint of the mare in stocks is critical to avoid movement during dissection of the perineal body.
  - Check the mare's tetanus toxoid vaccination status. Administer a booster as necessary.

COMMENTS

Client Education

- Advise clients to evaluate the VC of all mares.
- If VC is less than ideal, a Caslick's vulvoplasty surgery is needed.
- Surgery may be necessary to obtain a pregnancy.

Patient Monitoring

- Suture removal 10 to 12 days after surgery to prevent the possibility of stitch abscess forming at the suture site.
- High probability of this VC becoming worse with age.
- Management option: place sutures within 48 hours following a confirmed ovulation. Suture removal can be delayed until the mare is brought into the barn for an early pregnancy check at 16 days post-ovulation; savings on labor cost.

Prevention/Avoidance

Select broodmares with excellent VC.

Possible Complications

- Primary contraindication to vulvoplasty: necessity to re-open the vulvar commissure about 5 to 10 days before parturition to prevent tearing of the perineum at delivery.
- It should be replaced (i.e., local block, incised, and sutured) immediately after foaling or breeding and confirmation of ovulation in the next season, depending on severity of VC abnormality.
- Place the Caslick's vulvoplasty following breeding as soon as ovulation has been confirmed:
  - Ensures the best uterine environment for the newly arriving embryo 6-days post-ovulation.
  - Do not wait until after the first pregnancy check to suture the mare. The unsutured vulva allows endometrial contamination to continue unabated and the embryo arrives into a more hostile uterine environment.
- Even if a mare will not be bred back after foaling, or she is not intended to be a broodmare, if her VC is less than ideal, a Caslick's vulvoplasty should be done, sutures removed in 10 to 12 days after it has healed, allowing her genital tract to remain protected from further irritation by air aspiration.

Expected Course and Prognosis

Without surgical correction, mares may remain infertile or abort during pregnancy.

Synonyms

- Windsucker
- Windsucking

Abbreviations

U/S   ultrasound, ultrasonography
VC   vulvar conformation

See Also

- Dystocia
- Endometrial biopsy
- Endometritis
- Perineal lacerations
- Vulvar conformation (Caslick's vulvoplasty)

Suggested Reading

Caslick EA. 1937. The vulva and vulvo-vaginal orifice and its relationship to genital health of the thoroughbred mare. *Cornell Vet* 27: 178–186.

Colbern GT, Aanes WA, Stashak TS. 1985. Surgical management of perineal lacerations and recto-vestibular fistulae in the mare: a retrospective study of 47 cases. *JAVMA* 186: 265–269.

Shipley WD, Bergin WC. 1968. Genital health in the mare. III. Pneumovagina. *VM/SAC* 63: 699–702.

Author: Walter R. Threlfall

chapter 52

Postpartum Care of the Mare and Foal

DEFINITION/OVERVIEW

- The initial evaluation and care of the postparturient mare and her foal are important to the early detection and treatment of postpartum diseases in the mare and identifying abnormalities in the foal that may be serious or fatal.
- Postpartum care of the mare and foal aims at ensuring health of both mare and foal through identification and elimination of risk factors for infection, poor mothering ability, and slow neonatal development.
- Postpartum evaluation should always include a thorough evaluation of the placenta.
- Normal postpartum period includes a normal lactation, involution of the uterus, and return to cyclicity within 10 days.

ETIOLOGY/PATHOPHYSIOLOGY

Postpartum Mare

- Foaling and immediate postpartum are extremely stressful periods for both mare and foal.
- Postpartum complications in the mare may arise from traumatic injuries to the genital tract (uterus, cervix, vagina, and vulva), urinary bladder, or complete or partial RFM.
- Some injuries are emergencies (e.g., uterine artery rupture and hemorrhage into the broad ligament, uterine tear, or uterine rupture).
- The postpartum mare is also predisposed to colic of non-genital origin (e.g., large colon torsion, urinary bladder necrosis, or rupture).
- A certain degree of uterine contamination is always present after foaling. Most mares with a normal, uncomplicated parturition will clear contaminants and return to normal reproductive function within 10 to 12 days.
- Intrapartum or postpartum complications may have severe implications for the life of:
  - The mare: hemorrhage, toxic metritis.
  - The foal: lack of normal maternal bond, FPT, and injuries caused by an agitated/painful mare.

Foal

- The immediate postpartum period presents major challenges and changes to the foal's physiology.
  - Rapid adjustment to extra-uterine life.
  - Ability to stand and nurse within a short time, to ensure adequate transfer of IgG through ingestion of colostrum.
- Early detection of problems is important for rapid implementation of therapy or decision making as to the viability of the foal and prevention of agonizing moments for the foal.
  - Traumatic injuries (rib fractures).
  - Abnormalities (e.g., contracted tendons, joint laxity, congenital defects).
- The most important risk factor resulting in infectious diseases in the newborn foal is FPT.
- FPT results from:
  - Failure to ingest or absorb IgG from colostrum.
  - The newborn's inability to stand and suckle within a few hours following birth.
  - Because of weakness, immature foals are at even greater risk.
  - Failure to supplement colostrum (from stock-piled, frozen colostrum or administration of concentrated plasma, IV) by owners/veterinarians when it is known that the mare has insufficient colostrum or the foal is weak and/or not standing early postpartum.

Placenta

- Placental evaluation is integral:
  - To the postpartum evaluation of the dam.
  - To make appropriate decisions regarding neonatal care.
- Evidence of partial or complete RFM warrants immediate action to prevent complications in the mare.
- Evidence of infectious placentitis warrants immediate action to prevent neonatal septicemia.

Systems Affected

- Reproductive, GI, and urinary in the mare.
- General health, multisystem in the neonate.

 SIGNALMENT/HISTORY

- All parturient mares and their foals should be evaluated; an essential component of immediate postpartum care.
- All postpartum mares within first 24 hours following foaling.

- Mares with an unobserved foaling, previous history of dystocia, abortion, premature placental separation, neonatal loss, prolonged pregnancy, agalactia, placentitis (high-risk pregnancy).
- Mares with a prior history of having an NI foal.
- If possible, all mares and foals should be examined immediately or within the first 12 hours post-foaling.
- An immediate examination is required if there are *any* postpartum complications.
- Examination of the postpartum mare should always weigh benefit versus risk.
  - Complications or injuries may result from disturbing the mare and foal.
  - Interference with maternal-neonate bonding.

 CLINICAL FEATURES

Mare

- History of prior foaling(s) and foaling conditions should be taken into account when examining the postpartum mare.
- Pregnancy length should be calculated from breeding records.
  - Gestation shorter than 325 days necessitates an in-depth evaluation of the foal.
  - If indicators for prematurity or dysmaturity are present, a critical assessment of the need for supplemental nursing care is essential.
- Examination of normal foaling mares should be brief. Determine general condition, temperature, pulse and respiration rates, mucous membrane color and CRT, degree of responsiveness, and maternal behavior.
- Udder should be examined to confirm the teats are patent and adequate colostrum is present. The mammary gland should be cleansed and a small quantity of colostrum collected and tested for quality.
- Examination of the external genitalia:
  - Presence of vulvar tears, swelling, or excessive discharge.
- Mares should be monitored for signs of colic, depression, or abnormal maternal behavior for the next few days postpartum.
- Complete vaginal examination, and TRP is warranted only if the mare is not too nervous or if there is a clinical indication (colic, depression, poor mothering ability).
- Postpartum mares that have experienced dystocia, or other immediate postpartum complications (e.g., RFM) should undergo a complete evaluation of the genital organs and be monitored closely for a few days.
- Postpartum care of the mare should include the opportunity for her to exercise to promote uterine involution.

Foal Evaluation

- Foals should be evaluated and monitored in the first few hours of life.
- Immediately after birth the foal should be stimulated to promote breathing:
  - Rubbing vigorously with a dry towel.
  - Clearing the nostrils and mouth.

- Normal foals:
  - Suckling reflex by 2 to 20 minutes after birth.
  - Assume sternal recumbency by 1 to 2 minutes.
  - Stand within 1 to 2 hours.
  - Nurse within 2 hours after birth.
  - Rectal temperature should be 37.2°C to 38.6°C (99°F to 101.5°F).
  - Heart rate should greater than 60 beats per minute immediately after birth and 80 to 130 beats per minute after 5 minutes.
  - Respiration rate should be 60 to 80 breaths per minute in the first 30 minutes of life and drop to 30 to 40 breaths per minute by 1 to 2 hours.
  - The chest should always be examined for evidence of rib fractures; the most common traumatic intrafoaling injury.
- Humidified oxygen should be available for respiratory resuscitation.
- Check for common congenital abnormalities:
  - Cleft palate
  - Contracted tendons
  - Excessive joint laxity
  - Prognathism
  - Umbilical and inguinal hernias
  - Atresia ani
  - Abnormalities of sexual differentiation
- The umbilical cord should be checked for abnormalities and disinfected with 0.5% chlorhexidine diacetate every 4 to 6 hours. Strong iodine solutions should be avoided because they cause tissue necrosis. Keep stall clean and change bedding often.
- Normal urination and defecation. Note both activity and frequency. Warm water or soap based enemas (60–120 mL) may be administered to facilitate meconium passage.
- Examination from a distance. At a few hours of age, assess foal's coordination and strength, ability to rise and nurse, and its responsiveness to stimuli.
- Adequate passive transfer of immunity (colostral antibodies) should be verified by 12 to 18 hours post-foaling.

Placenta

- Evaluation is an important component of postpartum care of the mare and foal.
- Evidence of incomplete passage of the placenta (partial RFM) warrants further detailed examination and institution of treatment of the postparturient mare.
- Evidence of placental edema, placentitis, or other placental abnormalities warrants further clinical evaluation of the foal and possible prophylactic broad-spectrum antimicrobial treatment.

Risk Factors

- Mare risk factors for postpartum complications include: age, a high risk pregnancy, dystocia, and foaling conditions.
- Foal risk factors include: documented abnormalities of gestation (e.g., placentitis, prolonged, or short pregnancy), dystocia, and maternal abnormalities (e.g., agalactia, poor colostrum quality).

DIFFERENTIAL DIAGNOSIS

Vaginal Discharge

- Lochia: normal postpartum to 6 days
- Postpartum metritis

DIAGNOSTICS

CBC/Biochemistry/Urinalysis

Mare

- CBC and biochemistry are indicated in any mare with a history of dystocia, RFM, or signs of colic.
- Urinalysis may be indicated for some mares.

Foal

- Determination of passive transfer of immunity status. May be determined as early as 8 to 12 hours postpartum. Serum sample to measure IgG concentration:
  - Greater than 800 mg/dL demonstrates adequate colostrum intake and absorption.
  - Less than 400 mg/dL indicates FPT due to poor colostral quality, poor ingestion, or poor absorption.
  - Partial transfer of Ig: 400 to 800 mg/dL.
  - If a foal is more than 24 hours old and has less than 400 mg/dL serum IgG, then initiate treatment with 1 L of plasma IV plus broad-spectrum antibiotics.
- CBC and biochemistry should be considered if the foal is not displaying normal behavior, is weak, or there was evidence of an abnormal placenta.

Other Laboratory Tests

Assessment of Colostrum Quality

- Physical properties: thick, sticky, yellow or gray-tinged.
- Biochemical:
  - Colostrometer, colostral specific gravity. Colostral specific gravity ≥1.06 correlates with IgG content of greater than 3,000 mg of IgG/dL (30 g/L).
  - Refractometer (alcohol or sugar): colostrum with level of 6,000 mg of IgG/dL (60 g/L). Reads at 16% with the alcohol, and 23% with the sugar refractometer.
- Quality parameters for saving colostrum (to be banked):
  - Colostrometer specific gravity greater than 1.07
  - If it is 16% using the alcohol refractometer
  - If it is 23% using the sugar refractometer
  - Collect 250 mL of colostrum for storage after the foal's first suckling.
  - Colostrum can be stored at −5°C for up to 18 months.

- Colostrum should be checked for isoantibodies.
  - Do *not* mix saved colostrum from multiple mares in a bag. If isoantibodies are detected, would prevent identification and use of the safe portions of the stored colostrum.
- If stored colostrum is needed for supplementation, thawing should be done carefully.
- Colostrum should be stored and thawed out in small quantities:
  - Small zip-lock baggies (nice method; they flatten well in the freezer; more uniform freezing and thawing).
  - Ice-cube trays (one cube is approximately 1 ounce, freeze then dump cubes into zip-lock bags.
  - Thaw in a warm water bath or in a microwave with defrost cycle (must not microwave too quickly or the protein coagulates and is destroyed).
- Foal should receive the equivalent of 1 g of colostral IgG per kg of body weight.

Imaging

U/S Mare

- Transabdominal U/S is indicated if the mare is depressed or colicky, suspected of having a bladder rupture, broad ligament hemorrhage, or uterine rupture.
- Transrectal U/S to evaluate uterine involution and quantity and quality of fluid in the postpartum uterus.
- Transrectal U/S evaluation of the broad ligament, vagina and urinary bladder.

U/S Foal

- U/S of the umbilicus or abdomen of the foal is indicated if it is colicky or a patent urachus is suspected.
- U/S of the thorax if rib fractures are suspected.

Other Diagnostic Procedures

Abdominocentesis

- Indicated in postpartum mares showing depression or colic.

Endoscopy

- Uterine endoscopy is indicated if a uterine tear is suspected.

Nursing Care

Mare

- If a mare was not given a tetanus toxoid booster vaccination 4 to 6 weeks prepartum, or if a mare has an unknown history of vaccination, she should be given a tetanus toxoid booster at term.
- Tetanus antitoxin is appropriate only if a mare is diagnosed with active tetanus. The potential exists to cause serum hepatitis.

- Deworming is indicated on the day of foaling or within a few days following foaling in mares not on a routine anti-parasite preventive program.

Foal

- If mare has not been vaccinated appropriately, tetanus toxoid should be administered at birth (pre-suckle) and again at 6 weeks and 12 weeks.
- Observe the pair from a distance for normal maternal and foal behavior.

Diet

- Feeding should be light to moderate, laxative feeds such as bran mashes.
  - To prevent constipation and colon impaction.

Activity

- Exercise to promote uterine involution: Postpartum mares confined to a stall because of health problems or foal concerns or illness or are predisposed to delayed uterine involution and metritis.
- Confined mares should be evaluated for uterine accumulation of intrauterine fluid. Proper therapeutic measure should be immediately instituted to facilitate clearance from the uterus (e.g., uterine lavage, oxytocin therapy).

Surgical Considerations

- RVF (foaling trauma)
- Some foal conditions: hernias, umbilical hemorrhage, patent urachus.

COMMENTS

Client Education

- Pregnant mare immunization and care.
- Colostrum management: Assessment of colostrum quality, harvesting, testing for risk of NI, storage, and use.
- Clients (stable managers or owners) are often the first care provider. Not all foalings are assisted or cared-for after-the-fact by a veterinarian.
  - Clients need to be familiar with normal foaling, normal mare and foal behavior, and essential and immediate pre- and postpartum care.
  - Educate these individuals to recognize postfoaling abnormalities and early indicators of foal health crisis.
  - Clients should be able to recognize the major foal abnormalities.
- Large stud farms routinely maintain an emergency kit available for personnel to supply respiratory resuscitation.

Prevention/Avoidance

- Preventive measure for pregnant mares: vaccination

Abbreviations

CBC   complete blood count
CRT   capillary refill time
FPT   failure of passive transfer
GI   gastrointestinal
IgG   immunoglobulin G
IV   intravenous
NI   neonatal isoerythrolysis
RFM   retained fetal membranes
RVF   rectovaginal fistula
TRP   transrectal palpation
U/S   ultrasound, ultrasonography

See Also

- Agalactia
- Broad ligament hemorrhage
- Cervical lesions
- Foal diseases (septicemia, congenital defects)
- Parturition
- Postpartum metritis
- RFM
- Rectovaginal tears
- Retained placenta
- Postpartum hemorrhage

Suggested Reading

Asbury AC, Lyle SK. 1993. Infectious causes of infertility. In: *Equine Reproduction.* McKinnon AO, Voss JL (eds). Philadelphia: Lea and Febiger; 381–391.

Dolente BA, Sullivan EK, Boston R, et al. 2005. Mares admitted to a referral hospital for postpartum emergencies: 163 cases (1992–2002). *J Vet Emer Crit Care* 15: 193–200.

Frazer GS. 2003. Postpartum complications in the mare. Part 1: Conditions affecting the uterus. *Eq Vet Educ* 15: 36–44.

LeBlanc MM, Tran T, Baldwin JL, et al. 1992. Factors that influence passive transfer of immunoglobulins in foals. *JAVMA* 200: 179–183.

Pierce SW. 2003. Foal care from birth to 30 days: A practitioner's perspective. *Proc AAEP* 13–21.

Author: Ahmed Tibary

Postpartum Metritis

chapter 53

DEFINITION/OVERVIEW

- Acute metritis resulting from RFM or uterine contamination after parturition or dystocia. Also known as Toxic Metritis.
- Marked by concurrent septicemia/endotoxemia and, possibly, laminitis.

ETIOLOGY/PATHOPHYSIOLOGY

- Subsequent to a difficult foaling, RFM, or heavy bacterial contamination of the uterus during foaling, coupled with septicemia/endotoxemia, the uterus is flaccid and thin-walled compared with a normal uterus (normal presentation is thickening walls and longitudinal rugae) as it rapidly involutes postpartum.
- Accumulated fluid and debris provide favorable conditions for bacterial growth, inflammation, and endotoxin release.
  - During gram-negative bacterial proliferation or death, aggregates of LPS are released.
  - If the protective mucosa is damaged, inflamed, or mechanically traumatized, LPS (endotoxins) reach systemic circulation and cause clinical signs.
- LPS are easily absorbed into maternal circulation (i.e., endotoxemia) because of the highly vascularized, inflamed, and thin-walled postpartum uterus.

Systems Affected

- Reproductive
- Hemic/Lymphatic/Immune
- Musculoskeletal

SIGNALMENT/HISTORY

- Postpartum mare
- Signs start with mild tachypnea, anorexia, abdominal pain or depression 12 to 24 hours after dystocia, RFM, or extensive intrapartum uterine contamination.
- Also can occur after normal delivery if a mare is confined to a stall (i.e., a foal with a limb deformity that necessitates restriction of its exercise).
  - Exercise aides in the clearance of postpartum debris and fluid accumulation.

Risk Factors

- Mares with a history of placentitis, RFM, dystocia, abortion, prolonged or assisted delivery, fetotomy, or C-section are at greater risk of postpartum metritis.
- Postpartum complications depend on the amount and type of bacteria in the reproductive tract. Postpartum metritis is often associated with a dirty foaling environment or excessive manipulation at parturition.
- Aerobic gram-negative and gram-positive bacteria such as *Escherichia coli, Pseudomonas aeruginosa, Klebsiella pneumoniae, Streptococcus zooepidemicus* and other β-hemolytic Streptococci, and *Staphylococcus* sp. are frequently involved.
- The gram-positive anaerobe *Bacteroides fragilis* resides in the external genitalia of mares and stallions and is periodically introduced into the uterus by coitus or genital pathologies such as pneumovagina and vagino/cervical damage. Spontaneous or iatrogenic (i.e., excess manipulation) mucosal breakdown and necrotic tissue create favorable conditions for this bacteria's overgrowth.
- Autolytic RFM, in concert with bacterial contamination, initially results in endometritis, which progresses to the deeper layers; the end result is metritis.
- Metritis, left untreated, can lead to systemic illness: septicemia, endotoxemia, and laminitis.

Historical Findings

See Signalment/History.

CLINICAL FEATURES

- Metritis may become evident by 12 to 24 hours postpartum.
- Mares present with signs of endotoxemia: fever, elevated pulse and respiratory rate, depression, anorexia, intermittent signs of colic or abdominal pain, increased CRT, and congested or toxic mucous membranes (Fig. 53.1).
- Uterus is poorly involuted upon palpation (Fig. 53.2): enlarged, flaccid, and baggy from accumulation of fetid, dark-red to chocolate-colored fluid. The fetid odor can be striking in its severity.
- U/S: Large amounts of fluid may accumulate in the uterus by 24 to 48 hours postpartum.
  - Degree of echogenicity generally relates to the amount of debris or inflammatory cells in the fluid, but "clear" fluid can be misleading (Figs. 53.3 and 53.4).
- Uterine wall is thin and atonic.
- Attachment of RFM usually at/in the previously nongravid horn. The RFM may either be a large portion of the total placenta and be evident hanging through the vulvae, or be limited to a small piece of the remaining placenta (Fig. 53.5).
- Signs of laminitis (e.g., bounding digital pulses, lameness) may appear 12 hours to 5 days postpartum (Figs. 53.6 and 53.7).

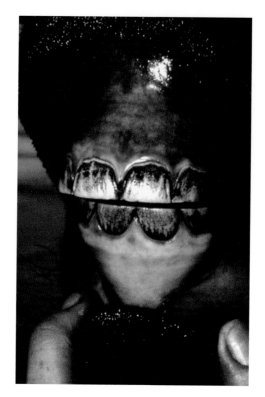

■ **Figure 53.1** Congested, toxic mucous membranes.
Image courtesy of P. R. Morresey.

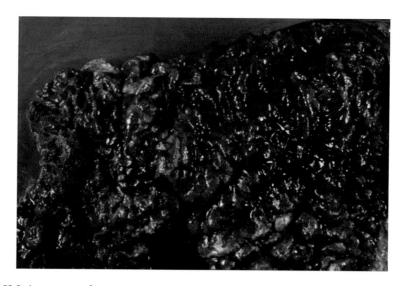

■ **Figure 53.2** Appearance of postpartum uterus at necropsy. Uterine involution was delayed and fetid, deep red material remained throughout the uterine lumen.
Image courtesy of P. R. Morresey.

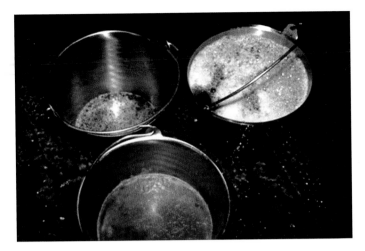

■ **Figure 53.3** Accumulated fluid flushed and collected from a mare affected by postpartum metritis. Image courtesy of P. R. Morresey.

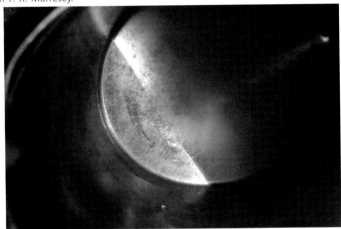

■ **Figure 53.4** Appearance of fluid accumulation can be misleading when it is red-tinted but less cellular. Image courtesy of P. R. Morresey.

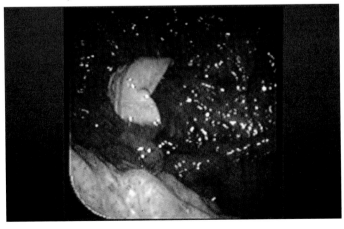

■ **Figure 53.5** A tag of retained fetal membranes could be visualized during an endoscopic examination of a mare affected by postpartum metritis.
Image courtesy of P. R. Morresey.

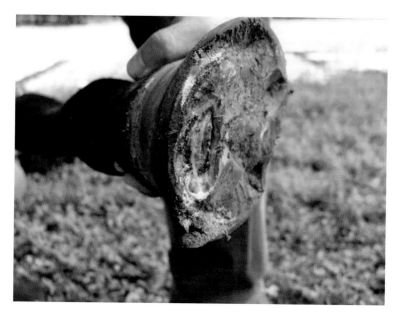

■ **Figure 53.6** Laminitis in a mare affected by severe metritis with P3 rotation evident through the sole of her foot.
Image courtesy of M. Porter.

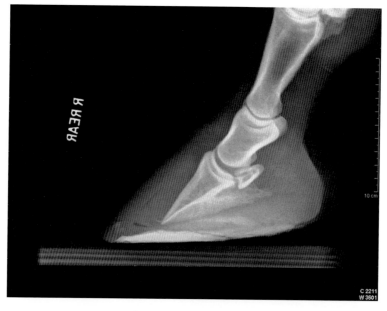

■ **Figure 53.7** Radiographic evidence of rotation, sinking, of P3.
Image courtesy of M. Porter.

DIFFERENTIAL DIAGNOSIS

Other Causes of Postpartum Abdominal Pain/Depression

- Normal uterine involution and placental expulsion.
- Uterine artery rupture, with or without internal hemorrhage: A clot forms between the myometrium and serosa. The uterus or broad ligament is enlarged and painful upon palpation. The hematocrit may be normal or decreased.
  - If the initial hemorrhage (eventual clot) fails to be contained by the broad ligament (its separated walls are under tension) or if undue pressure is applied to it during examination or transrectal palpation, the broad ligament may rupture.
  - Abdominocentesis, if done to diagnose abdominal pain of uncertain origin (assuming broad ligament hematoma was not on a rule-out list), may reveal increased RBCs, PMNs, and some bacteria.
- Uterine torsion
- Uterine rupture may be difficult to identify at TRP. Abdominocentesis reveals PMNs, bacteria, and elevated protein.
- Rupture of the cecum or right ventral colon: strong abdominal contractions during parturition can rupture or bruise the large bowel if it is distended by gas or ingesta or if it becomes trapped between the uterus and the pelvis. Abdominocentesis reveals ingesta in the peritoneal cavity.

Other Causes of Postpartum Vaginal Discharge

- Normal postpartum lochia: until 6 days postpartum, odorless, dark red-brown vaginal discharge associated with a palpably normal, involuting uterus, with thickening and corrugation (i.e., TRP description) of the uterine wall.

DIAGNOSTICS

- CBC/TP: Marked leukopenia (less than or equal to 2,000 cells/µL) with toxic PMNs and left shift. Response to treatment is evaluated by the return of WBCs to normal values (5000–12,000 cells/µL).
- Fibrinogen may increase to or more than 500 mg/dL during the acute phase, but usually returns to normal values (less than or up to 400 mg/dL) 2 to 3 days after the WBC count returns to the normal range.

Other Laboratory Tests

- Bacterial identification: Obtain a sample of uterine contents using a guarded swab. Plate the sample on Blood and McConkey's agar. Blood agar will support growth of gram-positive, select gram-negative, and some yeasts, whereas McConkey's will only support growth of gram-negative organisms. Incubate plates at 37°C and examine at 24 and 48 hours.

- For anaerobes, streak swabs onto two Wilkins-Chalgren anaerobe agar plates and incubate in an atmosphere of 10% hydrogen, 10% carbon dioxide, and 80% nitrogen at 37°C and examine at 24 and 48 hours.
- Because diagnosis of *Bacteroides fragilis* is difficult, when conditions are present that support its growth (i.e., necrotic tissue, lacerations), assume it may be contributory.
- The presence of large numbers of mixed flora is expected from a uterine swab taken from normal postpartum mares in the first week, but possibly as long as 14 days postpartum.
- Collect a uterine culture before instituting antibiotic therapy, if possible, but do not wait for culture results before beginning treatment.
  - Initiate treatment immediately with broad-spectrum antibiotics, metronidazole, intravenous fluids, and anti-inflammatory/anti-endotoxic drugs if metritis is suspected based on clinical signs, CBC, history of dystocia, RFM (especially if retained more than 8–12 hours), or contamination/trauma has occurred.
  - Adjust therapy when the culture and sensitivity results are available, switching to other, more appropriate antibiotics, if indicated.

Pathological Findings

- Postpartum acute inflammatory response extending from the endometrium to the deeper regions, that is, stratum compactum, stratum spongiosum, to and including the myometrium (full-thickness, uterine wall disease).
- Contrast with endometritis and routine uterine infections/reaction in the mare, which are limited to the endometrium and luminal infections.

 THERAPEUTICS

- Endotoxemia is prevented or treated by intravenous fluids for circulatory support and anti-inflammatory or anti-endotoxic drugs.
- Administer systemic, broad-spectrum antibiotics and metronidazole to control uterine bacterial overgrowth and to prevent endotoxemia.
- Only after the mare is medically stable, should the source of infection (i.e., RFM, infected uterine fluid) be addressed; a critical point in the management of this condition. Uterine manipulation in the face of acute postpartum metritis (fever, systemic illness), may guarantee absorption of endotoxins from the uterus; and increase the likelihood of death by endotoxemia.
- Once medically stable, evacuate bacteria and inflammatory debris from the uterine lumen by uterine lavage with large volumes of warm saline solution. Six to 12 L is infused at each treatment period through a sterile nasogastric tube or large diameter uterine flush catheter; uterine contents are then siphoned off, and the lavage is repeated until the recovered fluid is clear. Repeat one to three times daily based on TRP and U/S findings. Administer oxytocin routinely to aid uterine evacuation or if fluid remains after lavage.

- Finding a thickened, corrugated uterine wall at this subsequent palpation indicates a positive response to treatment, indicating that uterine involution is beginning and uterine health may be finally be regained or at least underway.
- Unresponsive mares have flaccid, thin uterine walls and accumulate large amounts of fluid between treatments. Treatment is discontinued when intrauterine fluid is clear or slightly cloudy.
- Begin with a smaller volume (1 L) if a uterine tear is suspected. Finding fluid accumulation ventrally within the uterine lumen is one indicator that a ventral tear is not present.

Drug(s) of Choice

Fluids

- Use polyionic solutions (e.g., Normosol).
- Estimate dehydration based on clinical signs (e.g., skin turgor), hematocrit (normal 32%–53%), and total protein (normal 5.7–7.9 g/dL).
- Calcium gluconate (125 mL of 23% solution) and oxytocin (40 IU) may be added to every other 5-L bag of Normosol.
- Mild colic or discomfort will result from uterine contractions stimulated by treatment.
- Discontinue or slow the rate of administration if severe signs of colic occur.

Systemic Antibiotics

- Potassium penicillin for gram-positive organisms: loading dose of 44,000 IU IV QID, followed by 22,000 IU IV QID daily.
- Combine with gentamicin for gram-negative organisms: 2.2 mg/kg IV QID or 6.6 mg/kg IV SID.
- For oral administration, use 15 to 30 mg/kg of trimethoprim sulfa (broad-spectrum) BID.
- Metronidazole, for anaerobes, should always be combined with IV or PO therapy: loading dose of 15 mg/kg PO, followed by 7.5 mg/kg PO QID or 15 to 25 mg/kg PO BID.

Uterotonic Drugs

- Oxytocin: multiple protocols have been proposed and used.
    - 10 IU IV or 20 IU IM after uterine lavage.
    - 40 IU added to intravenous fluids.
    - 10 IU IV QID

NSAID Therapy for Anti-Inflammatory/Anti-Endotoxin Effect

- Flunixin meglumine (Banamine): anti-endotoxic/anti-inflammatory dose, 1.1 mg/kg IV or IM, BID.
- Polymyxin B: administer 6000 U/kg or 1.5×10^6/550 kg IV in 1 L of sterile saline over 30 to 60 min; recommended BID for 1 to 3 days.

- Lidocaine and Pentoxifylline appear to inhibit or down-regulate the acute pro-inflammatory cytokine response to endotoxins.
  - 2% Lidocaine: initial slow bolus 1.5 mg/kg followed by constant rate infusion of 0.05 mg/kg per hour
  - Pentoxifylline: 8.5 mg/kg BID, PO.

Precautions/Interactions

- NSAIDs may cause bone marrow dyscrasia and GI ulceration.
- Aminoglycosides can be nephrotoxic and ototoxic; ensure good hydration during treatment.
- Polymyxin B: potentially nephrotoxic at therapeutic doses.
- Dehydration and NSAID administration may potentiate the nephrotoxicity associated with aminoglycosides and polymixin B.
- Metronidazole can decrease appetite in a number of circumstances. If it decreases appetite, then milk production in postpartum mares could be affected.
- Lidocaine: monitor for toxic effects such as muscle fasciculation or collapse.

Alternative Drugs

Use of DMSO is controversial: minimal effects on clinical signs of induced endotoxemia in horses.

Activity

- Exercise aides in evacuation of uterine luminal fluid.
- Turn out twice a day, if no signs of laminitis.

 COMMENTS

Do not wait for signs of endotoxemia to develop. Start aggressive prophylactic therapy after a difficult dystocia or RFM are present more than 12 to 24 hours. Draft breeds are even more susceptible to sequelae of RFM; aggressive treatment should begin by no more than 6 hours postpartum.

Client Education

- Practice good hygiene during mare's parturition, whether or not assistance is necessary.
- Early detection and treatment of RFM.
- Perform detailed reproductive and physical evaluation of mare after every parturition, especially after difficult parturition or RFM.

Patient Monitoring

- Monitor CBC every 48 to 72 hours for signs of endotoxemia or response to treatment.

- Monitor for signs of laminitis by early and repeated evaluation of digital pulses, signs of shifting weight, and radiographs of the distal phalanx to rule-out rotation or sinking of P3.
- Monitor for postpartum constipation or postsurgical or dystocia ileus. Mineral oil (0.5–1.0 gallon) or bran mash may be used to prevent or treat ileus; fluid therapy also is helpful.

Prevention/Avoidance

Practices that may provide beneficial include supportive care and delay or thwart laminitis from developing: icing of hooves or the use of soft stall bedding (e.g., sand or wood shavings).

Possible Complications

- Delayed uterine involution
- Mare often recumbent: assist her remaining sternal by support with bales; adjust her position multiple times per day to avoid developing pressure sores
- Septicemia/endotoxemia
- Laminitis
- Death

Expected Course and Prognosis

- Prognosis depends on severity, duration, and secondary complications caused by metritis.
- Rapid response to therapy indicates a favorable prognosis.
- Laminitis after endotoxemia carries a guarded to grave prognosis.

Synonyms

- Metritis/laminitis/septicemia complex
- Toxic metritis

Abbreviations

BID	twice a day
CBC	complete blood count
CRT	capillary refill time
GI	gastrointestinal
NSAID	nonsteroidal anti-inflammatory drug
IM	intramuscular
IV	intravenous
LPS	lipopolysaccharide
P3	third phalanx
PMN	polymorphonuclear leukocyte/WBC

PO	per os (by mouth)
RBC	red blood cell
RFM	retained fetal membranes
QID	four times a day
SID	once a day
TP	total protein
TRP	transrectal palpation
U/S	ultrasound, ultrasonography
WBC	white blood cell

See Also

- Delayed uterine clearance
- Dystocia
- Endometritis
- Retained fetal membranes
- Uterine torsion

Suggested Reading

Asbury AC. 1993. Care of the mare after foaling. In: *Equine Reproduction*. McKinnon AO, Voss JL (eds). Philadelphia: Lea & Febiger; 976–980.

Mackay RJ. 1996. Endotoxemia. In: *Large Animal Internal Medicine*, 2nd ed. Bradford P Smith (ed). St. Louis: Mosby-Year book.

Ricketts SW, Mackintosh ME. 1987. Role of anaerobic bacteria in equine endometritis. *J Reprod Fertil Suppl* 35: 345–351.

Threlfall WR, Carleton CL. 1986. Treatment of uterine infections in the mare. In: *Current Therapy in Theriogenology*. Morrow DA (ed). Philadelphia: WB Saunders; 730–737.

Turner RM. 2007. Postpartum problems: The top ten list. *Proc AAEP* 53: 305–319.

Author: Maria E. Cadario

chapter 54

Pregnancy Diagnosis

DEFINITION/OVERVIEW

- Pregnancy: the condition post-fertilization of an embryo or fetus developing and maturing *in utero*.
- Pregnancy diagnosis: determination of a pregnant state based on clinical signs, laboratory and physical findings, including TRP and U/S, hormonal evaluations.

ETIOLOGY/PATHOPHYSIOLOGY

Systems Affected

- Reproductive
- Other systems may be affected in abnormal pregnancy.

SIGNALMENT/HISTORY

- Nonspecific. Puberty occurs between 12 and 24 months in equine females.
- Pregnancy may occur anytime after puberty until advanced age in mares.
- History of having been mated.

Risk Factors

- An inherent risk to the mare results from the examination technique itself (TRP). Although risks associated with TRP may be overblown, rectal tears are nonetheless a possibility.
- They may be more likely to occur with a novice or impatient/hurried palpator, result from palpations done with inadequate restraint of the mare, or secondary to rapid movements of the mare during the procedure (i.e., falling, kicking).
- Their incidence can also increase in mares with a stovepipe rectum (some Arabian mares), horses with abdominal adhesions from a prior infection, or colic episode that has affected the terminal colon or rectum.

- It is essential that sufficient time be allowed to remove fecal material from the rectum, and achieve sufficient relaxation to allow lateral movement by the palpator to comfortably palpate both uterine horns, ovaries, and cervix.

Historical Findings

- Failure of a mare that has been bred to return to estrus 16 to 19 days post-ovulation may indicate a pregnancy is present (a presumptive diagnosis).

 CLINICAL FEATURES

Physical Examination Findings

- Early in pregnancy, little external physical change may be noted.
- The earliest alterations in the TRP may occur by 14 to 16 days gestation and a presumptive diagnosis may be based on uterine findings (excellent tone in the uterine horns), coupled with ovarian findings in early pregnancy (15 to 20 days: there are often no follicles larger than 25 mm), and cervical changes (not only closed, but remarkably narrow and may be very elongate, for example, palpates as a number 2 pencil).
- As pregnancy advances, most mares will develop recognizable abdominal distention and weight gain.
- In the final 2 to 4 weeks prior to parturition, most mares will have increased development of the mammary gland with secretion of fluid from the nipples ranging from thin and straw-colored to sticky and creamy.

 DIFFERENTIAL DIAGNOSIS

Other causes of failure to cycle:

- Seasonal anestrus: TRP and U/S reveal little ovarian activity; uterine and cervical tone is flaccid.
- Behavioral anestrus: serial TRP or U/S will distinguish mares in estrus from those in diestrus or pregnancy.
- Prolonged luteal life span: evidence of a CL detected by U/S examination of the ovary or progesterone assay. Responds to PGF$_2\alpha$ treatment.
- Granulosa-thecal cell tumor: abnormally enlarged, multicystic ovary and small contralateral ovary. Confirmed with elevated serum inhibin concentrations.
- Chromosomal abnormalities (gonadal dysgenesis, testicular feminization): confirm by karyotype determination.

Other U/S findings resembling early pregnancy:

- Uterine/lymphatic cysts: U/S examination of the mare prior to breeding and pregnancy can aid in determining presence, number, size, and shape of lymphatic cysts; a small uterine map (uterine horns and body) can be drawn on each mare's TRP record and easily referenced at the time of the early pregnancy examinations.

- This permanent record of cystic structures can be beneficial in distinguishing lymphatic cysts from early embryonic vesicles throughout the season and serial pregnancy examinations.
- Update the mare's record and her *cyst map* at the start of each breeding season to note the changing appearance and number of cysts as a mare ages.
- Aging mares will frequently develop multiple lymphatic cysts.

 # DIAGNOSTICS

Hormonal Assays

Progesterone Assay

ELISA and RIA for serum or milk progesterone concentrations:
- Elevated concentrations of progesterone at 18 to 21 days post-ovulation imply that functional luteal tissue is present.
- This is a presumptive, but not diagnostic, test for pregnancy.
- Progesterone assay may be a useful adjunct to other methods of early pregnancy diagnosis (i.e., TRP without U/S). Confirmation of pregnancy, using an assay such as estrone sulfate or total estrogens, is advisable if early pregnancy was diagnosed solely by a progesterone assay.

eCG Assay

- eCG is a hormone secreted by endometrial cups in the pregnant mare uterus.
- Endometrial cups form between approximately 34 and 37 days gestation, when chorionic girdle cells (fetal trophoblasts) actively invade the endometrial epithelium.
- The cups attain maximum size and hormone output between 55 to 70 days gestation.
- Endometrial cups regress between 80 to 120 days gestation; secretion of eCG ceases at that time.
- eCG is measured using an ELISA.
- False-positives occur if fetal death occurs after endometrial cups have formed.
- The cups can persist up to 3 to 4 months after a mare has lost a pregnancy, either a nonviable fetus *in utero* or fetal loss (early abortions often not noted).
- False-negatives occur in samples evaluated:
  - Before the formation of endometrial cups (less than 36 days of gestation).
  - After the regression of the cups (more than 120 days of gestation).

Estrogen Assay

- Estrogens are secreted by the feto-placental unit.
- Total estrogens or estrone sulfate (conjugated estrogen) can be measured from plasma or urine to diagnose pregnancy after Day 60 using RIA. This is a test that can be used to monitor pregnancy activity in wild bands of mares: observation of mustangs from a distant hill, ID location of urination, collection of urine soaked sand/soil after horses have moved away from watering hole/tank.

- Estrone sulfate concentrations in milk are diagnostic for pregnancy after day 90 in the mare.
- Fetal death, and subsequent compromise to the feto-placental unit, results in an immediate decline in estrogen concentrations.

Imaging

- Transrectal U/S: Pregnancy diagnosis can be determined as early as 9 days after ovulation, with a 5 MHz transducer and a high quality U/S scanner.

Days 13 to 15 days post-ovulation

- an optimal time to scan for early pregnancy. The embryonic vesicle is an anechoic, spherical yolk sac that averages between 12 and 20 mm in height.
- Not only is the detection of an embryonic vesicle more reliable by 14 to 15 days, but it is still pre-fixation. Twin embryonic vesicles can also consistently be located at this time.
- Early diagnosis of twin pregnancies increases the probability of successfully reducing twins to a singleton pregnancy using the manual reduction technique (Figs. 54.1, 54.2, 54.3, and 54.4).

Days 18 to 24 post-ovulation

- The U/S appearance of the vesicle becomes more triangular by day 18 when the embryonic vesicle becomes less turgid.

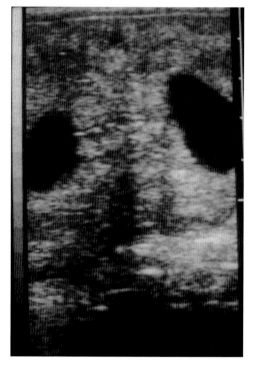

■ **Figure 54.1** Ultrasound of early pregnancy check in the mare, bicornual twins (transducer rotated 90 degrees).

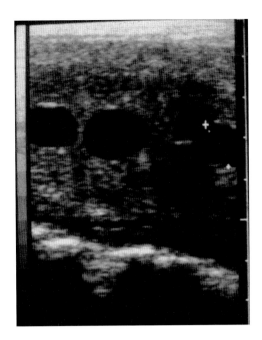

■ **Figure 54.2** Ultrasound of early pregnancy check reveals unicornual pregnancy plus a small lymphatic cyst (cyst is identified between the two "+" markers).

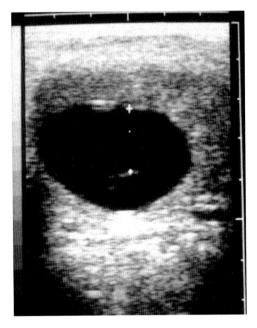

■ **Figure 54.3** Ultrasound of early twins; subtle overlap of unicornual twins could be missed in the absence of a deliberate, complete examination.

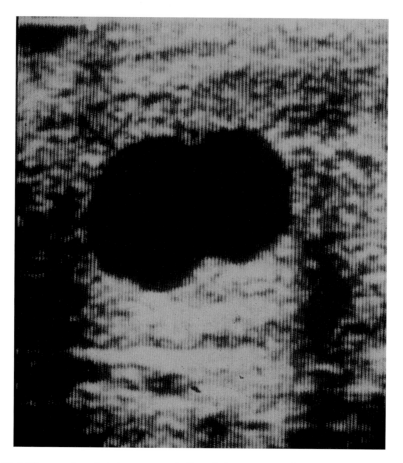

■ **Figure 54.4** Ultrasound, early twin assessment. If ovulations were synchronous (no more than 48 hours apart), there is a high likelihood these will reduce prior to 25 days' gestation.

- The embryo proper often can be visualized by day 20 to 21 and a heartbeat can be seen as early as 24 days, and certainly should be evident on most U/S machines by 25 days.
- The allantoic sac is visible ventral to the embryo by day 24.

Days 25 to 48 post-ovulation

- As the allantois develops and the yolk sac regresses, the embryo appears (during U/S examinations) to be lifted from the ventral aspect of the vesicle to a dorsal location.
- The embryo is visualized mid-vesicle by 28 to 30 days and is in the dorsal aspect of the vesicle by day 35 (Figs. 54.5 and 54.6).
- The umbilical cord forms and attaches at the dorsal aspect of the vesicle around day 40.
- As the cord elongates, the fetus migrates toward the ventral aspect of the allantoic sac (Fig. 54.7).
- Descent to the ventral wall is normally complete by day 48.

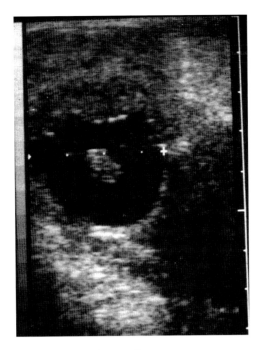

■ **Figure 54.5** Singleton pregnancy, 30 days ultrasound assessment.

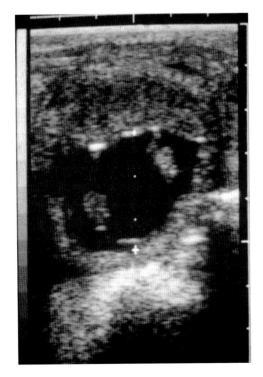

■ **Figure 54.6** Ultrasound of a continuing 28-day twin pregnancy with two embryos, each with a heartbeat (28 days). Necessitates action to reduce prior to development of endometrial cups (which develop between days 34–37).

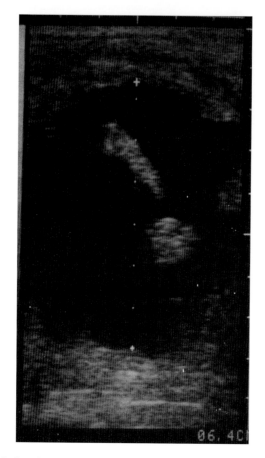

■ **Figure 54.7** Ultrasound of singleton pregnancy at 44 days' gestation. Normal appearing umbilical cord and fetus.

Other Diagnostic Procedures

Behavioral Assessment

A mare teased to a stallion should begin to show signs of behavioral estrus 16 to 18 days after ovulation if she is not pregnant. Response of a mare to a stallion is a non-specific indicator of pregnancy. This method should be used only as an adjunct to more reliable means such as TRP and U/S.

False-Positive

- Failure to show estrus even as she returns to heat.
- Pregnancy loss occurs after formation of endometrial cups.
- Prolonged luteal activity but not pregnant.

False-Negative

- Mare continues to exhibit signs of behavioral estrus when pregnant.

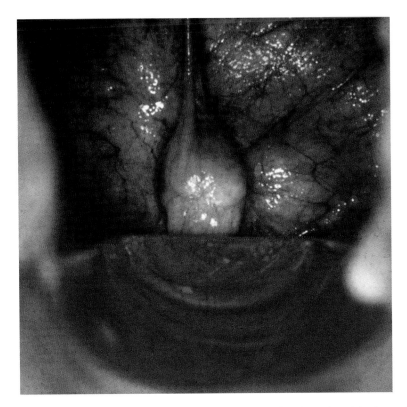

■ **Figure 54.8** Vaginal speculum examination of a closed cervix (dorsal frenulum of cervix is also readily visible).

Vaginal Speculum Examination

- Under the influence of progesterone, the cervix is tightly closed, pale and dry (Fig. 54.8)
- This test is not diagnostic for pregnancy because a functional CL in a cycling mare has the same effect on the cervix.
- Often, a speculum examination is used as an adjunct to TRP of the reproductive tract.

TRP of the Reproductive Tract

15 to 18 days post-ovulation
- Tubular tract becomes toned, and the T or V shape of the uterine bifurcation is often distinctly palpable.
- Palpation of a vesicular bulge in the uterine horn has been reported as early as day 15; however, palpation of a true ventral bulge at this stage is difficult in all but maiden mares with small uterine horns.
- The cervix is generally tightly closed, narrow, and elongated.
- Both ovaries are often actively producing follicles during early pregnancy.
- False diagnosis of pregnancy based on TRP findings may occur at this stage due to EED or persistent/prolonged luteal activity.

25 to 30 days of gestation
- Uterine tone is very distinct (elevated) and the cervix is narrow and elongated.
- Follicular activity is present.
- A bulge the size of a small hen's egg can be appreciated at the caudoventral aspect of a uterine horn, adjacent to the uterine bifurcation.
- The uterine wall is slightly thinner over the fluid-filled, resilient vesicle.

35 to 40 days of gestation
- Uterus still demonstrates increased tone, the cervix is closed and elongated and the ovaries active.
- A bulge about the size of a tennis ball can be noted at the base of the uterine horn on the side of pregnancy.
- Uterine tone begins to drop at/around the enlarging bulge.
- Greatly increased uterine tone is still present in the nonpregnant horn.

45 to 50 days of gestation
- Palpable bulge increases to softball size.

60 to 65 days of gestation
- Vesicle begins to expand into the uterine body, and the palpable bulge resembles the shape of a child-sized football (Fig. 54.9).
- Wall of the uterine horn is distinctly thinner at this stage and the pregnancy begins to lose some of its resiliency.
- Good uterine tone is often maintained in the nongravid horn and the tip of the gravid horn.

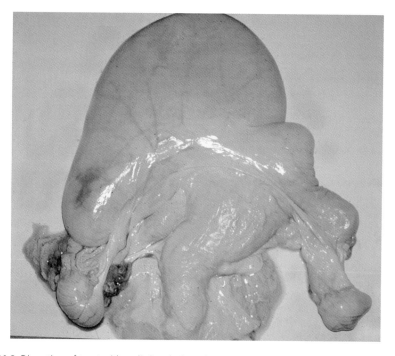

■ Figure 54.9 Dissection of tract with a distinct bulge of pregnancy in the left uterine horn.

- The increasing size of the pregnancy begins to pull the uterus ventrally.

75 to 120 days of gestation

- Pregnancy occupies more of the uterus and uterine tone diminishes. It expands dorsally and resembles the size of a basketball.
- The pregnant uterus can be confused with a full urinary bladder.
- To distinguish the two, the fluid-filled uterus can be traced back to the closed cervix at the caudal aspect of the uterine body.
- Additionally, as the uterus continues to drop deeper into the abdomen, the ovaries are drawn ventrally and toward the midline.
- Occasionally the fetus may be ballotted during the latter aspect of this time period; however, it may not be possible or noticeable.

150 to 210 days of gestation

- Uterine descent into the ventral abdomen is complete; ovaries are often found at the midline.
- The fetus may consistently be ballotted within the fluid-filled uterus.

250 days of gestation

- Tremendous fetal growth occurs from approximately 8 months to term.
- Ratio of the fluid volume of the pregnancy to the fetus decreases.
- Fetal growth is rapid and it occupies a greater percentage of the uterus late in gestation.

Fetal Sexing

Determination of fetal gender is best accomplished between 60 and 70 days of gestation. The technique is useful in both horses and cattle, but high-resolution U/S equipment and experience are necessary for accurate identification of fetal gender.

- Fetal sex is determined by locating the position of the genital tubercle during its developmental migration.
- The genital tubercle is the precursor to the clitoris in females and the penis in males.
- The genital tubercle is located on the fetus's ventral midline and is imaged as a hyperechoic, bilobed structure that is approximately 2 mm in diameter.
- The tubercle migrates from between the rear legs caudally toward the tail in female fetuses and cranially toward the umbilicus in male fetuses.
- The location and orientation of the fetus must be determined.
- Fetal position can be determined by locating the mandible, which points ventrally and caudally.
- The heart is imaged on the ventral midline of the thorax.
- Examining the fetus cranially to caudally, the abdominal attachment of the umbilicus is located.
- Immediately caudal to the umbilical attachment is the male genital tubercle.
- The female tubercle is best visualized at the caudal most aspect of the fetus under the tailhead. The optimal image of the female tubercle appears within a triangle formed by the tailhead and the distal tibias or hocks.

U/S findings from day 70 to 130 days

- Days 70 to 75, the fetus can be visualized using transrectal U/S. There will be some variation depending on the mare's age and parity. At this time, the weight of the developing pregnancy pulls the uterus over the brim of the pelvis.
- 95 days gestation, the fetus may move more dorsally within the pregnant uterus and can be imaged to determine fetal gender.
- From 95 to 130 days gestation, gender can be determined by locating external genital structures:
  - Mammary gland, teats and clitoris in the female.
  - Penis, prepuce and scrotum in the male.

COMMENTS

Client Education

- Pregnancy palpations and U/S are essential, especially early, to determine if there is more than one dominant follicle, if a double ovulation has occurred, to examine for the presence of twins at an early pregnancy evaluation, or if there is no pregnancy and the mare will need to be rebred on a subsequent estrus (to avoid missing an estrus, especially a mare that fails to tease in strongly).
- Prior ovulations may be confirmed by a thorough ovarian U/S examination: double ovulations may occur one from each ovary or two on one side.
- Reduction of twins is most effective if done early (manual reduction/crush technique), preferably by 15 to 18 days gestation. Reduction is easier when the conceptus is small; creates less of an endogenous release of prostaglandin from the endometrium.

Patient Monitoring

- Pregnant mares are routinely examined in the last trimester of gestation to verify fetal viability.
- The most common method of pregnancy diagnosis at this stage is TRP with ballottement of the fetus.
- Transabdominal U/S may be used to measure fetal parameters such as fetal heart rate, aortic diameter, fetal activity, and fetal fluid quality.

Possible Complications

- Large lymphatic cysts may interfere with early transuterine migration and block the early establishment of pregnancy (Fig. 54.10). Cysts greater than 25 mm diameter should be reduced prior to breeding a mare.
- Embryonic or fetal loss, twins, placentitis, abortion, ruptured prepubic tendon, abdominal wall herniation, hydrallantois, hydramnion, uterine torsion, uterine rupture, prolonged gestation, or dystocia (Fig. 54.11).

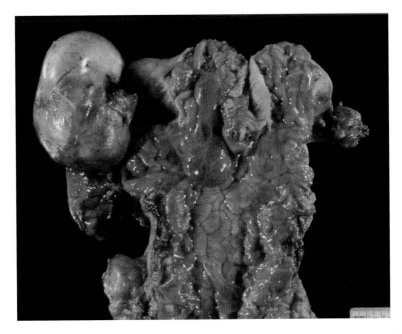

■ **Figure 54.10** Dissection of a large lymphatic cyst within the left uterine horn, the same side as the dominant follicle (left ovary).

Expected Course and Prognosis

A normal, viable fetus born at term gestation.

Abbreviations

CL	corpus luteum
eCG	equine chorionic gonadotropin
EED	early embryonic death
ELISA	enzyme-linked immunosorbent assay
PGF	natural prostaglandin
RIA	radioimmunoassay
TRP	transrectal palpation
U/S	ultrasound, ultrasonography

See Also

- Abortion, induction of (elective termination)
- Abortion (spontaneous infectious, noninfectious)
- Conception failure
- Early embryonic death/EED
- Dystocia and parturient complications
- Placenta (basics, insufficiency, placentitis)
- TRP

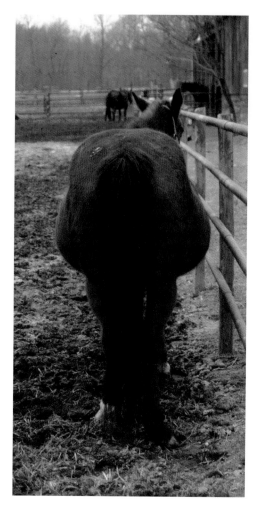

■ **Figure 54.11** A mare near term gestation. Despite her pear-shaped appearance as viewed from the rear, this was a normal pregnancy and she delivered without complication.

- Twinning
- Fetal sexing, early
- Fetal sexing, mid to late gestation

Suggested Reading

Ginther OJ. 1992. *Reproductive Biology of the Mare*, 2nd ed. Cross Plains, WI: Equiservices.
Ginther OJ. 1986. *Ultrasonic imaging and reproductive events in the mare*. Cross Plains, WI: Equiservices.
McKinnon AO. 1993. Diagnosis of pregnancy. In: *Equine Reproduction*. McKinnon AO, Voss JL (eds). Philadelphia: Lea & Febiger; 501–508.

Authors: Carla L. Carleton and Margo Macpherson

chapter 55

Premature Placental Separation

DEFINITION/OVERVIEW

Premature disassociation or detachment of the CA membrane from the endometrium before delivery of the term fetus.

- The CA membrane is responsible for supplying the fetus with oxygen and nutrients and for removing its waste products.
- With premature detachment of this membrane (e.g., late Stage 1, early Stage 2 of parturition), the fetus will die from hypoxia if immediate delivery assistance is unavailable

ETIOLOGY/PATHOPHYSIOLOGY

Etiology of premature separation is proposed to be due to alterations in the CA membrane in the area of the internal os of the cervix or abnormal attachment of the CA membrane to the endometrium at any point.

- Either of these predispose to PPS. PPS occurs secondary to cervical relaxation (i.e., hormonal, ascending infection, cervical incompetency) and development of low-grade placentitis.
- It may also originate from the GI tract via blood-borne origin. The bacteria compromise the normal relationship of the chorioallantois with the endometrium.

Systems Affected

Reproductive

SIGNALMENT/HISTORY

- Incidence increases significantly with induction of parturition, with particular impact caused by select agents used to induce.
- Incidence is less than 1% in medium-size to large breeds of horses but reportedly higher in miniature horses.
- All breeds of horses have been reported to have this condition.

Risk Factors

Miniature horses are at a higher risk than other breeds. Induction of parturition may increase PPS dependent on the agent used. Oxytocin is the safest of the induction agents available. Older mares also have a higher occurrence of PPS.

 CLINICAL FEATURES

- This condition is an emergency. Once the placenta separates, no oxygen is reaching the fetus. Because of the abrupt reduction in oxygen delivery to the fetus, immediate delivery assistance is essential. As soon as the CA membrane protrudes through the vulvar lips (common name is "red bag"), assistance must be rendered (Fig. 55.1).
- Although its initial occurrence may occur at any parity, a history of previous PPS is often found.
- Closely observe at term any mare with a history of PPS. Physical examination findings are normal. The CA membrane, when presented at the vulva, may appear to be

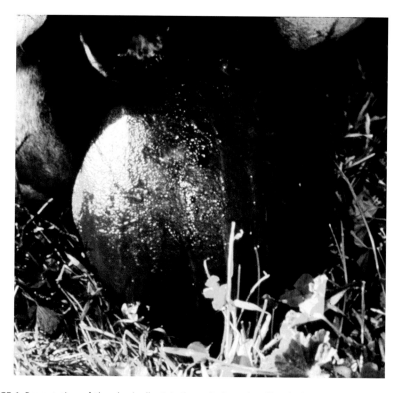

■ **Figure 55.1** Presentation of the chorioallantois through the vulvar lips during Stage 2 of parturition. With separation of the chorioallantois from the uterine body (and potentially more of the uterine surface), the fetus will quickly be in a hypoxic crisis.

characteristically red, velvety, and roughened. This condition only occurs at the end of gestation.

DIFFERENTIAL DIAGNOSIS

- Evagination of the vaginal wall must be differentiated from PPS because the treatment for PPS involves incising the CA membrane. This would be a costly error if vaginal wall were mistaken for the CA.
- Eversion of the urinary bladder may be misidentified as chorioallantois (Fig. 55.2). Its incision would be unfortunate and lead to additional serious health sequelae for the mare.
- Prolapse of the vaginal wall, lacerations of the vaginal wall, and prolapse of intestines must also carefully be differentiated from the placenta before making any incisions.

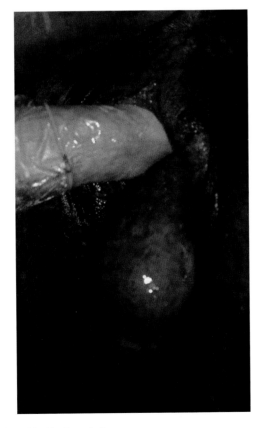

■ **Figure 55.2** Eversion of the bladder in a draft mare.
Image courtesy of C. L. Carleton.

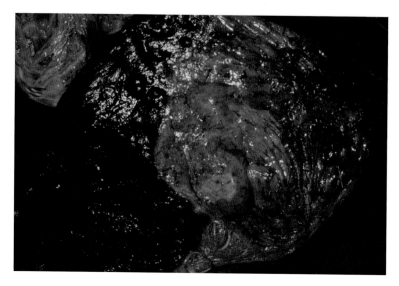

■ **Figure 55.3** Thickened chorioallantois. The fetus, unable to tear through the cervical star, exited through a portion of the uterine body of the placenta (postpartum examination of the placenta).
Image courtesy of C. L. Carleton.

DIAGNOSTICS

U/S examination of the prepartum mare may reveal an area of detachment of the placenta cranial to the cervix. This could also be an indication of a mare at risk for placentitis (Fig. 55.3). Intrapartum appearance of the CA membrane protruding through the vulvar lips (i.e., "red velvet" or "red bagging") is diagnostic for PPS and is an emergency.

COMMENTS

Oxytocin is contraindicated.

Client Education

Clients should be knowledgeable of the appearance and sequence of a normal parturition. Even if they only have videos to view they will be better prepared if or when something goes wrong. Knowing the sequence in which membranes appear and general knowledge regarding the appropriate order of events is important prior to delivery.

- With normal parturition, the first membrane observed at the vulvae should be smooth and white, opaque, or pale pink. Any reddish or roughened protruding membrane indicates a problem requiring immediate action.
- This is a true emergency. Because of fetal hypoxia, insufficient time is available to seek outside assistance and still deliver a live foal.

■ A normal placenta examined when freshly delivered serves as an excellent teaching tool to educate clients regarding what is normal and abnormal. If PPS is observed and the client cannot or will not tear the chorioallantois and assist in delivery, instruct the client to walk the mare until the veterinarian arrives. Although this is not nearly as desirable as providing immediate assistance in tearing the membranes and removing the fetus, it may reduce abdominal contractions somewhat and decrease further separation for a short time.

Patient Monitoring

Mares do well after delivery. The potential problem is with the fetus and its inability to exchange oxygen on placental separation or it has been delivered dead. The neonate, if alive when delivered, can suffer permanent damage from oxygen deprivation that occurred during delivery. Oxygen should be available if at all possible or the use of a funnel over the nose to force air into the lungs if there is any difficulty in the neonate's ability to exchange oxygen.

Prevention/Avoidance

There is no known prevention for PPS. Observation of parturition for any signs of PPS or any abnormality, especially in mares with a history of previous delivery involving PPS, is always encouraged.

Possible Complications

■ Oxytocin administration to the mare is contraindicated before the fetus has been delivered. There are no specific complications in the mare other than delayed parturition with possibly a dead fetus.
■ Fetal death is caused by lack of oxygenation. A dummy foal postpartum may also be the result of decreased oxygenation during delivery.

Expected Course and Prognosis

Delayed delivery of fetus with probable fetal death.

Synonyms

■ Red bag
■ Red bagging
■ Red velvet

Abbreviations

CA   chorioallantoic
GI   gastrointestinal
PPS   premature placental separation
U/S   ultrasound, ultrasonography

See Also

- Dystocia
- Prolonged pregnancy

Suggested Reading

Asbury AC, LeBlanc MM. 1993. The placenta. In: *Equine Reproduction*. McKinnon AO, Voss JL (eds). Philadelphia: Lea & Febiger; 513.

Roberts SJ. 1986. In: *Veterinary Obstetrics and Genital Diseases: Theriogenology*. Woodstock, VT: Author; 251–252.

Whitwell KE, Jeffcott LB. 1975. Morphological studies on the fetal membranes of the normal singleton foal at term. *Res Vet Sci* 19: 44–55.

Author: Walter R. Threlfall

chapter 56

Prepubic Tendon Rupture

DEFINITION/OVERVIEW

Prepubic tendon rupture occurs when the prepubic tendon separates from its attachment to the pubis.

ETIOLOGY/PATHOPHYSIOLOGY

The weight of the mare's abdomen, plus the enlarging fetus, increasing quantity of fetal fluids and membranes, and the accumulation of ventral abdominal edema, place sufficient pressure on the prepubic tendon's pelvic attachment that it surpasses the tendon's attachment load limit. Therefore, separation occurs to any of the following degrees: partial tear, half, or full rupture. The abdominal wall falls ventrally as the tendon tears away from the pubis. The degree of ventral movement of the abdominal wall is dependent on the degree of separation.

Systems Affected

- Muscular
- Reproductive
- GI
- The primary systems affected are the muscular system permitting the tear to occur and the reproductive system, which many times is responsible for the increased weight within the abdomen. The GI system may also be involved if it becomes trapped in the hole provided by the rupture.

SIGNALMENT/HISTORY

Risk Factors

- The occurrence of this condition is low.
- No known genetic link.
- All breeds and breeding ages, dependent on how large the abdomen becomes.
- Older mares are at an increased risk.
- Rupture usually occurs in late gestation or near-term due to excessive weight of the fetus, uterine fluid and membranes, and ventral edema.
- The male's prepubic tendon may rupture after severe trauma, but this is much less common.

Historical Findings

- Late in gestation, carrying twins, hydrops conditions.
- Usually present with an abdomen that has slowly enlarged; its excessive size is quite noticeable.
- Discomfort is associated with abdominal size; difficulty breathing, short shallow respirations, or reluctance to lie recumbent.
- The area in front of and involving the udder appears lower (more ventral) than normal. This can be a dramatic alteration of appearance of the ventral belly conformation.
- Prepubic tendon rupture can occur abruptly following severe trauma (e.g., after being hit by a car).

 ## CLINICAL FEATURES

Dependent edema of the ventral abdomen; may extend to and involve the mare's legs. A characteristic appearance of the ventral abdomen after rupture finds the udder and surrounding area much more ventral than its normal location.

- It has a distinct appearance when viewed from the side. The ventral abdominal line appears flat with no rise in the flank region by the udder.
- The udder loses its normal orientation on its anterior aspect, slanting steeply down, lying at a lower point than its posterior aspect. The normal definition between udder and abdominal wall is absent.
- TRP of the rupture may not be possible while the mare is pregnant due to the presence of the fetus and fetal fluids. The intestines can be identified immediately below the skin (i.e., outside the abdominal musculature indicating rupture of the tendon or abdominal wall has occurred).

 ## DIFFERENTIAL DIAGNOSIS

Abdominal wall rupture with a tearing of the muscles near the prepubic tendon, but without an actual separation of the prepubic tendon from the pubis. This may be impossible to distinguish from actual tendon rupture.

 ## DIAGNOSTICS

- History usually places the mare at least mid-gestation with a history of possible twins, hydrops, or a singleton fetus, and the abdomen larger than normal for some time.
- Physical examination usually reveals dependent edema of ventral abdomen, which may involve the legs.
- The mare's side profile is flat from the front limbs to, and including, the udder (Figs. 56.1 and 56.2). The normal definition between the udder and the abdominal wall is absent.

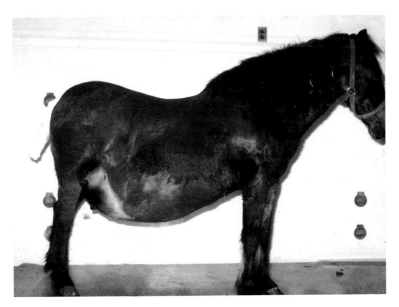

■ **Figure 56.1** Complete rupture of the prepubic tendon. Normal contours of belly wall to mammary gland have been lost. The mare has lost the ability to undergo active labor; no abdominal press is possible.

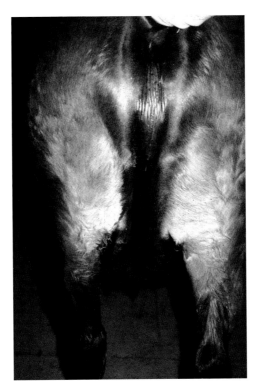

■ **Figure 56.2** Rear view of complete rupture of the prepubic tendon; it demonstrates lengthening of the vulva and loss of normal mammary architecture.

- The intestines may be palpated immediately underlying the skin in the absence of the abdominal wall. Only skin separates the intestines from the outside of the mare. Abdominal U/S examination may confirm abdominal viscera immediately under the skin near the udder.

 THERAPEUTICS

Dependent on the degree of prepubic tendon tearing determined postpartum and the mare's value, her remaining reproductive life will be limited to ET, if repair is possible at all. With complete rupture, repair is usually not possible. ET may also be unrewarding. These mares are not candidates to carry subsequent pregnancies.

Appropriate Health Care

With complete rupture, the mare loses her abdominal press (i.e., she cannot undergo normal, active labor). She cannot expel the fetus at term (she has lost abdominal musculature) and is also unable to develop normal uterine contractions. Once assisted delivery is complete, a better more realistic assessment can be made if there are realistic surgical options.

Activity

Restrict exercise to hand walking; attempt to prevent additional tearing of the ruptured tendon. Belly wraps of the mares can be employed but may be of little value depending on the degree of tearing.

 COMMENTS

Client Education

Extreme pressure and weight on the abdominal wall, usually from excessive uterine size, exceeds the physiologic limit that the attachment can withstand. Because this occurs primarily late in gestation, the owner must understand that the mare has acquired an impaired ability to participate in active labor due to the absence of an intact abdominal wall. Advise owners to seek veterinary help if a mare's abdominal size exceeds that of a normal pregnancy.

- Multiparous mares, older mares, mares with twins or triplets, hydrops, or any other condition that increases size and weight of the pregnant uterus will increase the likelihood of prepubic tendon rupture.

Patient Monitoring

Close observation is essential. Ensure assistance will be available at parturition as these mares will not be able to have normal abdominal contractions during labor. Changes in diet may be indicated to reduce additional abdominal bulk, if possible.

Patient Monitoring

- Keep mare off surfaces that may contribute to her falling or contribute to further damage (e.g., slippery, angled, or uneven). Attempt to prevent the mare from rolling, if possible. Close observation for signs of intestinal obstruction, parturition, or dystocia is indicated in these mares.
- Consider the use of trusses or supportive devices to prevent the rupture from worsening (at least attempt to slow its progression) until delivery, while being careful not to create problems by transferring all of the weight to her back.
- In addition to the increased pressure on her ventral abdomen, abdominal contents lose lateral/ventral support and lose their normal orientation and ability to move ingesta normally.

Prevention/Avoidance

Consider or recommend termination of pregnancy in seriously at-risk mares before the prepubic tendon ruptures completely, especially if excessive abdominal size or ventral dependent edema is present late in gestation.

Possible Complications

Avoid any medications to treat the prepubic tendon rupture that could have an effect on the fetus. The goal of treatment of the mare is medical stabilization and preparation and observation for an observed, but more preferably, an induced parturition. Diuretics (e.g., furosemide) may be used to reduce edema in dependent areas. Phenylbutazone can be used but only if the possibility of ulcer induction in the foal has been considered. Mares may die prepartum or postpartum from GI complications or rupture of the uterine or middle uterine arteries.

Expected Course and Prognosis

- These mares have a high probability of survival, if managed properly. Many of the mares with partial ruptures do well after delivery without surgical repair, if they are not rebred.
- Do not rebreed any mare with a partial prepubic tendon rupture because it will continue damaging the remaining tendon as the weight of the subsequent pregnancy increases.
- If she has a partial rupture, her reproductive future can be continued as an embryo donor, if ET foals are allowed by the particular breed association.

Abbreviations

ET   embryo transfer
GI   gastrointestinal
TRP   transrectal palpation
U/S   ultrasound, ultrasonography

See Also

■ Dystocia

Suggested Reading

Löfstedt R. 1993. Miscellaneous diseases of pregnancy and parturition. In: *Equine Reproduction*. McKinnon AO, Voss JL (eds). Philadelphia: Lea & Febiger; 596–603.

Roberts SJ. 1986. *Veterinary Obstetrics and Genital Diseases: Theriogenology*. Woodstock, VT: Author; 229–230, 347–352.

Tulleners E, Fretz P. 1983. Prosthetic repair of large abdominal wall defects in horses and food animals. *JAVMA* 192: 258–262.

Author: Walter R. Threlfall

chapter 57

Prolonged Diestrus

DEFINITION/OVERVIEW

Persistence of a CL post-ovulation such that the normal return to estrus is delayed.

ETIOLOGY/PATHOPHYSIOLOGY

- After ovulation, the CL forms and begins progesterone production. In the mare, a CL is unresponsive to $PGF_2\alpha$-induced luteolysis for the first 5 days after ovulation.
- Endogenous $PGF_2\alpha$, produced by the endometrium, is released approximately 14 to 15 days post-ovulation to initiate luteolysis in the nonpregnant mare.
- The life span of the CL is prolonged when $PGF_2\alpha$ release is inhibited or when the CL fails to respond to $PGF_2\alpha$ that is released.

Systems Affected

Reproductive

SIGNALMENT/HISTORY

Mares of any age and breed.

Historical Findings

Failure to return to estrus at the expected time interval in the cycling mare.

CLINICAL FEATURES

- The general physical examination is usually normal.
- TRP may reveal some ovarian activity (complete inactivity could indicate anestrus and is addressed elsewhere), a normal or enlarged uterus, and a closed cervix.
- Transrectal U/S may allow a CL to be visualized. If a mare is prone to multiple ovulations, more than one CL may be identified. A mature CL appears as a round or tear drop shape, uniformly hyperechoic area within the ovary. The periphery of a recent ovulation may appear as described, but the center of the CH/CL is often hypoechoic

or mottled. Transrectal U/S should also be used to evaluate the uterus for lymphatic cysts, luminal fluid accumulations, or pregnancy.

- Vaginoscopy can confirm TRP findings regarding the degree of cervical relaxation or the presence of uterine or cervical discharge.

 # DIFFERENTIAL DIAGNOSIS

- The diagnosis is based on finding a normal, nonpregnant, diestrus reproductive tract coupled with a history of failing to show estrus behavior more than 2 weeks post-ovulation and a serum progesterone concentration of greater than 4 ng/mL. This assumes some ovarian activity has previously been observed and is therefore not being mistaken for anestrus. Regular teasing, serial TRP, and U/S are the cornerstones to proper interpretation of the reproductive cycle of an individual mare.
- Idiopathic or spontaneous CL persistence has been associated with normal diestrus ovulations (after day 10 of the cycle), which results in an immature CL being present at the time of normal luteolysis (day 14 to 15). Persistent CL has also been related to fescue ingestion.
- CL function continues in the presence of a conceptus. Pregnancy can occur without any history of a scheduled breeding, if access to any stallion/colt is remotely possible in the mare's environment. Therefore, it is essential to palpate a mare before doing any invasive vaginal procedures (uterine culture or biopsy) or administering prostaglandin to short-cycle a mare in a prolonged diestrus.
- Maternal recognition of pregnancy occurs by day 14 post-ovulation. Embryonic death after this time results in a delayed return to estrus (i.e., a longer than expected inter-estrus interval). If embryonic death occurs after the formation of endometrial cups (35 to 40 days post-ovulation), the mare will not return to estrus until the cups regress and production of eCG by the cups ceases (day 120 to 150 post-ovulation).
- Because endogenous $PGF_2\alpha$ is of endometrial origin, endometritis, pyometra, or other decline of uterine health can result in ineffective prostaglandin formation or release. Pyometra and endometritis are typically diagnosed on the basis of TRP, U/S, uterine culture, and biopsy.
- A history of a normal foal heat followed by reproductive quiescence can either be due to prolonged diestrus or lactational anestrus. Ovarian activity as assessed by TRP or U/S and serum progesterone concentration assays allow differentiation. A CL may persist following the first (foal heat) ovulation. This may be more likely in mares that are in less than optimal body condition or suffering a caloric deficit.
- Iatrogenic/Pharmaceutical
  - Administration of progestin compounds will suppress behavioral estrus. Clinically the mare will appear to be experiencing a prolonged diestrus.
  - NSAIDs can potentially interfere with endometrial $PGF_2\alpha$ release and result in prolonged luteal activity. There is no evidence that chronic administration at recommended therapeutic dosages inhibits the spontaneous formation and release of $PGF_2\alpha$ from the endometrium.

- GnRH agonist (deslorelin) implants used to stimulate ovulation have been associated with prolonged interovulatory intervals. The effect is more profound if $PGF_2\alpha$ is used during the diestrus period in an attempt to "short-cycle" the mare.

DIAGNOSTICS

- Serum progesterone concentrations. Basal levels of less than 1 ng/mL indicate no mature luteal tissue is present. Mature CL function is associated with levels greater than 4 ng/mL.
- Serum eCG levels may be useful in cases of suspected EED after endometrial cup formation, especially if there is no evidence of pregnancy at the time of the examination.
- Uterine cytology, culture, and endometrial biopsy are useful to diagnose and treat pyometra and endometritis.

THERAPEUTICS

- If deslorelin was used to stimulate ovulation, consider removing the implant 48 hr after administration (post-ovulation) on subsequent cycles.
- Prolonged diestrus: if the presence of a CL is confirmed, treat with $PGF_2\alpha$. Pregnancy should first be definitively ruled out. Luteolysis is the goal of treatment, whether the release of endogenous $PGF_2\alpha$ is accomplished with uterine manipulation or exogenous $PGF_2\alpha$ is administered to the mare.
- Endogenous $PGF_2\alpha$ release can be stimulated by intrauterine infusion of sterile saline at ambient temperature or not warmer than 48°C (120°F). Maintain aseptic technique, use a 500- to 1000-mL volume.
- Endometrial biopsy or uterine culture may infrequently stimulate endogenous $PGF_2\alpha$ release.

Drug(s) of Choice

- $PGF_2\alpha$ (Lutalyse® [Pfizer], 10 mg, IM) or its analogs are used to stimulate luteolysis. Mares with a functional CL typically exhibit estrus 2 to 4 days post-injection and ovulate 6 to 12 days after treatment.
- Two doses of $PGF_2\alpha$ given 14 to 15 days apart are useful if TRP cannot easily or safely be accomplished. This regimen ensures that immature/nonresponsive luteal tissue present at the time of the first injection has ample time to mature and be able to respond to the second $PGF_2\alpha$ injection.

Precautions/Interactions

Horses

- $PGF_2\alpha$ and its analogs are contraindicated in mares with asthma, COPD, or other bronchoconstrictive disease.

- Prostaglandin administration to pregnant mares can cause CL lysis and abortion. Carefully rule out pregnancy before administering this drug or its analogs.
- $PGF_2\alpha$ causes sweating and colic-like symptoms due to its stimulatory effect on smooth muscle cells. If cramping has not subsided within 1 to 2 hours, symptomatic treatment should be instituted.
- Antibodies to hCG can develop after treatment. It is desirable to limit its use to no more than two to three times during one breeding season. The half-life of these antibodies ranges from 30 days to several months; they typically do not persist from one breeding season to the next.
- Deslorelin implants have been associated with suppressed FSH secretion and decreased follicular development in the diestrus period immediately following use, leading to a prolonged interovulatory period in nonpregnant mares. Implant removal by 48 hours post-ovulation may decrease this possibility.
- Altrenogest, deslorelin, and $PGF_2\alpha$ should not be used in horses intended for food purposes.

Humans

- $PGF_2\alpha$ or its analogs should not be handled by pregnant women or persons with asthma or bronchial disease. Any accidental exposure to skin should be washed off immediately.
- Altrenogest should not be handled by pregnant women, or persons with thrombophlebitis or thromboembolic disorders, cerebrovascular disease, coronary artery disease, breast cancer, estrogen-dependent neoplasias, undiagnosed vaginal bleeding, or tumors that developed during the use of oral contraceptives or estrogen-containing products. Any accidental exposure to skin should be washed off immediately.

Alternative Drugs

Cloprostenol sodium (Equimate® [Schering-Plough Animal Health], 250 µg, IM), is a prostaglandin analog. This product is used in similar fashion as the natural prostaglandin, but it has been associated with fewer side effects. It is not currently approved for use in horses.

 COMMENTS

Patient Monitoring

- Serial (three times weekly) teasing, TRP, and U/S is recommended to evaluate the mare's reproductive tract for evidence of estrus.
- Serum progesterone concentrations, measured twice weekly for 2 weeks post-administration of $PGF_2\alpha$, can be used to determine the effectiveness of treatment or persistence of functional luteal tissue.

Possible Complications

Prolonged nonpregnant periods or infertility are possible.

Synonyms

- eCG, PMSG (pregnant mare serum gonadotropin)

Abbreviations

CH   corpus hemorrhagicum
CL   corpus luteum
COPD   chronic obstructive pulmonary disease
eCG   equine chorionic gonadotropin
EED   early embryonic death
FSH   follicle stimulating hormone
GnRH   gonadotropin releasing hormone
hCG   human chorionic gonadotropin
IM   intramuscular
NSAID   nonsteroidal anti-inflammatory drug
PGF   natural prostaglandin
TRP   transrectal palpation
U/S   ultrasound, ultrasonography

See Also

- Abnormal estrus intervals
- Anestrus
- EED
- Endometritis
- Abnormal estrus intervals
- Pregnancy diagnosis
- Pseudopregnancy
- Pyometra

Suggested Reading

Daels PF, Hughes JP. 1993. The abnormal estrous cycle. In: *Equine Reproduction.* McKinnon AO, Voss JL (eds). Philadelphia: Lea & Febiger; 144–160.

Hinrichs K. 2007. Irregularities of the estrous cycle and ovulation in mares (including seasonal transition). In: *Current Therapy in Large Animal Theriogenology*, 2nd ed. Youngquist RS, Threlfall WR (eds). St. Louis: Saunders Elsevier; 144–152.

Löfstedt RM. 1986. Some aspects of manipulative and diagnostic endocrinology of the broodmare. *Proc Soc Therio* 67–93.

Sharp DC. 1996. Early pregnancy in mares: Uncoupling the luteolytic cascade. *Proc Soc Therio* 236–242.

Van Camp SD. 1983. Prolonged diestrus. In: *Current Therapy in Equine Medicine.* Robinson NE (ed). Philadelphia: WB Saunders Co; 401–402.

Author: Carole C. Miller

chapter 58

Prolonged Pregnancy

DEFINITION/OVERVIEW

A gestation exceeding the normal range for the mare (320–355 days) is considered a prolonged gestation. It may appear to be lengthened by abnormal characteristics of the fetus. It is not rare for the gestational length to fall outside this range. No statistics are available regarding incidence of prolonged gestation. It is not a major reproductive problem.

ETIOLOGY/PATHOPHYSIOLOGY

- Multifactorial elements combine to create the individual variation, placental function or dysfunction, and hormonal changes seen from mare to mare.
- It may also involve damage to the endometrium, thus reducing the nutrient supply to the fetus. The placenta is still able to sustain fetal life but results in fetal growth retardation.
- It may also be related to fetal pituitary or adrenal function.

Systems Affected

- Reproductive
- Endocrine

SIGNALMENT/HISTORY

Risk Factors

- Prolonged gestation can affect mares of all breeds and breeding ages.
- Hormonal abnormalities are most commonly incriminated as causal with pituitary or adrenal gland involvement.
- It does not appear to be a mare problem; mares can be bred again with little concern for recurrence.

CLINICAL FEATURES

- Prolonged gestation in the equine differs from other domestic species, in which it is linked with iodine deficiency, increased progesterone, and inheritance. This is not the case with the mare.
- It may be due to abnormal fetal pituitary and adrenal development or by lack of hypothalamic maturity at term. Usually appears to be a fetal problem, so historical information may have limited value.
- The uterus may or may not be larger than normal. If the fetus is dead or dies postpartum, a necropsy should be done to determine if its adrenal, pituitary glands, and hypothalamus are normal.

DIFFERENTIAL DIAGNOSIS

- Prolonged pregnancy with a hydrops is invariably shorter than the lengthened gestation associated with a fetus having a higher center defect. Hydrops will also have a larger abdomen than a prolonged gestation due to fetal cause.
- Prolonged pregnancy with a hydrops is invariably shorter than the lengthened gestation due to a fetus that has a higher center defect.
- Hydrops amnion (caused by a defective fetus [it has some degree of segmental aplasia of its GI tract that impairs swallowing of amniotic fluid]) will result in the mare having a slower enlarging abdomen than that observed with a hydrops allantois (the result of abnormal placentation, an endometrial defect).
- Known breeding and ovulation dates facilitate differentiation.

DIAGNOSTICS

- The mare exhibits no abnormalities unless excessive uterine fluid has accumulated.
- Examination of the fetus postpartum usually reveals a dead or weak fetus, smaller than normal, and it may appear undernourished.
- An accurate history combined with TRP of an overdue mare (with an outwardly normal appearance), with a smaller than normal fetus, is probable cause for the prolonged gestation leans toward a fetal origin.
- A peritoneal tap can be performed to determine the location of excessive fluid accumulation to differentiate prolonged pregnancy from hydrops.
  - Hydrops amnii are the result of a fetal swallowing defect and excessive fluid accumulates within the amniotic sac.
  - Hydrops allantois is the result of a uteroplacental defect and excessive fluid accumulates within the allantoic cavity.

- U/S examination: to determine the location of excessive fluid.
  - The endometrium may be thickened.
  - Fetal extremities may be smaller than normal.
  - Perform an endometrial biopsy on the mare when she is no longer pregnant to determine the status of her endometrium before rebreeding.

Pathological Findings

- The fetus is expected to be smaller than normal and has a low probability of survival. If dead, fetal necropsy should always be performed.
- The means to prevent or avoid a prolonged pregnancy are unknown because the major causes involve abnormal fetal pituitaries, adrenals, or hypothalamus.

 # THERAPEUTICS

Parturition induction is an option. However, it is essential that the breeding date is accurate, and that records can confirm its accuracy, to avoid inducing a preterm, nonviable foal.

 # COMMENTS

Client Education

- Remind owners that fetal survival after a prolonged gestation is in question. The actual circumstances of survival may not be known until after delivery.
- Provide routine care for the mare during the postpartum period. Emphasize to owners that prolonged pregnancies can occur and that most affected mares have normal foals.
- Remind owners that gestational length may fall outside the normal range and still be normal for that individual.
- There are no drugs that are indicated during the pregnancy.

Patient Monitoring

- Mares should be monitored once a pregnancy is suspected to be "overdue." It is advisable not to take action unless the pregnancy goes beyond her expected due date, especially in the absence of external evidence of advanced gestation and approaching parturition (mammary development, relaxation of soft tissues around her tail head, etc.).
- A pluriparous mare should be close to her previous duration of "term gestation" in which she delivered a normal foal before considering inducing parturition.
- There may be considerable variation with time of year (winter versus summer foaling).

Prevention/Avoidance

- Do not breed the mare, this only occurs with pregnancy.
- The means to prevent or avoid a prolonged pregnancy are unknown because the major causes involve abnormal fetal pituitaries, adrenals, or hypothalamus.

Possible Complications

- Prolonged pregnancy could result in dystocia due to the increase in fetal size and over stretching of the uterus.
- However, because the fetus is usually smaller than normal, not associated with anky-losis of joints, dystocia is usually not a problem.

Expected Course and Prognosis

- Normal postpartum examination of the mare is always indicated.
- The fetus is expected to be smaller than normal and has a low probability of survival.
- If dead, fetal necropsy should always be performed.

Abbreviations

TRP   transrectal palpation
U/S   ultrasound

See Also

- Parturition induction
- Postpartum care, mare and foal

Suggested Reading

Vandeplassche M. 1980. Obstetrician's view of the physiology of equine parturition and dystocia. *Equine Vet J* 12: 45–49.

Author: Walter R. Threlfall

chapter 59

Pseudopregnancy

DEFINITION/OVERVIEW

- Condition existing after the loss of a pregnancy between 15 to 140 days of gestation.
- Affected mares fail to show estrus (type I, early loss) and genital tract tone (although not uterine horn diameter) is consistent with that of pregnancy.
- Type II occurs after formation of endometrial cups and persists until these cups regress.

ETIOLOGY/PATHOPHYSIOLOGY

Characterized by two types, I and II; that occur during different stages of gestation.

Type I

- Occurs when the conceptus is lost between days 15 and 36 of gestation.
- Recognition of pregnancy normally occurs by 12 to 14 days after ovulation. The embryo blocks uterine release of prostaglandin and signals the CL to maintain its function and to continue progesterone production; prolonged luteal phase.
- TRP: Uterine and cervical tone, mimic that of pregnancy.

Type II

- Occurs when pregnancy is lost between 37 and 140 days of gestation.
- Production of eCG by the endometrial cups (Fig. 59.1) is an independent process that does not require a viable fetus to continue.
- Characterized by the continued eCG production until the endometrial cups regress (Fig. 59.2).
- Production of eCG begins at approximately 36 to 37 days of gestation in a normal pregnancy and continues until approximately 120 to 140 days.
- Source of eCG in mares is the endometrial cups of the placenta (*see* Fig. 59.1).
- The major function of eCG is to stimulate development of accessory CLs, which provide additional progesterone for pregnancy maintenance from day 40 to approximately 120 to 140 days of gestation.

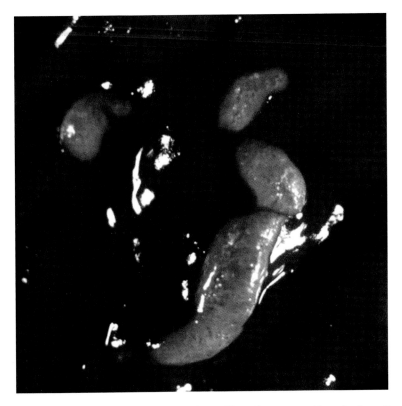

■ **Figure 59.1** Close-up of endometrial cups—pale color and irregular—arranged in a circular pattern mirroring the chorionic girdle previously in gestation.

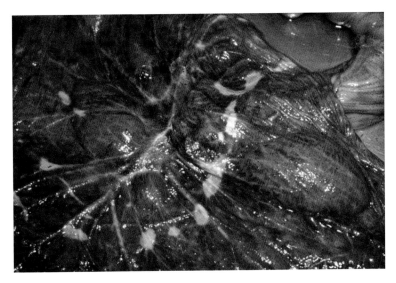

■ **Figure 59.2** A placenta from a mid-gestation abortion still showing evidence of the former location of the endometrial cups. Persistent cups and equine chorionic gonadotropin production are responsible for prolonging a pregnancy following the demise of the fetus.

Systems Affected

Reproductive

SIGNALMENT/HISTORY

- Ten to 15% of general broodmare population less than 15 to 18 years old (Type I).
  - Type I: stress (e.g., colic); embryo defects; negative energy deficit.
- Occurrence may be much higher (25%) in old mares, 18 to 20+ years (Type II).
  - Type II: stress; uterine disease (e.g., DUC, lymphatic stasis, chronic endometritis, fibrosis); body pregnancy.
- No overt clinical signs other than lack of conceptus in uterus, as detected at TRP and U/S.
- Occurs in all breeds.

Risk Factors

Type II: aged mares

CLINICAL FEATURES

- TRP or U/S: Absence of a conceptus in the uterus.
- TRP: Uterine and cervical tone, mimic that of pregnancy.
- Mare may demonstrate one of two distinct reproductive behavior patterns:
  - Recurrent periods of estrus with follicular development, coupled with anovulatory luteinization of follicles (ovum is retained). These are not fertile estrus periods.
  - Continued progesterone production or prolonged periods of anestrus with small, inactive ovaries. Anestrus persists until the endometrial cups regress (90 to 150 days). There is no effective way to eliminate the cups prematurely.

DIAGNOSTICS

Imaging

U/S

- Identification of retained CL (continued luteal function), after a pregnancy has been lost.
- Type I: inappropriate embryonic vesicle size (i.e., reduced conceptus volume) for known gestational length; increased echogenicity of the vesicle, and loss of normal embryonic architecture.

Other Diagnostic Procedures

TRP

- Palpable bulge of pregnancy disappears because of fluid resorption.
- Other characteristics of early pregnancy remain: tightly closed, narrow and elongated cervix, and excellent uterine tone.

Pathologic Findings

Chronic endometrial fibrosis and endometrial cysts, particularly in type II aged mares.

 # THERAPEUTICS

Drug(s) of Choice

- $PGF_2\alpha$ to lyse the existing CL and initiate ovarian activity; as a single treatment.
- Exogenous progestogens (Regu-Mate® for 15 days) to induce renewed cyclic activity, followed by $PGF_2\alpha$ on the final day of ReguMate to increase treatment efficacy.

Appropriate Health Care

- For both Types I and II: breeding management practices/techniques to decrease the incidence of EED.
- Proper breeding hygiene: washing of mare and stallion.
- AI, using appropriate semen extender.
- Pre- and postbreeding intrauterine infusions or flushes.
- Postovulatory uterine treatment: antibiotic or oxytocin.

 # COMMENTS

Client Education

See Appropriate Health Care.

Patient Monitoring

- Monitor pregnancy via TRP and U/S.
- It is an off-label use, but a frequent reason cited for using exogenous progesterone is for "pregnancy maintenance" in the mare.

Expected Course and Prognosis

- Prognosis for mare is good.
- Pregnancy has been terminated.
- Likelihood for recurrence is good in some aged mares suffering from chronic, irreversible uterine disease (e.g., fibrosis; endometrial/lymphatic cysts).

Synonyms

- False pregnancy
- Pseudocyesis
- Spurious pregnancy

Abbreviations

AI   artificial insemination
CL   corpus luteum
DUC   delayed uterine clearance
eCG   equine chorionic gonadotropin
EED   early embryonic death
TRP   transrectal palpation
U/S   ultrasound, ultrasonography

See Also

- Abnormal estrus intervals
- Abortion, induction of
- Abortion, spontaneous, noninfectious
- Anestrus
- Conception failure
- EED
- Endometritis
- Pregnancy
- Pregnancy diagnosis

Suggested Reading

England GCW. 1996. Problems during pregnancy. In: *Allen's Fertility and Obstetrics in the Horse.* Sutton JB, Swift ST (eds). London: Blackwell Science Ltd; 127–129.

Ginther OJ. 1992. *Reproductive Biology of the Mare: Basic and Applied Aspects.* Cross Plains, WI: Equiservices; 228–229.

Lefranc AC, Allen WR. 2004. Nonpharmacological suppression of oestrus in the mare. *Eq Vet J* 36: 183–185.

McKinnon AO. 1993. Reproductive examination of the mare. In: *Equine Reproduction.* McKinnon AO, Voss JL (eds). Philadelphia: Lea & Febiger; 297.

Author: Carla L. Carleton

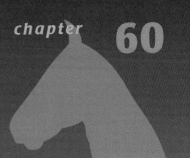

Pyometra

chapter 60

DEFINITION/OVERVIEW

Accumulation of a large volume of purulent exudate within the uterine lumen.

ETIOLOGY/PATHOPHYSIOLOGY

- Impaired drainage of uterine fluids.
- Frequently a sequel to metritis, cervicitis, or cervical adhesions or trauma.
- Associated with severe endometrial inflammatory changes, loss of epithelium, and permanent gland atrophy.
- May result in prolonged luteal phase due to the inability of endometrium to produce or release $PGF_2\alpha$.
- Signs of systemic disease (e.g., anorexia, weight loss, and depression) are rare.

Systems Affected

Reproductive

SIGNALMENT/HISTORY

- Aged pluriparous mares are predisposed to recurrent uterine infections because of anatomic defects and failing mechanical uterine defense mechanisms.
  - Poor VC
  - Pendulous uterus
- Cervical/uterine trauma or adhesions.
- Aging: repeated uterine stretching associated with pregnancy results in a uterus suspended low in the abdomen, predisposing to fluid accumulation and increased risk for pyometra.

Risk Factors

Noninfectious

- Mechanical impairment preventing normal uterine drainage.
- Physical obstruction of the cervical canal that inhibits uterine evacuation (e.g., trauma, cervical fibrosis/induration that prevents either complete closure or dilation and obstruction of the cervical lumen by adhesions).

- Extra-uterine impairment caused by abdominal adhesions to the uterus may prevent the uterus from involuting or evacuating completely.
- Chronic uterine distention also impairs ability of the uterus to contract and evacuate its contents.
- Age and parity: multiparous, more than 14 years of age.
- Conformational abnormalities: history of postpartum metritis/cervicitis; history of cervical laceration, trauma, or incomplete cervical dilation.

Infectious

- Bacteria do not cause pyometra in the mare, they are opportunists.
- Most common isolates: *Streptococcus zooepidemicus*, *Escherichia coli*, *Actinomyces* sp., *Pasteurella* sp., and *Pseudomonas* sp.
- Chronic infection with *P. aeruginosa* or fungi may predispose the mare to developing a pyometra.

Historical Findings

- The mare may cycle regularly or remain in a prolonged diestrus.
- Prolonged diestrus is associated with a decreased ability of the uterus to secrete endogenous PGF$_2\alpha$ because of extensive endometrial destruction.
- Watery, milky, or purulent vaginal discharge may be continuous, intermittent (i.e., open pyometra) or absent (i.e., closed pyometra) depending on cervical patency, stage of the estrous cycle, and uterine clearance (Fig. 60.1 and 60.2).

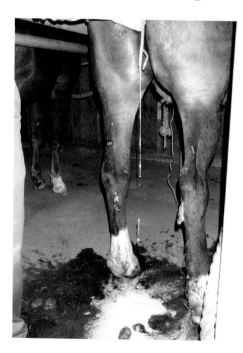

■ **Figure 60.1** Relatively watery consistency of pyometra discharge from a 24-year-old Quarterhorse mare with a recurrent vaginal discharge.
Image courtesy of A. Tibary.

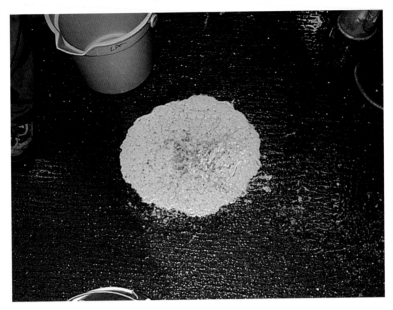

 Figure 60.2 Thick, caseated discharge from a 15-year-old Arabian that developed a pyometra following dystocia, fetotomy, or cervical/vaginal adhesions.
Image courtesy of A. Tibary.

- Contact dermatitis and alopecia of the inner thighs and hocks may be evident (Fig. 60.3).
- Can be an incidental finding on routine examination.

CLINICAL FEATURES

- External conformation may be normal.
- Chronic or intermittent purulent vaginal discharge.
- TRP reveals an enlarged, fluid-filled uterus that may be further described with U/S (Figs. 60.4 and 60.5). A large fluid volume (0.5–60 L) may accumulate within the uterine lumen.
- Intrauterine fluid can be categorized by its presence, quantity, and quality.
- Depending on the amount of accumulated debris and inflammatory cells, the exudate may be moderately to highly hyperechoic.
- Digital cervical examination often reveals adhesions, constrictions, or other abnormalities.
- Culture and cytology results show bacteria and fungi similar to those associated with infectious endometritis. Bacterial isolation ranges from a mixed population of organisms to no bacterial growth.
- Presence of variable amounts of PMNs is a consistent finding.

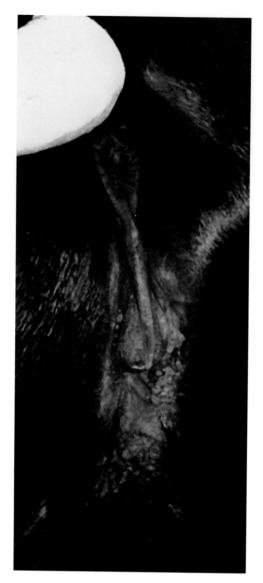

■ **Figure 60.3** Ulcerations and alopecia on the perineum of a standardbred mare with a chronic pyometra. Image courtesy of C. L. Carleton.

 DIFFERENTIAL DIAGNOSIS

Endometritis

- Accumulation of fluid within the uterine lumen due to infectious cause or PMIE.
- Cervix may be tight in young or old maiden mares but has no adhesions.
- Luteal phase usually shortens due to premature release of $PGF_2\alpha$.

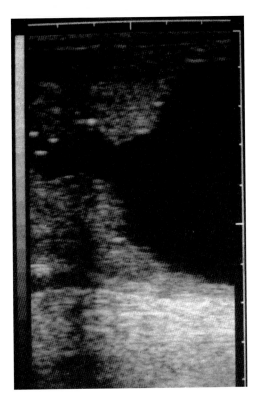

■ **Figure 60.4** Ultrasound image of a dilated uterine horn. The hypoechoic nature of the intrauterine fluid was not reflective of the fluid collected with uterine evacuation of the content. Image courtesy of C. L. Carleton.

Pregnancy

- The uterine walls of a pregnant mare demonstrate a characteristic tone and responsiveness.
- The uterine walls of a mare with a pyometra may become thickened. The purulent exudate causes the uterus to feel doughy.
- U/S findings provide additional differentiating characteristics. Uterine fluid with a pyometra usually has a characteristic appearance: hyperechoic, flocculant, echo-dense, but it can appear hypoechoic (*see* Figs. 60.4 and 60.5).

Pneumouterus

- Associated with abnormal VC and poor uterine tone, a result of or resulting in wind-sucking and pneumovagina.
- Poor tone of the vestibulovaginal sphincter allows air to pass through the cervix and into the uterus. This most commonly occurs during estrus because of vulvar/cervical relaxation and also after administration of sedatives (e.g., acepromazine).

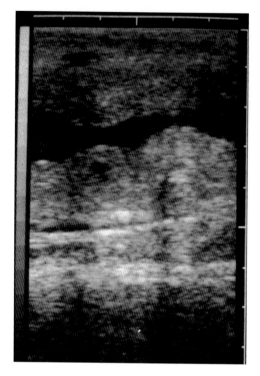

■ **Figure 60.5** Ultrasound image of the uterine body of a pyometra mare. Demonstrates the thickness of the wall that frequently develops with a chronic infection.
Image courtesy of C. L. Carleton.

Mucometra

Mucoid exudate accumulation associated with hormonally induced cystic endometrial hyperplasia in old mares is a rare condition.

Placentitis

- May be characterized by a purulent vaginal discharge in a pregnant mare.
- Ascending placentitis occurs late in gestation and is localized at the cervical star.
- Premature mammary development also may be present.

Distended Bladder

Distinguish the uterus from the bladder by the ability to locate ovaries or trace along either the uterine horns or the cervix during TRP.

Other Causes of Vaginal Discharge

See Endometritis.

DIAGNOSTICS

CBC may reveal a mild normocytic, normochromic anemia, or neutropenia in some mares.

Other Laboratory Tests for Infectious Causes

Bacteria

- Endometrial cells and intraluminal contents may be obtained by scraping the endometrial surface with the swab tip or cap (if using a Kalayjian culture swab). The sample is then stained with Diff-Quik. The presence of neutrophils indicates active inflammation.
- Evaluation of the endometrial contents for bacteria is obtained using a guarded swab.
  - The sample should be cultured in blood agar and McConkey's at 37°C and examined at 24 and 48 hours.
  - Blood agar will support growth of Gram-positive, select Gram-negative, and some yeasts.
  - McConkey will support only the growth of Gram-negative organisms.
  - Both agar mediums should be used.

Yeasts

- Samples obtained for bacterial culture can also be used to isolate *Candida* and *Aspergillus* sp. because these organisms grow in blood agar.
- Branching hyphae can be identified in stained smears or wet mounts.
- For fungal-specific culture, the sample is inoculated in Sabouraud's agar and incubated for 4 days at 37°C.

Other Diagnostic Procedures

Endometrial Biopsy

- An important prognostic tool.
- Collect the initial sample before treatment.
- Evacuate uterine content before performing the biopsy to lessen what is a slight likelihood of rupturing/penetrating the uterine wall during the procedure.

Endoscopy

- May reveal intrauterine adhesions that preclude effective uterine drainage.
- Purulent exudate may be attached to the walls or found free in the uterine lumen.

Pathological Findings

- Wide range of findings, depending on the severity and duration of the condition.
- Especially pronounced in old mares with severe endometrial inflammatory changes or glandular atrophy.

- Atrophy may be permanent and confers an extremely poor prognosis for the mare's reproductive life.

 # THERAPEUTICS

- Administer a luteolytic dose of PGF$_2\alpha$ if a persistent CL is suspected, to aid with cervical relaxation and subsequent drainage of uterine content.
- Mechanical evacuation of purulent contents by repeated uterine lavage (daily or alternate days) using a NG tube and large volumes of warm saline.
- Follow lavage with administration of an ecbolic drug (oxytocin or PGF$_2\alpha$).
- The uterus is then infused with antibiotics based on results of culture and sensitivity.
- Note: Antibiotics should be infused 45 to 60 minutes after oxytocin administration to avoid their being prematurely evacuated.

Drug(s) of Choice

- See Endometritis.
- PGF$_2\alpha$, dinoprost tromethamine (Lutalyse; 5–10 mg total, IM)

Precautions/Interactions

- See Endometritis.
- Infuse fluid for uterine lavage carefully into the distended and friable uterus, beginning with relatively low volumes to avoid rupture.

Surgical Considerations

- If the option is to forego further breeding when faced with a chronic pyometra or if the mare is unresponsive to recommended care, treatment may be left undone. A hysterectomy, although not often used, is an option.
- If hysterectomy is performed, the uterus must be emptied as completely as possible before surgery.
- Life-threatening complications after hysterectomy have decreased significantly due to improved surgical techniques.

 # COMMENTS

- Pregnancy can be achieved in few of the treated mares.
- Mares with chronic uterine inflammation or anatomical problems may require the use of ART to obtain a pregnancy (e.g., oocyte transfer, *in vitro* fertilization, ICSI).

Patient Monitoring

- TRP and U/S to evaluate response to treatment: uterine size and tone; amount of intrauterine fluid.

■ Endometrial biopsy or endoscopy after treatment to characterize or visualize the endometrium, evaluate response to treatment, and develop a prognosis.

Possible Complications

■ Contamination of abdomen during surgery (if hysterectomy is attempted) can cause peritonitis.

Expected Course and Prognosis

■ Recurrence is common.
■ A chronic condition: prognosis for fertility is poor due to endometrial damage.
■ The prognosis for fertility is grave in cases with severe uterine or cervical adhesions.
■ Cervical adhesions may obliterate the cervical lumen and keep it from opening and closing properly.

Abbreviations

CBC   complete blood count
CL   corpus luteum
ICSI   intracytoplasmic sperm injection
IM   intramuscular
PGF   natural prostaglandin
PMIE   postmating induced endometritis
PMN   polymorphonuclear neutrophil
TRP   transrectal palpation
U/S   ultrasound, ultrasonography
VC   vulvar conformation

See Also

■ Cervical lesions
■ Endometritis/delayed uterine clearance
■ Postpartum metritis
■ Vulvar conformation

Suggested Reading

Hughes JP, Stabenfeldt GH, Kindahl H, et al. 1979. Pyometra in the mare. *J Reprod Fertil Suppl* 27: 321–329.
Murray WJ. 1991. Uterine defense mechanisms and pyometra in mares. *Compend Contin Educ Pract Vet* 13: 659–663.
Rotting AK, Freeman DE, Doyle AJ, et al. 2004. Total and partial ovariohysterectomy in seven mares. *Equine Vet J* 36: 29–33.

Author: Maria E. Cadario

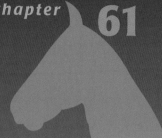
Rectal Tears

DEFINITION/OVERVIEW

- Tearing of one or more layers of the rectal wall most often occurs as the contents of the abdominal cavity and pelvic canal are examined per rectum.
- Successful management of rectal tears requires good communications with the owner and rapid referral of horses with severe tears.

ETIOLOGY/PATHOPHYSIOLOGY

- The length of the rectum is approximately 25 to 30 cm.
- Anatomically it is divided into cranial (or peritoneal) and caudal (or retroperitoneal) segments.
  - The *peritoneal segment* is suspended dorsally by the mesorectum and extends from the terminal small colon to the peritoneal reflection.
  - The *retroperitoneal segment* extends from the peritoneal reflection to the anus and is attached to surrounding pelvic structures by connective tissue and muscular bands.
  - The *peritoneal reflection* is located approximately 15 to 20 cm cranial to the anus in an adult, light breed horse.
- Most tears occur at or cranial to the pelvic inlet (i.e., greater than 25–30 cm cranial to the anus), therefore cranial to the peritoneal reflection.
- Tears are typically oriented longitudinally in the dorsal aspect of the rectum between the 10:00 and 2:00 o'clock positions.
- This is felt to be an inherently weaker area of the rectal wall because it is devoid of serosa and large blood vessels perforate the muscular layers.
- Complete tears of the rectal wall cranial to the peritoneal reflection communicate directly with the abdominal cavity.
- Tears caudal to the peritoneal reflection extend into the retroperitoneal space.

Systems Affected

- GI
- Urogenital
- Musculoskeletal

SIGNALMENT/HISTORY

- Although young horses, 1 to 5 years of age, are most often affected, rectal tears may occur in horses of all ages.
  - Rare relative to the total number of examinations conducted per rectum in horses.
  - Accounts for 7% and 20% of liability claims involving medical or surgical procedures on horses, respectively.
- Proportionally higher incidence among:
  - Male than female horses examined per rectum.
  - Arabian than Quarter Horses examined per rectum.
- The examiner may:
  - Feel a sudden release of pressure and relaxation of the rectum.
  - Be able to palpate the abdominal organs directly.
  - Not be aware a tear occurred but finds blood on the palpation sleeve or on feces when removed from the rectum.
  - Even small amounts of blood on the sleeve or feces indicate mucosal damage has occurred and warrants appropriate precautions be taken to prevent further damage.
- Rectal tears can occur while palpating a horse per rectum regardless of the examiner's level of experience.
- The majority of tears occur when the rectal wall contracts around the examiner's hand or forearm. However, it is difficult to penetrate a healthy rectal wall with one's fingertips during an examination.
- Other documented, but less frequent, causes of rectal tears include:
  - Ischemic vascular disease of the rectal wall.
  - Misdirected stallion penis, also known as *false entry*.
  - Parturition/dystocia
  - Accidents associated with utilizing an enema or forceps to remove meconium.
  - Sand impactions
- Signs vary with the severity of the rectal damage.
  - Occasionally the first evidence a tear has occurred is when the horse develops signs of colic associated with fecal contamination of the abdomen, usually within a few hours after an examination was performed.
  - Signs of severe damage are attributable to septicemia, endotoxic shock, and peritonitis.
  - Signs include anxiety or depression, anorexia, increased heart and respiratory rates, fever, sweating, pawing, and abdominal discomfort.

Risk Factors

- Age
- Gender
- Breed
- Inadequate or improper restraint
- Inadequate examiner experience

- Poor technique
- Prior damage to the rectal wall

DIFFERENTIAL DIAGNOSIS

- When clinical signs develop, without previous evidence a tear has occurred, other causes that should be ruled out include: septicemia, endotoxemia, and peritonitis.

DIAGNOSTICS

- When a rectal tear is suspected, the examiner should immediately disclose the situation to the owner and evaluate the severity of the tear without causing further damage.

CBC/Biochemistry/Urinalysis

- Peripheral neutrophil and plasma protein values may decrease initially because of effusion of WBC and exudation of protein into the peritoneal cavity.

Other Laboratory Tests

- WBC count and protein concentration will increase in peritoneal fluid as peritonitis progresses.
- Bacteria or fecal material may also be observed in peritoneal fluid.

Other Diagnostic Procedures

- When a tear is suspected, it is advisable to establish baseline values for temperature, pulse and respiratory rates, abdominal paracentesis, and hematologic parameters as soon as possible.
- When a tear occurs, peristalsis should be stopped with sedation, caudal epidural anesthesia, or administration of an anticholinergic agent to allow safe evaluation of the area.
- Once peristalsis is stopped, feces are carefully evacuated from the rectum.
- Use of a glass (clear) speculum may facilitate visual evaluation of the tear.
- The tear and surrounding tissue should also be evaluated by gentle, manual palpation to determine the extent of the damage.

Pathologic Findings

- Classification of rectal tears is based on severity, the tissue layers involved, and the location of the tear.

Classification of Rectal Tears

Grade 1 Tears

- Involve only the mucosa
- Involve mucosal and submucosal layers

Grade 2 Tears

- The muscularis is torn, but the mucosal and submucosal layers remain intact.
- A mucosal-submucosal hernia may develop.

Grade 3 Tears

- The mucosal, submucosal, and muscularis layers are perforated, leaving only serosa (*3a* tears) or mesentery (*3b* tears) as a barrier to the peritoneal cavity or retroperitoneal space.

Grade 4 Tears

- All rectal wall layers are perforated.
- The rectal lumen communicates with the peritoneal cavity or retroperitoneal space.

 THERAPEUTICS

- Specific medications used may vary with the severity of the case and financial limitations of the owner.
- The seriousness of the situation, how the case is managed, and appropriate treatment are based on:
  - Size of the tear
  - Its distance from the anus
  - Position on the rectal wall
  - Layers involved
  - Time interval between occurrence and initiation of treatment
- From the outset, the examiner should clearly communicate to the owner the nature of the injury and its (potential) seriousness to the horse's health.
- Initiate an appropriate therapeutic plan.
- Monitor the horse's vital signs, hydration status, fecal character, and for tenesmus and signs of colic.

Grade 1 Tears

- Generally do not require aggressive treatment.
- Extensive mucosal defects require suturing.
- Antibiotics and NSAIDs should be administered prophylactically.
- Fecal softeners (i.e., DSS, MgOH, mineral oil) and a laxative diet are also indicated.
- Wounds normally heal within 7 to 14 days, but palpation should be avoided for 20 to 30 days.

Grade 2 Tears

- On rare occasion, when a rectal diverticulum develops, a horse will present with signs of colic and straining to defecate.

- Evacuate the rectum and further evaluate the defect.
- Attempt management with fecal softeners and diet.
- The diverticulum may need to be ablated surgically.

Grade 3 and 4 Tears

- Treatment is difficult but immediate recognition and treatment may improve the prognosis.
- The practitioner must initiate an appropriate therapeutic plan and refer the case quickly and safely to a surgical facility.
- Broad spectrum antibiotics and NSAIDs.
- Prevent straining and peristalsis.
- Pack the rectum (a 3-inch stockinette packed with 0.25–0.5 kg of moistened cotton, sprayed with a dilute, "weak tea" color iodine solution, and lubricated with surgical gel) to prevent further tearing and contamination of the peritoneal cavity with fecal material (this step may vary depending on the surgical facility used).
- Administer initial dose of fecal softeners before shipping the horse.

Drug(s) of Choice

Sedation

- Xylazine (0.33–0.44 mg/kg) and butorphanol (0.033–0.066 mg/kg), IV.
- Detomidine (0.01–0.02 mg/kg) and butorphanol (0.044–0.066 mg/kg), IV.

Caudal Epidural Anesthesia

- Lidocaine or mepivacaine (0.22 mg/kg).
- Xylazine (0.17 mg/kg) diluted with saline to a volume of 10 mL.
- Xylazine (0.17 mg/kg) and lidocaine (0.22 mg/kg) in a 10-mL volume.

Anticholinergics

- N-butylscopolammonium bromide or Buscopan (0.3 mg/kg), IV.
- Propantheline bromide (0.014–0.07 mg/kg), IV.
- Atropine (0.01–0.1 mg/kg), IM or SC.

Broad-Spectrum Antibiotics

- Penicillin (22,000 IU/kg) every 6 hours, IV.
- Gentamicin (6.6 mg/kg) every 24 hours, IV.
- Metronidazole (15 mg/kg) every 6 hours, IV.

NSAIDs

- Flunixin meglumine (0.25–1.0 mg/kg) every 12 hours, IV.

Tetanus Prophylaxis

- Tetanus toxoid

Precautions/Interactions

- Avoid aminoglycosides and anti-inflammatories in severely dehydrated individuals.
- Monitor hydration status closely when the horse is on aminoglycoside antibiotics and NSAIDs concurrently.

Alternative Drugs

- Antibiotics may be adjusted based on culture and sensitivity results of peritoneal fluid.

Appropriate Health Care

- Maintain normal health care as long as clinical signs allow.
- Pay particular attention to tetanus prophylaxis.

Care

- Monitor vital and clinical signs.
- Maintain hydration
- Laxative diet until recovery is complete.
- Fecal softeners as needed.

Diet

- Initially, withhold feed until after surgery.
- Promote soft feces.
- Avoid stemmy hay or forage.
- Feed oily bran or pelleted mashes.

Activity

- Hand walking or turnout exercise is acceptable, as long as clinical signs permit and access to grazing is consistent with a laxative diet.

Surgical Considerations

- Not all rectal tears are amenable to surgical repair.
- Grade 4 tears have a grave prognosis unless presented for surgery immediately upon recognition and the tear is small.
- Surgical management is directed toward repair of the defect with or without fecal bypass.
- Peritoneal lavage is indicated in cases of severe peritonitis.
- In cases of severe tears, euthanasia may be a better choice than unrealistic heroic attempts at surgical repair.

COMMENTS

Client Education

- Clear and frank communications about the extent and seriousness of the injury as well as the need for immediate and aggressive treatment.

Patient Monitoring

- Vital signs
- Fecal consistency
- Reevaluate minor tears allowed to heal by second intention to ensure complete healing.
- Periodically recheck Grade 2 tears to ensure a diverticulum does not develop.

Prevention/Avoidance

- Use plenty of palpation lubricant.
- Invert plastic palpation sleeves to minimize irritation from the plastic seam.
- Completely evacuate the rectum of feces.
- Do not attempt to palpate through feces.
- Do not attempt to palpate through a taut rectal wall (e.g., pneumorectum).
- Do not push or palpate against peristaltic waves.
- Intra-abdominal structures should only be palpated when sufficient manure has been cleared from the rectum, that the examiner's hand can be inserted safely beyond that depth, and withdrawn to that level, ensuring sufficient relaxed rectal tissue to perform the exam.

Possible Complications

- Mesorectal or retroperitoneal fecal contamination can lead to extensive cellulitis and abscessation.
- Retroperitoneal fistula
- Delayed wound healing
- Laminitis
- Rectal stricture
- Mucosal-submucosal hernia
- Peritoneal adhesions
- Chronic colic
- Death

Expected Course and Prognosis

- Prognosis is generally better for dorsal rectal tears than ventral tears.
- A survival rate of 82% or better is reported for minor mucosal-submucosal tears.
- However, survival drops to 44% to 77% for Grade 3 and early, well-managed Grade 4 tears.

- Depending on the nature of the tear, the complete course or treatment and recovery may take up to 3 months or more.
- Prognosis is poor to grave for horses with Grade 4 tears that involve peritoneal contamination with fecal material.

Summary of Steps for Handling a Rectal Tear

- Client Communication
- Establish baseline vital signs.
- Stop peristalsis and straining.
- Assess rectal tear.
- Contact referral center.
- Initiate appropriate therapeutic plan.
- Ship horse to referral center, if indicated.
- Report situation to liability insurance carrier.

Abbreviations

BSE   breeding soundness examination
CBC   complete blood count
DSS   dioctyl sodium sulfosuccinate
GI   gastrointestinal
IM   intramuscular
IV   intravenous
MgOH   magnesium hydroxide
NSAIDs   nonsteroidal anti-inflammatory drugs
SC   subcutaneous
WBC   white blood cell

See Also

- Transrectal palpation
- BSE, mare

Suggested Reading

Baird AN, Freeman DE. 1997. Management of rectal tears. *Vet Clin North Amer Eq Pract* 13(2): 377–392.

Blikslager AT, Roberts MC, Mansmann RA. 1996. Critical steps in managing equine rectal tears. *Compend Contin Educ Pract Vet* 18(10): 1140–1143.

Sayegh AI, Adams SB, Peter AT, et al. 1996. Equine rectal tears: Causes and management. *Compend Contin Educ Pract Vet* 18(10): 1131–1139.

Spensley MS, Markel MD. 1993. Management of rectal tears. In: *Equine Reproduction*. McKinnon AO, Voss JL (eds). Philadelphia: Lea & Febiger; 464–470.

Authors: Gary J. Nie and Carla L. Carleton

chapter 62

Retained Fetal Membranes

DEFINITION/OVERVIEW

Fetal membranes are defined as retained if they have not been passed within 3 hours postpartum. The placenta can be completely or partially retained (small to moderate portion) within the uterus (Fig. 62.1).

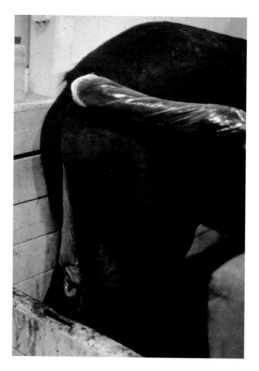

■ **Figure 62.1** Common appearance of retained fetal membranes in a postpartum mare. The placenta is commonly gathered up in knots to prevent it from dragging on the stall floor.
Image courtesy of C. L. Carleton.

ETIOLOGY/PATHOPHYSIOLOGY

- One etiology for RFM that has been suggested to be pathological sites of adherence between the endometrium and chorion with the first pregnancy or previous pregnancy that may recur during future pregnancies.
- Infections between the endometrium and chorion have also been incriminated.
- Any debilitating condition such as excessive fatigue, poor conditioning, unhygienic environment, or advanced age may increase the occurrence of RFM.

Systems Affected

- Reproductive
- Endocrine

SIGNALMENT/HISTORY

- All breeds of horses.
- All females of breeding age.
- There does not appear to be a genetic influence for this condition.
- No affect attributed to breeding by AI versus natural (i.e., live) cover the previous year.
- No affect due to sex of foal or birth of a weak or dead fetus.

Risk Factors

- The most common postpartum condition in mares; incidence of 2% to 10%.
- Incidence is reported to increase after dystocia or C-section, in draft mares, hydrops pregnancy, and after a prolonged pregnancy.

Historical Findings

- Prior incidence of RFM increases the likelihood of another retention of the membranes; true of partial or complete failure to pass the fetal membranes.
- Increased occurrence following dystocia due to any cause.
- Prolonged pregnancy or abortion increase likelihood of RFM.
- Incidence increases in mares older than 15 years.
- No effect attributed to previous reproductive status (i.e., maiden, barren, or foaling) the previous year.

CLINICAL FEATURES

- The portion of RFM visible at the vulvar lips is an unreliable indicator of the proportion that may yet be attached (retained) within the uterus (Figs. 62.2 and 62.3).

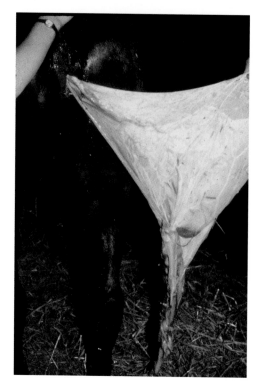

■ **Figure 62.2** The chorioallantois and amnion will change color, especially the exposed portions, with retention. This image is of amnion in a mare recently postpartum.
Image courtesy of C. L. Carleton.

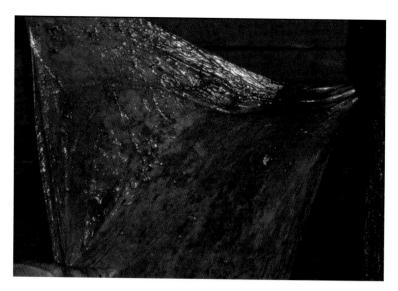

■ **Figure 62.3** Amnion color change due to oxidative change.
Image courtesy of C. L. Carleton.

- As mares move about immediately postpartum, portions of the membranes may be torn or break free.
- A careful look through stall bedding may yield the balance of the placental membranes and decrease the concern regarding a retained portion.

DIFFERENTIAL DIAGNOSIS

- Uterine infection
- Delayed or failure of normal postpartum uterine involution.

DIAGNOSTICS

- TRP is the primary diagnostic tool.
- Include in the assessment: uterine size and tone; the amount of fluid in the uterus, if any.
- Vaginal examination may be necessary, but it is not always essential; dependent on the condition of the placenta and the uterus.

THERAPEUTICS

Drug(s) of Choice

- Treatment of RFM is primarily with oxytocin and is always the first treatment if the placenta has been retained less than 24 hours. Its effectiveness is optimal when administered early (up to or fewer than 3 hours) postpartum.
- Oxytocin treatment should be initiated beginning at less than 3 hours postpartum if membranes have not passed.
  - The treatment can be repeated every 60 to 120 minutes for the first 21 hours postpartum.
- Prostaglandin therapy should also be considered if the placenta is still retained more than 18 hours.
- Once the placenta is retained longer than 18 hours, the treatment may change to intrauterine with irritants or antibiotics used and possibly systemic antibiotics.
  - If intrauterine antibiotics have already been instituted to treat RFM, systemic antibiotics are not necessary unless systemic disease develops.
- Flushing the uterus with warm saline or water solutions can have great value if a portion of the placenta is retained.
- Insufflation of the RFM with fluid placed within the lumen of the membranes (only useful if the RFM are largely intact): fluid, preferably isotonic saline solution (alternatively LRS or water), is placed into the uterus within the innermost aspect of the fetal membranes, sufficiently to expand the uterus and stimulate uterine activity.

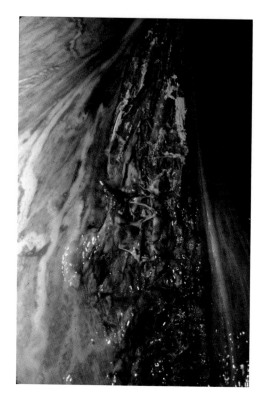

■ **Figure 62.4** A full examination of the placenta once passed is of value. This necrotic plaque was on the amnion. Placental abnormalities reflect the neonate's prepartum intrauterine environment and may serve as a warning to monitor more closely a neonate's heath.
Image courtesy of C. L. Carleton.

- Proper preparation of the mare includes tail wrap, tied or held to one side, sterile tube and appropriate technique to minimize further contamination of the uterus during this procedure.
- The fetal membranes are gathered at the exposed (external to the vulvae) portion and tied outside of the vulvae to maintain the saline within the uterus and placenta for a brief time. This creates uterine expansion, stretching the myometrium or endometrium to facilitate release of the microvilli.
- Cost of this larger-volume treatment may be more expensive, but it yields a modest increase in benefit, especially if oxytocin alone is ineffective.

Appropriate Health Care

Administer oxytocin postpartum to all mares with a history of RFM. Such mares are at higher risk for recurrence. Examine the placenta in its entirety after passage to determine that all portions of the placenta are present (Fig. 62.4).

Diet

There are no changes in diet indicated because of RFM.

Activity

Affected mares may exercise normally.

 COMMENTS

Client Education

- RFM is a postpartum condition and is a failure to expel the fetal membranes normally.
- The incidence usually increases with induction of parturition.
- RFM is relatively common and should be treated if membranes do not pass by 3 hours postpartum.
- It is advisable for owners to have their own stock of oxytocin, administering 10 units if needed, but beginning no sooner than 3 hours after foaling.
- Older mares have a higher incidence of RFM on some farms.

Patient Monitoring

- The owner should monitor the vulvar area and the stall for fetal membrane passage as well as changes in the mare's activity in case she begins to develop laminitis.
- Note any alterations of appetite and defecation as well as lactation.
- Once RFM has been diagnosed, TRP may ascertain whether uterine involution is progressing normally. Uterine tone should at least be good (with normal involution the size of the uterus rapidly decreases, resulting in an increase in uterine tone).

Prevention/Avoidance

- The only way to eliminate this condition from occurring is not to breed a mare or prevent pregnancy from progressing past 90 to 120 days of gestation.
- Exercise and dietary supplementation with selenium may have some value.
- Avoid pasturing mares on fescue infected pasture or hay within at least the final month of gestation.

Possible Complications

- One of the most prevalent complications of RFM, especially in draft mares, is laminitis. Monitor feet/hooves for increased heat and pain. Medications to reduce the effects of laminitis may be indicated in select cases.
- Higher doses of oxytocin may lead to uterine prolapse. Oxytocin may induce uterine cramping causing the mare to go down, and she could unintentionally harm her foal.

- Septic (i.e., toxic) metritis or metritis.
  - A mare with septic metritis will have systemic signs and be obviously ill.
  - A mare with metritis may not exhibit any signs until it is time to re-breed the mare.

Expected Course and Prognosis

- Of mares treated with oxytocin for RFM, over 90% pass the RFM without any other problem within a few hours, and their prognosis is excellent.
- RFM passed without secondary involvement have no affect on conception at foal heat breeding.
- Affected mares treated with intrauterine antibiotics have higher rates of conception but also higher rates of pregnancy termination.

Synonyms

- Retained afterbirth
- Retained placenta

Abbreviations

AI   artificial insemination
LRS   lactated Ringer's solution
RFM   retained fetal membranes
TRP   transrectal palpation

See Also

- Dystocia

Suggested Reading

Alexander RW. 1971. Excessive retainment of the placenta in the mare. *Vet Rec* 89: 175–176.
Burns SJ, Judge NG, Martin JE, et al. 1977. Management of retained placenta in mares. *Proc AAEP* 381–390.
Provencher R, Threlfall WR, Murdick PW, et al. 1988. Retained fetal membranes in the mare. A retrospective study. *Can Vet J* 29: 903–910.
Threlfall WR. Retained placenta. In: *Equine Reproduction*. McKinnon AO, Voss JL (eds). Philadelphia: Lea & Febiger; 614–621.
Threlfall WR, Carleton CL. 1986. Treatment of uterine infections in the mare. In: *Current Therapy in Theriogenology*, 2nd ed. Morrow DA (ed). Philadelphia: W. B. Saunders; 730–737.
White TE. 1980. Retained placenta. *Mod Vet Pract* 61: 87–88.

Author: Walter R. Threlfall

chapter 63

Superovulation of the Mare

DEFINITION/OVERVIEW

- Mares usually only ovulate one follicle per cycle. Increasing the number of ovulations, or inducing "superovulation," could increase the efficiency and decrease the cost of ET in horses.
- Superovulation may also be beneficial in some cases of mare or stallion subfertility. Increasing the number of oocytes ovulated may increase the probability of fertilization in mares bred with a limited number of spermatozoa.

ETIOLOGY/PATHOPHYSIOLOGY

- Mares typically have one or occasionally two follicular waves during a given estrous cycle.
- A follicular wave begins when a group of follicles "emerge" from a pool of small follicles over a period of several days.
- This group develops in response to endogenous FSH during the common growth phase.
- Follicles increase in size at approximately 3 mm per day during this period.
- Follicular divergence or deviation occurs at the end of the common growth phase when the largest follicle of the wave reaches 22 to 25 mm in diameter and begins to secrete estradiol and inhibin.
- These hormones (estradiol and inhibin) feed back to the anterior pituitary to suppress the secretion of FSH.
- Smaller follicles in the wave are still critically dependent on FSH support for continued development and subsequently regress as FSH levels decline.
- The dominant follicle continues to develop, mature, and eventually ovulate in response to secretion of LH from the pituitary.
- This mechanism of follicle selection limits the number of ovulations in most equine estrous cycles to one.
- The goal of superovulation therapy is to administer exogenous FSH, beginning just prior to or at the time of follicular divergence and rescue or prevent regression of the subordinant follicles.

Systems Affected

Reproduction

SIGNALMENT/HISTORY

There are no breed differences.

DIAGNOSTICS

Transrectal U/S

- Monitoring follicular growth patterns by transrectal U/S is critical to determine the optimal time to start eFSH therapy, evaluate response to therapy, and determine when to administer an OIA.

THERAPEUTICS

Drug(s) of Choice

- eFSH (Bioniche, Inc., Athens, GA).
- hCG (Chorulon®, Intervet, Millsboro, DE).
- Cloprostenol sodium (Estrumate®, Schering-Plough Animal Health Corp., Union, NJ).

Superovulation Protocol

- Administer FSH (i.e., 12.5 mg eFSH or 0.5 mg reFSH) IM BID beginning approximately 5 to 7 days after ovulation when the largest follicle is 18 to 20 mm in diameter.
- Administer prostaglandins (i.e., 250 µg cloprostenol sodium, the day after the onset of eFSH therapy to cause luteolysis.
- Discontinue FSH treatment when the diameter of the largest follicle is 35 mm.
- Allow the mare to coast without any hormone therapy for 36 hours.
- Administer hCG (2,500 IU, IV) to induce ovulation.

Precautions/Interactions

- More days of therapy will be required if treatment is administered when follicles are less than 20 mm in diameter.
- If a single follicle is at least or larger than 30 mm in diameter at the onset of therapy it is unlikely that additional follicles will successfully be recruited to develop and ovulate.

Alternative Drugs

- A recombinant eFSH (EquiPure FSH™, AspenBio Pharma Inc., Castle Rock, CO) is currently in early testing and may become available in the future.

 COMMENTS

Client Education

- Success of eFSH therapy in inducing multiple ovulations is lower in older mares.

Patient Monitoring

- Achieving pregnancy: ovulations induced following eFSH therapy are fertile.

Possible Complications

- Some mares fail to develop multiple large follicles in response to eFSH therapy.
- Some eFSH treated mares fail to ovulate after administration of hCG or deslorelin.
- Follicles that fail to ovulate may either regress or form hemorrhagic follicles that eventually luteinize.

Expected Course and Prognosis

- An average of three to six large follicles will develop after 3 to 4 days of eFSH therapy.
- Eighty-five percent to 95% of the large follicles will ovulate in response to hCG.

Abbreviations

BID	twice a day
eFSH	equine follicle stimulating hormone
ET	embryo transfer
FSH	follicle stimulating hormone
hCG	human chorionic gonadotropin
IM	intramuscularly
IV	intravenously
LH	luteinizing hormone
OIA	ovulation inducing agent
reFSH	recombinant equine follicle stimulating hormone
U/S	ultrasound, ultrasonography

See Also

- Abnormal estrus intervals
- Ovulation failure
- Ovulation, induction of

- Ovulation, synchronization of
- Estrous cycle, manipulation of

Suggested Reading

Niswender KD, Alvarenga MA, McCue PM, et al. 2003. Superovulation in cycling mares using equine follicle stimulating hormone (eFSH). *J Eq Vet Sci* 23: 497–500.

McCue PM. 1996. Superovulation. *Vet Clinics North Am, Eq Pract: Diagnostic Techniques and Assisted Reproductive Technology.* 12: 1–11.

Welch SA, Denniston DJ, Hudson JJ, et al. 2006. Exogenous eFSH, follicle coasting and hCG as a novel superovulation regime in mares. *J Eq Vet Sci* 26: 262–270.

Author: Patrick M. McCue

chapter 64

Teratoma

DEFINITION/OVERVIEW

The teratoma is a congenital tumor of the gonad derived from the germ cells. It is well differentiated and characterized by multiple tissue types. Teratomas contain somatic structures that can derive from all embryonic germ cell layers including ectoderm (i.e., hair, teeth), neuroectoderm (i.e., nerves, melanocytes), endoderm (i.e., salivary gland, lung), mesoderm (i.e., fibrous, adipose, bone, muscle), and nervous and adipose tissue (nearly always present).

ETIOLOGY/PATHOPHYSIOLOGY

Teratomas are a congenital tumor.

Systems Affected

Reproductive: tumor is in the place of normal reproductive tissue. May be concurrent with other gonadal neoplasia including carcinoma and granulosa cell tumor. Abdominal pain has resulted from traction (by the weight of the tumor) on supporting structures of the affected gonad.

SIGNALMENT/HISTORY

- Teratomas are congenital. Horses of any age may display signs because of the physical presence of a teratoma (e.g., colic).
- Young males: usual presenting age is 1 to 2 years. May result in a cryptorchid testis as its presence in the fetus/fetal gonad precludes normal testicular descent.
- Females: usually discovered in place of an ovary during a routine reproductive examination.

Risk Factors

Tumor of congenital origin

Historical Findings

Female

- Incidental finding during routine reproductive examination. Colic has been reported with larger ovarian teratomas (small colon torsion in a foal, caused by traction pressure on supporting structures).

Male

- Can present in a scrotal location (descended), but the frequency of its being a teratoma increases when the testis is cryptorchid (undescended). Due to the alteration of normal scrotal dynamics, a teratoma may decrease spermatogenesis or induce tubular atrophy of the contralateral testicular tissue.

 CLINICAL FEATURES

Female

Palpable abnormality in place of the ovary

Male

Scrotal enlargement due to testicular mass or as a cryptorchid testis

 DIFFERENTIAL DIAGNOSIS

Female

- Ovarian hematoma
- Granulosa theca cell tumor
- Dysgerminoma
- Ovarian carcinoma
- Fibroma
- Ovarian abscess

Male

- Seminoma
- Sertoli cell tumor
- Interstitial cell tumor
- Carcinoma
- Testicular hematoma
- Fibroma

DIAGNOSTICS

U/S

- Female: couple with TRP when possible. Teratomas appear as abnormal paraovarian masses that are solid and multilocular. Echogenicity will be heterogenous, with shadowing due to calcified structures.
- Male: Heterogenous mass.

Endocrinology

- Lack of endocrine abnormalities that are usually associated with other causes of an enlarged gonad.

Pathological Findings

Characteristic histological findings of multiple differentiated tissue types with a single tumor.

 THERAPEUTICS

Surgical removal of tumor mass by ovariectomy or hemi-castration.

 COMMENTS

Client Education

Removal of tumor leads to complete resolution of clinical signs.

Possible Complications

Although usually benign in nature, there are reports of malignant transformation and metastasis throughout the abdominal cavity.

Expected Course and Prognosis

Surgical removal is curative.

Abbreviations

TRP   transrectal palpation
U/S   ultrasound, ultrasonography

See Also

- Large Ovary Syndrome

Suggested Reading

Allison N, Moeller RB Jr, Duncan R. 2004. Placental teratocarcinoma in a mare with possible metastasis to the foal. *J Vet Diagn Invest* 2: 160–163.

Buergelt CD. 1997. *Color Atlas of Reproductive Pathology of the Domestic Animals*. St. Louis: Mosby-Year Book; 55–56, 106–107.

Catone G, Marino G, Mancuso R, et al. 2004. Clinicopathological features of an equine ovarian teratoma. *Reprod Domest Anim* 39: 65–69.

Gurfield N, Benirschke K. 2003. Equine placental teratoma. *Vet Pathol* 40: 586–588.

Jubb KVC, Kennedy PC, Palmer N. 1993. *Pathology of the Domestic Animals*, 4th ed. San Diego: Academic Press; 3: 368, 510.

Lefebvre R, Theoret C, Dore M, et al. 2005. Ovarian teratoma and endometritis in a mare. *Can Vet J* 46: 1029–1033.

Author: Peter R. Morresey

chapter 65

Transrectal Palpation

DEFINITION/OVERVIEW

- TRP is a highly valuable technique for examining the reproductive tract of the horse.
- The technique is performed alone or in combination with other equipment to gather diagnostic information for management, treatment selection, or establish prognoses.
- The technique is of most value when applied in a safe and systematic manner.

ETIOLOGY/PATHOPHYSIOLOGY

Systems Affected

- Urogenital
- GI

SIGNALMENT/HISTORY

- Routinely and frequently employed in equine reproduction practice.
- Need is recognized for diagnostic and prognostic information about the reproductive tract.
- Any horse of sufficient size to allow safe examination of the reproductive tract per rectum regardless of age, gender, or breed.
- Most often examinations are conducted in mares, but stallions are also palpated in some circumstances.
- Common times to examine by TRP:
  - Estrus
  - Diestrus
  - Anestrus
  - Nymphomania
  - Stallion-like behavior in a mare
  - Colic TRP to identify portion of GI tract that may be affected.

Risk Factors

- Useful throughout most of gestation for diagnosing and assessing pregnancy.
- Care should be taken not to damage the early embryonic vesicle during TRP of the uterus, if pregnancy is suspected.
- Risks of injury to the horse, handler, or examiner are associated with the procedure.
- TRP is contraindicated in young horses that have not reached sufficient body size to permit a safe examination.

Risks for the Horse

- Age
- Gender
- Breed
- Inadequate or improper restraint
- Inadequate examiner experience
- Poor technique
- Prior damage to the rectal wall

Risks for the Handler or Examiner

- Inadequate or improper restraint
- Inadequate or poorly constructed facilities for examinations

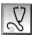 **DIFFERENTIAL DIAGNOSIS**

In many cases it is helpful to know the horse's history and behavioral signs.

 DIAGNOSTICS

Laboratory Tests

Endocrine assays may be used to support the findings of a TRP.
- Progesterone assay
- Conjugated estrogens (estrone sulfate).
- eCG

U/S

Diagnostic U/S is an indispensable adjunct to TRP in most situations.

Diagnostic Procedures

A systematic examination is conducted of the ovaries, uterus, and cervix.

Required Materials

- Shoulder length palpation sleeve
- Palpation lubricant (e.g., carboxymethylcellulose)
- Halter
- Lead rope

Optional Materials (Recommended To Be Used or Available)

- Tail wrap
- Tail tie
- Stocks (particularly important to limit lateral motion of the mare).
- Twitch
- Sedation
- Anticholinergic agent
- Local anesthetic
- Water source

Routine Procedures/Techniques

- Ready the horse for TRP with the minimum amount of restraint necessary for the safety of the examiner, handler, and horse.
- Its tail is wrapped and tied out of the way to prevent tail hairs from being introduced through the anus and potentially causing a laceration.
- Invert a plastic palpation sleeve to prevent its seam from causing a laceration, or use a seamless latex sleeve (reusable, usually has a surgical glove glued to the arm portion, better fit on one's hand). Lubricate the sleeve by taking a generous handful of lubricant and distribute lubricant to the level of the elbow.
- With a well-lubricated sleeve, one finger at a time is introduced into the anus starting with the index finger, ultimately coning all four fingers and thumb, as the entire hand is passed through the anal sphincter.
- Once the hand is in the rectum, feces are gently and completely removed to the extent of the examiner's reach.
- Additional lubricant is reapplied to the hand as needed.
- Feces are carried from the rectum through the anal sphincter in the examiner's hand and discarded.
- Do not apply force against peristaltic waves in the rectum, instead allow them to pass over the hand and arm, or withdraw a brief distance caudally (partial accommodation, rarely necessary to completely remove one's hand) until the wave passes.
- If the horse strains excessively with its abdominal muscles, additional restraint may be necessary, with or without a local anesthetic, to reduce the sensitivity of the rectal mucosa.
- Once the fecal matter within reach is removed, the hand is positioned in the rectum and on the midline with the palm facing down; the examiner's elbow at this point will be approximately at the level of the anus.

- In most cases the examiner's hand should be cranial to the uterus. With sufficient relaxation of the mare, this permits rectal tissue to be brought caudally to the reproductive tract for palpation, instead of trying to palpate the structures by stretching the rectum cranially to the tract.
- Patience is essential; less activity with one's hand provides greater information (i.e., an overly active hand and rapid movements during palpation merely induces more peristalsis and yields less useful information). The free hand should remain in gentle contact with the mare (i.e., tail, rump, flank) and provide comfort to the mare and information to the examiner if the horse is remaining tense and may decide to react badly. One must, of course, keep a watchful eye on the horse's head and other behavior to anticipate any approaching undesirable reaction.
- The examiner's cupped hand is gently retracted caudally and ventrally until the cranial uterine body or horns are located.
- Keeping the hand cupped, each uterine horn is carefully palpated from body to tip.
  - The uterus is evaluated for size, symmetry, and consistency.
  - The uterine wall relaxes as it develops some degree of edema during estrus (influenced by the absence of progesterone and presence of estradiol) and becomes toned during diestrus and early pregnancy (the influence of progesterone).
- Slightly craniodorsad from the tip of the uterine horn, the ipsilateral ovary is located.
  - The ovary is evaluated for size, shape, and follicular structures (i.e., number, size, and location).
  - Though follicular structures can be found at any stage of the estrous cycle, a large, dominant follicle should be present during mid- to late estrus.
  - The CL is not discernible on palpation of the ovary. The ovarian tunic prevents a "luteal crown" from developing during diestrus as happens in the cow.
- The hand is cupped again to follow the uterine horn across the cranial body to the contralateral horn and ovary.
- To finish the examination, the hand is opened at the cranial uterine body with the palm facing down. The fingers are swept back and forth while feeling the length of the uterine body with the pads of the fingers.
- At the caudal end of the uterine body, the fingers define the cervix for its length, width and degree of relaxation. Its external os can readily be defined.
  - The examiner's wrist will be at or just inside the anus when feeling the caudal end of the cervix.
  - The cervix relaxes and widens during estrus (the absence of progesterone), while becoming more tubular with increased tone during diestrus and pregnancy (the presence of progesterone).
- Once the arm is fully retracted, examine the palpation sleeve closely for evidence of blood before discarding it (especially if using disposable sleeves).

Pathologic Findings

Palpable Ovarian Abnormalities

- Ovarian tumors
- Ovarian hematomas

- Anovulatory follicles
- Abnormally small ovaries

Palpable Uterine Abnormalities

- Pyometra
- Large lymphatic cysts
- Neoplasia, most commonly leiomyoma
- Hematomas
- Abscesses

Palpable Cervical Abnormalities

- Failure to relax during estrus.
- Failure to close when more than 48 hours post-ovulation.
  - This is justification to evaluate the cervix per vagina to rule out the presence of a cervical tear.

 # THERAPEUTICS

Drug(s) of Choice

Sedation or administration of an anticholinergic agent may be necessary to facilitate proper restraint and safe conditions for TRP.

Sedation

- Xylazine (0.2–1.1 mg/kg), IV.
- Xylazine (0.33–0.44 mg/kg) and butorphanol (0.033–0.066 mg/kg), IV.
- Detomidine (0.01–0.02 mg/kg), IV.
- Detomidine (0.01–0.02 mg/kg) and butorphanol (0.044–0.066 mg/kg), IV.

Anticholinergics

- N-butylscopolammonium bromide or Buscopan® (0.3 mg/kg), IV.
- Propantheline bromide (0.014–0.07 mg/kg), IV.

Local Anesthetic

- Lidocaine (50 mL), 2%, infused into the rectum.

Precautions/Interactions

- Although sedation may be necessary to make the horse more tractable to TRP, over-sedation can cause instability and increase the risk to horse, handler, and examiner.
- Some horses may display signs of abdominal discomfort due to the generalized effects of propantheline bromide on the GI tract.

Appropriate Health Care

General health care appropriate for the region in which the horse is located.

Nursing Care

It is advisable to rinse the feces and lubricant off the perineum following TRP to avoid skin irritation.

Activity

No limit on activity unless complications develop from the procedure.

Surgical Considerations

None, unless a rectal tear occurs.

 COMMENTS

Client Education

- Inform the owner of the risks associated with TRP.
- Advise the owner to observe the horse for the few hours post-TRP for signs associated with a rectal tear.

Patient Monitoring

- The procedure is associated with some risk of damage to the rectal wall, therefore the horse should be observed within a few hours of TRP for clinical signs consistent with a rectal tear.

Prevention/Avoidance

- Not often performed in nonbreeding horses unless required for prepurchase or a medical or surgical condition.

Possible Complications

- Rectal tear

Expected Course and Prognosis

- In the vast majority of cases, TRP is a minimally invasive procedure that progresses without incident or complication.

Abbreviations

CL   corpus luteum
eCG   equine chorionic gonadotropin

GI   gastrointestinal
IV   intravenous
TRP   transrectal palpation
U/S   ultrasound, ultrasonography

See Also

- Breeding soundness examinations
- Breeding management
- Pregnancy
- Behavior abnormalities
- Large Ovary Syndrome
- Rectal Tears

Suggested Reading

Ley WB, Santschi EM. 1999. Examination and surgery of the uterus. In: *Large Animal Urogenital Surgery*. Wolfe DF, Moll HD (eds). Baltimore: Williams & Wilkins; 115–136.

Shideler RK. 1993. Rectal palpation. In: *Equine Reproduction*. McKinnon AO, Voss JL (eds). Philadelphia: Lea & Febiger; 204–210.

Authors: Carla L. Carleton and Gary J. Nie

chapter 66

Twin Pregnancy

DEFINITION/OVERVIEW

The simultaneous intrauterine production of two or more embryos or fetuses.

ETIOLOGY/PATHOPHYSIOLOGY

- The majority of multiple pregnancies in the mare are twins.
  - Most twins are dizygotic and result from double ovulations.
  - Early twin vesicles behave similarly to a singleton conceptus.
  - The vesicles undergo transuterine migration until 15 days of gestation, when fixation occurs in one or both uterine horns at approximately day 16 to 17 of gestation.
  - Approximately 75% of twin vesicles fix in the same horn (unicornual) (Figs. 66.1, 66.2, and 66.3).

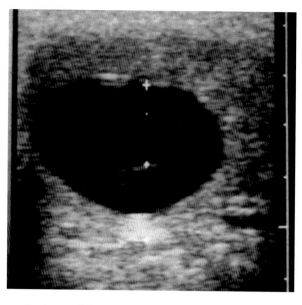

■ **Figure 66.1** Unicornual twins, careful assessment is critical at an early check to avoid missing the overlap of twin vesicles. Image courtesy of C. L. Carleton.

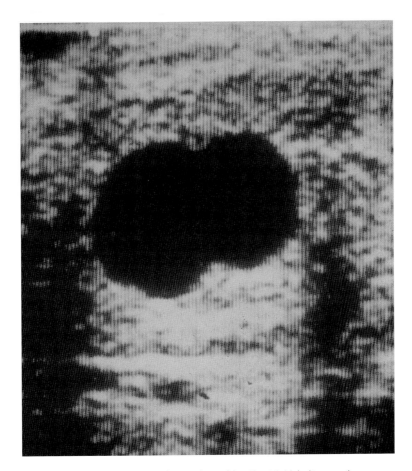

■ **Figure 66.2** Unicornual twins, slight overlap, easier to identify at initial ultrasound. Image courtesy of C. L. Carleton.

- Approximately 75% of unicornual twin pregnancies less than 40 days of age undergo natural reduction to one embryo.
  - The remaining embryo develops normally to term as a singleton.
  - If natural reduction of one embryo fails to occur by 40 days of gestation, there is a strong probability that the twins will continue to develop, only to abort later in gestation (Figs. 66.4 and 66.5).
- Bicornual twins do not undergo natural reduction. Instead, the twins usually develop through the last trimester of gestation, at which time abortion is common (Fig. 66.6).

Systems Affected

Reproductive

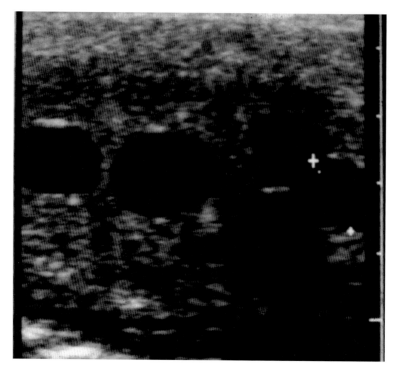

■ **Figure 66.3** Unicornual twins, side-by-side, in addition to a small lymphatic cyst to the right (indicated by the + markers, to the right). A reminder to create a *cyst map* on a mare's record prior to breeding at the beginning of a season; it eliminates the uncertainty of crushing a pregnancy by mistake and leaving the cyst behind. Image courtesy of C. L. Carleton.

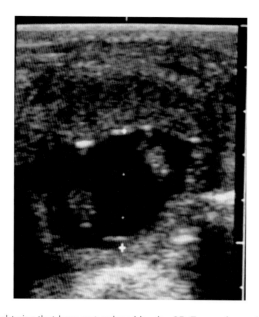

■ **Figure 66.4** Unicornual twins that have not reduced by day 25. Two embryos, both with heartbeats were present.
Image courtesy of C. L. Carleton.

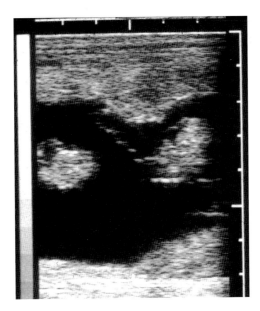

■ **Figure 66.5**   Unicornual twins failing to reduce early in gestation. More common with asynchronous ovulations (ovulations occurring more than 48 hours apart at the same estrus).
Image courtesy of C. L. Carleton.

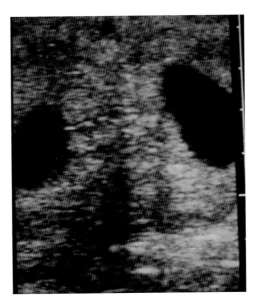

■ **Figure 66.6**   Bicornual twins (transducer turned 90 degrees to capture both in the image). These are the easiest twins to reduce by crush techniques (in opposite horns).
Image courtesy of C. L. Carleton.

 # SIGNALMENT/HISTORY

- The incidence of twin pregnancy is related to age, breed, and reproductive status.
- Higher incidence of double ovulations in some breeds of horses.

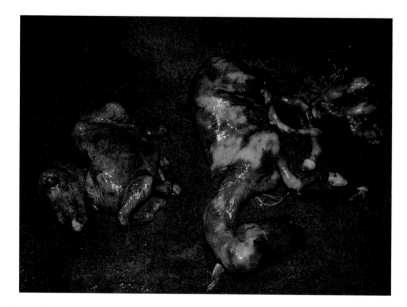

■ **Figure 66.7**   The most common outcome of a twin pregnancy not addressed early in gestation, abortion of both.
Image courtesy of C. L. Carleton.

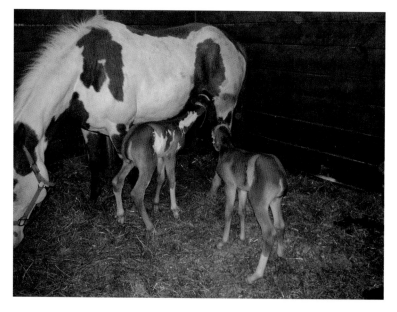

■ **Figure 66.8**   Successful full-term delivery of twins (unassisted) from a mare not checked early in gestation.
Image courtesy of C. L. Carleton.

■ Twin pregnancy occurs more frequently in older mares, barren mares, thoroughbred, and draft breeds.
■ Arabians, Quarter Horses, ponies, and primitive breeds are reported to have a lower incidence of twin pregnancy.

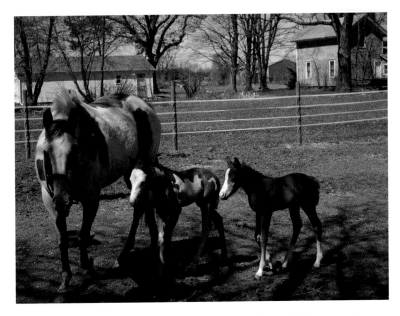

■ **Figure 66.9** Viable twins requiring supplemental feeding only during first 2 weeks of life. Image courtesy of C. L. Carleton.

Risk Factors

- Breed, age, and reproductive status.
- Twinning is undesirable in the mare and routinely ends in abortion (Fig. 66.7). Less than 0.005% result in the birth of viable twins (both surviving) (Figs. 66.8 and 66.9).

                    CLINICAL FEATURES

- Mares that develop twin pregnancies tend to have twins in subsequent pregnancies.
- Ovulation and fertilization of multiple ova in most cases. Rare incidence of monozygotic multiple pregnancies have been reported.
- Survival of twins to term is most likely if the uterine space is evenly shared between the two fetuses (Fig. 66.10). Unfortunately there is no way to facilitate that division.

Management of twins prior to day 40 of gestation:

- Twins detected during transuterine migration of the conceptus (days 9–15) are best managed by crushing one embryonic vesicle. There are two techniques:
  - One vesicle is manipulated transrectally to the tip of a uterine horn. Pressure is placed on the vesicle and it is crushed (Fig. 66.11), or
  - Using U/S, confirm the approximate distance from the bifurcation of the uterine horns to the vesicle, entrap the vesicle between the thumb (dorsally) and at least 2 fingers (ventral aspect) where it lies. As gentle pressure around the vesicle is

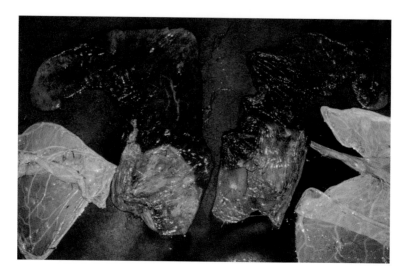

■ **Figure 66.10**   Placental division most often observed in mares successfully carrying twins to term. Each twin occupied one uterine horn and split the difference of the uterine body. The large avillous area represents placental contact.
Image courtesy of C. L. Carleton.

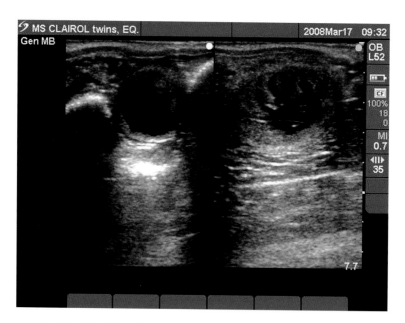

■ **Figure 66.11**   Crushing of a twin. *Left*: pre-crush; *Right*: disruption of the vesicle (yolk sac).
Image courtesy of C. L. Carleton.

increased, the perimeter of the sphere will be evident. Continue increasing pressure on the vesicle until its disruption has been felt as a slight "popping sensation" with a successful crush. Immediately follow-up with U/S to confirm vesicle disruption has been accomplished (Fig. 66.12).

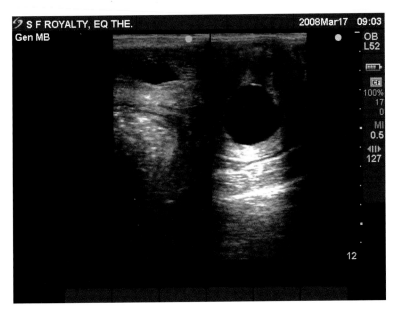

■ **Figure 66.12**   Successful twin crush. Always confirm by ultrasound that the yolk sac has been disrupted. Pre-crush on the *right*, post-crush on the *left*.
Image courtesy of C. L. Carleton.

- The remaining vesicle survives in approximately 90% of the cases.
- The crush technique is useful for twins in the transuterine migration (mobility) phase and bicornual twins prior to 30 days of gestation. The earlier it can be done (15–20 days), the greater will be the success. There will be less endometrial prostaglandin release with crushing of smaller vesicles. Larger vesicles (30+ days) require greater pressure, thus more prostaglandin release.
- After 30 days of gestation, fluid released from the crushed vesicle tends to disrupt the remaining pregnancy.
- Unicornual twins are usually both destroyed when crushing of one vesicle is attempted.
- Always confirm the success of the crush by an U/S examination immediately after the crush, confirm dispersal of fluid from its former spherical shape.

Management of twins after day 40 of gestation:

- Management of twin pregnancies in the fetal period (at least, or longer than, day 40) is further complicated by the formation of endometrial cups.
- Pregnancy loss once endometrial cups have formed has been shown to cause irregular estrous cycles or to delay a return to fertile cycles.
- Consequently, maintenance of a singleton pregnancy following a reduction procedure is critical to the reproductive success of the mare for a reduction done later than day 40.

Alternate methods of twin management that have been attempted include:

- Dietary restriction: In one study, mares with twin pregnancies (diagnosed by TRP) were limited to poor quality grass hay early in gestation (days 21–49 of gestation).

- One viable foal (reduction had occurred) was delivered in 56% (23/41) of the cases examined.
- Surgical removal of one twin: Surgical removal of one twin was attempted in seven unicornual and eight bicornual twins at 41 to 62 days of gestation.
  - None of the unicornual twins survived.
  - Five of eight bicornual twin pregnancies were successfully reduced to a singleton.
- Intracardiac injection of KCl: Using transcutaneous U/S one fetal heart is located and fetal death is caused by intracardiac injection of KCl.
  - The technique has been successful in approximately 50% of the cases attempted.
  - This procedure is most useful from 115 to 130 days of gestation.
- Transvaginal allantocentesis: Transvaginal U/S has been used to aid in identification of the allantoic sac in one twin fetus, pass a needle into the allantois, and aspirate the allantoic fluid.
  - Aspiration of the fluid causes collapse of the vesicle and fetal death.
  - To date, this technique has been successful in approximately 30% of the attempted cases.
  - The technique is most applicable for bicornual twins.

 DIFFERENTIAL DIAGNOSIS

Differentiating Similar Signs

- Uterine (lymphatic) cysts can be confused with developing embryonic vesicles causing an improper diagnosis of twin pregnancy.
- Differentiation of uterine cysts from embryonic vesicles may be simplified by recording the location, size, and shape of uterine cysts prior to pregnancy.
- If records are unavailable from a prior season, reexamine the mare in 2 days. The vesicle of pregnancy will demonstrate a noticeable increase in U/S diameter; the diameter of a uterine/lymphatic cyst will not increase in that limited period of time.
- Differentiation of an embryonic vesicle from a uterine cyst may also be confirmed with observation of an embryonic heartbeat present at 24+ days of gestation.

 DIAGNOSTICS

Other Diagnostic Procedures

TRP of the Reproductive Tract

- Pregnancy diagnosis by TRP at 25 to 30 days of gestation is characterized by distinct, increased uterine tone and a narrow, elongated cervix.
- By days 25 to 30, a bulge the size of a small hen's egg can be appreciated at the caudoventral aspect of a uterine horn, adjacent to the uterine bifurcation.

- If twin vesicles of pregnancy are bicornual in location, it may be possible to diagnose twin pregnancies at this time (two ventral bulges, one to either side of the bifurcation of the uterine horns).
- If the vesicles of pregnancy are unicornual in location, it is impossible to determine the presence of twin pregnancy using TRP alone, but an experienced practitioner may note the bulge of pregnancy seems to be larger than anticipated.

Imaging

Transrectal U/S

- U/S examination of the reproductive tract early in gestation allows for prompt diagnosis and treatment of twin pregnancies and is an opportune time to also examine both ovaries; determine if two CL's are present (may be one on each, or two on one ovary).
- Pregnancies may be detected as early as day 9 of gestation, however, twin pregnancies may differ in age by as much as 2 days.
- Due to the possible differences in age and size of twin pregnancies, U/S diagnosis of twins is recommended between 13 and 15 days of gestation.
- The embryonic vesicle(s) at this time is an anechoic, spherical yolk sac that averages between 12 and 20 mm in height.
- Twin vesicles are highly mobile between day 6 (embryo entry into the uterus) to days 15 to 16 (the period of transuterine migration until fixation) and can be located adjacent to one another or in different locations within the uterus.
- To properly determine if twin vesicles are present, it is critical to scan both uterine horns and the uterine body to the cervix, sequentially; with at least two full sweeps across the tract.

Transabdominal U/S

- Transabdominal U/S is useful for diagnosing twin pregnancies more than 75 to 100 days of gestation.
- Diagnosis is generally made by identification of two fetal heartbeats.

 THERAPEUTICS

Drug(s) of Choice

- Flunixin meglumine (1 mg/kg, IV) is often administered at the time of attempted twin reduction to prevent prostaglandin release from the uterus and subsequent lysis of the CL.
- Exogenous progestins (altrenogest, 1 mL per 50 kg BW [0.044 mg altrenogest per kg BW], PO, SID) at double the recommended dose (2 mL per 50 kg) may be administered when twin reduction is attempted:
  - to maintain uterine and cervical tone following uterine manipulation
  - to counter the effects of possible fetal fluid release into the uterine lumen.

Diet

See Alternate Methods, above.

 COMMENTS

Client Education

- Importance of TRP in the periovulatory period (before and after breeding and insemination), and noting if there is more than 1 ovulation during an estrus.
- Emphasis of early (latest 16 days following ovulation), serial evaluations of a high-risk mare:
  - Multiple ovulations
  - Prior history of twinning.
  - Breeds with higher incidence of twinning.
  - Suspicious appearance of vesicle of pregnancy at the initial examination; warrants follow-up U/S at least 2 and 4 days later.
- Earlier reduction of twins (less than 16 days, prior to fixation) increases likelihood of success and continuation of remaining embryo/fetus to term.

Patient Monitoring

- After any method of twin reduction is performed, it is useful to monitor the progress and viability of the remaining embryo or fetus using U/S.
- It is critical to monitor the mare for embryo or fetal death if the mare is being treated with exogenous progestins.
- Once weekly U/S examinations are warranted for the first 3 weeks following the procedure.
- Less frequent examinations (i.e., once monthly) after the initial examinations, would be useful to monitor fetal progress.
- The mare can also be monitored for signs of abortion such as mammary development, vulvar discharge, or fetal expulsion.

Prevention/Avoidance

- Serial, complete TRP and maintenance of individual records for broodmares.
- Record sizes of all follicles larger than 30 mm on both ovaries during estrus (average growth is 5 to 6 mm/day) to account for ovulation or regression.
- Double ovulation: the earliest indicator of mares at higher risk for developing twins.
- Early diagnosis of pregnancy in mares from families with a history of twinning, or one known to have twinned in a prior pregnancy (same season or prior years).
- Earlier reduction is associated with greater success in achieving a singleton pregnancy.

Possible Complications

Embryonic or fetal loss, abortion, or dystocia.

Expected Course and Prognosis

Success associated with each reduction technique:
- Ninety percent success with early crush of a bicornual twin.
- Fifty percent with KCl intracardiac injection between days 115 and 130 of gestation.
- Twenty percent to 30% transvaginal aspiration of allantoic fluid from one of bicornual twins.

Abbreviations

BID   twice a day
BW   body weight
CL   corpus luteum
KCL   potassium chloride
IV   intravenous
PO   per os (by mouth)
SID   once a day
TRP   transrectal palpation
U/S   ultrasound, ultrasonography

See Also

- Abortion
- Early embryonic death
- Dystocia and parturient complications
- Placenta, placentitis

Suggested Reading

Ginther OJ. 1986. *Ultrasonic Imaging and Reproductive Events in the Mare*. Cross Plains, WI: Equiservices.
Ginther OJ. 1992. *Reproductive Biology of the Mare*, 2nd ed. Cross Plains, WI: Equiservices.

Authors: Carla L. Carleton and Margo L. Macpherson

chapter 67

Urine Pooling/Urovagina

DEFINITION/OVERVIEW

- Reflux of urine from the urethral orifice into the vagina and possibly the uterus; secondary to vaginal collection of urine; it is an abnormal circumstance. Vaginally retained urine enters the uterus when the cervix relaxes (during estrus or winter anestrus) or subsequent to the irritation, inflammation, and cervical relaxation caused by the presence of the urine.
- The presence of urine in the uterus may cause subfertility, infertility, and permanent endometrial, cervical, or vaginal damage. The mare may exhibit infertility or loss of pregnancy secondary to urine pooling.

ETIOLOGY/PATHOPHYSIOLOGY

- Urine pooling results from an altered position of the urethral orifice in its relationship to the vulvar commissure, vestibule, and vestibular sphincter.
- This changed anatomical relationship leads to incomplete voiding and, therefore, retention of urine within the vestibule and vagina.

Systems Affected

- Reproductive
- Urinary

SIGNALMENT/HISTORY

Inherited predisposition for poor VC and, thus, the altered location of the urethral orifice (to a more cranial position) may influence the frequency of this condition. May also develop secondary to loss of body condition and vaginal fat.

Risk Factors

- Incidence of urine pooling may increase with age, parity, and worsening VC.
- Occurs in all breeds, but mares with the least muscled perineal area (Thoroughbreds) have the highest incidence.
- The greatest incidence is reported in older pluriparous mares. With increasing age, the VC often deteriorates.

- This condition is frequently associated with:
  - An elevation and cranial tilting of the dorsal vulvar commissure accompanied by cranial displacement of the anal sphincter.
  - Frequently coupled with relaxation of the vestibule, which elevates the caudal urethral opening and permits urine to reflux into the cranial vagina.
  - Inherited conformational traits
  - Multiparous mares
  - Possible tendency for soft-tissue supporting structures of the vestibule, including the vestibular sphincter, to decrease their tonicity with age.
  - Old mares have a higher occurrence of this condition, and thin mares may be more predisposed to urine pooling.
- Urine pooling is most severe when the mare is in estrus and vestibular tissues are relaxed. If there is increased inflammation in the endometrium and longer term exposure, endometrial fibrosis may occur.

Historical Findings

- Mare continues to void urine after the main act of urination. May include dribbling of urine or frequent squatting and voiding even though the mare has just urinated. This behavior may appear similar to a mare in estrus.
- Urine scalding of the rear legs may also indicate improper/abnormal voiding of urine.
- On examination of the vestibular or vaginal wall, moderate to severe inflammation may be present.

 CLINICAL FEATURES

- There are few to no outward signs other than some urine possibly observed on the rear legs or the discharge of urine following a normal urination.
- The sole complaint may be subfertility or infertility. These mares may be bred multiple cycles but do not conceive or remain pregnant if conception were to occur.
- Sometimes when the stallion dismounts he may have urine or calcium carbonate crystals evident on the glans and shaft of the penis.
- Vaginal examination with a speculum will indicate moderate to severe inflammation of the vestibule, vaginitis, and scalding of the external os of the cervix, plus the presence of urine.
- Transrectal U/S examination may reveal luminal fluid within the uterus.

 DIFFERENTIAL DIAGNOSIS

Urine pooling must be differentiated from vaginitis due to other causes:
- Finding urine in the vagina is the first evidence that may provide conclusive evidence of urovagina.

- Pneumovagina can also cause severe inflammation of the vaginal wall, but in the absence of urine, as well, "urine burns" of the vaginal wall are absent.
- Differentiating urine from purulent material in the uterine lumen may be slightly more difficult, but urine will also be present in the vagina as well as in the uterus.

 ## DIAGNOSTICS

- U/S determination of urine is diagnostic, as is the visualization of urine in the vagina.
- Relative dorsal displacement of the external urethral os, combined with a downward slant (i.e., caudocranial) of the vagina towards the cervix, is helpful in arriving at the diagnosis of urine pooling.
- Carefully evaluate the spatial relationship of the urethral opening in relation to the dorsal and ventral vulvar commissure, vestibular sphincter, and vagina.

 ## THERAPEUTICS

- The primary method of treating this condition is surgical. The techniques are based on:
    - Elevation of the vestibular sphincter to prevent urine from moving forward
    - Extending the urethra caudally; thus the urine is voided from a more caudal location in the vestibule, increasing the likelihood it will be voided normally from the vestibule
- Another method that has been successful in thin mares is to increase their BCS above average, approaching the maximum score possible. This is generally not recommended for broodmares, but it has corrected the problem in some mares not worth the cost of surgical correction. Its success is attributed to deposition of fat in the pelvic area, ventral to the vaginal and anterior vestibular wall and thereby elevates the floor. The elevation of the vaginal and vestibular floor assists in moving urine caudally, emptying the vestibule.

Appropriate Health Care

- Broodmare perineal conformation should be evaluated prior to purchase. If severe compromise is present, perhaps seek out a better candidate for purchase if she is to be a broodmare. Mares affected by urine pooling and other perineal problems are not good broodmare purchase candidates.
- Once the problem exists, early diagnosis and treatment will be of great value in preventing permanent damage to the endometrium.

Nursing Care

There is no nursing care for this problem unless surgery is performed. With surgery, postoperative care is dependent on the technique used and recommendations of the surgeon.

Surgical Considerations

- Urethral extension is based on posterior relocation of the urethral orifice. The technique includes undermining strips of the vaginal wall, folding the left and right mucosal strips medially, and suturing them on the midline. This creates a caudal extension of the urethra; following surgery, the urethra is longer than it was preoperatively. The external urethral opening has been moved closer to the vulvae and urine exits more easily without reflux. Surgical repair is the only permanent means of correction.
  - The Pouret technique is utilized for repair of those mares with poor VC too extreme to be corrected by a Caslick's vulvoplasty alone. The Pouret technique is a transection of the perineal body. The pie-shaped dissection of the perineal body begins between the anal sphincter and the dorsal vulvar commissure, widest caudally (the wedge is in a flat plane from left to right), dissecting cranially. The distance (depth) to be separated is determined by the degree of correction required. With the dramatic division of the rectum from the vagina, the vagina slides ("falls") more caudally. The vulva in turn lies more caudal and ventral, thus also moving the urethral orifice more caudal. The anal sphincter remains in its approximate preoperative position. This not only aids with pneumovagina, but it decreases the possibility of urine pooling. Restraint to prevent mare movement during the procedure is critical to avoid dissection outside of the plane of the perineal body (dorsally lies the rectum, ventral to the plane of dissection lies the vagina).
  - A third technique is the Monin vaginoplasty. This intent of this technique is to build a dam on the ventral floor using ventral vestibular and vaginal tissue immediately cranial to the vestibular sphincter. The dam is to restrict urine from moving forward from the vestibule into the vagina. It has limited success and usually is torn at the time of the subsequent delivery.

 COMMENTS

Client Education

- In the absence of systemic signs (which I have never observed), systemic therapy is neither justified nor necessary. Flushing the urine from the uterus and vagina before insemination may increase the likelihood of conception but does not prevent subsequent, vaginal and cervical irritation, or urine accumulation and pregnancy loss.
- Urine pooling (i.e., the urethral orifice being drawn forward) becomes more extreme with increased weight of the uterus, fetus, placenta, and fluids later in gestation; subsequently pulls the entire vestibule further cranial and ventral.
- If poor vulvar and vestibular conformations are secondary to loss of vaginal fat (e.g., mare that is cachectic, thin, poor conditioning), urine pooling may be a slight problem and may resolve as the mare gains weight. Increasing fat within the pelvic cavity may elevate the vestibular floor in relationship to the ventral vulvar cleft and may provide some relief to thin mares. This is considered to be a temporary solution,

however, because the condition most likely will recur as the mare increases in age, parity, or experiences any subsequent weight loss.

Patient Monitoring

Mares should be carefully evaluated following any of the corrective techniques to be certain the technique was successful.

Prevention/Avoidance

There is no specific way to prevent this condition, but it can be diminished by not breeding the mare. Furthermore, examination of broodmare candidates before purchasing would be of value but seldom practiced. Conformation of the perineal area is inherited.

Possible Complications

The major complications of this condition are infertility and vaginitis. There is rarely any systemic involvement. It is localized to the reproductive tract.

Expected Course and Prognosis

Early recognition and treatment may assist in avoiding permanent damage to the vagina and endometrium. Without medical management (increasing mare's body condition/ weight) or surgical correction, mares will continue to pool urine. As the condition progresses, irritation increases as well as urine accumulation in the vagina and uterus.

Synonyms

- Urovagina
- Vesicovaginal reflux

Abbreviations

BCS body condition score
U/S ultrasound
VC vulvar conformation

See Also

- Vulvar conformation

Suggested Reading

McKinnon AO, Beldon JO. 1988. Urethral extension technique to correct urine pooling (vesicovaginal reflux) in mares. *JAVMA* 192: 647–650.
Shires GM, Kaneps AJ. 1986. A practical and simple surgical technique for repair of urine pooling in the mare. *Proc AAEP* 51–56.

Author: Walter R. Threlfall

chapter 68

Uterine Inertia

DEFINITION/OVERVIEW

Primary Uterine Inertia

- Failure of the myometrium to contract. May be associated or related to conditions, such as lack of exercise, over-conditioning, chronic illnesses, twinning, uterine disease, and aging.
- Can result in abnormal uterine contractions and failure to deliver the fetus and RFM.
- To increase the likelihood of delivering a live fetus with either type of uterine inertia, it is advisable to assist mares, once the condition has been diagnosed.

Secondary Uterine Inertia

- Usually follows prolonged labor without expulsion of the fetus and exhaustion of the myometrium.
- More common than primary uterine inertia.
- To increase the likelihood of delivering a live fetus with either type of uterine inertia, it is advisable to assist mares, once the condition has been diagnosed.

ETIOLOGY/PATHOPHYSIOLOGY

- Primary uterine inertia may result from the failure of the myometrium to respond to hormonal stimulation, a lack of hormonal release, or deficiency of hormonal receptors for oxytocin, estrogen, or $PGF_2\alpha$.
- The exact cause of secondary inertia is more easily understood, exhaustion of the myometrial muscle fibers occurs with a prolonged labor.
  - The major cause of secondary uterine inertia is dystocia.
  - Lack of exercise has been incriminated repeatedly as a cause.
  - The benefits observed in fit mares appear to be related to less fatigue during delivery and a shortened time to parturition possibly due to improved body tone and abdominal strength.
  - Over-conditioning and excess weight increase the likelihood of uterine inertia, as does restricted exercise during pregnancy.
  - Older mares are also prone to uterine inertia.

Systems Affected

- Reproductive
- Endocrine

SIGNALMENT/HISTORY

Risk Factors

- There does not appear to be any genetic link to these conditions.
- Incidence: Secondary uterine inertia occurs in less than 1% of foaling mares.
- All breeds and any female of breeding age.
- Incidence (primary or secondary) increases with age.
- Uterine inertia only occurs at parturition or shortly thereafter.

Historical Findings

- Mares in prolonged dystocia frequently are affected with secondary uterine inertia.
- Often a history of prolonged labor, followed by an absence of labor.

DIFFERENTIAL DIAGNOSIS

- Dystocia of other causes
- Colic

DIAGNOSTICS

- Determine the degree of uterine contractions by TRP, and vaginally, the space between the uterus and fetus.
- Observations of the mare's expulsive efforts are also beneficial.
- During examination of the uterus, determine if productive contractions are occurring.

THERAPEUTICS

- With primary uterine inertia, assisting with the delivery of the fetus is followed by the administration of oxytocin to assist the uterine contractions.
- On diagnosing secondary uterine inertia, no correction is possible prior to resolution of the dystocia. Priority: remove the fetus and permit the uterus to return to normal.
- Oxytocin should not be administered prior to delivery because it will cause uterine contractions around the fetus, compounding delivery problems.

- Foaling mares require assistance if normal delivery times for Stages 1 and 2 are exceeded.
  - The window of time for successful delivery (i.e., delivery of a live foal) is very short in the mare (70 minutes for Stage 2).
  - After removal of the fetus, oxytocin (10 IU, IM) is the hormone of choice.

Drug(s) of Choice

- Avoid high doses of oxytocin; they are unnecessary and may cause excessive contractions and the possibility of uterine prolapse.
- PGF$_2\alpha$ enhances uterine contractions.
- Regardless, do *not* attempt correction of uterine inertia before the fetus is delivered, and only then treat with low doses (10 IU, IM) of oxytocin.

 COMMENTS

Patient Monitoring

- Postpartum uterine examinations are essential to monitor treatment progress.
- Determine if involution is proceeding normally after oxytocin administration.
- Confirm that all fetal membranes have been passed.

Prevention/Avoidance

- Exercise and proper nutrition play important roles in preventing primary uterine inertia although their exact mechanism is unknown.
- Secondary uterine inertia occurs most often. It may be impossible to prevent unless parturition is observed and assistance rendered as soon as dystocia is observed and prior to development of secondary uterine inertia.

Possible Complications

- Administration of oxytocin prior to fetal delivery can result in strong segmental contractions, making fetal delivery yet more difficult.
- Administration of too high doses of oxytocin may result in possible uterine prolapse.
- RFM are much more common in cases of uterine inertia. There is also an increase in delayed uterine involution following parturition. Both RFM and delayed uterine involution may result in uterine infection or inflammation, and a further delay in rebreeding, or result in infertility.

Expected Course and Prognosis

- Prognosis is excellent with proper treatment.
- It may be warranted to skip breeding on foal heat and wait to the next heat, or short cycle the mare to save reproductive time. Reserve making the final decision regarding

foal-heat breeding until examination of the uterus near to or at the time just prior to breeding. The reason is because some mares recover quickly.

Abbreviations

IM   intramuscular
PGF   natural prostaglandin
RFM   retained fetal membranes
TRP   transrectal palpation

Suggested Reading

Roberts SJ. 1986. *Veterinary Obstetrics and Genital Diseases—Theriogenology*, 3rd ed. Woodstock, VT: Author; 347–352.

Author: Walter R. Threlfall

chapter 69

Uterine Torsion

DEFINITION/OVERVIEW

Clockwise or counterclockwise torsion or twisting of the uterine horns at the uterine body that can, but usually does not, extend caudally to involve the cervix.

ETIOLOGY/PATHOPHYSIOLOGY

- A lengthening of the broad ligament during gestation and possible influence by previous pregnancies that permits the uterus (due to decreased broad ligament suspension) to twist around itself.
- This lengthening may result from repeated stretching during previous gestations, rapid movement of the fetus, or rolling or falling and turning of the mare, with one occurring faster than the speed with which the other is rotating.

Systems Affected

Reproductive

SIGNALMENT/HISTORY

- No hereditary predisposition for uterine torsion but for a possible link with large abdominal size.
  - All breeds with deeper bodies or larger abdomens are most affected.
  - All mares of breeding age that are pregnant are predisposed to uterine torsion because the condition is not reported in the nonpregnant mare.
  - Increased occurrence in pluripara mares, but primipara mares can be affected.
  - If the supporting tissue (i.e., broad ligament) is longer in some animals because of genetics, this could support that theory of hereditary predisposition.
- Conditions during which there would be less ingesta within the abdomen.
- Either instance allows more space for a torsion if the additional circumstances occur that put a mare at risk.

- Although there is an infrequent occurrence of this condition in mares, it can occur anytime during the last 6 months of pregnancy, but it usually occurs between 6 and 9 months.
- The condition should be corrected when first diagnosed.
- The later in gestation uterine torsion occurs, the more serious the consequences can be for both the mare and the fetus.

Historical Findings

- The mare can exhibit a variety of clinical signs, depending on the stage of gestation when the torsion occurs.
- Mares may present with signs of slight to mild colic, be inappetent, depressed, or exhibit a general decrease or increase in activity, apprehension, sweating, and increased urination.

 CLINICAL FEATURES

- Depending on stage of gestation, the mare may exhibit a tense abdomen with an increased auscultation and increased respiratory rate.
- TRP examination reveals twisting of the broad ligament and body of the uterus or cervix.
- A reliable TRP finding confirming torsion is one broad ligament crossing to the opposite side. One broad ligament will cross over the uterine body and the opposite broad ligament will lie under the uterine body.
- Vaginal examinations are less valuable in mares (compared with cows) because vaginal involvement is less common in mare uterine torsions.
- Also torsions of the mare's uterus are less common at term gestation than in the cow.
- However, if the torsion does occur at term, the mare may fail to show signs of labor because the fetus is unable to enter the pelvic canal and cervix (i.e., setting up the circumstance for an absence of Ferguson's reflex, by virtue of no point pressure contacting the cervix). Therefore, fetal death may occur from placental separation without the owner's knowledge of the mare being in labor.

 DIFFERENTIAL DIAGNOSIS

- Intestinal colic: rule out by TRP examination of the uterus and broad ligaments.
- Onset of a normal parturition.
- Keep in mind that the majority of mare uterine torsions occur prior to term. History is of value, as well as TRP and possible vaginal examination, if indicated.

- TRP examination of the broad ligaments will determine the direction (clockwise or counterclockwise) of torsion. Knowledge of direction is essential to proper resolution.

 # DIAGNOSTICS

- Transabdominal U/S examinations, if necessary, aid in the determination of fetal viability.
- The uterus is rotated clockwise or counterclockwise; increased tension on the broad ligament; the uterine wall may exhibit increased tone.
- Although counterclockwise torsion is more common than clockwise torsion, never assume this to be the case as clockwise torsions do occur.

 # THERAPEUTICS

Options for resolution and prognosis:
- Rolling to correct uterine torsion. Unlike uterine torsion in a cow, in which rolling can be accomplished without anesthesia, the mare must be placed under general anesthesia. This alone makes this procedure much more difficult. It usually is not indicated, unless sufficient help is available and the mare is less than 9 months of gestation.
    - Multiple assistants are required to roll the mare rapidly in the direction of the torsion.
    - The mare is dropped on the side toward which the torsion turns. A mare with a clockwise torsion (as viewed from the rear of the mare) would be placed down on her right side. A mare with a counterclockwise torsion would be laid down on her left side. The mare is then rolled rapidly over her back with the idea of rolling the mare faster than the rotation of her uterus.
    - Contraindications for rolling a mare as she approaches term are uterine artery rupture or uterine wall tears; more common in mares than cows that are rolled to "undo" a torsion.
    - Assistance may be required following the procedure until the mare recovers from anesthesia.
- Laparotomy is the technique more successful and commonly used to resolve a mare's uterine torsion.
    - Minimal assistance is required: the surgeon and horse handler. Uterine repositioning is very successful, especially when gestation is 9 months or less.
    - As the mare approaches term, additional help may be required, including the possibility of a second incision to permit another surgeon to work from the opposite flank because of the size and weight of the fetus and fetal fluids.
    - If the torsion occurs at term, a C-section may be required to deliver the fetus and save the mare.

- C-section is usually not necessary because most torsions occur before the onset of labor.

Drug(s) of Choice

- Xylazine (1.1 mg/kg IV), followed 5 to 10 minutes later with morphine (0.1 mg/kg, IM or 0.05–0.12 mg/kg IV), detomidine HCl (0.02–0.04 mg/kg IV or IM), or drug of choice for heavy sedation.
- Following this, the prepped area can be infiltrated prior to incision with 2% carbocaine to effect.

Appropriate Health Care

An accurate diagnosis is extremely important in the correction of uterine torsion before the fetus dies. If left untreated, a torsion of greater than 180 degrees compromises the blood supply to the fetus and uterus, and fetal death may occur, especially if the mare is approaching term.

Activity

After correction of the torsion, stall rest of the mare is indicated; hand-walking multiple times per day until parturition is appropriate. Prevent the mare from running or having the opportunity to roll (strong recommendation) until parturition.

Surgical Considerations

- Laparotomy is the more common and successful means to manage a mare's uterine torsion. Requires minimal assistance to reposition the uterus if the gestation is no more than 9 months.
- As the mare approaches term, additional help may be required, including the possibility of a second incision to allow a second surgeon to work from the opposite flank (necessitated by the increased size and weight of the fetus and fetal fluids).
- If one incision is sufficient, it must be of adequate length to allow the surgeon to pull the ventral aspect of the uterus into proper position. It is easier to pull the uterus from the ventral aspect than it is to push the uterus and fetus from its dorsal aspect.
- If a second incision is necessary, it is made in the opposite flank. A second surgeon pulls the dorsal aspect of the uterus as the primary surgeon applies traction to the ventral aspect of the uterus. The two combined efforts provide the rotation necessary to return the uterus to its normal orientation (left horn to the left, right horn to the right).
- If the torsion occurs at term gestation, a C-section may be required to deliver the fetus and save the mare. This can be performed at the time the uterine torsion is corrected, but it is important to correct the torsion before incising the uterus to

extract the fetus. Subsequent uterine suturing is also easier with the properly oriented uterus. Usually a C-section is only necessary with a term fetus and delivery must be immediate, or if the fetus is dead and vaginal delivery is not possible. C-section is usually not necessary because most torsions occur before the onset of labor.

- Procedural comments:
  - A grid incision in the flank usually provides insufficient area for manipulation. Therefore, an incision of the abdominal muscles is necessary. One hand is moved ventrally under the uterus, a hock or other fetal extremity is grasped, and then pulled toward the incision.
  - At first, the uterus will be difficult to move, but as it begins to return to its normal position, movement becomes easier. It may be necessary to get the uterus "swinging" back and forth before being able to return it to its proper position. Once uterine detorsion passes the halfway point, it will easily move the remainder of the distance.
  - If one person is incapable of returning the uterus to its normal position, a second incision can be made on the opposite side of the mare. Both surgeons' efforts, in tandem, pull (rotate) the uterus to its normal position.
  - Refer to Drug(s) of Choice for dosing recommendations: xylazine administered IV, followed 5 to 10 minutes later with intravenous morphine, detomidine, or drug of choice can be used for heavy sedation. Following this, the prepped area can be infiltrated prior to incision with 2% carbocaine, to effect.

 COMMENTS

Client Education

- As with any condition of pregnant mares, subtle changes in the mare's demeanor or behavior may indicate abnormal gestation and immediate assistance should be sought.
- Bedding changes in the stall may reduce rolling, cross-tying would be beneficial if the mare will tolerate this procedure. Any other managerial option that may discourage the mare from rolling in the stall will be of value.
- The mare's diet should permit access to free-choice hay to help keep the abdomen as full as possible and thus reduce the space for a torsion to occur. Quality of the hay is not as important as quantity.

Patient Monitoring

- Frequent monitoring following correction of uterine torsion, to include close, daily observation and TRP of the broad ligaments and uterus.
- Examination of the uterus at 1- to 2-week intervals is indicated until it appears that recurrence is unlikely.
- For mares at term and in labor, recurrence of this condition after delivery has not been reported.

Prevention/Avoidance

- The only definite way to avoid this condition is not to breed the mare.
- Limiting exercise is one possible method to reduce the likelihood of the mare falling or rolling, but it is rarely indicated or warranted. Limited exercise also creates other problems such as an increase in difficult deliveries because of restricted exercise.
- Available free-choice hay may reduce the occurrence of abdominal colic.

Possible Complications

- Confirm the diagnosis as rapidly as possible, especially if the mare is near term, to save the fetus.
- As the mare approaches term pregnancy: uterine artery rupture or uterine wall tears are more common with the rolling technique than when this procedure is used to relieve torsion in cows.
- Uterine torsion can result in prolonged delivery and fetal death.
- Be certain of the direction of the torsion's rotation. Otherwise, during "correction," the condition may actually be made worse.
- Administration of the suggested agents for sedation or anesthesia should not be detrimental to fetal viability at any stage of gestation.

Expected Course and Prognosis

- Correction of uterine torsion before term requires follow-up examinations.
- Although recurrence is uncommon, it has been reported even with the best of post-corrective care.

Abbreviations

HCl   hydrochloride
IM   intramuscular
IV   intravenous
TRP   transrectal palpation
U/S   ultrasound, ultrasonography

See Also

- Dystocia
- Premature placental separation
- Stages of normal parturition

Suggested Reading

Guthrie RG. 1982. Rolling for correction of uterine torsion in a mare. *JAVMA* 181: 66–67.
Perkins NR, Robertson JT, Colon LA. 1992. Uterine torsion and uterine tear in a mare. *JAVMA* 201: 92–94.

Vaughan JT. 1986. Equine urogenital systems. In: *Current Therapy in Theriogenology*, 2nd ed. Morrow DA (ed). Philadelphia: W. B. Saunders; 756–775.

Wichtel JJ, Reinertson EL, Clark TL. 1988. Nonsurgical treatment of uterine torsion in seven mares. *JAVMA* 193: 337–338.

Youngquist RS. Equine obstetrics. 1986. In: *Current Therapy in Theriogenology*. Morrow DA (ed). Philadelphia: W. B. Saunders; 699.

Author: Walter R. Threlfall

Vaccination Protocols, Mare

chapter 70

DEFINITION/OVERVIEW

Before vaccinating the mare, certain considerations need to be addressed:
- The dam's vaccination status, the mare's foaling date, her geographical location, likelihood of being transported and moved off-farm (i.e., showing, breeding, production sale, and so on), the client's budgetary constraints, morbidity/mortality associated with individual diseases for which vaccines are available, and the efficacy of different vaccine products.
- Timing is based on her need for protection against endemic disease as well as ensuring there is adequate passive immunity for the neonate after it ingests colostrum soon after foaling.
  - In general, mare vaccinations usually allow for annual vaccinations (once a year).
  - However, when a mare foals early in the year, certain vector-transmitted diseases may require that the mare be vaccinated once to provide high antibody levels in colostrum and a second time (later in the year) to provide the mare with optimal protection.
- All vaccinations presently marketed are safe for pregnant mares, but vaccination during the first trimester of pregnancy should be avoided if possible, to reduce the slight risk of early pregnancy loss or of impacting fetal organogenesis (teratogenic effect).
- However, if the mare is unvaccinated or her vaccinal history is unknown, core vaccines need to be administered to offer protection against known endemic diseases.
- In the face of a known disease outbreak, core vaccines may prevent severe illness or death of the mare.

ETIOLOGY/PATHOPHYSIOLOGY

Systems Affected

- Hemic
- Lymphatic
- Immune

SIGNALMENT/HISTORY

Risk Factors

- Do not give tetanus antitoxin to mares because there is an increased risk of developing serum hepatitis (Theiler's Disease).
- When an injury occurs, if it has been more than 6 months since her prior tetanus protection, the mare should be administered a booster injection of tetanus toxoid and be placed on appropriate antibiotics.

CLINICAL FEATURES

- All North American mares should be vaccinated against: tetanus, EEE,WEE, WNV, and rabies where it is endemic. These vaccines are considered core due to their demonstrated efficacy, safety, and low risk of side effects. In unvaccinated individuals, these diseases usually result in death. In addition, rabies is a zoonotic disease. If unvaccinated or with an unknown history, mares are usually administered a series of vaccinations similar to the recommendations for foals (See foal vaccination chapter). In addition, pregnant mares should be vaccinated several times with a killed vaccine for EHV-1 and EHV-4 when they are pregnant to reduce the risk of an abortion storm.
- Diseases included are in order of their importance, morbidity/mortality/frequency of exposure or relationship to equine health:

Tetanus

- The dam needs to receive an annual vaccination 4 to 6 weeks prior to foaling.

EEE/WEE

- Annual vaccination is required 4 to 6 weeks prior to foaling.
- If insects are present year round, vaccination may be necessary semiannually. Vaccine immunity lasts no more than 6 to 8 months.
  - Early foaling mares in the northern regions of North America will need to be vaccinated 4 to 6 weeks before foaling and then be administered a booster vaccination during the summer to ensure she remains protected for the entire mosquito season.
  - In the southern areas of North America, mares are routinely vaccinated twice a year.

VEE

Recommendations for VEE mirror those for EEE/WEE in areas where it is present or outbreaks have been reported.

- Present in Mexico, South and Central America; therefore, equids residing in the southern United States are potentially at greater risk for exposure.

WNV

- The protocol employed is dependent on the product chosen. Currently four products are licensed for protection against WNV.
  1. Inactivated vaccine: The timelines for vaccination mirror those for the encephalitides. If starting a vaccination series in an unvaccinated mare, optimal protection is not achieved until 3 to 4 weeks after the booster has been administered.
  2. Canary pox vaccine: Vaccination follows the protocol for EEE/WEE. If starting a series in an unvaccinated mare, some protection is achieved after the initial vaccination with optimal protection after administration of the booster vaccine.
  3. Flavivirus chimera vaccine: Vaccination follows the protocol for EEE/WEE. In the unvaccinated mare, one vaccination provides protection. In an unvaccinated mare during the vector season, this is the vaccine of choice.
  4. DNA vaccine: This vaccine uses purified DNA plasmids to stimulate an immune response. Annual vaccination provides a 12-month duration of immunity. In unvaccinated mares, an initial vaccine is given with a booster vaccination 4 weeks later, followed by annual vaccination. It is not currently being marketed.
- Annual vaccination may be administered using any of the aforementioned products without concern for the product used the previous year.

Rabies

- The dam needs to receive an annual vaccination 4 to 6 weeks prior to foaling. However, if there is concern about vaccinating the late-term pregnant mare, the rabies vaccine may be given after foaling and will provide adequate colostral antibodies for subsequent foalings.
- Because rabies is zoonotic and fatal, all horses in or traveling to endemic areas should be protected.

Herpes/Rhinopneumonitis

- EHV-1 and EHV-4.
- Most often results in respiratory disease, rather than its abortive (EHV-1, rarely EHV-4) or neurologic form (EHV-1). However, because abortions can both be sporadic or an abortion storm, vaccination is recommended using a killed product.
- Herpes viruses persist and can recrudesce during periods of stress (e.g., foaling, transport, introduction of new horses, and so on).
- Recommendations for vaccination require that the vaccine be given at 5, 7, and 9 months of gestation; however, I have had EHV-1 abortions occur at 5 months, vaccination may be started as early as 3 months of gestation. Efficacy of the vaccine is no better than 80% (i.e., vaccinated animals may still develop disease).
- No vaccine protects against the neurologic form of EHV-1. Older animals may be at greater risk of developing neurologic Herpes.

Influenza

- The dam needs to receive an annual vaccination 4 to 6 weeks prior to foaling.
- There are two types of vaccine, an inactivated form and an intranasal MLV.
  - Many companies market an inactivated vaccine. Calvenza® (Boehringer-Ingelheim) is an inactivated product that can be used either IM or intranasally.
  - A MLV vaccine is also available and is called Flu-avert® (Intervet).

Strangles

- Vaccination for Strangles should only be considered for mares where there is a high likelihood for exposure, such as large breeding farms.
- There are two types of vaccine, an inactivated form (cell wall derivative, Strepguard) and an intranasal MLV (Pinnacle).

Rotavirus

- Administered to pregnant mares at 8, 9, and 10 months of gestation to provide colostral protection for the foal.

Botulism (If Endemic)

- Mares are vaccinated 4 to 6 weeks prior to foaling to prevent Shaker Foal Disease. If the mare received no prior vaccinations, she will require a series of three vaccinations given at monthly intervals, with the last to be administered 1 month prior to foaling.
- Although multiple toxins exist, the vaccine only contains the B-toxin which is predominant in the southeast and west coast.

PHF

- The current vaccine contains only one strain of *Neorickettsia risticii*. Multiple inactivated, whole cell vaccines of this strain exist.
- However, of the more than 14 strains of *N. risticii*, the vaccine is not protective against these other strains.
- If the vaccine is to be used, vaccinate 4 to 6 weeks prior to foaling. Booster vaccinations are typically administered every 3 to 4 months during vector season.

EVA

- Modified live vaccine (Arvac®) produced by Pfizer Animal Health.
- Appropriate for mares being bred to a known positive stallion (semen shedder).
- The vaccine should be given no less than 3 weeks prior to breeding (live cover or AI).
- EVA can persist in frozen and cooled semen.
- If the mare is intended for export, vaccine administration may be contraindicated because some countries prohibit entry of horses with a titer against EVA. Confirm a

country's status for imported horses or horses in transit: may range from acceptance of horses only with no titer or those with stable or falling titers. That also means that breeding to an EVA shedding stallion should be avoided.

- Vaccinated mares should be isolated from nonvaccinated animals and all pregnant mares for at least 3 to 4 weeks.

 # DIAGNOSTICS

Strangles or WNV: may test for high titer before electing to vaccinate.

 # THERAPEUTICS

Precautions/Interactions

Strangles: the development of purpura hemorrhagica is possible either from disease or of vaccine origin.

Appropriate Health Care

- If a mare reacts to a certain vaccine, first assess the risk of disease/complications versus the benefit of the vaccine.
- If vaccination is deemed necessary, initially, select a different company's vaccine because the adjuvant will be different. If the mare still reacts to the vaccine and the vaccine is a combination product, vaccinate the mare with the individual component vaccines.
- In addition, premedicating the mare with flunixin meglumine may be warranted.

 # COMMENTS

Client Education

Because muscle soreness may occur post-vaccination, do not vaccinate within 7 to 10 days of showing. Also, to reduce the risk of the mare developing multiple sore muscles, limit the number of vaccines given at one time to no more than two or three products and give any subsequent vaccines at least 1 week later.

Possible Complications

- Abscessation at injection site.
- Clostridial myositis has been reported post-vaccination.

Abbreviations

AI	artificial insemination
EEE	eastern equine encephalitis
EHV	equine herpes virus
EVA	equine viral arteritis
IM	intramuscular
MLV	modified live virus
PHF	Potomac Horse Fever
VEE	Venezuelan equine encephalitis
WEE	western equine encephalitis
WNV	West Nile Virus

See Also

May refer to specific diseases against which vaccinations are to be protective.

Suggested Reading

AAEP Vaccination Guidelines, revised 2008. www.aaep.org/vaccination_guidelines.htm.

Foote CE, Love DN, Gilkerson JR, et al. 2004. Detection of EHV-1 and EHV-4 DNA in unweaned Thoroughbred foals from vaccinated mares on a large stud farm. *Eq Vet J* 36: 341–345.

Holyoak GR, Balasuriya UB, Broaddus CC, et al. 2008. Equine viral arteritis: Current status and prevention. *Therio* 70(3): 403–414.

www.boehringer-ingelheim.com/corporate/products/animal_health_horse_01.htm

www.intervet.ca/products/flu_avert__i_n__vaccine/020_product_details.asp

http://merial.com/

http://pfizer.com/products/animal_health/animal_health.jsp

Author: Judith V. Marteniuk

chapter 71

Vaginal Prolapse

DEFINITION/OVERVIEW

A displacement of all or part of the vaginal wall caudally through the vulvae.

ETIOLOGY/PATHOPHYSIOLOGY

- Predisposing factors: relaxation of the vaginal wall or vulvar lips, such as occurs near parturition. Relaxation at either location permits the possibility of vaginal wall protrusion. Furthermore, the increased abdominal pressure caused by the pregnancy places additional pressure on the vaginal wall.
- A previous dystocia may have damaged or weakened the perineal area, including the vagina and vulva, adding to the possibility of vaginal prolapse.
- The incidence is low and there appears to be no genetic link.

Systems Affected

Reproductive

SIGNALMENT/HISTORY

All breeds and all females of breeding age are affected.

Risk Factors

- Vaginal prolapse is often secondary to other abnormalities, conditions that predispose mares to everting part of the vaginal wall.
- This may cause straining and additional tissue protrusion and injury.
- Usually occurs immediately postpartum.

Historical Findings

There is history of the mare straining. Clients often report of seeing tissue protrude during these episodes of straining.

CLINICAL FEATURES

- The vaginal wall protrudes through the vulvae. It may become damaged due to exposure, with the damage permitting paravaginal fat to protrude through the already prolapsed wall. This protruded fat may complicate/add to the existing straining and result in further prolapse.
- The protruding tissue has a characteristic pink to red color, depending on the length of time it has been outside the body. The color can change to dried and necrotic with the passage of time and further damage.
- Differentiating vagina from the bladder, intestines, uterus, cervix, and vestibule is essential before initiating treatment.

DIFFERENTIAL DIAGNOSIS

- Eversion of the urinary bladder, uterus, or cervix (Fig. 71.1).
- Vaginal tears through which paravaginal fat or intestines is protruding.
- Eversion of the vestibular wall occurs more frequently than a vaginal prolapse (closer proximity to the vulvar opening).

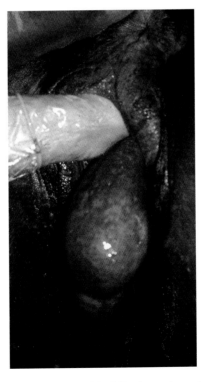

■ **Figure 71.1** Prolapse (eversion) of the urinary bladder following prolonged postpartum straining in a Belgian mare. Image courtesy of C. L. Carleton.

DIAGNOSTICS

Critical to a proper diagnosis is the careful visual and digital examination to differentiate vaginal wall from other prolapsed tissues.

 ## THERAPEUTICS

- The first consideration of therapy is to achieve reduction of the prolapse (i.e., return tissues to their normal anatomic location) and terminate subsequent expulsive efforts. This is critical to a permanent resolution.
- Treatment must include reduction of inflammation, if it is present, and it usually is.
- There is no restriction of activity, unless the activity increases abdominal pressure.
- Any protrusion of tissue through the vulvar lips requires immediate attention and correction.
- A Caslick's vulvoplasty may help prevent further vaginal irritation and thus, decrease the likelihood of additional straining and tissue damage. Vulvoplasty, however, does not prevent recurrent prolapse from continued straining because mares may strain and tear the perineal tissue (see Chapter 73).

Appropriate Health Care

Epidural anesthetic may be indicated to reduce straining early on. This may be combined with the application of local, nonirritating antibiotics in the early stages of resolution/recovery.

Surgical Considerations

Replacement of the tissue and retention is superior to attempted excision of excess tissue. Removal may cause scaring and reduction in the size of the vestibular canal for the next foaling.

 ## COMMENTS

Client Education

If anything is protruding from the vulva at a time other than at foaling, or it appears abnormal, the client should call her or his veterinarian immediately.

Patient Monitoring

At reexamination, conduct a careful and gentle assessment of previously affected tissues to prevent renewed irritation and initiating a subsequent bout of straining.

Prevention/Avoidance

- Early treatment is indicated for any condition (e.g., vaginal damage or irritation) that may initiate straining and result in eventual prolapse of the vaginal wall.
- Once recognized, early initiation of treatment of prolapsed vaginal tissue is critical to limit tissue trauma.

Possible Complications

Possible complications of prolapsed vagina include infections and abscessation of or within the vaginal wall.

Expected Course and Prognosis

- Rapid recovery if the inciting cause is removed and the vaginal tissue returned to its normal position and protected from further irritation.
- Satisfactory recovery if further damage can be avoided.
- The time to diagnosis and treatment is extremely important to the degree of recovery of this condition.

See Also

- Dystocia
- Postpartum care, mare and foal
- Vaginitis and vaginal discharge
- Vulvar conformation

Suggested Reading

Cox JE. 1987. *Surgery of the Reproductive Tract in Large Animals.* Liverpool: Liverpool University Press; 127–143.

Author: Walter R. Threlfall

chapter 72

Vaginitis and Vaginal Discharge

DEFINITION/OVERVIEW

- Vaginitis can be the result of any condition that causes inflammation of the vagina, with or without infection.
- Vaginitis may result in a vulvar discharge but generally does not.
- It may be indicative of a venereal disease (Fig. 72.1) but usually is not.

ETIOLOGY/PATHOPHYSIOLOGY

- The first consideration is determination of the source of the discharge (Fig. 72.2). Establish if it originates from the vagina, vestibule, or the urethra.
- Pneumovagina is one of the major causes of vestibular and vaginal inflammation. Pneumovagina is primarily caused by abnormal VC. It may also occur in fillies or mares in training or racing because of incomplete vulvar closure.

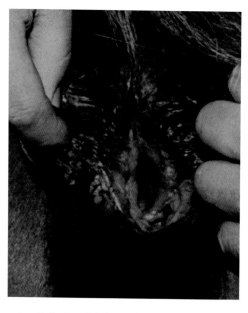

■ **Figure 72.1** Equine herpes virus-3, Equine Coital Exanthema.

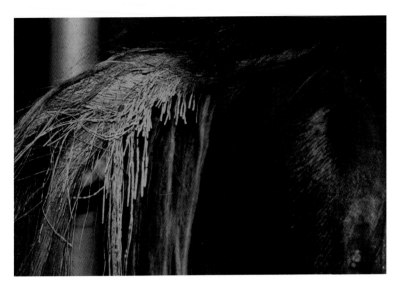

■ **Figure 72.2** Chronic discharge on a mare's tail; an unusual presentation. Image courtesy of C. L. Carleton.

■ Breed differences increase the incidence in mares with poor body condition (i.e., little fat) or less muscle in the perineal area. Thoroughbreds will have more of a problem with pneumovagina than will Quarter Horses.

Systems Affected

■ Reproductive
■ Urinary

    # SIGNALMENT/HISTORY

Risk Factors

■ There is definite possibility for inheritance of poor VC, which can result in vaginitis due to inflammation or infection.
■ Incidence of vaginitis increases with age and parity/number of parturitions.
■ It occurs in all breeds, especially females of breeding age.
■ A summary of causes or associations responsible for vaginitis and vulvar discharge include: poor VC, trauma at parturition, vaginal breeding injury, pneumovagina, and multiparous broodmares.

Historical Findings

Infertility or subfertility often accompanies mares with a history of vulvar discharge and vaginitis. The discharge may be present periodically throughout the estrous cycle.

CLINICAL FEATURES

- A normal discharge may be noted on a mare's vulvar lips, especially when she is in estrus. During estrus and in particular when she is being teased, the mare urinates frequently and often repeatedly in small amounts. This results in evacuation of calcium carbonate crystals, a predominant component in equine urine sediment. The calcium carbonate crystals often accumulate at or on the ventral vulvar commissure (a normal finding).
- Abnormal discharges can be of mucoid or fluid consistency and may be malodorous. Their color can range from white to yellow to brown. It must be remembered that mares may have vaginitis without any external discharge or signs.
- When discharges are secondary to infection or inflammation, there may be discharge on the tail and perineum and fluid in the vagina or uterus. There will also be hyperemia of the vaginal mucosa (see Fig. 72.2).
- Abrasions, ulcerations (*see* Fig. 72.2 and Fig. 72.3), and lacerations of the vaginal or vestibular wall or perineum may be present. Recent or chronic adhesions or fibrin

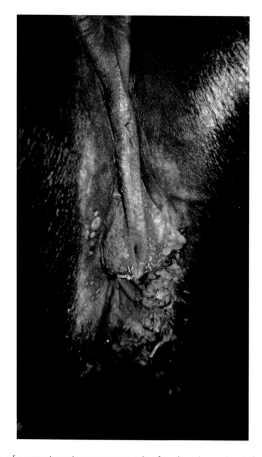

■ **Figure 72.3** Ulceration of a mare's perineum as a result of a chronic uterine infection.

deposition may be present in longer term infections or inflammation of the vagina or vestibule. Large amounts of discharge may be adhered to the tail or attract flies during summer months. Discharges may be evident only when the mare is more excitable, being ridden or worked.

DIFFERENTIAL DIAGNOSIS

- Uterine disease/infection
- Urinary tract infections
- Vaginitis and vulvar discharge can be linked with uterine contamination and result in metritis, endometritis, or pyometra (Fig. 72.3).
- Vaginal/vulvar tumors or metastases (Figs. 72.4, 72.5a, b, and c).

DIAGNOSTICS

Careful speculum examination per vagina is the best means to establish a definitive diagnosis.

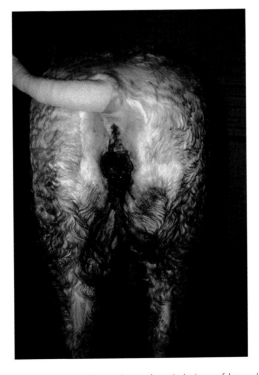

■ **Figure 72.4** Vulvar discharge of a mare with erosive melanotic lesions of her vulvae.

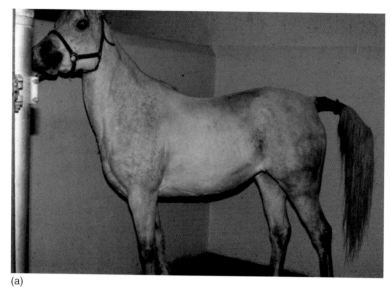

(a)

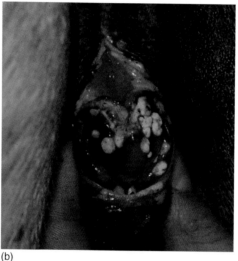

(b)

■ **Figure 72.5** Aged mare presented for unusual appearance of her vulva and clitoris. Owners thought she had an infection *(a)*. Clitoral appearance of aged mare, minimal discharge *(b)*. Primary tumor of aged mare, osteosarcoma, metastasized to the genital tract *(c)*.
Images courtesy of C. L. Carleton.

THERAPEUTICS

- The cause of vaginitis or vulvar discharge must be determined before treatment can be initiated.
- If only vaginitis is present (i.e., not secondary to injury), treatment need only halt the chronic contamination, and inflammation should subside. Systemic antibiotics

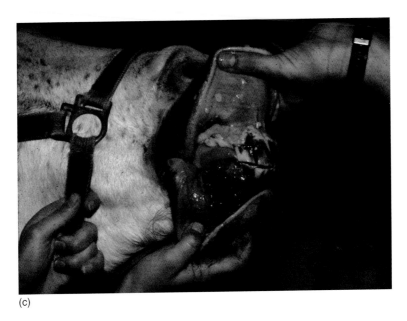

(c)

■ **Figure 72.5** continued

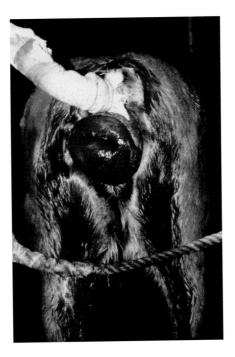

■ **Figure 72.6** Rectal prolapse, postpartum Belgian mare.

have no value. Local therapy with antibiotics can be useful, if indicated. Chronic vaginitis, especially postpartum, can lead to severe straining and in its extreme, chronic (if unattended) presentation, rectal prolapse (Fig. 72.6) or bladder eversion (Figs. 72.7a and b).

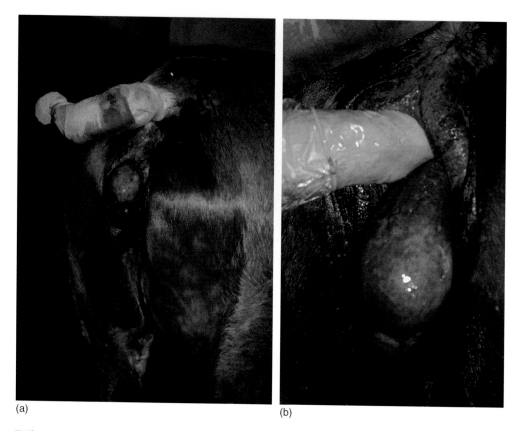

(a)   (b)

■ **Figure 72.7** Bladder eversion, postpartum Belgian mare *(a)*.
Bladder eversion (close-up), postpartum Belgian mare *(b)*.
Images courtesy of C. L. Carleton.

■ A Caslick's vulvoplasty is the surgical procedure by which deficits of VC are repaired (see Chapter 73). It reduces further contamination of the genital tract. If indicated after vulvoplasty, nonirritating, local application of antibiotics may reduce the mare's discomfort. This is usually unnecessary because inflammation decreases rapidly once the source of irritation has been eliminated.

Activity

Mares should be examined during exercise and/or during estrus, because the problem may be more obvious at these times. However, the best method to diagnose the condition is to visually examine the vestibule and vagina for indications of inflammation.

Surgical Considerations

The surgical correction of choice is the Caslick's vulvoplasty. It greatly reduces the probability that vaginitis and vaginal discharge will occur or continue (see Chapter 73).

COMMENTS

Client Education

- Essential to educate clients regarding the problems attributable to poor VC, vaginitis, and vaginal discharge.
- These latter conditions can lead to severe uterine infections even in pleasure horses and may even render that animal unusable as a pleasure horse (e.g., as may occur with cases of chronic pyometra).

Patient Monitoring

- Reexamination and removal of sutures approximately 2 weeks following vulvoplasty is indicated.
- If a Caslick's vulvoplasty has not been done in the past, the mare's VC should be examined at least annually to determine if it is still providing adequate protection of her genital tract from ascending infection or contamination.
- There are significant variations between breeds relative to VC. A significant percentage of the predominant U.S. racing breeds (thoroughbreds, standardbreds) are known for their less than stellar VC.
- VC decreases with age, parity, foaling trauma, prior Caslick's repairs (depending on the procedure used, the degree of scar tissue in the vulvae may make subsequent repairs more challenging), and so on.
- Preventing problems by timely addressing ascending inflammation is much superior to treatment after the fact.

Prevention/Avoidance

- A Caslick's vulvoplasty or other cosmetic repair of the vulva is indicated whenever a defect is present (See Fig. 73.5).
- Mares born with poor VC have an increased likelihood of vaginitis and are not ideal broodmare candidates. Surgical repair should be performed as soon as the defect is observed. There are breed and individual mare predispositions for vulvar abnormalities.
- Any postpartum injury to the genital tract should also be repaired as soon as possible postpartum.

Possible Complications

- If left untreated, vaginitis or vestibular inflammation or infection may result in infertility, endometrial damage, or vaginal adhesions.
- May prevent pregnancy or cause premature termination of pregnancy as well as result in placentitis.

Expected Course and Prognosis

- If treated early in the course of disease, excellent resolution and normal fertility should be expected.
- Uterine culture and biopsy are recommended if a vaginitis or inflammation of the vestibule has been present; ensure the uterus has not become inflamed or infected in the interim, to prepare the broodmare for optimal reproductive health.

Abbreviations

VC   vulvar conformation

See Also

- Dystocia
- Endometritis
- Metritis
- Pneumovagina/Pneumouterus
- Vulvar conformation

Suggested Reading

Ricketts SW. 1991. Vaginal discharge in the mare. In: *Equine Practice*. Boden E (ed). Philadelphia: Bailliere Tindall; 1–26.

Authors: Walter R. Threlfall and Carla L. Carleton

chapter 73

Vulvar Conformation

DEFINITION/OVERVIEW

- The quality or grade of a mare's VC is determined by the anatomic orientation of the anal sphincter to the vulvae and pubis. This orientation impacts directly on the mare's reproductive health and affects her ability to maintain a healthy uterus and to carry pregnancies to term. The vulva is the first line of defense in keeping foreign substances, including bacteria, out of the reproductive tract.
  - Good VC implies the dorsal commissure of the vulva is at or below the level of the pubis. This generally is coupled with vulvae that have an effective side-to-side seal and are not slanted cranially, effectively protecting the genital tract from fecal contamination or aspiration of air (Fig. 73.1).

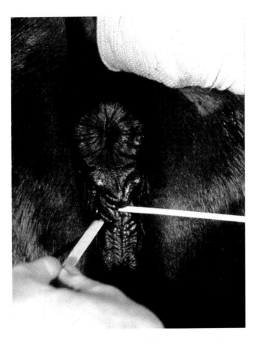

■ **Figure 73.1** Assessment of vulvar conformation, good (left marks dorsal commissure, right marks floor of pubis).
Image courtesy of W. R. Threlfall.

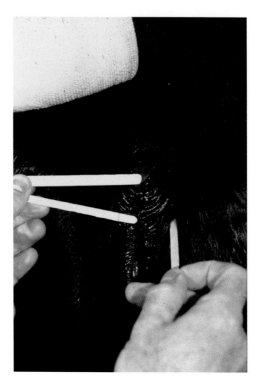

■ **Figure 73.2** Assessment of vulvar conformation, Fair (left marker indicates the extent that the dorsal commissure lies dorsal to the pubis, which is indicated by the marker to the right.).
Image courtesy of W. R. Threlfall.

- Fair VC implies the dorsal vulvar commissure is elevated above the floor of the pubis or the vulvae slope anteriorly, permitting pneumovagina or fecal contamination of the vestibule (Fig. 73.2).
- Poor VC implies the dorsal vulvar commissure is elevated above the pubis. This usually is accompanied by an obvious anterior slant of the vulvae. Fecal contamination of the vestibule occurs frequently to continually (Figs. 73.3a, b, and c).
- Problems with VC account for a major portion of equine subfertility and infertility including placentitis.

 ETIOLOGY/PATHOPHYSIOLOGY

Factors predisposing mares to poor VC include:
- Breed of mare as well as individual conformation of each mare. Breeds or individuals with less muscle in the perineal area, perineal lacerations, and underweight mares are all at greater risk.
- Genetics can influence VC (mother/daughter) and should be considered when selecting broodmares. This is particularly important if farm-born fillies are to be the source

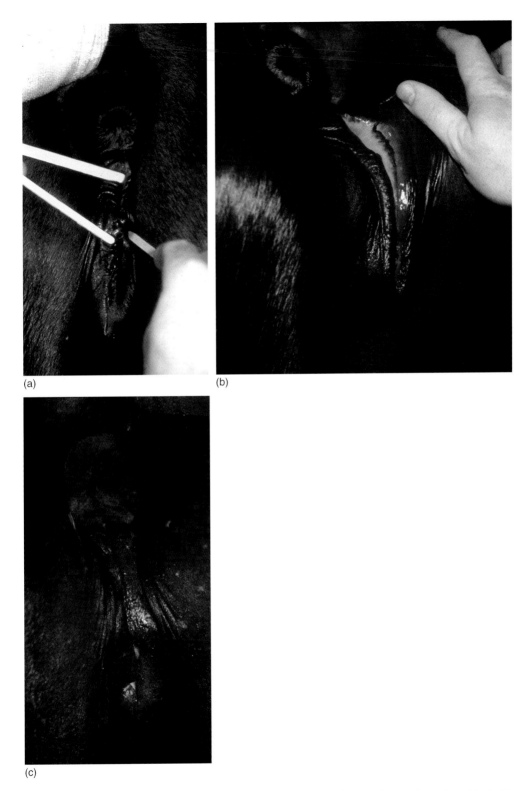

(a)

(b)

(c)

■ **Figure 73.3** Assessment of vulvar conformation, Poor *(a)*; example of poor vulvar conformation with significant forward slant lying above the floor of the pubis *(b)*; example of poor vulvar conformation *(c)*, due to a cranial slant compounded by loss of integrity of lateral seal of the vulvae.
Image *a* courtesy of W. R. Threlfall; images *b* and *c* courtesy of C. L. Carleton.

of replacement stock. Mares with good VC have fewer reproductive problems. Inherited poor VC can become a significant problem. Perineal lacerations resulting from abnormal fetal posture or position at parturition, or fetal extremities pushed dorsally during Stage 2 of parturition (causing the fetus' feet to tear into the wall of the vagina or vestibule) can also be detrimental to VC.

Systems Affected

Reproductive

SIGNALMENT/HISTORY

- Decreases in the grade or ability of the vulva to protect the genital tract from ascending infection or inflammation can occur in all breeds and at any breeding age.
- The incidence of poor VC increases significantly in older, pluriparous mares.

Risk Factors

- Inheritance (dam/daughter) of VC.
- No specific risk factor to the mare other than compromising her ability to carry a healthy pregnancy to term.
- Increased occurrence of placentitis in mares with poor VC.
- Posterior presentation of a fetus might be linked with an increased incidence of perineal lacerations. Fetal posture and position can change within minutes of birth, so a previous examination for fetal position and posture has little predictive value.
- Abnormal VC is extremely common, especially in some breeds, (e.g., thoroughbred and standardbred). The more muscular breeds or certain families within breeds have less of a problem with less-than-ideal VC.

Historical Findings

- A history of subfertility or infertility exists in many of these mares because of failure to conceive or EED or abortion.
- In addition to the presence of endometritis, vaginitis or cervicitis may also be present.

CLINICAL FEATURES

Compromised VC is fairly easy to identify and quantify.
- Assessment of each broodmare's VC should be noted on her record at the start of each breeding season and again at the fall pregnancy examination. This condition can worsen with age.

- Physical examination to determine the degree of less than ideal VC. Poor VC may result in gross/histopathologic changes of the tubular genital tract. TRP of the reproductive tract may reveal enlargement of uterine horns, increased uterine size, intraluminal fluid accumulation, and aspiration of air (e.g., pneumovagina, pneumouterus).
- If severe, hyperechoic echogenicities identified at U/S examination may be evidence of fecal or air aspiration into the uterine lumen.
- Vaginal examination using sterile lubricant and a sterile vaginal speculum may reveal inflammation, discharge (e.g., endometritis, cervicitis, or vaginitis), urine pooling, or adhesions (if chronic). Other physical parameters of the mare are usually normal.

DIFFERENTIAL DIAGNOSIS

- Recto-vaginal laceration
- RVF
- Perineal laceration (first, second, or third degree)

DIAGNOSTICS

- Determining the location of the dorsal VC in relation to the floor of the pubis is critical to the diagnosis and resolution of this condition.
- Careful palpation of the vestibule, vagina, and rectum aid in identifying lacerations.
- RVF may be small and not readily identifiable but results in sufficient contamination of the uterus to have a negative effect on fertility.

THERAPEUTIC

No systemic antibiotics are indicated to treat poor VC. Selection of local anesthetic to accomplish the repair is at the discretion of the surgeon.

Appropriate Health Care

- Determine that a laceration does not extend into the peritoneal cavity (rare, but possible with a perineal laceration or RVF). Systemic antibiotics seldom are indicated. Local medication is rarely indicated.
- Repair more severe lacerations of the vulva before attempting rebreeding. Generally it is best to wait until the area has a good bed of granulation tissue (30–60 days). Increase the mare's antibody protection by administering a tetanus toxoid booster, especially if her vaccinal status is not current or is unknown. There are no dietary changes required unless perineal surgery is attempted.

Activity

Activity with poor VC is unrestricted, but pneumovagina or pneumouterus may be evident or heard by the sound elicited when affected mares are trotting/running.

Surgical Considerations

- Surgical correction for poor VC (vulvoplasty or episioplasty) was first described by Dr. E. A. Caslick in 1937.
- First, wrap and tie the mare's tail away from the field of surgery and thoroughly clean the perineal area with cotton and soap.
- Carbocaine or other local anesthetic is infiltrated into the mucocutaneous junction of the vulva; approximately 6 to 12 mL typically is used to infiltrate both sides of the vulva (Fig. 73.4). With local infiltration of anesthetic, the suture line will appear puckered slightly when sutures are in place. Sufficient tension needs to be placed, so that once the anesthetic is absorbed, the tissue edges will remain in contact for first intention healing.
- The tissue edges are freshened before suturing, either by:
  - Strip removal: very narrow strip of tissue is cut away from the edge of the each vulvar lip (usually with scissors), or by
  - Split-thickness technique: incising (number 10 scalpel blade) at the mucocutaneous junction along the line dilated with local anesthetic (i.e., no tissue is removed).

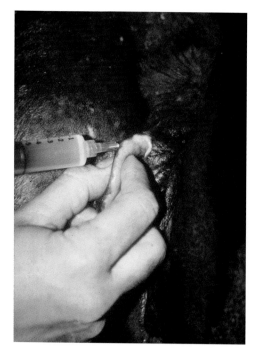

■ **Figure 73.4** Local anesthetic is placed along the mucocutaneous junction. The block is shallow, just along the edge of the junction; a deep local block is not necessary.
Image courtesy of C. L.Carleton.

The incised line on the mucocutaneous junction, dilated with anesthetic, separates up to or less than 1 cm wide as the vulvar lip is elevated/slightly lifted while being incised. The horseshoe shaped incision reaches from right vulvar lip, dorsally in an arch over the top of the vulvar commissure, continuing to the left vulvar lip (Figs. 73.5a, b, and c). The lateral aspects (skin to middle of the deepest point of the incision) of the right and left vulvar lip incision are closed (Fig. 73.5d). Create an appropriately thin but protective barrier to prevent further fecal and air contamination.

- The latter technique is tissue-sparing and preferred for the long-term reproductive welfare of the mare. Over the reproductive life of a mare, the split-thickness technique serves to prolong the normal elasticity of the vulvar lips needed during labor by minimizing prior, annual vulvoplasty-induced scarring. The adage often quoted is, "Once a Caslick's, always a Caslick's." VC doesn't improve from one year to the next, but an annual repair of the VC as necessary post-foaling, can permit the mare to carry the next pregnancy by minimizing or eliminating fecal and air contamination of her genital tract.
- Both described techniques are in common use and considered acceptable.
- Suture patterns may vary: Ford interlocking pattern allows adjustment of tension along preplaced sutures (Fig. 73.5e); simple interrupted sutures may result in gaps and small fistulas (increased likelihood to form gaps); simple continuous sutures may also more evenly distribute tension along the suture line, and so on. Staples are expensive and unnecessary but may be useful as a temporary closure for a day or two postpartum to minimize genital tract contamination until breeding in a mare with the worst VC.
- A quick check when the procedure is completed to confirm the integrity of suture placement, that no "gaps" exist that may preclude good closure, takes but seconds (Fig. 73.6). If necessary an additional simple interrupted or mattress suture can be placed while the local block remains.
- Use nonabsorbable suture material or staples, with removal in about 10 to 12 days.
  - Often commercial stud farms will leave sutures in place until the broodmare is examined at her early pregnancy check (16 days). It saves labor (one extra trip to the barn). If pregnant, the sutures are removed. If not pregnant, sutures remain until after the subsequent AI, to disrupt the vulvoplasty as little as possible. If the mare is to be bred live cover, a breeding stitch may be placed at the ventral limit of the vulvoplasty to protect it from being completely disrupted during cover. The latter presumes the remaining vulvar cleft is sufficient to accommodate the stallion's penis. If it is not, the vulvoplasty needs to be opened (partial) prior to live cover.
  - At the time of suture/staple removal, evaluate the surgical site for the presence of small fistulae through which contamination may continue.
- It is a mistake not to place the vulvoplasty post-breeding as soon as ovulation has been confirmed (preferably within 48 hours of ovulation). The time of greatest pregnancy loss in the mare occurs in the first 50 days of gestation. To leave the mare's genital tract unprotected from her poor VC as soon as possible, puts the first 15 to 20 days of her pregnancy at much higher risk for EED, due to fecal and air aspiration, contamination, and inflammation.

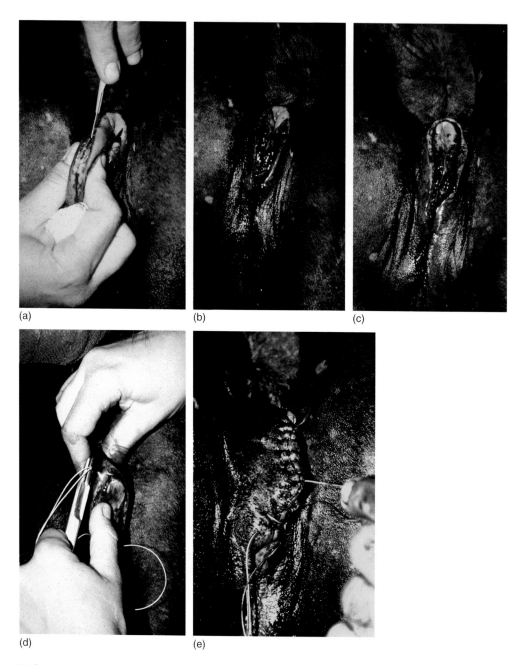

(a)　　　　　　　　　　　(b)　　　　　　　　　　　(c)

(d)　　　　　　　　　　　(e)

■ **Figure 73.5** Incision being placed along the mucocutaneous junction. Rest the hand holding the scalpel on the back by the tailhead of the mare as the incision is made. If the mare moves, the blade moves with her *(a)*. Incision is first made along the left and right vulvar margins *(b)*. Rather than forming a sharp point at the dorsal commissure, continue the incision in a rounded horseshoe, to lessen likelihood of a fistula forming at the time of suturing *(c)*. Begin suturing at the dorsal commissure, not below that limit. Decreases likelihood of a small dorsal fistula forming *(d)*. Preplace sutures for the entire limit of the Caslick's vulvoplasty. Then, adjust tension from top to bottom, to even tension, and decrease fistula formation along length of the vulvoplasty *(e)*. Images courtesy of C. L. Carleton.

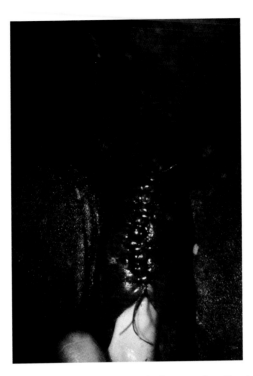

■ **Figure 73.6** Completed vulvoplasty: quick assessment of adequacy of seal/tension. Image courtesy C. L. Carleton.

- The Pouret technique is another surgical option only considered for cases of very poor VC. In cases of severe/extremely poor VC, it may be necessary to dissect the perineal body in a caudal (widest) to cranial (complete the dissection in a narrower point) flat plane, creating a pie-shaped wedge. It permits the genital tract, ventral to the rectum, to slide caudally and slightly ventral; out of the line of fecal contamination as well as aspiration of air; only the skin is closed (i.e., no deep reconstruction of dissected tissue) between the anal sphincter and dorsal vulvar commissure. The degree/depth of dissection determines the degree of correction that is attained.
  - Restraint of the mare in stocks is critical to avoid movement during dissection of the perineal body.
  - Check the mare's tetanus toxoid vaccination status. Administer a booster as necessary.

COMMENTS

Client Education

- It is always important to emphasize the value of closely observing mares leading up to and during foaling, with attention to normal times and events in each stage. Many lacerations occur before a foaling problem is noticed, even with trained attendants.

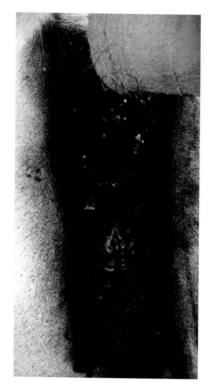

■ **Figure 73.7** Perineal melanoma lesions.
Image courtesy of C. L. Carleton

■ Melanoma is often first identified on the perineum. Increase your client's awareness of additional health concerns for a broodmare extending beyond mere assessment of VC and angle of slant (Fig. 73.7).

Patient Monitoring

Suture removal 10–14 days after surgery to prevent the possibility of stitch abscesses at the suture site is recommended.

Prevention/Avoidance

Select broodmares with excellent VC.

Possible Complications

Placing a Caslick's vulvoplasty is the necessity to reopen the vulvar commissure from 5 to 10 days prepartum to prevent the perineum from tearing at delivery. Caslick's vulvoplasty should be replaced (i.e., incised and sutured) immediately after foaling or breeding and confirmation of ovulation in the next season, depending on severity of her VC abnormality.

Expected Course and Prognosis

Without surgical correction, many of these mares with fair to poor VC will remain infertile, subfertile, or abort during pregnancy.

Synonyms

- Wind sucker

Abbreviations

AI   artifical insemination
EED   early embryonic death
RVF   recto-vaginal fistula
TRP   transrectal palpation
U/S   ultrasound
VC   vulvar conformation

See Also

- Dystocia
- Endometrial biopsy
- Endometritis
- Perineal lacerations, fistulas
- Pneumovagina/Pneumouterus
- Urine pooling
- Vulvar conformation

Suggested Reading

Aanes WA. 1964. Surgical repair of third degree perineal lacerations and recto-vaginal fistulas in the mare. *JAVMA* 144: 485–491.

Caslick EA. 1937. The vulva and vulvo-vaginal orifice and its relationship to genital health of the thoroughbred mare. *Cornell Vet* 27: 178–186.

Colbern GT, Aanes WA, Stashak TS. 1985. Surgical management of perineal lacerations and recto-vestibular fistulae in the mare: a retrospective study of 47 cases. *JAVMA* 186: 265–269.

Heinze CD, Allen AR. 1966. Repair of third-degree perineal lacerations in the mare. *Vet Scope* 11: 12–15.

Shipley WD, Bergin WC. 1968. Genital health in the mare. III. Pneumovagina. *VM/SAC* 63: 699–702.

Stickle RL, Fessler JF, Adams SB, et al. 1979. A single stage technique for repair of rectovestibular lacerations in the mare. *J Vet Surg* 8: 25–27.

Authors: Walter R. Threlfall and Carla L. Carleton

chapter 74

Abnormal Scrotal Enlargement

DEFINITION/OVERVIEW

A condition causing the gross appearance of the scrotum to deviate from normal size and texture (e.g., scrotal enlargement and/or asymmetry).

ETIOLOGY/PATHOPHYSIOLOGY

- Equine scrotum and associated contents are positioned on a horizontal axis between the hind limbs of the animal and are relatively well protected from external insult.
- Scrotal skin is thin and pliable and its contents freely movable within the scrotum.
- Blunt trauma (i.e., breeding accident, jumping) is the most common cause of scrotal abnormality.
- Trauma can result in scrotal hemorrhage, edema, rupture of the tunica albuginea, hematocele, hydrocoele, and inflammation.
- Similar signs can occur with inguinal or scrotal herniation, torsion of the spermatic cord, or neoplasia.

Systems Affected

Reproductive

SIGNALMENT/HISTORY

- Intact male horses
- Any age
- Incidence and prevalence is dependent on the cause of enlargement, whether traumatic, vascular, infectious, noninfectious, or neoplastic.

Risk Factors

- Breeding activity
- Large internal inguinal rings
- Systemic illness
- Extremes of ambient temperature (hot or cold)

Historical Findings

- Gross changes in the size of the scrotum (usually acute).
- Pain (generally colic-like symptoms).
- Reluctance to breed, jump, or walk.
- Extreme environmental temperatures (hot or cold).

 CLINICAL FEATURES

Physical Examination Findings

- Increased scrotal size (unilateral or bilateral).
- Abnormal testicular position.
- Abnormal scrotal temperature (too warm or cold).
- Edema/engorgement of scrotum or contents.
- Scrotal laceration
- Derangements in systemic parameters (elevated heart rate, respiratory rate, inappetance, CBC abnormalities).
- Any combination of abnormalities may be present and not all signs are present in every animal.

Causes

Most Common

- Trauma, may include testicular hematoma/rupture.
- Inguinal/scrotal hernia
- Torsion of the spermatic cord (i.e., testicular torsion).

Inflammatory/Infectious Causes

- EIA
- EVA/EAV
- Orchitis/epididymitis

Neoplasia

- Primary scrotal: melanoma, sarcoid.
- Testicular neoplasia: seminoma, teratoma, interstitial cell tumor, Sertoli cell tumor.

Other Causes

- Noninflammatory scrotal edema.
- Hydrocoele/Hematocoele
- Varicocoele
- See also: Abnormal Testicular Size

DIFFERENTIAL DIAGNOSIS

Differentiating Causes

- Onset/duration of problem
  - Acute: traumatic injury, torsion of spermatic cord, herniation, or infection.
  - Chronic: neoplasia, temperature-induced hydrocoele/edema, varicocoele, or infection.
- History of recent breeding, semen collection or trauma.
- Palpation of the caudal ligament of the epididymis (attaches epididymal tail to caudal testis and aids in the determination of testicular orientation).
- Palpation of the inguinal rings.
- U/S (see Imaging)

 ## DIAGNOSTICS

CBC/Biochemistry/Urinalysis

- Inflammatory or stress leukocyte response
- Increased fibrinogen
- Results of serum biochemistry profile and urinalysis are usually normal

Other Laboratory Tests

EVA

- SN or CF
- Acute and convalescent serum samples
- Virus isolation from serum or seminal plasma, but if a stallion is seropositive, carrier state is confirmed by virus isolation from semen. Titer alone is inconclusive; validates exposure (vaccinal or prior disease exposure). Approved laboratories expect a frozen sample of semen to accompany serum to confirm shedding or non-shedding status.
- Semen is the best sample for diagnosis (freeze portion of ejaculate immediately after collection) and send to an approved lab (with serum samples).
- Must send samples to an approved laboratory.

EIA

- AGID or ELISA, the Coggins test.

Imaging, Scrotal U/S

Examination of scrotal contents may reveal:
- Bowel with inguinal or scrotal herniation.
- Rupture of the testis or tunica albuginea:
  - Accumulation of hypoechoic fluid in scrotum with loss of discrete hyperechoic tunica albuginea around testicular parenchyma.

- Hypoechoic appearance of contents will gradually contain echogenic densities with the formation of fibrin clots.
- Engorgement of the pampiniform plexus or testicular congestion with torsion of the spermatic cord
  - Doppler can verify loss of blood flow to the testis.
- Hypoechoic dilation of venous plexus of spermatic cord with varicocoele.
- Hypoechoic accumulation of fluid within the vaginal cavity with hydrocoele.
- Loss of homogeneity in testicular parenchyma with neoplasia.
  - May see areas of increased or decreased echogenicity or be variable throughout.

Other Diagnostic Procedures

- Needle aspirate and cytology: differentiate hydrocoele from recent hemorrhage.
- Neoplasia: diagnosed using fine needle aspirate or biopsy.

Pathological Findings

Dependent on etiology

THERAPEUTICS

Treatment is directed at the cause of scrotal enlargement.
- Management of inflammation is a primary concern with abnormal scrotal enlargement.
- Sexual rest is indicated for all causes of scrotal enlargement.

Drug(s) of Choice

- Anti-inflammatory therapy (phenylbutazone, 2–4 mg/kg, PO or IV, BID or flunixin meglumine, 1 mg/kg, IV, BID) is indicated in all cases.
- Diuretics (furosemide, 0.5–1 mg/kg, IV) may be useful in managing scrotal edema.
- Antibiotic therapy should be considered in cases of scrotal laceration or scrotal hemorrhage.
- Tetanus toxoid should be administered for scrotal trauma or prior to surgery.

Appropriate Health Care

Inpatient or Outpatient treatment:
- Acute scrotal enlargement warrants hospitalization for treatment and care.
- Chronic scrotal enlargement may or may not warrant hospitalization; it is etiology dependent.

Nursing Care

- Cold therapy (i.e., cold packs, ice water baths, water hose) for acute scrotal trauma is implemented only in the absence of testicular rupture.

- Testicular tunics must be intact.
- Cold therapy sessions should not exceed 20 minutes and can be repeated every 2 hours.
- Scrotal massage with emollient salve: useful to reduce scrotal edema and ischemic injury.
- Fluid removal should be considered with hydrocoele.
  - Use only an aseptically placed needle or an intravenous catheter.
  - Excess fluid accumulation may cause thermal damage to the testes acts to insulate; has a negative effect on testicular temperature regulation.
- Administration of intravenous fluids is dependent on systemic status of the horse.

Diet

- Diet modification is necessary only with secondary ileus or as a preoperative consideration.

Activity

The need to restrict activity depends on the etiology of scrotal enlargement.

Surgical Considerations

Hemi-castration is the treatment of choice for:
- Torsion of the spermatic cord, if the duration of vascular compromise has caused irreversible damage or gonadal necrosis.
- Unilateral inguinal or scrotal herniation
- Testicular rupture
- Unilateral neoplasia
- Varicocoele
- Nonresponsive hydrocoele/hematocoele.

Primary repair of scrotal laceration is required to protect scrotal contents.
- Repair generally fails due to extensive scrotal edema associated with traumatic injury.

 COMMENTS

Client Education

- Fertility may be irreversibly impaired with acute scrotal trauma.
- Semen evaluation should be performed 90 days after nonsurgical resolution of scrotal enlargement.
- Compensatory semen production may occur in the remaining testis of a horse undergoing hemi-castration.
- Following removal of a neoplasia, examine carefully for evidence of metastatic tumor growth (serial examinations).

Patient Monitoring

Semen collection and evaluation 90 days after complete resolution of cause or surgery.

Possible Complications

- Infertility
- Endotoxemia
- Laminitis
- Scrotal adhesions
- Death

Abbreviations

AGID   agar gel immunodiffusion
BID   twice a day
BSE   breeding soundness examination
CBC   complete blood count
CF   complement fixation
EAV   equine arteritis virus
EIA   equine infectious anemia
ELISA   enzyme-linked immunoadsorbent assay
EVA   equine viral arteritis
IV   intravenous
PO   per os (by mouth)
SN   serum neutralization
U/S   ultrasound, ultrasonography

See Also

- Abnormal testicular size
- Abnormal stallion semen
- BSE, stallion
- Semen collection, methods
- Semen collection, routine semen evaluation
- Semen evaluation, abnormal stallion

Suggested Reading

Love CC. 1992. Ultrasonographic evaluation of the testis, epididymis and spermatic cord of the stallion. In: *The Veterinary Clinics of North America: Equine Practice. Stallion Management.* Blanchard TL, Varner DD (eds). 8: 167–182.

Varner DD, Schumacher J, Blanchard T, et al. 1991. *Diseases and management of breeding stallions.* Goleta: American Veterinary Publications.

Author: Margo L. Macpherson

chapter 75

Abnormal Testicular Size

 ## DEFINITION/OVERVIEW

Any condition causing the gross appearance of a testis to deviate from normal size and texture (e.g., testicular enlargement, reduction, or asymmetry).

 ## ETIOLOGY/PATHOPHYSIOLOGY

- The testes and epididymides are positioned in a horizontal orientation between the hind limbs of the horse and are freely movable within the scrotum.
- The scrotum and contents, although relatively protected from external insult, are at increased risk for injury during breeding or athletic activity.
- Acute enlargement of a testis occurs after trauma (Figs. 75.1a, b, c, and d), torsion of the spermatic cord (Figs. 75.2a and b), or orchitis/epididymitis.
  - Origin may be bacterial, viral, autoimmune, or parasitic.
- Testicular neoplasia is uncommon in the horse.
  - Seminoma, teratoma, Sertoli cell tumor, interstitial cell tumor.
  - Of these, seminoma is the most frequently reported testicular tumor of the stallion (Figs. 75.3a and b). The incidence of teratoma is increased with retained/cryptorchid testes.
  - Most equine testicular tumors arise from germ cells, including seminomas and teratomas.
  - The effect of neoplasia on testicular size (increase or decrease) may be insidious.
- Hypoplastic and degenerative testes are smaller than normal (Figs. 75.4a and b).
- Testicular degeneration can be transient or permanent.
  - An acquired condition, degeneration may arise from thermal injury, infection, vascular insult, hormonal disturbances, toxins, and age.
- Testicular hypoplasia is an irreversible condition.
  - Hypoplastic testes are incompletely developed.
  - Condition is usually congenital.
  - Suspected causes include genetic aberrations, teratogens, cryptorchidism (Fig. 75.5), and postnatal insult.

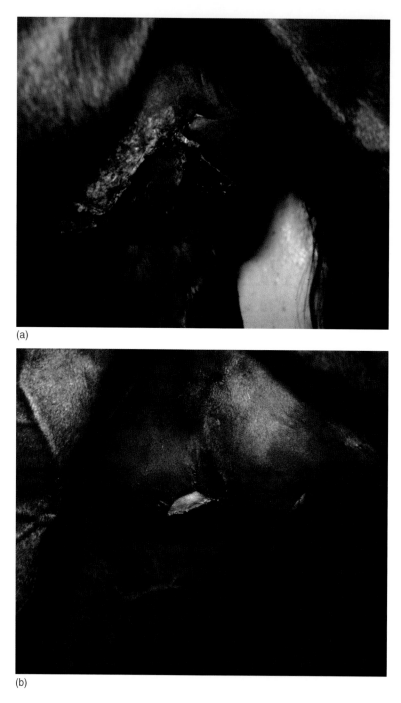

(a)

(b)

■ **Figure 75.1** Stallion with grossly enlarged scrotum after a direct kick during a live cover. Bottom of scrotum lost to necrosis and edema. Owner declined requests to castrate stallion *(a)*. Stallion presented months after kick injury with significant scarring and permanent fibrosis of testes to scrotum. Limited intrascrotal testicular motion *(b)*. Scar on ventral aspect of stallion's scrotum. Required stallion be protection from environmental extremes, frostbite in winter and excessive summer heat to maintain semen quality *(c)*. Scar tissue formation also prevented full extension of penis after healing. Collected by AV, semen quality remained adequate to breed 2 mares per ejaculate *(d)*.
Images courtesy of C. L. Carleton.

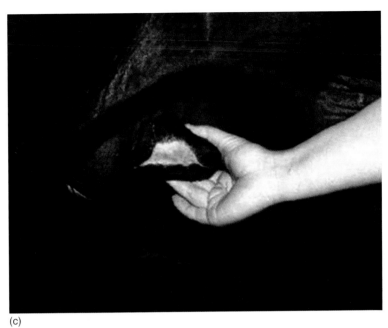

(c)

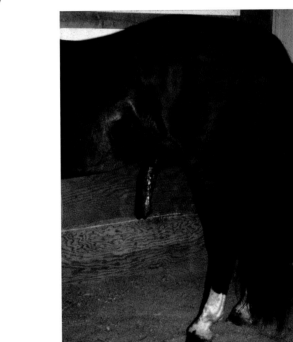

(d)

■ **Figure 75.1** continued

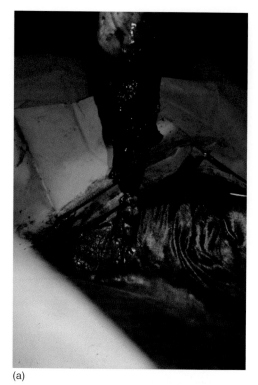

(a)

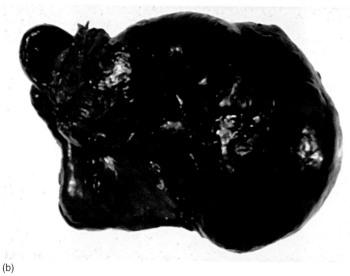

(b)

■ **Figure 75.2** Intraoperative view of spermatic cord torsion *(a)*. Necrotic, devascularized testis from chronic spermatic cord torsion *(b)*.
Image courtesy of C. L. Carleton.

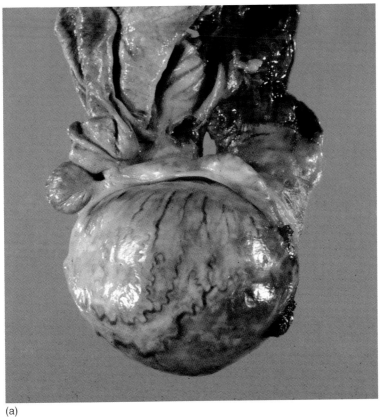

(a)

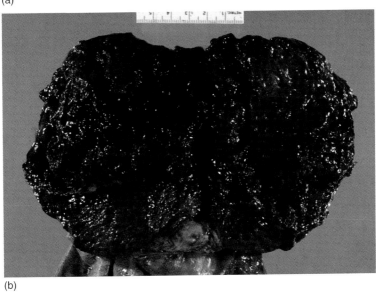

(b)

■ **Figure 75.3** Seminoma, unilateral *(a)*. Cross-section of testis affected by a seminoma. Remaining functional testicular stroma is in ventral aspect of the image (slight brownish region of remaining stroma) *(b)*.
Image courtesy of C. L. Carleton.

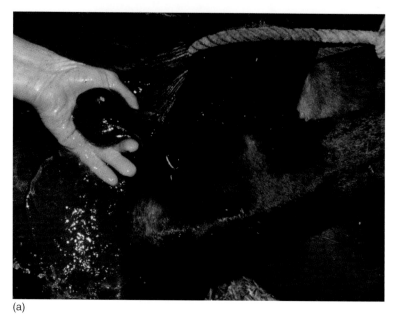

(a)

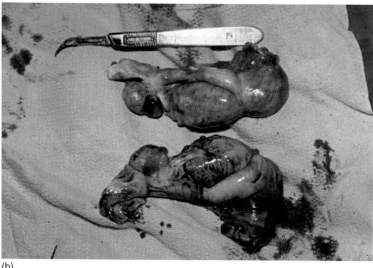

(b)

■ **Figure 75.4** Hypoplastic testes of a 3-year-old standardbred stallion *(a)*. Hypoplastic testes after castration of the stallion *(b)*.
Images courtesy of C. L. Carleton.

Systems Affected

- Reproductive
- Metastases from primary testicular neoplasia:
  - Respiratory
  - GI
  - Lymphatic

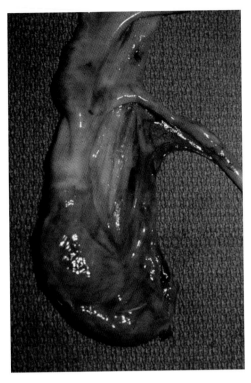

■ **Figure 75.5** Intra-abdominal cryptorchid testis, small and soft appearance is typical.

 ## SIGNALMENT/HISTORY

Intact male horses:
- Any age, prepubertal testes are small and can be misdiagnosed as pathologically hypoplastic.
- Testicular growth increases rapidly from 12 to 24 months of age in horses.
- Testes may take 4 to 5 years to reach full size and maturity.

Risk Factors

- Breeding activity
- Systemic illness
- Temperature extremes
- Anabolic steroid use

Historical Findings

- Recent history of breeding or semen collection.
- Gross changes in the size of a testis.
- Reduced fertility
- Pain (generally colic-like symptoms).

- Reluctance to breed, jump or walk.
- Cryptorchidism is commonly associated with testicular hypoplasia.
- Male equine hybrids (mules or hinnys) often have hypoplastic testes.

 CLINICAL FEATURES

Physical Examination Findings

- Increased or decreased scrotal size.
- Increased or decreased testicular size.
- Abnormal testicular texture (too soft or firm).
- Abnormal testicular position.
- Abnormal scrotal temperature (too warm or cold).
- Edema/engorged scrotum or contents.
- Derangements in systemic parameters (elevated heart rate, respiratory rate, inappetent, and CBC abnormalities).

Causes

- Three most common:
  - Trauma
  - Cryptorchidism
  - Torsion of the spermatic cord
- Testicular degeneration
- Testicular hypoplasia
- Testicular hematoma/rupture
- Neoplasia:
  - Seminoma
  - Teratoma
  - Interstitial cell tumor
  - Sertoli cell tumor
- Orchitis/epididymitis:
  - Bacterial infection
  - EIA
  - EVA
  - Strongylus edentatus infection
  - Autoimmune

 DIFFERENTIAL DIAGNOSIS

Differentiating Similar Signs

- Scrotal enlargement due to scrotal hydrocoele/hematocoele and scrotal or inguinal hernia may be confused with testicular enlargement (Fig. 75.6).

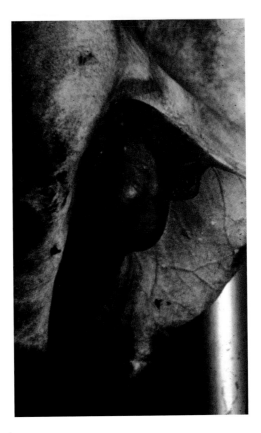

■ **Figure 75.6** Scrotal hernia.

- U/S examination and measurement of the testes is the best means of differentiating the pathologies.

Differentiating Causes

- Duration of problem:
  - Acute: traumatic injury, torsion of spermatic cord, infection.
  - Chronic: cryptorchidism, neoplasia, infection, or testicular degeneration/hypoplasia.
- History of recent breeding or trauma.
- Palpation of the caudal ligament of the epididymis (attaches epididymal tail to caudal testis and aids in the determination of testicular orientation).
- Testicular hypoplasia is usually congenital, while testicular degeneration is acquired.
- U/S (see Imaging)

DIAGNOSTICS

CBC/Biochemistry/Urinalysis

- Inflammatory or stress leukocyte response.
- Eosinophilia may be an indicator of a parasitic infection.
- Increased fibrinogen
- Serum biochemistry profile and urinalysis are usually normal.

Other Laboratory Tests

EVA

- SN or CF
- Requires acute and convalescent serum samples.
- If stallion is seropositive, carrier state is determined with virus isolation from the ejaculate.
- Freeze a portion of the ejaculate and send to lab with serum samples.
- Must send samples to an approved laboratory.

EIA

- AGID or ELISA, the Coggins test.

Testicular Degeneration

- Endocrine profile (LH, FSH, testosterone, estrogens) from pooled samples obtained hourly for a minimum of four samples (due to pulsatile release of hormones).
- Abnormal elevation of FSH and low total estrogen concentration are indicative of testicular degeneration.

Imaging

Scrotal and Testicular U/S

Testicular parenchyma should appear uniformly echogenic. Aberrations that may be identified by U/S include:
- Rupture of the testis or tunica albuginea:
  - Hypoechoic fluid accumulates in the scrotum with loss of discrete hyperechoic tunica albuginea around testicular parenchyma.
  - Hypoechoic appearance of contents will gradually be replaced with echogenic densities as fibrin clots form.
- Engorgement of the pampiniform plexus or testicular congestion with torsion of the spermatic cord.
  - Doppler can verify loss of blood flow to the testis.
- Loss of homogeneity in testicular parenchyma with neoplasia:
  - Neoplasia results in heterogeneity (usually a circumscribed area) in the testicular parenchyma.

- May see areas of increased or decreased echogenicity or appear variable throughout.

Other Diagnostic Procedures

- Needle aspirate and cytology: diagnose or differentiate recent hemorrhage or neoplasia.
- Testicular histopathology: diagnose or differentiate neoplasia and testicular degeneration or hypoplasia.
- Semen evaluation is useful in the diagnosis of testicular degeneration or hypoplasia
  - Oligospermia
  - Azoospermia
  - Premature release of spermatids

Pathological Findings

If neoplastic, etiology is dependent on histopathologic diagnosis.

 # THERAPEUTICS

Treatment is directed at the cause of testicular abnormality.

Drug(s) of Choice

- Anti-inflammatory therapy (phenylbutazone, 2–4 mg/kg, PO or IV, BID or flunixin meglumine, 1 mg/kg, IV, BID) is indicated in most cases.
- Antibiotic therapy should be considered in cases of orchitis or epididymitis and testicular trauma.
- Tetanus toxoid should be administered after testicular trauma and/or prior to surgery.
- Antiparasitic therapy for Strongylus edentatus infection (ivermectin, 0.2 mg/kg, PO, every 30 days until resolution of lesions).

Appropriate Health Care

Inpatient versus Outpatient
- Most causes of testicular enlargement require hospitalization for treatment or resolution.
- Horses with testicular degeneration that are not systemically ill may be managed on the farm.
- Horses with hypoplastic testes can be managed on an outpatient basis.

Nursing Care

- Cold therapy (i.e., cold packs, ice water baths, water hose, or hydrotherapy) is indicated for acute orchitis or epididymitis.
- Cold therapy sessions should not exceed 20 minutes and can be repeated every 2 hours.

- Sexual rest is indicated in most cases until resolution of the problem.
- Administration of intravenous fluids is dependent on systemic status of the horse.

Diet

Modification is necessary only with cases of secondary ileus or as a preoperative consideration.

Activity

Restriction depends on cause of the testicular aberration.

Surgical Considerations

Hemi-castration is the treatment of choice for:
- Torsion of the spermatic cord, if the duration of vascular compromise has caused irreversible damage or gonadal necrosis.
- Testicular rupture.
- Unilateral neoplasia or any condition causing irreparable damage to testis or testes.

 COMMENTS

Client Education

- Fertility may permanently be diminished.
- Testicular degeneration and subsequent reduction in semen quality can be transient or permanent, depending on the inciting cause.
- Testicular hypoplasia is a permanent condition.
- Horses with neoplasia should be examined carefully for evidence of metastatic tumor growth.
- Compensatory sperm production may occur in the remaining testis of a horse undergoing hemi-castration.
- Serial semen evaluations are beneficial to monitor fertility status of horses following testicular insult and treatment.
  - Semen should be evaluated 75 to 90 days after complete resolution of testicular insult.

Patient Monitoring

Semen collection and evaluation 90 days after complete resolution of testicular problem or surgery.

Possible Complications

- Infertility/subfertility
- Endotoxemia

- Laminitis
- Scrotal adhesions
- Death

Expected Course and Prognosis

Dependent on etiology

Abbreviations

AGID	agar-gel immunodiffusion
BID	twice a day
CBC	complete blood count
CF	complement fixation
EIA	equine infectious anemia
ELISA	enzyme-linked immunoadsorbent assay
EVA	equine viral arteritis
FSH	follicle stimulating hormone
GI	gastrointestinal
IV	intravenous
LH	luteinizing hormone
PO	per os (by mouth)
SN	serum neutralization
U/S	ultrasound, ultrasonography

See Also

- Cryptorchidism
- Abnormal scrotal enlargement

Suggested Reading

Brinsko SP. 1998. Neoplasia of the male reproductive tract. In: *Vet Clinics North Am Eq Pract.* Savage CJ (ed). *Neoplasia.* 14: 517–533.

Love CC. 1992. Ultrasonographic evaluation of the testis, epididymis and spermatic cord of the stallion. In: *Vet Clinics of North Am Eq Pract: Stallion Management.* Blanchard TL, Varner DD (eds). 8: 167–182.

Varner DD, Schumacher J, Blanchard T, et al. 1991. *Diseases and Management of Breeding Stallions.* Goleta: American Veterinary Publications.

Authors: Margo L. Macpherson and Carla L. Carleton

chapter 76

Anatomy, Reproductive, Stallion Review

DEFINITION/OVERVIEW

- A review of the normal reproductive anatomy of the stallion.

Prepuce

- See Figures 76.1a and b.
- The prepuce is formed by an external lamina (continuation of the skin) and an internal lamina that is attached to the penis at the proximal end (nearer the scrotum) of the free part of the penis.
- Absent stimulation, the penis is retracted within the preputial cavity.
- The preputial orifice (ostium) presents as a preputial fold of the internal lamina.
  - One of its surfaces faces the internal preputial lamina
  - The other surface faces the penis, forming the preputial ring.

Penis

- See Figure 76.2.
- Penis type is bulbocavernous.
- The free (distal) part of the penis ends with the *glans penis*.
- The interface between the free part of the penis and the glans (*collum glandis*) is easily differentiated or defined and is readily visible on gross examination.
- The urethra opens at the distal end (urethral orifice or urethral ostium) in a well-defined urethral process.
- The urethral process is surrounded by the *fossa glandis* ventrally and by the urethral sinus dorsally.
- The penile urethra is located ventrally along the length of the penis and is surrounded by the CSP.
- The CCP surrounds these structures over the entire dorsal aspect of the penis.
- The bulbospongiosus muscle and retractor penis muscle lie ventral to the urethra.
- The CCP is divided into *cavernae* by the *trabuculae* of the *tunica albuginea*.
  - It overlaps with the dorsal process of the glans penis at the distal tip of the penis.
- The penile blood supply is provided primarily by the cranial artery of the penis (branch of the external pudendal artery), the middle artery of the penis, and the dorsal artery of the penis (branch of the internal pudendal artery).

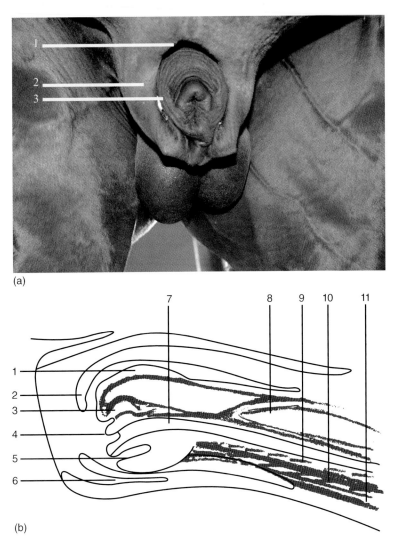

■ **Figure 76.1** Anatomy of the stallion prepuce: *A*, normal appearance of the stallion prepuce: (1) preputial cavity; (2) preputial orifice; and (3) preputial fold. *B*, Detailed anatomy of the prepuce and content: (1) glans penis; (2) preputial fold; (3) urethral sinus; (4) external urethral ostium; (5) fossa glandis; (6) preputial cavity; (7) urethra; (8) corpus cavernosum penis; (9) corpus spongiosum penis; (10) bulbospongiosus muscle; and (11) retractor penis muscle.

Scrotum

- See Figure 76.3.
- The scrotum is globular in shape and slightly pendulous. The latter is dependent on age and breed.
- A distinct raphé, evident on its ventral aspect, divides the scrotum into two distinct sacs each containing a testicle and its associated structures.

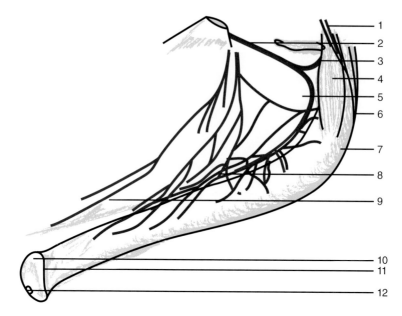

■ **Figure 76.2** Anatomy of the stallion penis: (1) internal pudendal artery and vein; (2) obturator artery and vein; (3) artery of the penis; (4) ischiocavernosus muscle; (5) middle artery and vein of the penis; (6) retractor penis muscle; (7) bulbospongiosus muscle; (8) cranial artery and vein of the penis; (9) superficial caudal epigastric vein; (10) corona glandis; (11) collum glandis; and (12) urethral process.

- Scrotal skin surface is smooth due to the presence of sweat, sebaceous glands, and the absence of hair.
- Scrotal layers include:
  - Skin
  - Tunica dartos muscle
  - Scrotal fascia
  - Parietal layer of the vaginal tunic.
- The tunica dartos muscle forms the septum separating the two sacs and is responsible for the changes of shape and position of the scrotum.

Testes

- See Figures 76.4a and b.
- The testes lie within the scrotal sacs, each with a horizontal long axis, with the epididymal tail positioned on their caudal aspect.
- The testicular parenchyma is encapsulated by the fibrous *tunica albuginea*, which projects into the testicular tissue and divides it into lobules.
- Each testis and associated epididymis is covered by the visceral layer of the vaginal tunic which adheres to the *tunica albuginea*.
- The narrow space formed between the visceral and the parietal layers of the vaginal tunic, called the vaginal cavity, communicates with the peritoneal cavity.

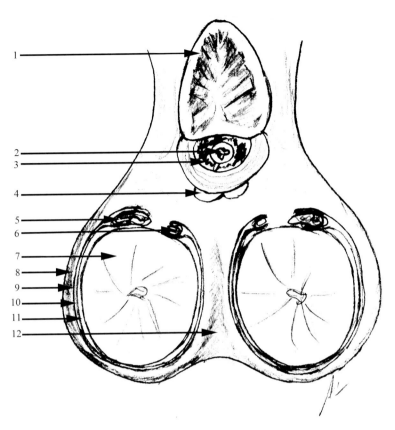

■ **Figure 76.3** Anatomy of the stallion scrotum and its content: (1) corpus cavernosum; (2) urethra; (3) corpus spongiosum; (4) retractor penis muscle; (5) body of the epididymis within the vaginal tunic; (6) ductus (i.e., vas) deferens within the vaginal tunic; (7) testis; (8) dartos; (9) parietal layer of the vaginal tunic; (10) visceral layer of the vaginal tunic; (11) tunica albuginea; and (12) median raphé of the testis.

- Testicular parenchyma is formed by the interstitial tissue and seminiferous tubules.
- The interstitial tissue is composed of Leydig cells, blood and lymphatic vessels, and fibroblasts.
- The seminiferous tubules are lined by the seminiferous epithelium (germinal cells) and Sertoli cells.
- Seminiferous tubules are composed of convoluted and straight portions (*tubuli seminiferi recti*).
- Straight tubules converge in the cranial two-thirds of the testis in the *reté testis* and penetrate the *tunica albuginea* to form an *extra-testicular reté*.
- Straight tubules fuse with one of 13 to 15 efferent ducts that lead to the epididymal duct in the epididymal head (*caput epididymis*).
- Stallion testes have a well-defined central vein.
- The volume (cm³) of the testicular stroma (grams of tissue of each testis) can be estimated from caliper measurements of each testis [[height × width × length] × 0.52).
  - This measurement is correlated with sperm production.

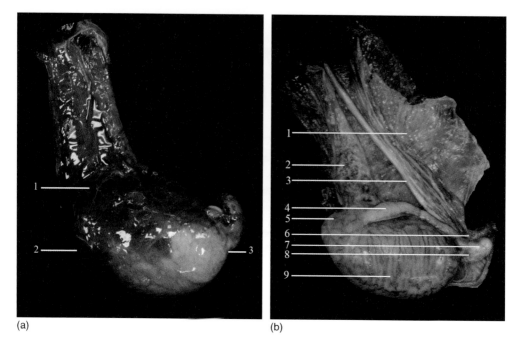

(a)   (b)

■ **Figure 76.4** Anatomy of the testis: *A,* left testis, lateral aspect: (1) cremaster; (2) cranial border; (3) caudal border with prominent cauda epididymis. *B,* Lateral aspect of the left testicle exposed: (1) vaginal tunic; (2) pampiniform plexus veins and testicular artery; (3) ductus deferens; (4) corpus epididymis; (5) caput epididymis; (6) ligament of the tail of the epididymis; (7) cauda epididymis; (8) proper ligament of the testis; and (9) testis.

Epididymis and Ductus Deferens

- The epididymal body lies on the dorso-lateral aspect of each testis.
- The epididymal tail (*cauda epididymis*) attaches to the caudal pole of the testis by the proper ligament.
- The tubular tract continues from the *cauda epididymis* to the *ductus deferens,* the excurrent duct that delivers mature spermatozoa to the *colliculus seminalis.*
- The *ductus deferens* dilates in its final portion as it nears the pelvic urethra.
  - These dilatations are called the *ampullae* of the *ductus deferens.*

Spermatic Cord

- The spermatic cords extend from the vaginal rings to the attached border of each testis.
- Each is enclosed by the parietal layer of the vaginal tunic.
- The *mesorchium* surrounds the testicular artery, *pampiniform plexus,* lymphatic vessels, nerves, and the deferent duct (*ductus deferens*).
- The cremaster muscle, that originates from the internal abdominal oblique muscle, attaches to the lateral and caudal border of the spermatic cord.
  - It provides upward and downward movement of the testis.
  - The distance testes are held from the body is to maintain thermoregulation (e.g., the testes are raised in cold weather, lowered/relaxed in warmer/hot weather).

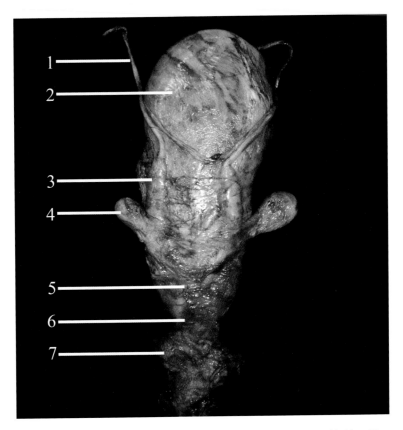

■ **Figure 76.5** Stallion internal genitalia en block: (1) ductus deferens; (2) urinary bladder; (3) ampulla of the ductus deferens; (4) seminal vesicle; (5) prostate; (6) pelvic urethra, pelvic portion of the penis; and (7) bulbourethral glands.

Internal Genitalia

- See Figures 76.5 and 76.6.
- The internal genital organs are composed of the pelvic urethra and the accessory sex glands (bulbourethral glands, prostate, seminal vesicles, and *ampullae*).

Bulbourethral Glands

- The bulbourethral glands are ovoid: 3 to 4 cm by 2 to 2.5 cm.
- Located on either side (slightly dorsolateral) of the pelvic urethra just as the penis courses caudally over the pubis.
- Enrobed in a thick muscular layer; they are only palpable if *grossly* abnormal in size.
- Each has several excretory ducts. These are visible, lying in a row, near the dorsal midline of the urethra, caudal to the *colliculus seminalis*.
- Provides the first ejaculatory fraction (clear, watery-like in nature).

Prostate

- The prostate gland measures 5 to 8 cm in length, 2 to 3 cm in width, and 1 to 3 cm in thickness.

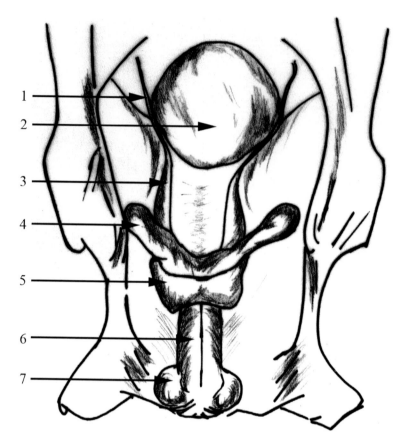

■ **Figure 76.6** Schematic representation of the internal genitalia in situ: (1) ductus deferens; (2) urinary bladder; (3) ampulla of the ductus deferens; (4) seminal vesicle; (5) prostate; (6) pelvic urethra, pelvic portion of the penis; and (7) bulbourethral glands.

- It is located dorso-laterally to the pelvic urethra and presents two lateral lobes connected by a thin transverse isthmus.
- As with the bulbourethral glands, it is enveloped by muscle and is not readily palpable.
- Multiple prostatic excretory ducts open on the lateral aspect of the *colliculus seminalis.*
- Its contribution is part of the second ejaculatory fraction.

Seminal Vesicles

- The seminal vesicles are located cranially and slightly lateral to the prostate.
- Thin-walled, pyriform, true vesicles/sac-like structures measuring 2 to 3 cm in diameter by 8 to 10 cm in length.
    - Compare these with the *vesicular glands,* the (vesicle-like) grape cluster, of the bovine.
- The base of the glands are covered by the genital fold of the peritoneum.

- Each seminal vesicle duct converges with the opening of the ipsilateral *ampulla* of the *ductus deferens*.
  - These are the common ejaculatory ducts lying on the left and right side of the pedicle that is the *colliculus seminalis* (visible within the pelvic urethra).
  - These ducts empty into the pelvic urethra.
- Its contribution provides the third ejaculatory fraction, the gel.

Ampullae of the Ductus Deferens

- The *ampullae* of the deferent ducts are dilations of the most caudal 10 to 15 cm of the *ductus deferens*.
- These lie medial to the seminal vesicles, almost midline on the floor of the pubis.
- Ampullae have a dual role:
  - They serve as the sperm reservoir.
  - The other major contributor to the second ejaculatory fraction, its *sperm-rich* portion.
  - Secretory role

Systems Affected

Reproductive

 COMMENTS

Abbreviations

CCP   corpus cavernosum penis
CSP   corpus spongiosum penis

See Also

- Abnormal scrotal enlargement
- Abnormal testicular size
- Breeding soundness examination, stallion

Suggested Reading

Amann RP. 1992. Functional anatomy of the adult male. In: *Equine Reproduction*, McKinnon AO, Voss JL (eds). Lea & Febiger; 645–667.

Chenier TS. 2009. Anatomy and physical examination of the stallion. In: *Equine Breeding Management and Artificial Insemination*, 2nd ed. Samper JC (ed). Philadelphia: Saunders Elsevier; 1–16.

Author: Ahmed Tibary

chapter 77

Breeding, Managing Penile Paralysis

DEFINITION/OVERVIEW

- Erectile dysfunction; loss of penile function (i.e., paralysis, priapism, paraphimosis) can end a stallion's career.
- Most commonly associated with trauma, pharmaceutical administration, and anesthesia.
- Condition can be temporary or permanent; management goal is to work toward resolution and achieving ejaculation to continue the stallion's breeding career.
- Loss of ability to feel the mare or AV, inability to ejaculate.
- Early treatment of cause or etiology is essential to increase his likelihood of recovery.
- Long-term dysfunction leads to:
  - Inability to retract the penis into the prepuce.
  - Inability to achieve a fully tumescent erection.

ETIOLOGY/PATHOPHYSIOLOGY

- Trauma: breeding accidents
- Promazine-based tranquilizers
- Following anesthesia: observed post-recovery
- Extreme emaciation, loss of body condition
- Sequela of EHV-1, neurologic disease, severe intoxications

Systems Affected

Reproductive

SIGNALMENT/HISTORY

- Postpubertal male, recent breeding activity.
- Stallion observed unable to retract penis into sheath or prepuce.
- Trauma related to breeding is most common cause.
- Return to service is a reflection of the degree of dysfunction.

- Collection of semen for AI may even be possible for horses with severe compromise of erectile function.

Risk Factors

- Any male equid capable of breeding activity.
- More commonly related to live cover activity than AV collections, although the latter is possible if the penis is not properly deflected or the stallion steps abruptly to one side or falls during collection.

 ## CLINICAL FEATURES

Physical Examination

- Paralyzed penis, with or without dependent edema (edema increases with time post-incident if the penis is not supported).
- Edema
- Evaluate for sensation perception, especially of the glans penis.
- Other lesions (i.e., laceration, excoriation) may develop in long-standing cases.

 ## THERAPEUTICS

- Challenge: maintaining health of the exposed penis.
- Dependent penis quickly becomes edematous; keratotic changes; cracked lesions on the surface.
- Maintain penis close to body wall and keep its surface moist.
- Bovine udder creams or 2% testosterone cream may be applied to the penile surface. Apply two to three times daily. Testosterone cream seems to result in a slight elevation in circulating testosterone levels, possible positive impact on libido enhancement.
- Use porous fabrics that allow urine to drain away.
- Note: porous materials made for support (netting materials) tend to score the penile surface.
- Alternative: stretch lace (fabric stores) finds a new use when applied as a bandage to support the penis, serves as a sling. The back (soft, nonlace) side will not score the penile surface. Dr. McDonnell recommends a 0.5 × 3 m piece to provide length for a sling and bow-tie at the horse's back. Urine passes rapidly through; avoids urine scald.

Drug(s) of Choice

- Enhance erection and ejaculation with pharmacologic aids.
- Pharmacologic induction of ejaculation:
  - Induced, *ex copula* ejaculation.
  - Imipramine hydrochloride (1 mg/lb, PO), 2 hours before xylazine (0.25 mg/lb, IV).

- Alternative method: detomidine and PGF$_2\alpha$.
- GnRH: 50 μg SC, every 2 hours and repeat 1 hour before breeding.
  - Results in a doubling of testosterone at the time of breeding.
  - Fifty percent of affected stallions will demonstrate improved arousal and sensation of the penis.
- Testosterone can be used in moderation:
  - Low levels only to boost sexual arousal and avoid adverse impact on spermatogenesis.
  - Dosage is 80 mg aqueous, SC, every other day.

Appropriate Health Care

- Recognize importance of creating a high libido situation to increase the likelihood of ejaculation when the stallion's sensory ability is compromised.
  - Create high level of sexual arousal when collecting semen ("encourage strong, stallion-like behavior").
  - House with mares, out of hearing and sight of other studs, tease to estrus mares.
- Maximize sensation and penile stimulation during live cover or AV collection.
  - In stallions without an erection and with compromised penile sensation, wet compresses or moist heat therapy packs applied to the base of the penis can stimulate a thrusting motion adequate for ejaculation.
  - Warm compresses applied to the glans penis may or may not help; dependent on sensation that remains at the distal penis.

Nursing Care

Refer to Appropriate Health Care.

Activity

Avoid further breeding activity until acute, traumatic lesions have healed.

 COMMENTS

Client Education

- Medical, supportive care must start soon post-injury to avoid the additional problems associated with accumulated edema, loss of sensation, and surface cracking.
- A necessity to confirm the readiness of mare for breeding (standing head for live cover) to protect the stallion from injury.

Patient Monitoring

- Proper penile support, replacement of penis into prepuce, application of emollient cream two to three times per day, serves to hasten recovery, if it is possible.

Prevention/Avoidance

- Fewer injuries related to controlled breeding programs in decreasing order of safety for the stallion are:
  - AV collections with a dummy mount (controlled circumstance). Deflection of penis to one side into a collector held AV can be safer for a stallion than a phantom with a built-in AV. If the built-in AV phantom's padding wears out or stallion steps sideways during a collection, the built-in AV placement can be unforgiving.
  - AV collections with a jump/mount mare (introduces possibility of mare movement during AV collection).
  - Hand-breeding in a paddock with or without a stud manager directing the stallion's penis into the mare's vulva.
  - Pasture breeding, no control over mare selection (readiness for breeding) or stallion's approach to mare, mare motion during cover, increased potential for kick injury.

Possible Complications

Permanent loss of function and inability to ejaculate.

Expected Course and Prognosis

- Approximately 80% of affected stallions were able to continue breeding by AI.
- If live cover is necessary (TB), manual stimulation and manual insertion by stud manager of the stallion's penis into the mare's vulva at the time of mounting may be effective.
  - First attempt and success will require the most effort.
  - Stallion learns that he can achieve ejaculation with assistance; effort needed to assist him lessens.
  - Most intense arousal of libido and effort, including pharmaceutical assists, may be possible to eliminate once a routine is established.

Synonyms

- Penile paralysis
- Erectile dysfunction

Abbreviations

AI	artificial insemination
AV	artificial vagina
EHV-1	equine herpes virus 1 (rhinopneumonitis)
GnRH	gonadotropin releasing hormone
IV	intravenous
PGF	natural prostaglandin

PO   per os (by mouth)
SC   subcutaneous
TB   Thoroughbred breed

See Also

- Breeding dummy/phantom, selection and fit
- Paraphimosis
- Phimosis
- Priapism

Suggested Reading

McDonnell SM, Turner RM, Love CC, et al. 2003. How to manage the stallion with a paralyzed penis for return to natural service or artificial insemination. *Proc AAEP* 49: 291–292

Author: Carla L. Carleton

chapter 78

Breeding Phantom/Dummy, Selection, Fit and Use

DEFINITION/OVERVIEW

- Breeding mount design and construction should be best matched to the stallion.
- Enhance his comfort and willingness to serve.
- Maximize breeding efficiency.
- Option that can be used for all breeds that permit registration of foals by AI.
- Allows collection of stallion semen in the absence of a mare in standing estrus.
- Means to lessen traumatic injuries to the stallion or mare during live cover; no kick injuries, but can increase risk with regard to AV handler.
- Prepare adequate surrounding area to enhance safety of collections.

ETIOLOGY/PATHOPHYSIOLOGY

Systems Affected

- Reproductive
- Musculoskeletal: accommodations/adjustments for the stallion to be trained and collected.

SIGNALMENT/HISTORY

Common, useful for collecting stallions of any breed that permits AI.

CLINICAL FEATURES

Design features to create a safe design for stallion, handler, and AV/semen collector.

Post/Leg Design

- Single leg: minimum 10-cm (4-in) diameter steel post; diameter can, of course, be constructed much more substantially (Figs. 78.1 and 78.2).
  - One pedestal may reduce entanglement if stallion falls or dismounts awkwardly.
  - May not tolerate same degree of impact and torque as a two-legged mount.

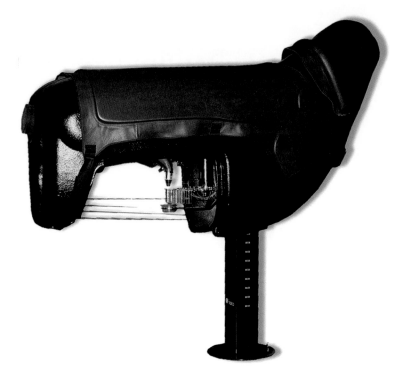

■ **Figure 78.1** Equidame®, computerized semen collection dummer.
Image courtesy Minitub®, Germany.

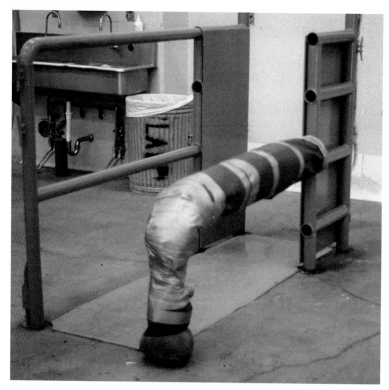

■ **Figure 78.2** One side of mare stocks adapted and padded for a miniature stallion collection dummy.

- Double leg: minimum 10-cm (4-in) diameter steel posts; diameter can, of course, be constructed much more substantially.
  - Can tolerate greater torque and pressure than single-post phantom design, especially if routinely collecting heavier horses, draft breeds (Fig. 78.3)
  - If concern arises for possible injuries due to a two-legged base, the area between the legs can be wrapped and padded. The padding may interfere with manual height adjustments.
- An adjustable height phantom that will not shift or make noise and startle the stallion during use is preferable to accommodate stallions of different size or ability. Can construct with hydraulic lift or manual adjustment (skid, tractor).
- Parameters for constructing a phantom: Preplace minimum 11 to 12-cm (4.5-in) diameter in-ground steel sleeves; proportionally larger than the post/leg size selected.
  - Minimum sleeve depth of 40 to 90 cm (24–36 in), with top of sleeve even with the floor/ground, preferably secured with cement around the perimeter of each.
  - Holes drilled fully through the pipe legs at approximate 10-cm (4-in) intervals (to adjust to/achieve height desired for collection), makes for uncomplicated adjustments, as needed, to accommodate different stallions.
  - Suitable strength/diameter pins (of greater length than the in-ground, sleeve diameter) can be inserted through pipe(s) when it needs to be raised or lowered.
  - Minimum 45 cm (18 in) depth of adjustable pipe(s) should remain within the buried sleeve when the phantom is at its highest point during use to maintain its stability.

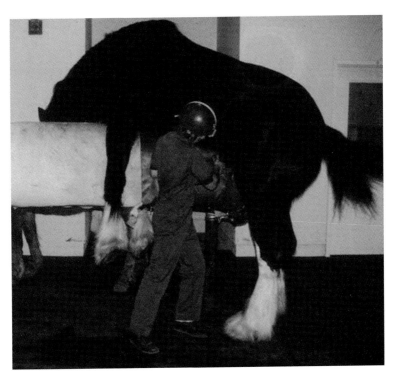

■ **Figure 78.3** Two-legged phantom, height adjustable, with welded frame to accommodate a range of stallions, Welsh ponies to draft stallions.

Width and Length of the Phantom

Width

- Width should be 45 to 46 cm (18 in), along body of phantom (Fig. 78.4).
- Common mistake of homemade phantoms is to use too large a discarded home hot water heater as the barrel of the phantom; added padding then creates an undesirable final width.
  - By the time padding has been applied and fixed around its perimeter, the width of the padded and covered phantom is as wide or wider than a mare the stallion might serve.
  - Phantom width should be less than the width of a live mare. With vigorous thrusting during collection, rub injuries, especially on the insides of the carpi, can be extreme, if using a too-broad phantom.
- Commercially produced phantom designs generally have taken safe, appropriate width into account and multiple commercial designs are available. Parameters in this chapter can serve as a guideline for selecting a suitable model.

Length

- A length of 2 to 2.5 meters (6–8 ft) is generally sufficient.
- Although a longer phantom may be desired, with training and teaching not to mount at a sharp angle to the phantom, the right stifle of the stallion will be "hooked" around the backend of the phantom and prevent his further forward motion (Fig. 78.5).

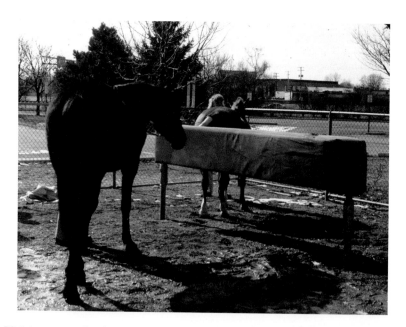

■ **Figure 78.4** Less conventional square dummy, little padding, but well-accepted by stallion. Vinyl covering was suitable for an outside, all-weather unit.

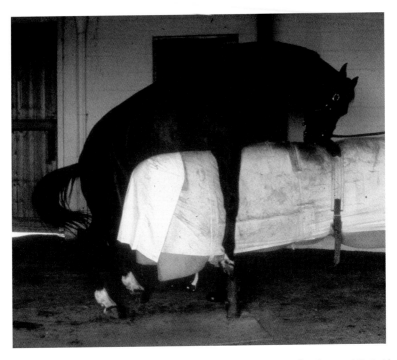

■ **Figure 78.5** Extended length phantom with canvas cover to aid gripping the dummy. Washable vinyl cover on collection end and bite straps to help stallion stabilize his mount.

Covering Material and Padding

- Smooth, well-fitted cover that can easily be cleaned (i.e., cotton and water, no chemicals) between collections and between stallions (Fig. 78.6).
- Distinct regions for different covering material:
  - Most posterior portion: may extend forward a distance of 45 to 90 cm (18–36 in); washable vinyl; covering the distance that can come into contact with the erect penis. Stitched, smooth seams: excess, darted material turned inward, toward the padding on the inside, away from contact with the penis.
  - More cranial portion of the cover can be a material that allows the stallion to grip the phantom with his forelimbs. A light or medium-weight fitted canvas cover over the padding is suitable to provide grip.
- Sufficient padding under the fitted cover to protect the stallion's forelimbs from rub injuries.
  - Least expensive: 10 to 15 cm thick (4–6 in) sheet of firm foam padding, wrapped over top, taped in place and well-secured before adding cover. It can easily be cut and fitted around the rounded posterior end of the mount and securely taped.
- Covering materials to avoid:
  - Synthetic fiber fabrics, all carpeting materials (i.e., difficult to clean; very abrasive during mounting and collecting); carpet burns, penile abrasions (Fig. 78.7).

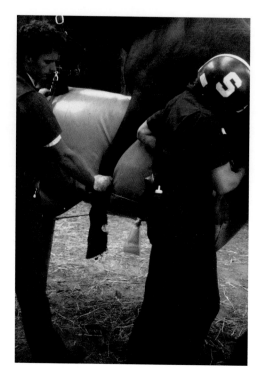

■ **Figure 78.6** Washable cover, single post dummy mare. Seams well turned in to avoid irritation to stallion's penis.

- Custom-fitted coverings:
  - Companies that make surgical and recovery pads for equine surgery recovery stalls can create custom covers for phantoms to desired specifications.
  - Custom covers for phantoms may also be ordered from local tent and tarpaulin companies.
  - Materials needed may vary dependent on permanent location of the mount, indoors or outside (weather resistant).

Additional Options

- Flat versus angled phantom: individual preference; no advantage of one or the other. The height at the mounting end is the most critical to the comfort and acceptance by the stallion.
- Added features (a head) to make a phantom appear more "mare-like" are unnecessary (Fig. 78.8). Remove, if possible, to avoid their causing injuries to handlers and stallion.
- Bite straps, grasping rigging:
  - Useful for horses that need to stabilize their stance when mounting/mounted.
  - Improve some stallion's ability to gain a more solid grip during a mount (*see* Fig. 78.5).

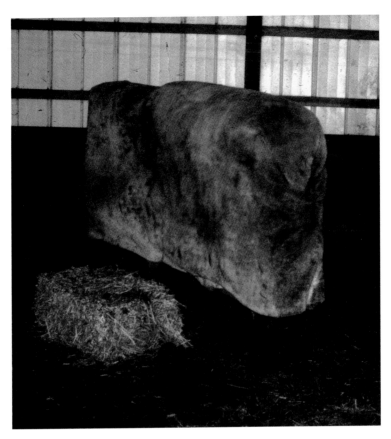

■ **Figure 78.7** Phantom covered with synthetic carpeting. Quite irritating to stallion's penis if the collector failed to divert stalloin's penis quickly into the AV.

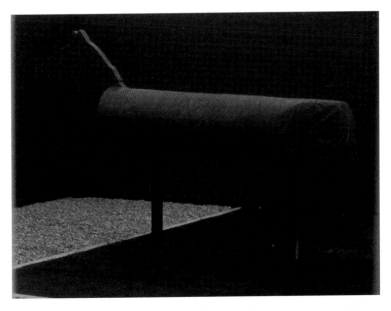

■ **Figure 78.8** A "headed" phantom placed in the middle of a collection pad surrounded by pea gravel. Note the cut-out to accommodate the larger bulk of the Lane type artifical vagina.

- Can be constructed of leather rolls that run parallel or perpendicular to the length of the phantom. If adjustable (leather belting), the bite strap can be moved to a location most beneficial for the stallion to grasp.
- Phantoms with a built-in AV carriage (self-service phantom):
  - May be useful for some stallions.
  - May be satisfactory if used with a calm stallion; can be a safe, one-person collection (*see* Fig. 78.1). The most elaborate systems can separate ejaculate fractions.
  - Potential for increased penile injury and behavior problems compared with AV that can be brought to the stallion or placed on the deflected penis.
  - Removes ability for the collector's stance to alter to shift weight applied to the middle of the AV or to apply additional pressure to the stallion's glans penis when a stallion is reticent to ejaculate.
  - If the phantom padding wears out or a vigorously mounting stallion impacts the mount with difficulty and misses the slot, injuries increase.

Footing around the Phantom

- Nonslip flooring: compressed, chipped rubber square or interlocking floor tiles: good footing, drains readily when placed on concrete flooring with drains. It is an expensive but safe, option. Of particular benefit for stallions that are hesitant, or have a tendency to slip or fall.
- Rubber matting: can create a safe collection area within a larger pen/yard (Fig. 78.9).
- Concrete: a less desirable option; horse may slip whether or not he is shod. Even if grooved, concrete can become slippery when wet. Unforgiving if the stallion falls.

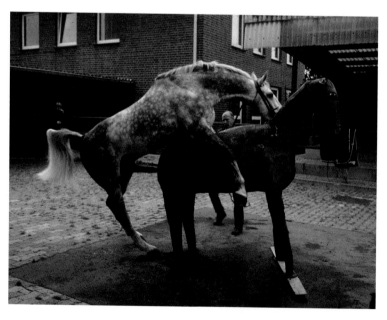

■ **Figure 78.9** An example of an extravagant, leather-covered phantom. More important was the non-slip underfooting to improve safety during collection.

- Dirt or sand: can be a less secure footing.
  - If very dusty, requires wetting before a collection to cut dirt and contamination.
  - Muddy and slippery when wet.
- Grassy paddocks: can be slippery when wet.

Location of the Phantom

- Adequate clearance on all sides and above to permit safe collection for stallion, stallion handler, and AV/collection person. Minimum 2 m on off side of phantom, 6 to 7 meters on near side, in front and behind phantom. More space is better.
- Eliminate laboratory/office doors with glass inserts; clear possible contact with electrical outlets on the walls or overhead fixtures. If designing a new breeding lab, face phantom away from windows and distractions introduced by traffic (people or vehicles).
- Consider covering cement or block walls with sheets of plywood or hang large pads, to cushion impact of horse's feet and legs if he kicks the wall.
- An inside collection facility is desirable:
  - All-weather, all-seasons collections.
  - If a stallion gets loose, he remains contained inside the facility.
  - Fewer distractions during collections, particularly useless when training a novice.

 COMMENTS

Client Education

- Once trained to use the phantom, a stallion may still require the presence of a tease mare in a nearby stocks or standing parallel to the phantom, to stimulate him to drop his penis and achieve an erection.
- Advantage that the mare usually needs not be in a standing, receptive stance.
- Collecting and freezing estrual mare urine in usable aliquots during the ovulatory season is advisable.
  - Twenty to 40 mL of estrual mare urine can be thawed and poured over the top of the phantom premount and encourage the stallion's demonstration of normal libido.
  - Especially helpful if collections are needed during the autumn and winter months (nonracing stocks, preseason BSE).
- Collection technique: preferable and safer for both stallion handler and AV/collector to be on the near (left) side of the stallion during a collection.
  - Off-side collections place the AV handler out of sight of the stallion handler (Fig. 78.10).
  - If a stallion becomes unruly, his head and neck can be pulled toward the stallion handler, which diverts the stud's rear end away from the person doing a near-sided semen collection.

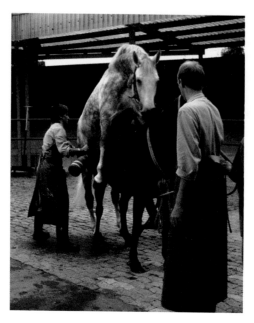

■ **Figure 78.10** There are inherent dangers when the stallion handler cannot see the collector on the opposite side of the phantom. Ideally both stud manager and artificial vagina or collection person should be on the near side and able to watch out for unpredictable stallion maneuvers.

Synonyms

- Breeding mount
- Dummy
- Dummy mare
- Dummy mount
- Mount
- Phantom mare

Abbreviations

AI	artificial insemination
AV	artificial vagina
BSE	breeding soundness examination
Near side	left side of the horse
Off or Far side	right side of the horse

Suggested Reading

McDonnell SM. 2001. How to select and fit a breeding dummy mount for stallions. *Proc AAEP* 417–420.

Mottershead J. Power-pole breeding phantom. Equine-Reproduction.com. www.equine-reproduction.com/articles/collection.htm.

Author: Carla L. Carleton

chapter 79

Breeding Soundness Examination, Stallion

DEFINITION/OVERVIEW

A method to determine the breeding potential of a stallion that includes:
- A thorough, detailed history.
- Physical examination
- Thorough examination and description of the reproductive organs (special techniques).
- Semen collection and evaluation.

BSE is not a measure of fertility. Its purposes are to:
- Evaluate a stallion for potential fertility or subfertility.
- Estimate sperm output to assist in the management of breeding.
- A systematic approach to reach a diagnosis of the causes of the stallion's infertility or subfertility.
- Prevent transmission of venereal diseases.

ETIOLOGY/PATHOPHYSIOLOGY

Multifactorial

- Factors that may affect stallion reproductive function include:
  - Failure of normal development of the reproductive system.
  - Behavioral problems
  - Acquired reproductive abnormalities.

General Factors Affecting Reproductive Development

- Sexual differentiation
- Testicular descent (cryptorchidism)
- Testicular development (hypoplasia)

Factors Affecting Semen Production (Spermatogenesis)

- General health of the stallion
- Testicular size and health
- Season
- Age

Factors Affecting Semen Delivery

- Reproductive behavior (libido)
- Erection failure
- Ejaculation failure

Factors Affecting Semen Quality

- General health of the stallion
- Testicular health
- Epididymal transport
- Environmental factors

Factors Affecting Semen Survival and Fertilizing Ability

- Genetics
- Local infections
- Hemospermia

Genetic Factors Affecting Fertility

- Breed
- Individual fertility, variations between stallions
- Specific fertility markers

Systems Affected

Reproductive

 SIGNALMENT/HISTORY

Historical Findings

- All stallions destined for breeding (natural or AI)
- Stallion with:
  - Visible abnormalities of the genital organs
  - History of infertility or subfertility
  - Detected seminal abnormalities
- Stallions recovering from a systemic illness

 CLINICAL FEATURES

General Comments

- BSE should be performed routinely at the beginning and end of each breeding season on all stallions.

Historical Findings

- Obtain complete history, including date of birth, feeding and training management, his preventive health program, and any previous health problems.
- Obtain complete breeding history, including number of seasons in service, number of mares bred (AI and natural cover), conception rate of bred mares (AI and natural cover), results of previous BSEs.

Physical Examination Findings

General Physical Examination

- Any conformation problems affecting mounting or ejaculation?
- Any signs of:
  - Congenital hereditary disease?
  - Systemic illness?
  - Chronic musculoskeletal problems?
  - Contagious disease?

Examination of the External Genitalia

The Scrotum and Its Contents (i.e., Inspection, Palpation, and Measurements)

- Examination of the external genitalia is generally easier after semen collection in a fractious stallion; take advantage of relaxation of the scrotum and testes after a collection.
- Inspect scrotal conformation:
  - Normal development and testicular descent.
  - Excessive swelling, asymmetry, or abnormal orientation.
  - Presence of lesions
- Palpate each testis for its:
  - Presence
  - Consistency
  - Orientation of the epididymal tail (spermatic cord torsion).
  - Presence of pain
  - Presence of fluid or abnormal scrotal content.
  - Symmetry of the testes
- Measure testicular size: Length × height × width (cm) of each testicle and total scrotal width (Figs. 79.1, 79.2, and Table 79.1).
  - To estimate sperm production

Examination of the Prepuce and Penis

- Prepuce and preputial orifice for lesions, abnormal discharge, or abnormal conformation.
- Penis after exteriorization:
  - After teasing (preferable) or,
  - After sedation, if necessary

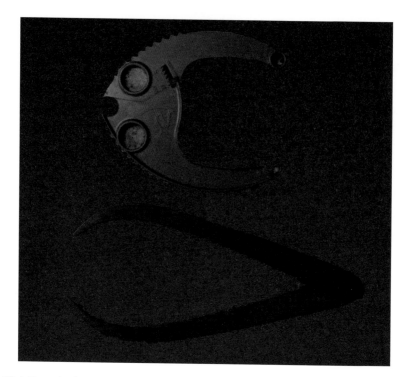

■ **Figure 79.1** Type of calipers used for testicular measurement in stallions.

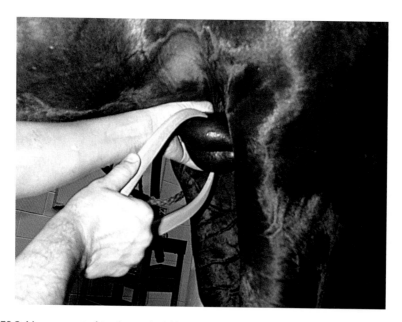

■ **Figure 79.2** Measurement of total scrotal width (TSW) using calipers.

TABLE 79.1 Testicular Measurements for the Estimation of Testicular Volume and Daily Sperm Production.

In the following equations: a, length; b, height; c, width; d, total scrotal width (all measurements should be in millimeters).
Testicular volume estimation = $4/3\pi$ $(a/2 \times b/2 \times c/2)$ or $0.533 \times a \times b \times c$
DSO = $[0.024 \times$ (volume of left testicle + volume of right testicle)$] - 0.76$
Or 0.066×10^9 TSW $- 3.36 \times 10^9$
DSO: 0.093×10^9 TSW $- 4.88 \times 10^9$
DSO = DSP $\times 0.87$

DSO, daily sperm output. TSW = total scrotal width.

- Special attention should be given to the presence of EHV-3 lesions (active vesicles or irregular scarred patches as evidence of prior active infection).

Evaluation of Reproductive Behavior

- Observe behavioral response of stallion in the presence of an estrus mare. Videotaping of the teasing (stallion to mare) is preferable and permits later analysis.
- Determine:
  - Latency to full erection
  - Latency to mount
  - Latency to intromission or ejaculation
- Semen evaluation (see other laboratory tests).
- Two ejaculates collected one hour apart should be evaluated for a routine BSE.

Examination of the Internal Genitalia and Associated Organs

- TRP
- Transrectal evaluation of the vaginal ring (internal inguinal ring).

DIAGNOSTICS

CBC/Biochemistry/Urinalysis

- Baseline data recommended for all stallions.
- Indications are based on physical examination findings and semen evaluation.

Other Laboratory Tests

Semen Volume

- Determine total gel-free ejaculate volume (most equine AVs are equipped with a collection bottle or bag with a nylon or cotton mesh, in-line, filter).

- Volume can be measured using graduated cylinders, bottles provided with the AV when it was purchased, or sterile specimen cups.
  - Precise volume is determined by using prewarmed (37°C) graduated cylinders.
- Determine the volume of gel in the filter (optional), the gel fraction.
- Precise determination of the gel-free ejaculate volume is important to determine the total sperm number in the ejaculate.

Semen Physical and Chemical Properties

- Determine pH using pH meter or pH paper:
  - Alterations in pH suggest urine contamination or alterations in the accessory sex gland fluid proprieties due to an infection.
- Note homogeneity of the ejaculate.
  - Precipitates or flocculant material may indicate reproductive disorders (seminal vesiculitis, urethritis, contamination, etc.).
- Record ejaculate color: normal should be grayish or white and translucent.
  - Abnormalities may be pink or bloody (hemospermia), or yellowish (urospermia).
- Note presence of debris; often due to presence of smegma (poor preparation of the stallion, inadequate cleaning of the penis).
- Note abnormalities of odor (urospermia).

Sperm Concentration

- Hemocytometer determination of concentration on a diluted sample of semen (1 : 100) is precise and provides a direct count of spermatozoa on the grid, but the process is tedious and time-consuming (approximately 10 minutes from start to finish).
- Densimeter determination of concentration (commercial equipment):
  - Precision depends on instrument quality, sample handling, and presence of contaminants in the ejaculate. These yield false high readings of samples containing debris or other cellular material.
  - Measurement of concentration is based on the percent transmittance (%T) of a beam of light through a sample. Low concentration sample is reflected by a high value %T, a concentrated sample a low %T.
  - The spectrophotometers thus also cannot be used to measure a sample's concentration if it has been extended with milk-based extenders.
- Determine the number of spermatozoa per mL.
- Determine the total number of sperm cells in the ejaculate:
  - $Volume_{mL} \times Concentration_{M/mL}$ = millions of sperm in an ejaculate.

Sperm Motility

- Evaluate raw and extended semen using a phase contrast microscope with heated stage.
- Motility should be evaluated immediately after collection.
- Semen should be maintained at body temperature.

- Anything in contact with the semen should be prewarmed to prevent cold shock (i.e., slides, coverslips, or pipettes).
- Ideally, all fields examined should be recorded for a permanent record.
- Motility should be evaluated on at least 10 fields at 200× to 400×.
- Estimate the percentage of TM as well as PM sperm cells.
- Objective determination of motility and other sperm motion parameters can be obtained with computerized systems (CASA); recommended for large stud farms and commercial semen freezing laboratories.
- Progressive motility less than 60% warrants further evaluation of the stallion.
- High rate of abnormal motility (backward or circular pattern) warrants evaluation of processing technique (induced cold shock) or morphologic abnormalities of the sperm.
- Serial motility evaluation of extended semen incubated at 37°C, may be indicated in some cases to determine longevity of semen.

Sperm Morphology

- Sperm morphology can be determined on stained smears using various techniques.
    - Most commonly used stain is eosin/nigrosin.
- Sperm morphology can also be determined under phase contrast on fixed samples (fixed in 10% phosphate buffered saline).
- Sperm morphology should be determined at high power under oil (1000×). High dry, 400×, is not acceptable to adequately evaluate individual sperm morphology.
- At least 100 sperm cells should be counted covering several fields. Counting 200 to 300 cells may be indicated to increase accuracy in some cases
- The frequency of normal cells and all types of abnormalities should be counted and recorded.
- Abnormalities are generally grouped into major/primary defects (related to infertility and thought to be due to abnormal spermatogenesis) and minor/secondary defects (abnormalities introduced within the excurrent duct or by semen processing [iatrogenic]).
- If the percentage of abnormalities is greater than 40%, additional testing may be required.
- Examination using Giemsa or DiffQuick® stain may be indicated to confirm the presence of abnormal cells (e.g., WBC, round/germinal cells [spheroids] and medusa cells).

Disease Testing

- EIA serology
- EVA serology: blood sampling, and also determine virus shedding status (virus in semen), if seropositive and unvaccinated.
- Bacteriology: urethral swab (pre- and post-ejaculation), semen, surface of penis or prepuce.
- Special samples for CEM: urethral fossa, urethral sinus, surface of the penis/prepuce, semen.

- Genetic testing:
    - HYPP (Quarter horses)
    - SCID (Arabians, Arabian crosses)
    - HERDA (Quarter horses)
    - JEB
    - GBED
    - OWLF (Paint)
    - Blood groups (prevention of erythrolysis)

Imaging

- U/S of testes and accessory glands may be indicated.
- Endoscopy of the urethra and evaluation of the colliculus seminalis and urinary bladder may be indicated.

Pathologic Findings

See infertility and specific reproductive disorders by organ.

 # THERAPEUTICS

Activity

Future sexual activity depends on the results of the BSE.

 # COMMENTS

Client Education

Emphasize the importance of BSE for all stallions at least once a year.

Precautions/Interactions

Age-Related Factors

- Prepubertal colts
- Overuse of a fertile horse before he is fully, sexually mature.
- Aged individuals (gonadal senescence).

Patient Monitoring

Depends on results of the routine BSE

Synonyms

- Breeding soundness examination
- Fertility evaluation

Abbreviations

AI	artificial insemination
AV	artificial vagina
BSE	breeding soundness examination
CASA	computer assisted semen analysis
CBC	complete blood count
CEM	contagious equine metritis, *Taylorella equigenitalis*
EAV	equine arteritis virus
EHV-3	equine herpes virus-3, equine coital exanthema
EIA	equine infectious anemia, also Swamp Fever, "Coggins test"
EVA	equine viral arteritis
GBED	glycogen branching enzyme deficiency syndrome
HERDA	hereditary equine regional dermal asthenia
HYPP	hyperkalemic periodic paralysis
JEB	junctional epidermolysis bullosa
OWLF	overo lethal white foal syndrome
PM	progressive motility
SCID	Severe Combined Immunodeficiency Disease
TM	total motility
TRP	transrectal palpation
U/S	ultrasound, ultrasonography
WBC	white blood count

Suggested Reading

Love CC. 2007. Reproductive examination of the stallion: Evaluation of potential breeding soundness. In: *Current Therapy in Large Animal Theriogenology*. Youngquist RS, Threlfall WR (eds). Philadelphia: Saunders/Elsevier; 10–14

Tibary A. 2006. Stallion reproductive behavior. In: *Current Therapy in Equine Reproduction*. Samper JC, Pycock J, McKinnon AO (eds). Philadelphia: Saunders/Elsevier; 174–184.

Author: Ahmed Tibary

Castration

chapter 80

DEFINITION/OVERVIEW

Surgical removal of the testes.

ETIOLOGY/PATHOPHYSIOLOGY

The testes are removed mainly to lessen stallion-like behavior or to remove testicular pathology.

System Affected

Reproductive

SIGNALMENT/HISTORY

Intact male horses of any age.

Risk Factors

- Diseased testis
- Trauma to scrotum or testis.
- Cryptorchidism
- Torsion of the testis
- Neoplasia
- Hydrocoele/hematocoele
- Orchitis/epididymitis

Historical Findings

- Normal testis size, shape, and consistency.
- Reduced fertility.
- Pain (spermatic cord torsion, testicular torsion).
- Failure to breed, walk, or jump without discomfort (performance affected).
- Testes of increased or decreased size, shape, and texture.

- Abnormal testis position.
- Enlargement in scrotum or contents.

DIAGNOSTICS

CBC/Biochemistry/Urinalysis

Laboratory parameters should be normal prior to routine castration.

THERAPEUTICS

Drug(s) of Choice

- Phenylbutazone (2–4 mg/kg PO or IV) is useful as an anti-inflammatory to help control swelling and pain post-operatively.
- Antibiotic therapy is not needed for a routine, uncomplicated castration.

Appropriate Health Care

Routine castration is managed as an on-farm procedure.

Nursing Care

- Stall confinement for complete recovery from anesthesia.
- Cold water therapy for 15 to 20 minutes SID for 3 to 5 days.

Activity

- Normal activity in the pasture.
- Forced exercise BID for 20 minutes for the first 10 to 12 days.

Surgical Considerations

- Two testes must be present in the scrotum. Castration of cryptorchid stallions is not a field procedure and should be referred to an appropriate surgical facility.
- Castration can be performed standing using local anesthesia or in lateral recumbency under general anesthesia. Standing castration has the advantage that recovery following surgery is faster and with less risk of injury during anesthetic recovery. Castration using general anesthesia, placing the animal in lateral recumbency, allows for greater safety for the surgeon, better exposure to the surgical site, and much better analgesia.
- Closed technique (vaginal tunic is not incised) versus open technique (vaginal tunic is opened and the testes are completely exposed) can be standing or under general anesthesia.

General Anesthesia

- Preoperative sedation with xylazine (1.0–1.1 mg/kg, IV).
- Butorphenol (0.01–0.02 mg/kg, IV) may be used combine with xylazine to achieve further sedation and analgesia.
- Induction with ketamine hydrochloride (2.2 mg/kg, IV), which provides 15 to 20 minutes of surgical anesthesia.
- Patient in lateral recumbency with the upper rear limb pulled lateral, exposing the testes.

Surgical Procedure/Technique

- Three 30-second scrubs of the scrotal area using betadine or chlorhexidine scrub.
- Following the second scrub, 2 to 3 mL of lidocaine is injected into each testis or spermatic cord to achieve further analgesia.
- Two incisions are made over the testes, 1 cm from the midline of the scrotum, and a 3- to 4-cm strip of skin is removed exposing the testes.
- Strip away the fascia from one exteriorized testicle to expose the spermatic cord to the inguinal ring.
- *Closed technique:* the emasculators are placed as close to the body wall as possible, removing as much of the cord as possible and emasculated.
- *Open technique:* the tunic over the testis is excised and the testis is exposed. The emasculators are placed close to the body wall on the artery, vein, and nerve of the exposed cord and are emasculated followed by the exposed tunic, which is emasculated close to the body wall.
- The other testis is removed using either the closed or open technique.
  - In large stallions, the mesorchium should be separated above the epididymis and the cord separated into the neurovascular and musculofibrous (i.e., cremaster muscle, vaginal tunic, and ductus deferens) portions before emasculation.
- Following emasculation, maintain hold on one side of the stump to keep it in view and observe it for any bleeding. If there is no bleeding from the site, the incision is inspected to ensure that it is open and will drain readily (to avoid serum accumulation).
- Remove any loose tags of fascia or fat protruding through the incision.
- Spray the area with an antiseptic solution and fly spray.

 COMMENTS

Client Education

- Six to 8 hours post-surgery the horse needs moderate exercise, 20 minutes BID (e.g., walking or at trot).
- See Complications.

Patient Monitoring

- The patient should be confined to a stall until anesthetic recovery is complete, after which time he must get 20 minutes of moderate, daily forced exercise BID.
- The surgical site should be monitored daily for hemorrhage, evisceration, excessive swelling, or infection.

Possible Complications

- Minor hemorrhage occurs through the skin, which should stop within 30 minutes.
- Treatment for excessive hemorrhage is identification and ligation of bleeding vessels.
- Excessive preputial or scrotal swelling results from poor drainage from the scrotum.
- Tranquilization, surgical scrub, and manually opening (stretching) the surgical site will facilitate drainage.
- Moderate forced exercise is the best means to ensure the surgical site will remain open and draining.
- Excessive preputial/scrotal swelling may also result from infection. If infected, antibiotics, anti-inflammatory therapy, and drainage of the site are indicated.
- Evisceration of the abdominal contents is an uncommon occurrence, which can be fatal if left untreated. The horse should be anesthetized and the intestinal contents cleaned and viable intestine replaced. The superficial inguinal ring should be sutured closed.
- Masculine behavior following castration is a reflection of learned behavior. Removal of the testes (verify by examining all tissues following emasculation) has eliminated the source of testosterone.

Synonyms

Gelding

Abbreviations

BID   twice a day
CBC   complete blood count
IV   intravenous
PO   per os (by mouth)
SID   once a day

Suggested Reading

Trotter GW. 1992. Castration. In: *Equine Reproduction*. McKinnon AO, Voss JL (eds). Philadelphia: Lea & Febiger; 907–914.

Author: Alfred B. Caudle

Castration, Henderson Technique

DEFINITION/OVERVIEW

Surgical removal of the testes.

ETIOLOGY/PATHOPHYSIOLOGY

The testes are removed to lessen stallion-like behavior or to remove testicular pathology.

System Affected

Reproductive

SIGNALMENT/HISTORY

Intact male horses of any age.

Historical Findings

Normal testis size, shape, and consistency.

DIAGNOSTICS

CBC/Biochemistry/Urinalysis

Laboratory parameters should be normal prior to routine castration.

THERAPEUTICS

Drug(s) of Choice

- Phenylbutazone (2–4 mg/kg PO or IV) is useful as an anti-inflammatory to help control swelling and pain postoperatively.

- Antibiotic therapy is not needed in a routine uncomplicated castration.
- Tetanus toxoid is a necessary and normal precautionary vaccination.

Appropriate Health Care

Routine castration is managed as an on-farm procedure.

Nursing Care

- Stall confinement for complete recovery from anesthesia.
- Cold water therapy for 15 to 20 minutes SID for 3 to 5 days.

Activity

- Normal activity in the pasture.
- Minimum of BID forced exercise for 20 minutes for the first 10 to 12 days.

Surgical Considerations

The reader is referred to the article: "How to Use the Henderson Castration Instrument and Minimize Castration Complications."
- Two testes must be present in the scrotum.
- The castration uses a closed technique under general anesthesia.

General Anesthesia

- Preoperative sedation with xylazine (1.0–1.1 mg/kg, IV).
- Butorphanol (0.01–0.02 mg/kg, IV) may be combined with xylazine to further sedation and analgesia.
- Induction with ketamine hydrochloride (2.2 mg/kg IV), which provides 15 to 20 minutes of surgical anesthesia.
- Patient in lateral recumbency with the upper rear limb pulled lateral and cranial to expose the testes.

Technique

- Three 30-second scrubs of the scrotal area using betadine or chlorhexidine scrub.
- After the second scrub, 2 to 5 mL of lidocaine is injected into each testis, for further analgesia.
- Two incisions are made over the testes, 1 cm from the midline of the scrotum, and a 3- to 4-cm strip of skin is removed to expose the testes.
- Strip away the fascia from one exteriorized testicle exposing the spermatic cord to the inguinal ring.
- Insert and secure the Henderson Instrument into a 14.4 volt cordless hand-drill with a 0.375 removable chuck (Fig. 81.1).
- Place the drill in a sterile shroud.
- Place the pliers of the Henderson on the spermatic cord proximal to the testicle (at the base of testis) (Fig. 81.2).

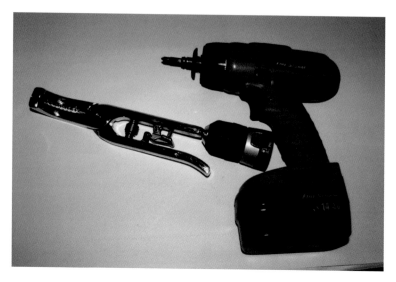

■ **Figure 81.1** The Henderson Instrument ready to be attached into a 14.4-v cordless hand-drill with a 0.375 removable chuck.

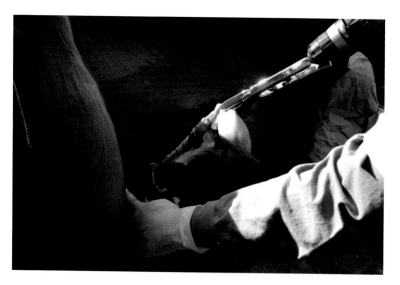

■ **Figure 81.2** The Henderson pliers placed on the spermatic cord proximal to the testicle (at the base of testis), demonstrating the twist of the cord just prior to its fracturing.

- Rotate (low torque setting) the Henderson in a clockwise direction slowly. Allow the tip of the Henderson Instrument to be drawn into the incision, approximately 2 cm, as it starts to rotate. As the spermatic cord twists, do not allow the instrument to go any further into the incision. The rotation can be moderately increased, as the cord starts to elongate just before it fractures. Once the cord fatigues and fractures, more tension can be placed on the cord to complete separation and removal of the testis. A tightly coiled cord is left behind which eliminates bleeding (Fig. 81.3).

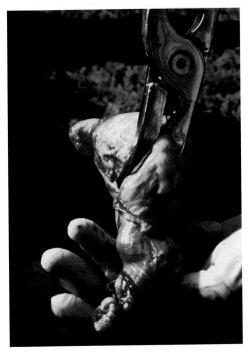

■ **Figure 81.3** The spermatic cord after it has fatigued and fractured. The tight coiling of the cord controls or eliminates bleeding.

- The first testis is removed from the instrument and the other testis is removed in a similar manner. The incision site is inspected for bleeders. Excess fascia or fat is removed. The incision is left open and sprayed with a topical antiseptic/spray bandage. The horse is allowed to stand and is put into a stall to complete anesthetic recovery.

 COMMENTS

Client Education

- The Equine Henderson Castration Instrument is a relatively new, approved procedure.
- The procedure reduces hemorrhage, swelling, and surgical time.
- See Complications

Patient Monitoring

- The patient should be confined to the stall until the anesthesia has completely worn off, after which time he must receive 20 minutes of moderate exercise twice daily for the first 10 to 12 days.

- The surgical site should be monitored daily for hemorrhage, evisceration, excessive swelling, or infection.

Possible Complications

- Hemorrhage
  - Excessive hemorrhage may occur if too much tension is put on the spermatic cord before it fatigues and fractures.
- Minor hemorrhage occurs from the skin but should stop within 30 minutes.
- Treatment for excessive hemorrhage should include identification and ligation of blood vessels.
- Excessive preputial or scrotal swelling results from poor drainage from the scrotum.
  - Tranquilization, surgical scrub, and manually opening the surgical site will allow drainage.
- Moderate forced exercise will help keep the surgical site open and draining.
- Excessive preputial or scrotal swelling may also result from infection. If infected: antibiotics, anti-inflammatory therapy, and drainage of the site are indicated.
- Evisceration of the abdominal contents is an uncommon occurrence, which can be fatal if not treated. The horse should be anesthetized, the intestinal contents cleaned and viable intestine replaced. The superficial inguinal ring should be sutured closed.
- Masculine behavior following castration (with the standard or Henderson Technique) is a learned behavior. As all sources of testosterone have been removed (testis along with 4–5 cm of spermatic cord), training should focus on altering/improving the gelding's behavior.

Synonyms

Gelding

Abbreviations

BID twice a day
CBC complete blood count
IV intravenous
PO per os (by mouth)
SID once a day

Suggested Reading

Reilly MT, Cimetti LJ. 2005. How to use the Henderson castration instrument and minimize castration complications. *Proc AAEP 51*.

Author: Alfred B. Caudle

chapter 82

Contraception, Stallion

DEFINITION/OVERVIEW

- By definition the aim or intent of contraception is to prevent fertilization.
- Contraception is an important step in the management of wild or feral equids.
- Contraception may be achieved by the elimination of sperm production or by preventing sperm from being delivered to the female genitalia.
- The ideal contraception technique should be safe for the patient, practical, efficacious, and economically viable.
- Means of contraception in the stallion can be divided into:
  - Hormonal techniques
  - Surgical techniques
  - Chemical castration

ETIOLOGY/PATHOPHYSIOLOGY

- Contraception can be achieved by altering the quantity and quality of sperm produced or by eliminating delivery of sperm in the ejaculate.
  - Suppression of spermatogenesis can be reversible (hormonal manipulation) or definitive (castration: surgical or chemical).
  - Elimination of sperm delivery during coitus can be achieved by surgical alteration such as vasectomy or caudal epididymectomy.
  - Reduced sperm delivery can be achieved by reducing libido.
- The most effective nonsurgical technique for contraception in the stallion is immunization against GnRH.
  - Immunization against GnRH is often referred to as immunological castration because circulating high levels of anti-GnRH antibodies cause a reduction in LH and a decrease in testosterone concentration.
  - In young stallions immunization against GnRH is reliable and causes reduction in libido, sperm production, testicular size, seminiferous tubule, and Leydig cell activity.
  - Treated young stallions have reduced libido, but this is not always observed in adult stallions.
  - Immunization against GnRH is reversible.

- Reduction of libido and semen quality in stallions may be achieved with chronic administration of altrenogest or progesterone.
  - Progestogen treatment is less efficacious as a contraception technique.
- Reduction of sperm quality and quantity may be achieved by administration of large doses of testosterone propionate.

Systems Affected

- Reproductive
- Central nervous system

DIAGNOSTICS

CBC/Biochemistry/Urinalysis

Unremarkable

Other Laboratory Tests

Antibodies Levels

Level of antibodies against GnRH to determine the efficacy of the immunization.

THERAPEUTICS

Progestogen Treatments

- Progesterone in oil may be administered daily (150 mg IM).
- Altrenogest daily (0.044 mg/kg PO).

Immunization against GnRH

- GnRH or LHRH vaccines are produced by conjugation of the peptide with a protein carrier such as serum albumin and adjuvant. The vaccine is given IM twice at a 4-week interval.
- Efficacy of this immunization depends on the age of the stallion. Older stallions are not as responsive as younger stallions.

Androgen Treatment

- Microencapsulated or silastic implants of an androgen treatment to the dominant stallion of a feral horse band has been used successfully to reduce the foaling rate in his mares.
- Treatment does not alter libido and social dominance.

Appropriate Health Care

Surgical procedures require postsurgical care.

Surgical Considerations

Complications from castration in adult stallions.

 COMMENTS

Expected Course and Prognosis

Good

Abbreviations

CBC   complete blood count
GnRH   gonadotropin releasing hormone
IM   intramuscular
LH   luteinizing hormone
LHRH   luteinizing hormone releasing hormone
PO   per os (by mouth)

Suggested Reading

Jaschke H. 1999. The sterilization of a stallion. *Wiener Tierärztliche Monatsschrift* 86: 423–424.
Stout TAE, Clenbrander B. 2004. Suppressing reproductive activity in horses using GnRH vaccines, antagonists or agonists. *Anim Reprod Sci* 82–83: 663–643.
Stout TAE. 2005. Modulating reproductive activity in stallions. *Anim Reprod Sci* 89: 93–103.

Authors: Ahmed Tibary and Jacobo Rodriguez

chapter 83

Cryptorchidism

DEFINITION/OVERVIEW

- Failure of one or both testes to descend completely into its associated scrotal sac (Fig. 83.1).
- Affected males are referred to as rigs, ridglings, originals, or if the testis is located in the inguinal canal, high flankers.
- False rig: a true castrate that retains some degree of stallion-like behavior.
- Complete abdominal cryptorchid: the testis and entire epididymis are contained within the abdomen.
- Incomplete abdominal cryptorchid: the testis and most of the epididymis are intra-abdominal, but the ductus deferens and cauda epididymis (i.e., epididymal tail) are located in the inguinal canal.
- Inguinal cryptorchid: the testis is located in the inguinal canal.
- Ectopic cryptorchid: the testis is subcutaneous and cannot be displaced manually into the scrotum.

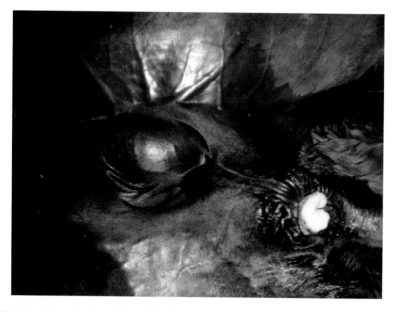

■ **Figure 83.1** One descended testis lies within the scrotum (preoperative image).

ETIOLOGY/PATHOPHYSIOLOGY

- Embryologically, testes develop adjacent to the kidneys and are situated in the dorsal abdomen.
- Normal descent: both testes descend ventrally through the abdominal cavity and inguinal canals into the scrotum sometime during the last 30 days of gestation or first 10 days after birth.
- There appears to be some genetic link/heritability, but this does not explain the entire population of individuals affected by cryptorchidism.
- Abnormal descent: failure to descend may result from faults in development of the gubernaculum, vaginal process, vaginal ring, inguinal canal, or testis, or from persistence of the testicular suspensory ligament.
  - Cryptorchidism: unilateral is more common, but may be bilateral.
  - Spermatogenesis of an abdominal testes is thermally suppressed with development arrested at the spermatogonia stage.
  - Unilateral cryptorchids have normal fertility.
  - Bilateral cryptorchidism results in sterility.
- If testes are retained in the inguinal canal, development may proceed to the primary spermatocyte stage.
- TRP of a retained testis:
  - If inguinal, the testis often is palpable.
  - If abdominal, the testis is difficult to locate by TRP (i.e., small and soft) (Figs. 83.2 and 83.3), but may be visualized at U/S.

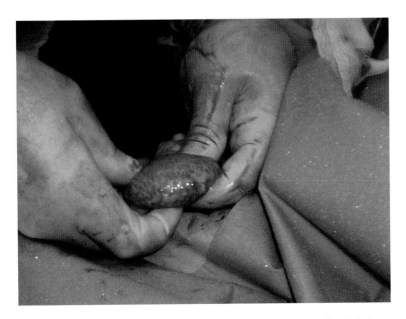

■ **Figure 83.2** Small and soft characteristic appearance of an abdominally retained testis being removed surgically (general anesthesia, in a surgical facility capable of intra-abdominal procedures).

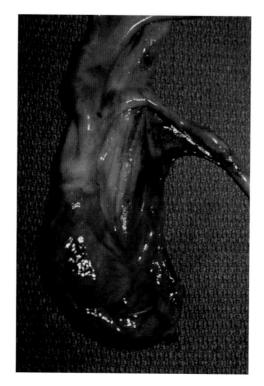

■ **Figure 83.3** Retained testis removed. Note the relationship of the size of the epididymis to the testis. Testicular size/development affected by abdominal body temperature.
Image courtesy of C. L. Carleton.

Systems Affected

Reproductive

 SIGNALMENT/HISTORY

- All breeds
- Absence of a palpable testis in the scrotal sac by 1 month of age is presumptive evidence of cryptorchidism. After 12 months, inguinal retained testes rarely enter the scrotum but, reportedly, have entered in horses as old as 2 to 3 years of age.
- Unilateral cryptorchidism is approximately 10-fold more prevalent than bilateral.
- The left testis is retained slightly more often affected than the right in horses, which contrasts with dogs and cats, in which the right testis is twice as likely as the left to be retained.
- Left testes more often are intra-abdominal; right testes are equally likely to be inguinal or abdominal.

Risk Factors

Cause unknown. There appears to be some poorly understood genetic link/heritability, but this does not explain the entire population of individuals affected by cryptorchidism.

- Higher incidence/risk: Quarter Horse, Percheron, Saddlebred, and pony breeds.
- Lower incidence/risk: Thoroughbreds, Standardbreds, Morgans, and Tennessee Walking horses.
- Cryptorchidism is relatively common in horses, with a higher prevalence compared with that reported in dogs and cats.
- Genetic research suggests a complex mechanism of inheritance involving several genes.
  - The decreasing incidence of cryptorchidism in certain lines of horses suggests that selective breeding influences the incidence.
  - Both autosomal dominant and autosomal recessive modes of inheritance have been proposed.
- In addition to genetics, other factors implicated in abnormal testicular descent include inadequate gonadotropic stimulation, intrinsically defective testes, and mechanical impediment of descent, all of which may, in turn, have a genetic basis.
- Cryptorchidism has been associated with intersexuality and abnormal karyotypes.

Historical Findings

- Stallion-like behavior in horses presumed to be geldings.
- Testes produce androgens regardless of location; even bilaterally affected individuals develop normal secondary sex characteristics and sexual behavior.
- Rarely associated with pain or other signs of disease.
- Isolated reports:
  - Torsion of the retained testis.
  - Intestinal strangulation in association with a retained testis.

 ## CLINICAL FEATURES

- Undescended testes are smaller and softer than scrotal testes.
- Absence of a palpable testis in the scrotal sac by 1 month of age is presumptive evidence of cryptorchidism.
- After 12 months, inguinal retained testes rarely enter the scrotum but, reportedly, have entered in horses as old as 2 to 3 years of age.

 ## DIFFERENTIAL DIAGNOSIS

- Bilateral cryptorchid stallion
- Cryptorchid hemicastrate

- Gelding
- True anorchidism, in which neither testis develops, is extremely rare.
- Monorchid animals, having failed to develop a second testis, have been described in isolated reports.

DIAGNOSTICS

- Complete history
- Behavioral observation
- A thorough visual examination and palpation of the scrotum and external inguinal region are often sufficient to provide a diagnosis.
- External deep inguinal palpation or TRP often requires tranquilization or sedation.

Other Laboratory Tests

Note: Endocrine assay is not reliable as a diagnostic tool in prepubertal males.

hCG Stimulation Test

- Administer hCG (10,000 IU IV), and collect blood samples as follows: baseline (pre-administration), 1 hour, 2 hour, and the final sample at 48 to 72 hours. Instances have been reported in which the response to hCG was significantly delayed (48–72 hours).
- Stallions and cryptorchids show a two- to threefold increase in serum testosterone levels.
- Geldings show no change in testosterone levels.

Serum Conjugated Estrogen Concentration

- Estrone sulfate
- Stallions and cryptorchids, greater than 400 pg/mL.
- Geldings, less than 50 pg/mL.
- Not reliable in horses less than 3 years and in donkeys of any age. Donkeys have no detectable conjugated estrogens.

Fecal Conjugated Estrogen Concentration

- Noninvasive technique.
- Estrogens are stable in feces for at least 1 week.

Serum Testosterone Concentration

- Stallion and cryptorchids, greater than 100 pg/mL.
- Geldings, less than 40 pg/mL.
- Unreliable in horses less than 18 months of age.
- Less reliable than hCG stimulation test and conjugated estrogen determination because of wide seasonal variation in basal concentrations.

Serum Inhibin Concentration

- Stallions, 1 to 3 ng/mL.
- Gelding, negligible.

Imaging

- Parenchyma of a cryptorchid testis is less echogenic and smaller than that of a normal descended testis.
- Percutaneous U/S may help to identify an inguinal testis.
- Transrectal U/S may help to identify an abdominal testis.

Laparoscopy

- Laparoscopy to identify an abdominal testis.
- Less invasive procedures usually are sufficient to diagnose the problem and often are used in conjunction with laparoscopic cryptorchidectomy.

Pathological Findings

- Thermally induced arrest of spermatogenesis in the retained, abdominal testis.
- Spermatocytogenic development may reach the primary spermatocyte stage if the testis is inguinal.
- Seminiferous tubule development is impeded.
- Elevated body temperature may induce interstitial cell hyperplasia.
- Testicular cysts and neoplasia (e.g., teratoma, interstitial cell tumor, seminoma, Sertoli cell tumor) have been reported. The incidence of teratoma increases in abdominally retained testes.

 # THERAPEUTICS

Currently, no consistently effective medical treatment is available.

Drug(s) of Choice

- One study indicated that administering 2500 IU of hCG, IM, twice weekly for 4 weeks, resulted in 50% of colts, in which one testis had been identified in the *inguinal canal* prior to initiation of treatment, were found to have the retained testis present in the scrotum following the final treatment.
- No change in testis location was noted in colts with abdominal cryptorchid testes.

Surgical Considerations

- Cryptorchidectomy via standard or laparoscopic approaches.
- Standard approaches:
  - Inguinal, parainguinal, paramedian, suprapubic, and flank.
  - Choice is dictated by the location of the testis.

- Laparoscopy can be performed with the horse standing or in dorsal recumbency.
  - Always remove the retained testis before the descended testis.
- Another, less reliable technique involves laparoscopic cautery and transection of the spermatic cord to induce avascular necrosis of the testis.
  - Revascularization can occur, with subsequent production of testosterone.
- Orchiopexy (i.e., surgical placement of a retained testis into the scrotum) is unethical.
- Surgical placement of a substitute, similarly shaped object (breast implant) is also unethical.

 COMMENTS

Client Education

Recommend castration of the cryptorchid individual.

Patient Monitoring

- Cessation of stallion-like behavior occurs concomitant with decreasing androgen levels and may require 6 to 8 weeks.
- Some stallions castrated at an older age or, after having bred mares, retain stallion-like behavior even after removal of all testicular tissue; a learned behavior.

Prevention/Avoidance

Recommend castration of the cryptorchid individual.

Possible Complications

- Complications are uncommon, usually those associated with cryptorchidectomy.
- Possible sequelae: infection, hemorrhage, adhesion formation, eventration, and incomplete castration.

Expected Course and Prognosis

Assuming the recovery from the cryptorchid surgery is uneventful, horses tend to return to a normal functional life as a gelding.

Synonyms

Lay terms include:
- High flanker (if the retained testis is inguinal)
- Originals
- Rigs
- Ridglings

Abbreviations

hCG   human chorionic gonadotropin
IM   intramuscular
IV   intravenous
TRP   transrectal palpation
U/S   ultrasound, ultrasonography

See Also

- Abnormal scrotal enlargement
- Abnormal testicular size
- Scrotal evaluation
- Semen evaluation, abnormal stallion
- Semen collection, routine semen evaluation

Suggested Reading

Brendemuehl JP. 2006. A comparison of the response to repeated human chorionic gonadotropin administration on serum testosterone in prepubertal Thoroughbred colts with descended and cryptorchid testicles, *Proc AAEP* 1–6.

Mueller POE, Parks H. 1999. Cryptorchidism in horses. *Equine Vet Educ* 11: 77–86.

Rodgerson DH, Hanson RR. 1997. Cryptorchidism in horses. Part I. Anatomy, causes and diagnosis. *Compend Contin Educ Pract Vet* 19: 1280–1288.

Rodgerson DH, Hanson RR. 1997. Cryptorchidism in horses. Part II. Treatment. *Compend Contin Educ Pract Vet* 19: 1372–1379.

Schumacher J. 2006. Reproductive system. In: *Equine Surgery*, 3rd ed. Auer JA, Stick JA (eds). St. Louis: Saunders-Elsevier; 775–810.

Authors: Jane Barber and Philip E. Prater

chapter 84

Dourine

DEFINITION/OVERVIEW

Dourine is a disease of exclusively of equidae, with natural infections reported only in horses and donkeys. The causative agent *Trypanosoma equiperdum* is transmitted only by direct venereal contact, with no vector host involved. The organism has a tropism for genital mucosa and cannot survive outside the host. Dourine causes significant debilitation of affected animals and as a result, predisposition to other diseases is significant. Dourine is a disease with a high mortality rate.

ETIOLOGY/PATHOPHYSIOLOGY

Dourine is considered to be endemic in Africa, Asia, and Central and South America. A low prevalence is reported in southeastern parts of Europe. Mortality is commonly reported to be approximately 50% with acute disease, however, up to 100% has occurred. Complicating diagnosis is that the organism is periodically unrecoverable from the urethra or vagina of infected animals. Additionally, transmission of the infectious agent to a susceptible animal is not certain even in situations where mating has occurred with known infected animals.

Systems Affected

- GI: weight loss and emaciation.
- Skin/Exocrine: edematous plaques in region of external genitalia and urticaria.
- Hemic/Lymphatic/Immune: peripheral lymphadenopathy, profound anemia.
- Musculoskeletal: progressive weakness
- Reproductive: abortion
- CV: dependent edema
- Neuromuscular: meningoencephalitis, progressive weakness, paresis, and paralysis.
- Ophthalmic: keratoconjunctivitis

SIGNALMENT/HISTORY

- Animals of breeding age are at risk in endemic environment.
- Clinical signs depend on strain of the infectious organism and the general health of the horse population.

- Incubation period: 1 week to 3 months, with approximately 50% mortality of affected animals due to acute disease in 6 to 8 weeks. Disease may last from 2 to 4 years.

Risk Factors

- Exposure to *T. equiperdum*: infection occurs across intact genital mucosal barriers.
- Asymptomatic carriers act as a herd reservoir of infection.
- Transport of horses from known-infected areas.
- Males may serve as noninfected mechanical carriers after breeding infected females.

Historical Findings

Characteristic cutaneous signs

CLINICAL FEATURES

Female

- Severe edematous vulvar and perineal swelling
- Mucopurulent vulvar discharge
- Frequent, painful attempts at urination because of vaginal mucosal irritation.
- Chronic cases develop urticarial subcutaneous plaques ("silver dollar lesions") on vulva and surrounding tissues. These may regress within hours or days to areas of depigmentation.
- Abortion, if pregnant

Male

- Edema of prepuce, urethral process, penis, testes, and scrotum. Paraphimosis may ensue.
- Plaques and depigmented lesions as in females.
- Inguinal lymph node enlargement.
- Intact male may present with urethral discharge.

DIFFERENTIAL DIAGNOSIS

- EHV-3: equine coital exanthema
- EIA
- EVA
- Endometritis: overtly purulent (e.g., CEM)

DIAGNOSTICS

CBC/Biochemistry

- Acute infection: leukocytosis; other inflammatory changes.
- Chronic infection: debilitating infection results in anemia and extensive multisystemic disease.

Cytology/Histopathology

- Causative organism is present in smears of body fluid or lymph node aspirates.
- Seminal fluid, mucus from prepuce, and vaginal discharges may also yield organisms.

Serology

- CF test is the most widely used and reliable test.
- Also available: AGID, IFA, and ELISA tests.

Pathological Findings

- Primarily emaciation with enlargement of lymph nodes, spleen, liver; periportal infiltrations in liver; and petechial hemorrhages in kidney.
- In the nervous form, the organism can be recovered from the lumbar and sacral spinal cord, sciatic and obturator nerves, and CSF.

 THERAPEUTICS

Treatment of affected animals is controversial due to the potential for a carrier state.

Drug(s) of Choice

Quinapyramine sulfate: 5 mg/kg, divided doses SC.

Alternative Drugs

- Diminazene: 7 mg/kg as 5% solution injected SC; repeat at half-dose 24 hours later.
- Suramin: 10 mg/kg IV, two to three times at weekly intervals.

Appropriate Health Care

- May be successful if treated early in the course of disease.
- Chronic cases in particular are unresponsive to treatment.

COMMENTS

Client Education

Recovered treated animals may become asymptomatic carriers.

Patient Monitoring

- Body weight and condition
- CBC
- Neurologic examination

Prevention/Avoidance

- Prohibit movement of horses from infected areas.
- Control breeding practices.
- Eradication: herd serology with slaughter of infected animals. Consecutive negative tests at least 1 month apart indicate freedom from disease.
- No vaccine is available.

Possible Complications

Multisystemic nature of the disease predisposes affected animals to multiple system failure.

Expected Course and Prognosis

- Incubation period: wide range from 1 week to 3 months.
- Course of disease: usually 1 to 2 months, but disease may last from 2 to 4 years. Approximately 50% of affected animals die of acute disease in 6 to 8 weeks. Mortality of up to 100% has been reported.
- Neurological: Hyperesthesia and hyperanalgesia, with hindquarter weakness progressing to ataxia.
- Anemia, wasting, and persistent intermittent pyrexia.

Abbreviations

AGID	agar gel immunodiffusion
CBC	complete blood count
CEM	contagious equine metritis
CF	complement fixation
CSF	cerebrospinal fluid
CV	cardiovascular
EHV-3	equine herpes virus-3
EIA	equine infectious anemia
ELISA	enzyme-linked immunosorbent assay

EVA   equine viral arteritis
GI   gastrointestinal
IFA   immunofluorescent assay
IV   intravenous
SC   subcutaneous

See Also

- Venereal diseases

Suggested Reading

Barrowman PR. 1976. Observations on the transmission, immunology, clinical signs and chemotherapy of dourine (Trypanosoma equiperdum infection) in horses, with special reference to cerebrospinal fluid. *Onderstepoort Vet Res* 43: 55–66.

Hagebock JM, Chieves L, Frerichs WM, et al. 1993. Evaluation of agar gel immunodiffusion and indirect fluorescent antibody assays as supplemental tests for dourine in equids. *Am J Vet Res* 54: 1201–1208.

Radositis OM, Blood DC, Gay CC. 1994. *Veterinary Medicine*, 8th ed. London: Balliere Tindall; 1220–1222.

Author: Peter R. Morresey

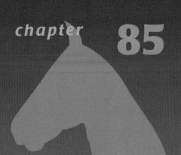

chapter 85

Hemospermia

DEFINITION/OVERVIEW

Contamination of an ejaculate with blood.

ETIOLOGY/PATHOPHYSIOLOGY

- Injury to the urethral process (from lacerations by tail hair, abrasion with the phantom during semen collection, cutaneous habronemiasis, squamous cell carcinoma).
- Lacerations to the glans or body of the penis.
- Tears in the urethral mucosa.
- Infection/inflammation of the accessory sex glands.

Systems Affected

Urogenital

SIGNALMENT/HISTORY

- General physical examination of the stallion at rest is usually unremarkable.
- Discoloration of semen ranging from pink-tinged to frank hemorrhage is the most common sign (Figs. 85.1 and 85.2).
- In live cover (natural breeding) situations, blood may be seen dripping from the penis on dismount (Fig. 85.3), at the vulvar lips of the mare following breeding, or mares may not become pregnant following breeding.
- Some stallions will concurrently have hematuria.
- Possible genetic link: Quarter Horse breed have tears in the urethral mucosa.

Causes

- Top most common:
  - Trauma: laceration of the urethral process, glans penis or body of penis (usually from tail hair); stricture of the urethra from chronic placement without monitoring/cleaning of a stallion ring (Fig. 85.4).
  - Urethral defects

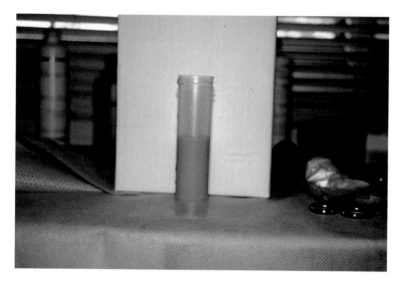

■ **Figure 85.1** Altered ejaculate color by introduction of blood at the time of ejaculation. Image courtesy of Ahmed Tibary.

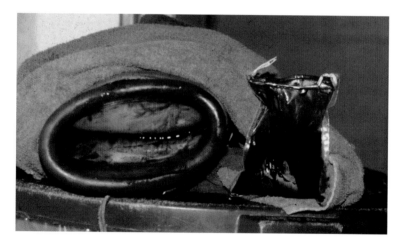

■ **Figure 85.2** Extreme case of hemospermia. Diagnosis determined the source to be a seminal vesiculitis. Image C. L. Carleton.

- Urethritis
- Infection/inflammation of the accessory sex glands.
- Neoplasia
  - Squamous cell carcinoma
  - Papilloma
- Cutaneous habronemiasis (Fig. 85.5).
- Active ulceration of penile surface (Fig. 85.6).

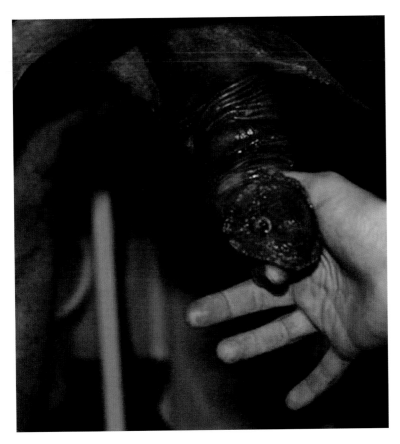

■ **Figure 85.3** Blood on or at the tip of a stallion's penis after dismount.
Image courtesy of C. L. Carleton.

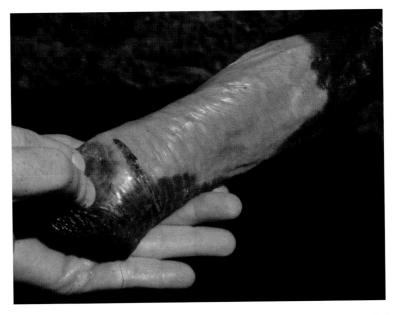

■ **Figure 85.4** Penile laceration on shaft. Exposure to mares and breeding had to be curtailed until healed entirely.
Image courtesy of C. L. Carleton.

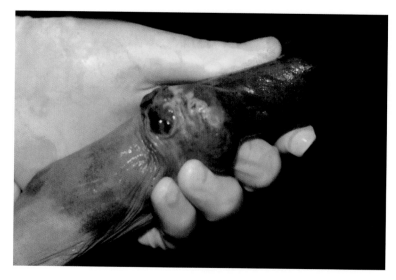

■ **Figure 85.5** Habronema lesion (the enlargement) on penile shaft.
Image courtesy of C. L. Carleton.

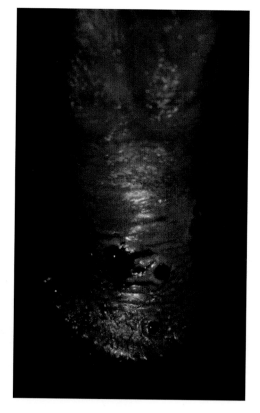

■ **Figure 85.6** Active ulcerations of equine herpes virus (EHV-3) also known as equine coital exanthema.
Image courtesy of C. L. Carleton.

Risk Factors

- Breeding activity (infection, lacerations to external penis).
- Hot, humid environmental conditions (cutaneous habronemiasis).

 DIFFERENTIAL DIAGNOSIS

Differentiating Causes

- Semen collected with an AV permits visualization of hemorrhage within the ejaculate.
- Fractionation of the ejaculate, using an open-ended AV; allows direct visualization of the ejaculate fractions, and may also aid in identifying from which portion of the ejaculate the hemorrhage originates.
  - Blood in the gel fraction likely originates from the SVs (Fig. 85.7).
  - WBCs predominate over RBCs with infections of the accessory sex glands.

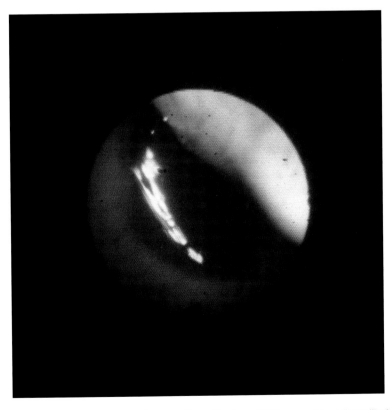

■ **Figure 85.7** Blood identified during endoscopy of a stallion's genital tract, clot is at the colliculus seminalis. Subsequent biopsies confirmed it to have originated from the seminal vesicles. Image courtesy of C. L. Carleton.

DIAGNOSTICS

CBC/Biochemistry/Urinalysis

- CBC and chemistry panel are generally unaffected.
- Urinalysis might reveal RBCs.

Imaging

- Transrectal U/S may be useful in diagnosing abnormalities of the SVs.
  - Normal SVs can vary significantly in appearance. They may range from flat in the nonaroused state (empty), to enlarged and filled with hypoechoic fluid after sexual stimulation.

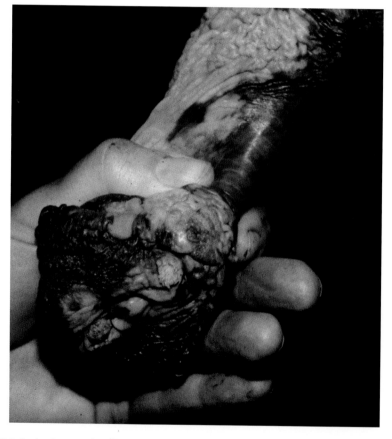

■ **Figure 85.8** Penis of an aged stallion presented for hemospermia. The disparate appearance of the lesions necessitated the collection of biopsies. Etiology of lesions was confirmed to be squamous cell carcinoma, *Habronema*, sarcoid, and papillomatosis.
Image courtesy of C. L. Carleton.

- Inflamed SVs may be thickened and filled with echogenic fluid.
- Note: Echogenic content in the lumen of the SVs does not always indicate pathology of the glands because some stallions produce normal gel that appears echogenic on U/S examination.
- Ancillary tests such as culture, cytology, and endoscopy should be considered for definitive diagnosis of accessory sex gland infection/inflammation.

Other Diagnostic Procedures

- Endoscopy: a useful tool to diagnose urethral abnormalities (urethritis, rents in the mucosa) and SV inflammation.
- Bacterial culture and cytology of semen are beneficial for determination of accessory sex gland infection.
- Biopsy and histopathology can be used to diagnose neoplasia or cutaneous habronemiasis (Figs. 85.8 and 85.9).

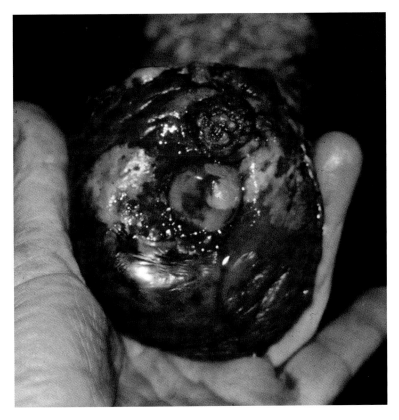

■ **Figure 85.9** Hemorrhage from penile lesions of aged stallion post-collection. Image courtesy of C. L. Carleton.

THERAPEUTICS

All conditions warrant sexual rest.
- Trauma: usually as an outpatient, palliative therapy aimed at hygiene and parasite control.
- Urethral defects:
  - Conservative approach: sexual rest (limited success).
  - Surgical approach: ischial urethrotomy and a minimum of 2 months sexual rest. Success rate is also limited.
- Urethritis: antibiotic therapy.
- Infection/inflammation of the accessory sex glands:
  - Antibiotic therapy (local, systemic).
  - Lavage of the glands (via endoscope using flush and biopsy channels).
  - Intrauterine infusion of semen extender containing appropriate antibiotics.
- Neoplasia:
  - Cryotherapy
  - Hyperthermia
  - Local excision
  - Reefing operation
  - Phallectomy
- Cutaneous habronemiasis:
  - Parasite control
  - Cryotherapy
  - Surgical removal of affected sites

Drug(s) of Choice

- Anti-inflammatory therapy (i.e., phenylbutazone, flunixin meglumine) is indicated in most cases.
- Antibiotic therapy is directed at the etiologic agent causing bacterial urethritis; culture and sensitivity to select the appropriate antibacterial.
- Systemic antibiotic therapy for SV infection is often ineffective due to poor diffusion of the drug into the affected area.
- Antibiotic of choice for systemic treatment is trimethoprim-sulfamethoxazole (15 to 30 mg/kg, PO, BID) if the identified organism is susceptible to it.
- Lavage of the glands and infusion of an antibiotic directly into the SVs may be a more effective treatment.
- Antiparasitic therapy for cutaneous habronemiasis (ivermectin, 0.2 mg/kg, PO, every 30 days until resolution of lesions).

Precautions/Interactions

- Trimethoprim-sulfamethoxazole at higher doses may cause colitis.
- Decrease the dosage or discontinue the drug if the horse shows signs of colitis (diarrhea).

Surgical Considerations

Refer to individual etiologies and treatment.

COMMENTS

Client Education

Sexual rest until problem is completely resolved is essential.

Patient Monitoring

Semen collection for identification of RBC or WBC in the ejaculate.

Possible Complications

- Infertility
- Urethral stricture or adhesions
- Adhesions of the SVs
- Ruptured urinary bladder

Expected Course and Prognosis

Dependent on etiology

Associated Conditions

Hematuria

Pregnancy

Blood in the ejaculate can be harmful to spermatozoa and thus conception rates may decrease.

Abbreviations

AV   artificial vagina
BID   twice a day
CBC   complete blood count
PO   per os (by mouth)
RBC   red blood cell
SV   seminal vesicle
U/S   ultrasound
WBC   white blood cell

See Also

- Breeding soundness examination, stallion
- Semen collection, methods

- Semen collection, routine semen evaluation
- Semen evaluation, abnormal stallion

Suggested Reading

Varner DD, Schumacher J, Blanchard T, et al. 1991. *Diseases and Management of Breeding Stallions.* Goleta: American Veterinary Publications; 257–340.

Voss JL, McKinnon AO. 1993. Diagnosis of pregnancy. In: *Equine Reproduction.* McKinnon AO, Voss JL (eds). Philadelphia: Lea & Febiger; 864–870.

Authors: Margo L. Macpherson and Carla L. Carleton

chapter 86

History Form, Stallion

DEFINITION/OVERVIEW

In order to understand the multitude of aspects that may affect a stallion's fertility, it is essential to review the impact of management decisions (i.e., vaccinations, anthelmintics, housing, level of performance), breadth of the stallion's activities/training, nutrition, exposure to pathogens, transportation, frequency of use, method of semen preservation, and so on, that impact his performance (positively or otherwise).

ETIOLOGY/PATHOPHYSIOLOGY

Systems Affected

Reproductive

SIGNALMENT/HISTORY

A comprehensive review of aspects affecting the stallion's health: management (i.e., vaccinations, anthelmintic administration), training, nutrition, and so on, as well as a detailed reproductive history in its many aspects, should accompany any *routine* stallion BSE (*See* Figure 86.1 at end of chapter).

Risk Factors

- Age (i.e., pubertal, mature, aging), when first used.
- Phantom/dummy mare collections, jump mare, live cover.
- Season and impact on fertility, semen parameters.
- Frequency of use, size of mare book.
- Methods of collection and potential for injury, infection.
- Genetic influence on individual fertility.

Historical Findings

- Breeding injuries
- Psychological damage from earlier injury.

- Other, non-reproductive factors that influence his reproductive health or ability (e.g., pasture breeding stallion with compromised vision or lameness; neurologic compromise, and so on).
- Results from any prior evaluations, including scrotal and testicular measurements, palpation, and U/S and TRP.

 CLINICAL FEATURES

- Primary use of breeding stallions in North America falls between February 15 (onset of the OBS) through the PBS (June, July), unless the stallion *shuttles* between northern and southern hemispheres.
- The February start of the OBS results from the use of the universal birth date of January 1 that is recorded for equine births occurring within a calendar year in the northern hemisphere. It is primarily employed by particular breeds (usually racing stock). The influence it has on equine breeding practices is not positive, in that breeding activity commences at a time of year when estrous cyclic activity is poorly established (most mares still in anestrus or vernal transition). The stallion is capable of breeding before most of his mares are synchronous (or have foaled in new season).

 COMMENTS

- The will to exert influence on the larger horse breeding industry is lacking and practices such as the universal birth date will continue. The OBS terminates while the PBS is just getting into full swing. Mare fertility, estrous cycles, and body condition are all enhanced by breeding during long days (the PBS), when pasture is available, and foals are less stressed by winter foaling conditions. The pressure for stallion's to cover their book of mares in a compressed period of time (OBS) creates its own frustrations.
- The point of early breeding is to have mares foaling as early as possible in the following calendar year.
  - Offspring of racing breeds are usually marketed at yearling sales the year after their birth.
  - Earlier born foals are larger, stronger, better developed and able to train and compete in the 2- and 3-year-old races, than foals born in May, June, and so on, against which they will compete.
  - Failing to enter the early breeding, early foaling, early training and racing schedule, would result in later born offspring. Because of the 5- to 6-month age differential, late foals (born in May, June, and later) are less developed at 2- and 3-year-old competitions.
- The potential for a stallion to be used at stud is often predicated on his earnings at 2 and 3 years of age. Early training methods of young horses can have negative consequences for the horse presented for a BSE in later years. Anabolic steroids are

contraindicated for stallions to be used for breeding. Anabolic steroid use (See Fig. 106.3) associated with testicular metabolic change is incompletely characterized at present, but it can interfere with normal endocrine feedback loops, result in decreased GnRH and LH, decrease sperm numbers, alter motility and morphology, and in some cases result in testicular degeneration.

■ A significant percentage of wastage has been documented in the thoroughbred breed extending from early breeding, conception, gestation, through parturition and weaning. A relatively small percentage of thoroughbreds actually reach training and are successful at the track. Breeding practices and pushing young horses to compete before they are sufficiently mature can contribute to these losses.

Abbreviations

BSE   breeding soundness examination
OBS   operational breeding season
PBS   physiologic breeding season
TB   thoroughbred breed
TRP   transrectal palpation
U/S   ultrasound

See Also

■ BSE, stallion
■ Nutrition, stallion
■ Reproductive efficiency, measures of
■ Semen, chilling of
■ Semen collection, techniques/methods
■ Semen collection, routine semen evaluation
■ Semen, cryopreservation, managing freezing ability
■ Semen evaluation: abnormalities
■ Spermatogenesis and factors affecting sperm production
■ Vaccination program, stallion

Suggested Reading

Chenier T. 1997. Physiology and endocrinology of stallions. In: *Current Therapy in Large Animal Theriogenology*, 2nd ed. Youngquist RS, Threlfall WR (eds). Philadelphia: Saunders; 3–9.

Jeffcott LB, Whitwell KE. 1973. Twinning as a cause of foetal and neonatal loss in the thoroughbred mare. *J Comp Pathol* 83(1): 91–106.

Jeffcott LB, Rossdale PD, Freestone J, et al. 1982. An assessment of wastage in thoroughbred racing from conception to 4 years of age. *Eq Vet J* 14(3): 185–198.

Love CC. 1997. Reproductive examination of the stallion: evaluation of potential breeding soundness. In: *Current Therapy in Large Animal Theriogenology*, 2nd ed. Youngquist RS, Threlfall WR (eds). Philadelphia: Saunders; 10–14.

Author: Carla L. Carleton

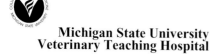

**Michigan State University
Veterinary Teaching Hospital**

STALLION HISTORY FORM

Date: _____ Age: _____

Weight, current: _____ kg
_____ lbs

Date purchased: _____

_____ Losing weight
_____ Gaining weight

Presenting Complaint: _____

PART ONE—NONREPRODUCTIVE INFO:

1. **GENERAL INFO:** *Use Medical Record PE/HX form for recording this info.

2. **IDENTIFICATION/INSURANCE INFO:**

Type of identification:

_____ Lip tattoo

_____ Freeze brand

Microchip (AVID or other?):

_____ #:

Insurance company: _____

_____ Neck tattoo

Registration   Name of Breed Association:
Number
_____ _____

Cross registration (QH & Paint, Hanoverian & Dutch, etc.): _____

3. **MEDICAL MANAGEMENT INFO:**

a. Vaccine/s

Type given & route of administration
(5-way [specify], rhino, PHF, WNV,
Rabies, etc.)

_____ (MLV, Killed, attenuated - if known)

_____

_____ Date given

Date of most recent Coggins

b. Anthelmintic/s

Type given (Panacur, Ivermectin, etc.)

_____

_____ Date given

_____ Frequency of administration

c. EVA status:

d. EPM status:
Evaluated: _____
Treated: _____

4. **ENVIRONMENT/MANAGEMENT INFO:**

Please check box or fill in blank to best describe patient's current environmental status:

_____ Pasture

_____ Racetrack

_____ Boarding facility

Stall time: _____

Hrs turned
out/day: _____

Hrs turned
out/night: _____

_____ Separate stud barn (Y/N)

_____ Breeding farm (Y/N)

Are mares housed near stallion (Y/N)?
Number of hours/day in stall:

■ **Figure 86.1** Stallion History Form.

Light therapy implemented (Describe wattage, type of bulb/system used):

Date that light therapy began:

_____ # hours under lights/24hr period:

List any current or previous disease conditions present at barn: _____

5. NUTRITIONAL/MEDICATION INFO:

Current feeding regimen (include amounts, cutting (1st, 2nd, 3rd) of hay, type of hay; concentrate (plain oats, sweet feed, custom mix, % protein; beet pulp, etc.):

Number of feedings per day (once, twice, etc.):

List any current medications/supplements:

List any previous injuries (non-repro & repro related)

List previous medications given, i.e. steroids, antibiotics, etc.

List any previous surgeries, dates, outcomes:

6. USAGE/FITNESS LEVEL:

Check performance level that best fits his current use:

_____ **High Level Performance**: (Racing, endurance training, dressage, polo)

_____ **Low Level Performance**: (Pleasure, trail riding)

PART TWO—REPRODUCTIVE INFORMATION:

1. BREEDING INFO:

Please check any of the following areas related to breeding that have been problematic:

_____	Libido	_____	Ejaculation	_____	Infections
_____	Mating ability	_____	Quality of sperm	_____	Disposition/behavioral vices
	Erection		Quantity of sperm		Breeding itself is difficult

Explain in detail:

Please check box which best describes the semen processing commonly used for breeding (fill in the blanks accordingl):

_____ *Live cover*

_____ *AI*

_____ Fresh (raw)

_____ Fresh, cooled

_____ Frozen

Type & brand of extender used:

Extender ratio commonly used (1:1, 1:2; dilution to 25 M/mL, 50 M/mL, etc.:

Type of AV:

_____ MO

_____ CO/Lane Method

_____ Other (describe):

■ **Figure 86.1** continued

_____

_____ Age at 1ˢᵗ service

_____ Date when last serviced a mare (prior to current examination):

2. SERVICING INFO:

MARES BRED by/SEASON:	Year	# Mares Bred	# Pregnant	# Live Foals Produced
Current yr: Prior years in reverse				

3. HEALTH INFO:

History of repro-related illness/es:	Describe:		
History of venereal infection:	Organism:		
	Treatment/therapy:		
	Abx (1)	Abx (2, or other):	Recheck?
Prior positive cultures (penis, urethra, diverticulum, prepuce), isolates? When?	Dose:	Dose:	Outcome?
	Tx frequency:	Tx frequency:	
	Route of Admin.	Route of Admin:	

4. RECORD KEEPING:

_____ Are breeding/performance records maintained (Y or N)   If yes, describe what parameters are routinely recorded:
_____ Previous fertility evaluation (Outcome, letters, reports)?   _____

If available, attach copy of earlier reports here: _____

5. GENERAL FARM MANAGEMENT:

A. Describe teasing methods used:
_____ Stallion to mare
_____ Mare to stallion
_____ Teaser pony
_____ Gelding
_____ How often?
_____ Who handles the stallion during teasing?
_____ Is stallion handler during breeding the same person who handles the stallion during the teasing (Y or N)
_____ Number of people involved with teasing
B. Describe method and frequency of pregnancy checks, schedule for earliest check post-breeding, etc.

_____ Who does the pregnancy evaluations?

6. BREEDING TECHNIQUE:

Frequency of breedings (collections/day/week)
_____ Is stallion servicing mares only on specific days/week (Y or N); please specify:

Who handles stallion during breeding?
_____ Trainer
_____ Farm manager
_____ Same person each time
_____ Owner
_____ Other (describe)   _____
_____ Are handlers patient (non-interfering) with stallion's expression of sexual interest? (Y or N)

Note any problem/s related to breeding management

■ **Figure 86.1** continued

Previous:

Current:

Is stallion washed pre-breeding: Y   N

Method/with what? _____   Frequency? _____

7.   LINEAGE INFO:

Note any congenital/heritable traits of this stallion:

_____ cryptorchidism
_____ wobbler
_____ other

8.   Additional comments, information, prior reports, that owner wishes to have included in the medical record?

■ **Figure 86.1** continued

chapter 87

Inguinal Herniation/Rupture

DEFINITION/OVERVIEW

- Inguinal herniation occurs when a portion of the intestine protrudes through the vaginal ring into the inguinal canal. If the intestine extends into the scrotum it is called a *scrotal hernia*. These terms are used interchangeably.
- Ruptured inguinal hernia occurs when the intestine herniates through the vaginal ring and then passes through a rent or tear in the parietal tunic so that it is positioned SC in the inguinal or scrotal area.
- Inguinal rupture is defined as intestine protruding through a rent in the peritoneum and abdominal fascia adjacent to the vaginal portion of the inguinal canal so that it is positioned SC in the inguinal area.

ETIOLOGY/PATHOPHYSIOLOGY

Congenital

- Inguinal herniation in foals is congenital and is generally an inherited condition from paternal genetics (Fig. 87.1).
- The genetic mechanisms of this condition are complex and not completely known. The complexity of inheritance may indicate that several genes are involved.
- May be unilateral or bilateral and usually reducible. The intestine is usually not strangulated and will self-correct by the time the foal is 3 to 6 months of age.

Acquired

- Usually in adult horses. The condition is most commonly associated with changes in inguinal canal integrity and increases in abdominal pressure after exercise or copulation.
- May be an increased incidence in Standardbreds, Tennessee Walking Horses, and American Saddlebreds.
- Acquired hernia or rupture usually results in strangulation of the small bowel. It is a surgical emergency.
- Acquired hernias are seen in foals and the result of extreme abdominal compressions of the dam during parturition (a peripartal etiology).
- Inguinal rupture typically results form trauma to the abdominal musculature and fascia.

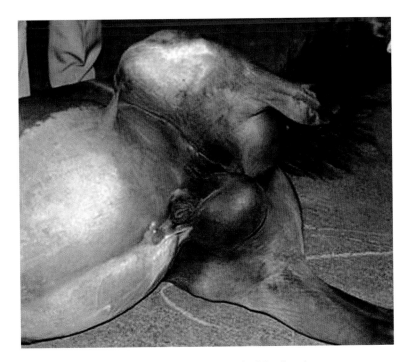

■ **Figure 87.1** Young colt presented for enlarged scrotum and mild colic pain.
Image courtesy of C. L. Carleton.

Systems Affected

- Reproductive: due to the defect in the integrity of the inguinal rings.
- GI: secondary involvement when bowel migrates through the inguinal rings and becomes strangulated; leads to ischemic necrosis of the bowel, systemic sepsis, and death, if uncorrected.

 ## SIGNALMENT/HISTORY

- Acquired condition usually in stallions, although the condition has been reported in geldings and mares.
- Congenital condition in foals from newborn to 6 months.
- Any breed but with an increased incidence in Standardbreds, Tennessee Walking Horses, and American Saddlebreds.

Risk Factors

- Although not well described, there may be some basis for a genetic predisposition from a sire line when stallions with this condition have been identified.
    - Congenital herniation is usually transferred from the sire.
    - The mechanism of inheritance has not been described completely.

- Congenital: mostly in foals.
- Acquired: mostly in stallions.

Historical Findings

Owners report signs of acute abdominal pain and associated signs of acute scrotal swelling.

 # CLINICAL FEATURES

- Swelling in the inguinal area, spermatic cord, or scrotum.
- Herniation in foals may be asymptomatic.
- Stallions with strangulated inguinal hernia or rupture will exhibit signs of colic after copulation.
- Colic signs are those associated with small intestinal obstruction (nasogastric reflux, distended small intestine per TRP).
- Acquired hernias may obstruct blood flow to the spermatic cord, resulting in edema of the external genitalia, testicular swelling and tenderness.
- Ruptured inguinal hernia or inguinal rupture may result in the skin over the affected area being cold, edematous, and macerated.
- TRP: distended small intestine and a loop of bowel descending through the vaginal ring of the inguinal canal.

 # DIFFERENTIAL DIAGNOSIS

- Varicocele: abnormally distended pampiniform plexus in the spermatic cord. Cord is thickened and has a "bag of worms" feel on digital palpation.
- Hydrocele: abnormal collection of fluid between the layers of the vaginal tunic of the peritoneum; results in a soft fluid swelling around the involved testicle.
- Hematocele: abnormal collection of blood within the vaginal tunic. Usually from a traumatic incident to the scrotum.
- Torsion of the spermatic cord: venous and arterial obstruction leading to testicular congestion, edema, and infarction. May result in signs of acute colic and enlargement of the scrotum and spermatic cord.

 # DIAGNOSTICS

CBC/Biochemistry/Urinalysis

- Hernia or rupture without intestinal strangulation generally produces no dramatic change in hematological or biochemical parameters
- Hernia or rupture with intestinal strangulation may result in:
  - Leukocytosis
  - Elevated total protein, HCT from dehydration and endotoxemia.

Other Laboratory Tests

Abdominocentesis: elevations in total WBC and total protein in peritoneal fluid (greater than 5,000 cells/uL and greater than 2.5 gm/dL, respectfully).

Imaging

U/S

- Gas dense echogenicity of the inguinal or scrotal area when bowel is incarcerated and distended in an inguinal hernia or rupture.
- Gas-filled loops of incarcerated bowel in subcutaneous tissue or scrotal tissue.

Pathological Findings

- Hernia: reducible, nonstrangulated bowel.
  - No pathologic findings.
- Hernia or rupture: incarcerated, strangulated bowel.
  - Varying degrees of ischemic necrosis of intestine.
  - Congestion of vasculature of intestine and spermatic cord.
  - Adhesion formation of intestine and peritoneum to inguinal or scrotal structures.
  - Histopathology associated with intestinal vascular congestion and ischemic necrosis.

 THERAPEUTICS

- As with any potential intestinal entrapment scenario, the most important consideration for the primary care veterinarian is determining whether the most appropriate treatment for the current condition is surgical or medical.

Drug(s) of Choice

- Drugs to combat shock and sepsis associated with devitalized intestine may be indicated.
- Administer balanced, isotonic intravenous fluids for treatment of endotoxemic shock.
- Administer broad-spectrum antibiotics for treatment of septic peritonitis.
  - Gentamicin sulfate (6.6 mg/kg, IV or IM, SID)
  - Amikacin sulfate (15 mg/kg, IV or IM, SID)
  - Ceftiofur (2.2–4.4 mg/kg, SC or IV, SID to TID)
- Administer anti-endotoxemic drugs.
  - Flunixin meglumine (0.5 mg/lb, IV, SID).

Appropriate Health Care

- Hernia: reducible, nonstrangulated bowel
  - Repeated, manual reduction may result in spontaneous closure.
  - Application of a truss support:
    - Sedate foal, place in dorsal recumbency.

- Reduce hernia and pack superficial inguinal ring area with rolled cotton.
- Maintain placement with elastic gauze and adhesive tape over the back and inguinal areas in a figure-eight fashion.
- Leave in place for 1 week.
- If hernia becomes incarcerated, surgical repair is necessary.
- Transrectal retraction of herniated loop of intestine. Grasp loop per rectum at the vaginal ring and apply gentle traction.
- Sedation and rectal relaxants (e.g., propantheline bromide) may be beneficial.
- Monitor health of bowel.
- Hernia or rupture: not reducible, strangulated bowel
  - See Surgical Considerations.

Nursing Care

- Repetitive manual reduction of hernia.
- Reapply truss, if necessary.
- Observe for signs of bowel incarceration.

Surgical Considerations

- Surgical correction of inguinal hernias is necessary when the:
  - Hernia cannot manually be reduced.
  - Intestines protrude into the subcutaneous tissue.
  - Hernia enlarges over time.
- Surgical correction of inguinal hernia with nonstrangulated intestine (Figs. 87.2 and 87.3):

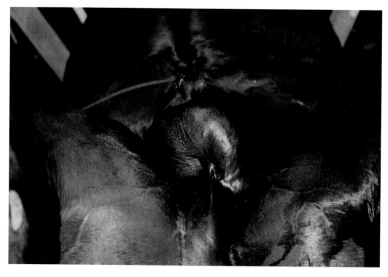

■ **Figure 87.2** Enlarged scrotum in dorsal recumbency for surgery. Mass is slightly reducible. Image courtesy of C. L. Carleton.

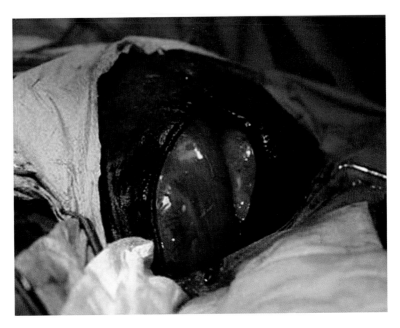

■ **Figure 87.3** Content of enlarged scrotum revealed. A reminder of why needles should not be placed in an enlarged scrotum without prior identification of content.
Image courtesy of C. L. Carleton.

- General anesthesia required in dorsal recumbency.
- Approach is over the superficial inguinal ring with blunt dissection to the testicle while in the vaginal tunic.
- With traction on the testicle, intestinal contents are "milked" back into the abdominal cavity (Fig. 87.4).
- Spermatic cord is ligated and the testis resected.
- Superficial ring is closed with absorbable suture in a simple interrupted pattern.
- Skin and subcutaneous tissue are closed for primary healing.
- Laparoscopic procedures have been described, necessitates a high degree of skill and additional equipment.
- Surgical correction of inguinal hernia or rupture with strangulated intestine:
  - Emergency measures are usually indicated if testicular or intestinal viability are in question.
  - Intravenous fluids and medications for shock may be necessary with incarcerated bowel.
  - Inguinal approach is used. Devitalized intestine can be resected. Resection and anastomosis is accomplished through a ventral abdominal incision.
  - Affected testis is removed.

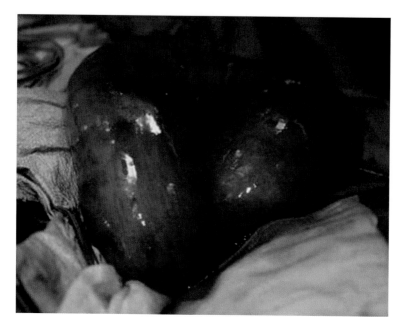

■ **Figure 87.4** Loop of bowel contained within scrotum. Tissue is still viable. Was replaced, colt castrated during same surgery, uneventful recovery.
Image courtesy of C. L. Carleton.

 COMMENTS

Patient Monitoring

- Postoperative CBC and biochemical monitoring for septic peritonitis.
- Manual palpation of inguina or scrotal area for swelling.
- Follow-up TRP.
- Follow-up U/S examination.
- Monitor for signs of endotoxemic shock.
- Monitor for peritonitis.

Prevention/Avoidance

- Palpate foal's inguinal area.
- Observe stallion for colic behavior after breeding.

Possible Complications

- Adhesion formation within the abdominal cavity.
- Observe postoperative for inguinal or scrotal swelling.
- Intestinal strangulation
- Septic peritonitis

Expected Course and Prognosis

- Inguinal hernia with reducible, nonstrangulated intestine: Good prognosis.
- Inguinal hernia or rupture with strangulated intestine: Prognosis depends on degree of intestinal incarceration, time, and devascularization.

Synonyms

- Inguinal rupture
- Ruptured inguinal hernia
- Scrotal hernia

Abbreviations

CBC   complete blood count
GI   gastrointestinal
HCT   hematocrit
IM   intramuscular
IV   intravenous
SID   once a day
SC   subcutaneous
TID   three times a day
TRP   transrectal palpation
U/S   ultrasound, ultrasonography
WBC   white blood cell

See Also

- Abnormal scrotal enlargement (includes spermatic cord torsion)
- Abnormal testicular size
- Anatomy review, reproductive, basic, stallion
- BSE, stallion
- Cryptorchidism

Suggested Reading

Schneider RK, Milne DW, Kohn CW. 1982. Acquired inguinal hernia in the horse: A review of 27 cases. *JAVMA* 180: 317.

Schumacher J. 2006. Reproductive system. In: *Equine Surgery*, 3rd ed. Auer JA, Stick JA (eds). St. Louis: Saunders-Elsevier; 775–810.

van der Velden MA. 1988. Ruptured inguinal hernia in new-born colt foals: A review of 14 cases. *Eq Vet J* 20: 178.

van der Velden MA. 1988. Surgical treatment of acquired inguinal hernia in the horse: A review of 51 cases. *Eq Vet J* 20: 173.

Author: Philip E. Prater

chapter 88

Nutrition

 DEFINITION/OVERVIEW

Stallion nutrition is the same as for any performance horse:

- Provision of a well-balanced ration consisting of predominantly good quality forage (preferably grass or grass/legume mix hay or good quality pasture, water, and salt.
- Obesity will adversely affect breeding performance and predispose the horse to laminitis or colic.
- Inadequate calorie intake will result in weight loss and perhaps loss of libido.
- Deficits of vitamins A, E, and perhaps C (stress induced deficit, not a normal dietary requirement) may adversely impact semen production.

Phases of Nutrient Concerns

Pre-Breeding

- Ensure adequate calorie and protein intake to maintain body condition at a score of 4 to 6 on the Henneke scale of 1 to 10.
- Adequate vitamin A (60 IU vitamin A/kg BW) and E (2 IU vitamin E/kg BW) should be provided at all times.
- Vitamins A and E are of critical importance in the 2 to 3 months prior to and during the breeding season when the horse is in active use.

Breeding Season

- Stallions are usually more active during the breeding season and have higher energy (Mcal/day) requirements.
- Increased energy intake may be necessary to maintain adequate body condition.
- Some stallions are stressed during breeding and may need supplemental Vitamin C (ascorbic acid, 0.01 g/kg BW, BID) to maintain semen quality and optimal immune function.

SIGNALMENT/HISTORY

Risk Factors

Improper nutrition will result in:
- Obesity
- Weight loss/emaciation
- Poor hair coat/hoof condition
- Poor semen production and quality

Historical Findings

- Some stallions are "hard keepers," whereas others are remarkably efficient.
- The challenge is to keep the weight on the former and to provide adequate minerals while avoiding obesity to the latter.

 # DIAGNOSTICS

- Weight loss emaciation: Clinical infection or illness, organ failure, toxicity.
- Poor hair coat or hoof condition: poor grooming or hygiene.
- Poor semen production and quality: Genetics.
- CBC/Biochemistry/Urinalysis
  - Use to rule out clinical infection or illness, organ failure, toxicity.
  - Blood concentrations of most nutrients do *not* reflect intake or dietary adequacy, especially with respect to calcium, phosphorus, and vitamins such as A and E.
- Other Laboratory Tests: If a nutrient imbalance is suspected, get the feed (i.e., hay, pasture, concentrates and supplements) analyzed at a feed or forage analysis laboratory to determine actual nutrient intake.

 # THERAPEUTICS

Appropriate Health Care

- Routine
- Semen evaluation at least 2 months before breeding season begins.

Diet

Pre-Breeding

- Free choice (2%–3% BW) good quality forage (hay or pasture), high fat (7%–10%) concentrates at less than 0.5% BW per feeding, if weight gain is needed.
- Possibly vitamin A (60 IU Retinyl compounds/kg BW) and E (2 IU alpha tocopherols/kg BW) supplements for 2 months before breeding.

Breeding Season

- Increase concentrate as necessary to maintain good body condition.
- Vitamin C (0.01 g/kg BW twice a day) may be beneficial for stallions that are extremely agitated during the season.
- Supplemental vitamin C is usually not necessary if the horse is at ease and quiet when not being used for actual breeding.
- Salt available free choice at all times.
- Electrolyte supplementation not necessary unless the horse is agitated and sweating excessively between breeding seasons.

Activity

- No restrictions
- Best if kept lean and fit.

 COMMENTS

Client Education

Disregard most of what is on the internet and in print in lay magazines.

Patient Monitoring

- Body Condition assessed weekly or biweekly.
- Age-Related Factors: Stallions older than 20 years old may need special senior-type feeds with higher digestibility and calorie content.

Prevention/Avoidance

Avoid
- Obesity
- Excessive weight loss.
- Excessive grain, especially sweet feeds.
- Over supplementation of fat soluble vitamins, herbal nutraceuticals.

Possible Complications

- Excess selenium will interfere with copper absorption or utilization and vice versa.
- Excessive Vitamin E will interfere with Vitamin A absorption and possibly vice versa.
- Excessive grain will predispose to obesity or colic.
- Obesity will predispose to laminitis or colic.

Abbreviations

BCS   body condition score
BID   twice a day

BW   body weight
CBC   complete blood count

See Also

- Nutrition, foals
- Nutrition, broodmare

Suggested Reading

Anonymous. Body condition scoring techniques. www.equineprotectionnetwork.com/cruelty/henneke.htm.

National Research Council. 2007. *Nutrient Requirements for Horses*, 8th ed. Washington, DC: National Academy Press.

Ralston SL. 1993. Analysis of feeds and forages for horses. www.rcre.rutgers.edu/pubs/publication.asp?pid=FS714.

Ralston SL. 1997. Diagnosis of nutritional problems in horses. www.rcre.rutgers.edu/pubs/publication.asp?pid=FS894.

Ralston SL. 2001. Feeding the "Easy Keeper" horse. www.rcre.rutgers.edu/pubs/publication.asp?pid=FS799.

Ralston SL. 2004. Hyperinsulinemia and glucose intolerance. In: *Equine Internal Medicine*, 2nd ed. Reed S, Bayly W, Sellon D (eds). St. Louis: Elsevier 1599–1603.

Rich GA, Breuer LH. 2002. Recent developments in equine nutrition with farm and clinic implications. *Proc AAEP* 48: 24–40.

Author: Sarah L. Ralston

chapter 89

Paraphimosis

DEFINITION/OVERVIEW

Prolapse of the penis and inner preputial fold with extensive penile and preputial edema and the inability to retract the penis into the prepuce.

ETIOLOGY/PATHOPHYSIOLOGY

- The anatomic location of the penis and prepuce affects how it reacts to injury. The effect of gravity magnifies the inflammatory reaction to an injury with the accumulation of edema or with the formation of a hematoma or seroma.
- As the penis and prepuce prolapse, further edema accumulates subsequent to the impedence of vascular and lymphatic drainage while in the prolapsed state.
- The inelasticity of the preputial ring further promotes fluid retention.
- Chronic prolapse may lead to penile or preputial trauma, balanoposthitis, or penile paralysis.

Systems Affected

- Reproductive: Prolapse of the penis and prepuce exposes them to trauma. Chronic paraphimosis may result in penile paralysis, fibrosis of the CCP, and an inability to achieve an erection.
- Urologic: Urethral obstruction may be the inciting cause of paraphimosis, or it may occur secondary to edema.

SIGNALMENT/HISTORY

- Predominantly occurs in stallions, but geldings can be affected.
- No breed predilection.
- Paraphimosis is unlikely to occur in the first month of life due to the persistent frenulum between the free portion of the penis and inner lamina of the preputial fold. The frenulum is present for a few days. No intervention should be attempted prior to 1 month of age should the frenulum persist.

Risk Factors

- The use of phenothiazine tranquilizers in stallions is contraindicated.
- Open-range stud management.
- Aggressive stallions.
- Poor management, unsanitary conditions, or malnutrition.

Historical Findings

- Acute cases often present as traumatic injury to the penis or preputial area.
- Chronic cases: Delay in presentation for veterinary care may occur if an owner believed an injury was minor and attempted care themselves, or the injury may only recently have become obvious because of its slow increase in size (e.g., a slow developing enlargement of the penis or preputial area such as seen with *Habronema* spp. infections or neoplastic growths).

 CLINICAL FEATURES

- Prolapse of the penis and prepuce with severe penile enlargement is readily apparent. Caudoventral displacement of the glans penis is common (Fig. 89.1). A careful visual and digital examination is necessary to properly define the nature of the injury (Fig. 89.2).
- Balanitis (inflammation of the penis), posthitis (inflammation of the prepuce), or balanoposthitis (inflammation of the prepuce and penis) may be present. Serous or hemorrhagic discharges on the surface of the penis and prepuce are common. Lacerations, excoriations, ulcerative lesions, or neoplastic masses may be evident.

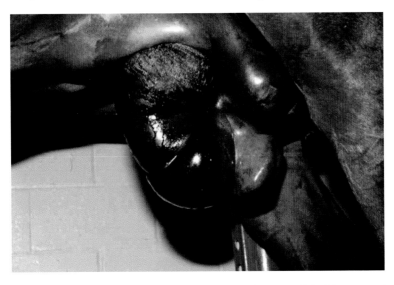

■ **Figure 89.1** Traumatic paraphimosis upon presentation 1 day after being kicked by a mare during natural service. Note the severe edema, bruising, hemorrhage, and caudal reflection of the glans penis. Image courtesy of C. L. Carleton.

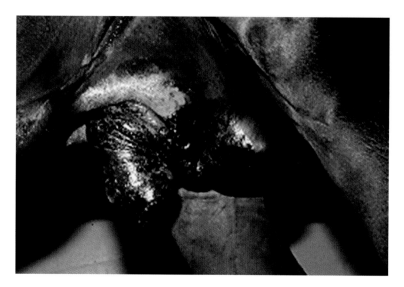

■ **Figure 89.2** Traumatic paraphimosis three days after therapy was initiated. Note the extensive bruising of the scrotum and prepuce. Excoriations of the exposed preputial surface are also visible. The problem completely resolved and the stallion returned to breeding service 12 weeks after the traumatic incident.
Image courtesy of C. L. Carleton.

- Hematomas, when present, are generally located on the dorsal surface of the penis and usually arise from blood vessels superficial to the tunica albuginea.
- TRP may reveal an enlarged urinary bladder indicative of urethral blockage.
- Chronic prolapse may lead to penile paralysis.

 DIFFERENTIAL DIAGNOSIS

General Comments

- Any injury or condition that leads to chronic protrusion of the penis or prepuce can lead to paraphimosis. The initial cause may be due to injury or disease, but because both lead to the accumulation of edema and leave surfaces exposed to further injury, the underlying cause must be determined whenever possible.
- Any traumatic incident (e.g., breeding trauma, lacerations, surgical intervention, may be the inciting cause of a paraphimosis).
- The presence of ulcerative or proliferative lesions warrants investigation to determine if the origin of the lesion is neoplastic, parasitic, or infectious in nature.
- Systemic signs indicative of neurologic or systemic disease include ataxia, depression, lymph node enlargement, or increased rectal temperature.

Noninfectious Causes

- Trauma: breeding injuries, fighting or kicks, improperly fitting stallion rings, falls, movement through brush or heavy ground cover, whips, or abuse.

- Priapism, penile paralysis, posthitis, or balanoposthitis.
- Postsurgical complication: castration or cryptorchid surgery.
- Neoplasia of the penis or prepuce: sarcoid, SCC, melanoma, mastocytoma, hemangioma, or papilloma.
- Debilitation or starvation.
- Spinal injury or myelitis.
- Urolithiasis or urinary tract obstruction.

Infectious Causes

- Bacterial: *Staphylococcus, Streptococcus.*
- Viral: EHV-1 (rhinopneumonitis), EHV-3 (equine coital exanthema), EIA, EVA.
- Purpura hemorrhagica: vasculitis as a sequela to infection or vaccine administration.
- Parasitic: *Habronema muscae, Habronema microstoma, Draschia megastoma, Onchocera* spp., *Cochliomyia hominivorax* (screw worm).
- Fungal: phycomycosis due to *Hyphomyces destruens.*
- Protozoal: *Trypanosoma equiperdum* (Dourine).

 DIAGNOSTICS

- Generally, there are no abnormal findings on standard diagnostic tests (CBC, biochemical profile) unless infectious agents, neoplastic disease, or severe debilitation is present.
- In some rare cases, urinalysis may indicate the presence of urolithiasis or cystitis.
- U/S findings are generally unrewarding. In other species, fibrosis of the CCP has been visualized in chronic cases on U/S examination.
- Cytology or biopsy of masses or lesions may be diagnostic in the case of parasitic, neoplastic, or fungal disease.
- Cultures of affected tissues if bacterial infection is suspected.
- EHV-1: Rising antibody titers from paired sera collected at a 14- to 21-day interval or virus isolation from nasopharyngeal swabs during the acute stage may be diagnostic.
- EHV-3: Rising antibody titers from paired sera collected at a 14- to 21-day interval, or the presence of eosinophilic intranuclear inclusion bodies in cytologic smears or virus isolation from lesions during the acute stage may be diagnostic.
- EIA: AGID test or ELISA (Coggins).
- EVA: Rising antibody titer from paired sera collected at a 14- to 21-day interval, virus isolation (EAV) from nasopharyngeal swabs in the acute phase, and virus isolation from semen.
- Protozoal: Identification of the causative agent in urethral exudates or serology (CF).

THERAPEUTICS

- The primary goals are to reduce the inflammation and edema and return the penis to the prepuce to improve venous and lymphatic drainage. The initial management of the patient is intensive and may require hospitalization to allow adequate physical restraint and patient access.
- Ensure urethral patency. Catheterize or perform a perineal urethrostomy, if necessary.
- Manually reduce the prolapse:
  - Elastic or pneumatic bandaging or sustained manual pressure applied along the free portion of the penis (stallion sedated and restrained in a stocks) may help reduce edema prior to attempting reduction.
  - Preputiotomy should be considered if the preputial ring is preventing successful reduction.
- Once reduced, the placement of a purse-string suture of umbilical tape around the preputial orifice, tightened to a one-finger opening to hold the penis within the prepuce, is beneficial to prevent recurrence, with the added benefit of maintaining pressure on the penis for sustained reduction of edema. Additional support can be gained by fitting the stallion with a "penile support," a sling of netting. It needs to cover the cranial aspect of the prepuce, but allow urine to drain to minimize urine scald.
- In clinical cases resistant to manual reduction, support remains of primary importance. Wrap the exposed penis and prepuce to reduce edema (Fig. 89.3). A support sling is essential (Fig. 89.4). Nylon slings should be used to raise and maintain the penis close to the ventral body wall; the use of netting (small perforations to allow the urine to drain) is recommended (Fig. 89.5).
- Local surgical resection, cryosurgery, or radiation therapy of neoplastic or granulomatous lesions should be pursued only after the edema is resolved.

Drug(s) of Choice

- NSAIDs including phenylbutazone (2–4 g/450 kg/day PO) or flunixin meglumine (1 mg/kg/day IV, IM, or PO) for symptomatic relief and to reduce inflammation.
- Systemic or local antibiotics, as indicated, to treat local bacterial infection and prevent septicemia.
- Diuretics: Furosemide (1 mg/kg IV, SID or BID), if indicated, in the acute phase for edema reduction.
- Specific topical or systemic treatments for parasitic, fungal, or neoplastic conditions, as indicated by results of diagnostic testing.

Precautions/Interactions

- Tranquilizers, particularly the phenothiazine tranquilizers, should be avoided in males to avoid drug-induced priapism.

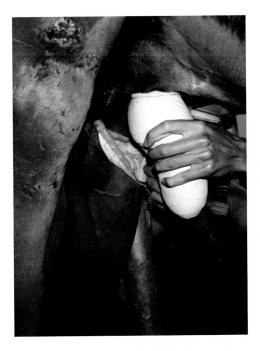

■ **Figure 89.3** A pneumatic bandage placed around the shaft of the penis to reduce penile and preputial edema.
Image courtesy of A. Tibary.

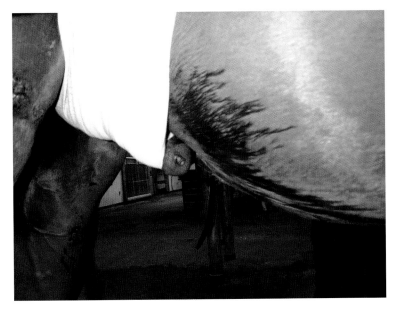

■ **Figure 89.4** The penis and prepuce are brought close to the ventral abdominal wall using a support bandage.
Image courtesy of A. Tibary.

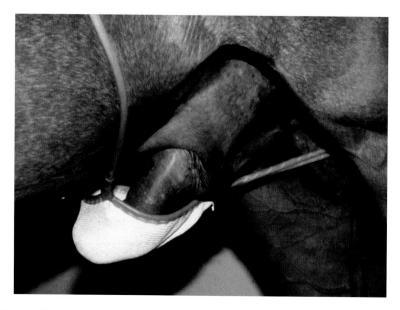

■ **Figure 89.5** Additional support is given to the penis and prepuce by use of a net sling.

- Nitrofurazone should not be used to treat horses intended for food.
- Diuretics are contraindicated if urinary obstruction is present. Their effectiveness in treating localized edema is doubtful.

Alternative Drugs

DMSO has been used topically (50/50 mixture by volume with nitrofurazone ointment) or systemically (1 g/kg IV as a 10% solution in saline, BID to TID for 3–5 days) to reduce inflammation and edema. Note: the parenteral administration of DMSO is not approved and is considered an extra-label use.

Nursing Care

- Hydrotherapy: Cold hydrotherapy should be applied for the first 4 to 7 days until edema and hemorrhage subside, then warm hydrotherapy can be used. Generally hydrotherapy is applied for 15 to 30 min BID to QID.
- Massage the penis and prepuce BID to QID to reduce edema.
- Topical emollient ointments should be applied as needed. Options include A&D ointment, lanolin, petroleum jelly, or nitrofurazone.

Activity

- Exercise: Confine and limit activity until after the active hemorrhage and edema subside, then slowly increase exercise to aid in the resolution of dependent edema.
- Avoid sexual stimulation in the early stages of therapy. It may be necessary to prevent exposure to mares for up to 4 to 8 weeks.

Surgical Considerations

Chronic refractory paraphimosis may require surgical intervention, including circumcision (reefing or posthioplasty), penile retraction (Bolz technique), or penile amputation (phallectomy).

 COMMENTS

Patient Monitoring

Initial management is intensive. Frequent evaluation is essential. Reduction of edema, coupled with the horse's ability to retain his penis in the prepuce, are good prognostic indicators.

Possible Complications

- Excoriations or ulcerations or further trauma of exposed skin surfaces
- Adhesions or fibrosis of tissues leading to the inability to achieve erection or urethral obstruction
- Chronic paraphimosis
- Continued hematoma enlargement indicates that a rent may be present in the tunica albuginea. The hematoma should be surgically explored.
- Penile paralysis
- Frostbite due to exposure
- Myiasis
- Infertility

Abbreviations

AGID	agar gel immunodiffusion
BID	twice a day
CBC	complete blood count
CCP	corpus cavernosum penis
CF	complement fixation
DMSO	dimethyl sulfoxide
EAV	equine arteritis virus
EHV-1	equine herpes-1 (equine rhinopneumonitis)
EHV-3	equine herpes-3 (equine coital exanthema)
EIA	equine infectious anemia (swamp fever)
ELISA	enzyme linked immunosorbent assay
EVA	equine viral arteritis
IM	intramuscular
IV	intravenous
NSAIDs	nonsteroidal anti-inflammatory drug
PO	per os (by mouth)

QID	four times a day
SCC	squamous cell carcinoma
SID	once a day
TID	three times a day
TRP	transrectal palpation
U/S	ultrasound, ultrasonography

See Also

- Viral diseases, infectious
- Penile lacerations
- Penile paralysis
- Penile vesicles/erosions
- Purpura hemorrhagica
- Priapism
- Venereal diseases

Suggested Reading

Clem MF, DeBowes RM. 1989. Paraphimosis in horses. Part I. *Compend Contin Educ* 11: 72–75.

Clem MF, DeBowes RM. 1989. Paraphimosis in horses. Part II. *Compend Contin Educ* 11: 184–187.

De Vries PJ. 1993. Diseases of the testes, penis, and related structures. In: *Equine Reproduction.* McKinnon AO, Voss JL (eds). Philadelphia: Lea & Febiger; 878–884.

Vaughan JT. 1980. Surgery of the penis and prepuce. In: *Bovine and Equine Urogenital Surgery.* Walker DF, Vaughan JT (eds). Philadelphia: Lea & Febiger; 125–144.

Vaughan JT. 1993. Penis and prepuce. In: *Equine Reproduction.* McKinnon AO, Voss JL (eds). Philadelphia: Lea & Febiger; 885–894.

Author: Carole C. Miller

chapter 90

Parentage Testing

DEFINITION/OVERVIEW

Two methodologies are routinely used:

Bloodtyping

- Testing for genetic markers; horse testing since the 1960s.
- Uses RBC surface antigen and RBC and serum proteins.
- RBC testing in horses uses similar methodology to determination of human blood groups, including ABO and Rh systems.
- Seven RBC systems are routinely tested in horses. Each system has one or more "factors."
- Ten biochemical markers are also tested. These markers consist of genetically variable proteins that exist with the RBC or in the serum.
- Thus, at least 17 systems are tested to generate a bloodtype.

DNA Testing

- DNA testing: since the mid-1990s DNA-based testing has supplanted blood typing as the method of choice for genotyping horses.
- DNA testing: Genetic system in current use involves microsatellites (small, repetitive elements within DNA).
  - These elements vary in size at a given locus.
  - Therefore, alleles of a microsatellite are defined by the size of these repetitive segments.
  - Microsatellite systems have been well-defined to genotype the horse; the sizes of each allele for a given marker have been assigned an alphabetical designation.
  - More than 17 blood group systems are necessary to generate a bloodtype, contrast this with as few as 12 microsatellite markers to yield the same or better efficacy.
  - A standard panel of 12 microsatellites detects 98% to 99% of incorrect parentages.

ETIOLOGY/PATHOPHYSIOLOGY

- Bloodtyping:
  - Method used for many years to identify individuals and determine parentage.
  - Because of the number of alleles that exist within each of these systems, bloodtyping can discriminate correctly between an incorrect parentage 96% to 98% of the time.
- DNA testing:
  - Because a foal inherits one allele from each parent, accuracy of parentage can be based on linking the alleles in the foal's with those of the parents.
  - Each allele present in the foal must be present in the parents, and,
  - One of the alleles present in each of the parents does indeed occur in the foal.
  - As in human parentage cases, parentage cannot be proven; it can only state that a parentage qualifies. Exclusion, however, can be proven.

Systems Affected

- Blood, if processed appropriately, see following text.
- DNA: hair bulbs are easiest to collect from the mane or tail.

CLINICAL FEATURES

- Bloodtyping: reagents to detect specific RBC Ag's are not commercially available.
  - Must be generated by injecting horses with RBC from other horses to induce Ab production.
  - Serum from immunized horses must be collected, screened, and processed to produce specific reagents.
  - In addition, the biochemical systems require at least four different methods to determine the biochemical genotype for one horse.

Disadvantages

- Very labor intensive and expensive.
- Both anticoagulant (EDTA or ACD) and serum tubes must be submitted for bloodtyping.
- Requires horse owner to schedule a farm visit to collect a sample, process and ship it properly to arrive at a lab in a "testable" condition.

Advantages

- Only bloodtyping can be used to determine stallion and mare compatibility to avoid NI.
- A genetic test for the Tobiano gene is now available, replacing the blood test.

DNA Testing

Advantages

- DNA can be extracted from nearly any tissue.
- DNA can be extracted from stored serum samples previously used for blood typing.
  - Owner can readily collect the sample for testing by submitting hair. Should be pulled from the mane or tail, grasped close enough to the crest or dock to ensure that the bulb from within the follicle remains attached to the hair shaft.
  - Bulbs are visible at the end of the hair shaft when held against a dark background.
  - Minimum 20 to 30 hairs to ensure sufficient workable bulbs have been collected and submitted.
  - Place hair in an individual envelope to avoid cross-contamination with samples from other horses.
  - Can be sent by regular postal service.
- Additional DNA tests are available for *color mutations* and *inheritable diseases*; the list will continue to grow.
  - Color mutation tests: Extension locus (chestnut), Agouti (bay), Cream, Sabino 1, Silver Dapple (chocolate), Gray, Champagne, and Tobiano.
  - Genetic diseases: HYPP (QH), GBED (QH), JEB (Belgian and Saddlebreds), SCID (Arabians) HERDA, PSSM, MH, RER, and OLWS. Note: there are separate JEB tests for Saddlebreds and Belgian horses, as the mutation causing disease is different between the two breeds.
  - Sample collection procedure: same as for DNA genotyping.

DIAGNOSTICS

Bloodtyping

- All factors are expressed codominantly.
  - The sire and dam's contributions to the foal's genotype are easily discerned.
  - If a foal possesses a factor not present in the sire or dam, the parentage is disqualified.
- Unlike biochemical markers (a straightforward inheritance pattern), RBC Ag's are inherited as phenogroups.
  - In a phenogroup, certain factors in a system are inherited in specific combinations with other factors. Parentage analysis for blood groups requires knowledge of these inheritance patterns.
- Table 90.1 provides a list of known equine blood group systems and genes found in each system.
- Table 90.2 provides the common biochemical marker systems and genes identified in each system.

TABLE 90.1 Equine Blood Group Systems and Genes Found in Each System.

A Blood Group		D Blood Group
a	a	ad
abdg	**K Blood Group**	adn
adf	a	bcm
adg	**U Blood Group**	cgm
b	a	cgmp
bc	**P Blood Group**	cfm
bce	a	cegimn
be	ac	cefgm
c	acd	cfgkm
cd	ad	
ce	b	de
e	bd	deo
Q Blood Group	d	dek
a	**C Blood Group**	dfk
abc	a	dgh
ac		
b		dk
c		dn

The lower case letters following a blood group are names of Ags in that system.
The combinations of Ags are the known alleles.

TABLE 90.2 Biochemical Marker Systems and Genes Identified in Each System.

ISAG	Biochemical Marker and Alleles of That System	ISAG	Biochemical Marker and Alleles of That System
Al	Albumin: A, B, I	Cat	Catalase: F, S
Es	Serum Carboxylesterase: F, G, I, L, M, O, R, S	CA	Carbonic Anhydrase: E, F, I, L, O, S
Tf	Transferrin: D, D2, E, F1, F2, F3, G, H1, H2, J, M, O, R, X	Plg	Plasminogen: 1, 2
Pi	Protease Inhibitor: E, F, G, H, I, J, K, L, L2, N, O, P, Q, R, S, T, U, V, W, X, Z	DIA	NADH Diaphorase: F, S
Xk	A1B Glycoprotein: F, K, S	MPI	Mannose Phosphate Isomerase: F,S
Gc	Vitamin D Binding Protein: F, S	AP	Acid Phosphatase: F, S
PGD	6-Phosphogluconate Dehydrogenase: D, F, S	ME	Malic Enzyme: F, S
Hb	A-Hemoglobin: A, AII, BI, BII	Hp	Haptoglobin: 1, 2
PGM	Phosphoglucomutase: F, V, S	Pep	Peptidase A: F, S
GPI	Glucosephoshate Isomerase: F, I, L, S		

ISAG, International Society of Animal Genetics, internationally recognized marker system abbreviations.

TABLE 90.3 An Example of How to Interpret and Use DNA Parentage Information.

Considerations are given to possible **inclusion** or **exclusion** of possible parentage based on the presence of microsatellites (small, repetitive elements within DNA).

In the example that follows, the possible foal types for system VHL20 given the sire's type of MO and the dam's type of NO are: MN, MO, NO, or O. The foal qualifies **in** this system.

For system AHT4, the possible qualifying foal types for sire type P (PP) and dam type KP are KP or P (PP). Both sire and dam are excluded in the AHT4 system, (i.e., therefore, their potential parentage is **excluded** by this system).

The dam is excluded in the ASB2, and the sire in the HMS6 system.

LEX3 is an X chromosome marker.

- An allele from the sire *and* the dam is only expected in fillies.
- In this case, either sire or dam qualifies in the LEX3 system, but not both of them together.
- Colts qualify in LEX3 by virtue of having an allele present in the dam only.

	Breed	**VHL20**	HTG4	**AHT4**	HMS7	**ASB2**	ASB17	AHT5		
Foal	GT	**NO**	LN	**N**	LO	**MN**	Q	J	RES	RUM35
Sire	GT	**MO**	LN	**P**	LO	**NO**	Q	J	RES	rum510
Dam	GT	**NO**	MN	**KP**	O	**O**	Q	J	RES	rum510
	EED	**HMS6**	ASB23	HGT10	HMS3	LEX33	HTG6	HTG7	HMS2	**LEX3**
Foal	GT	**LP**	S	KR	P	KR				**HO**
Sire	GT	**OQ**	S	OR	P	KR				**O**
Dam	GT	**LQ**	S	KO	PQ	R				**LO**

- Table 90.3 is an example of how to interpret and apply DNA parentage information.

Pathologic Findings

Refer to testing for genetic diseases (*see* Risk Factors)

 ## COMMENTS

Client Education

Refer to Risk Factors, Sample Collection.

Abbreviations

ACD   acid citrate dextrose
EDTA   ethyl diacetyl tetraacetic acid
GBED   glycogen branching enzyme deficiency
HERDA   hereditary equine regional dermal asthenia

HYPP	hyperkalemic periodic paralysis
JEB	junctional epidermolysis bullosa
MH	malignant hyperthermia
NI	neonatal isoerythrolysis
OLWS	overo lethal white syndrome
PSSM	polysaccharide storage myopathy
QH	Quarter Horse
RBC	red blood cell
RER	recurrent exertional rhabdomyolysis
SCID	severe combined immunodeficiency disease

Suggested Reading

Slovis NM, Murray G. 2001. How to approach whole blood transfusions in horses. *Proc AAEP* 266–269.

Snook C. 2001. Update on neonatal isoerythrolysis. In: *Recent Advances in Equine Neonatal Care.* Wilkins PA, Palmer JE (eds). Ithaca: IVIS; Document No. A0416.1201.

Authors: Kathryn Graves and Ahmed Tibary

chapter 91

Penile Lacerations

DEFINITION/OVERVIEW

Any wound to the penile epithelial surface.

ETIOLOGY/PATHOPHYSIOLOGY

Trauma may occur in response to breeding accidents, improperly fitted stallion rings, kicks, jumping injuries, masturbation, or improper surgical technique (Figs. 91.1 and 91.2).

Systems Affected

- Reproductive
- Urinary

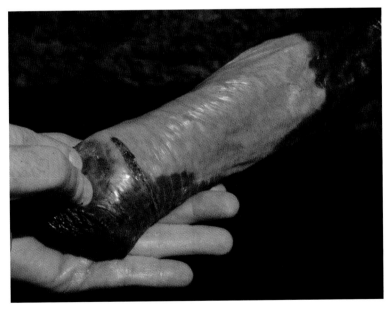

■ **Figure 91.1** Relatively minor laceration sustained by a stallion while maintained in his stall. Complete healing is necessary before cover (live or artificial vagina) can be done.
Image courtesy of C. L. Carleton.

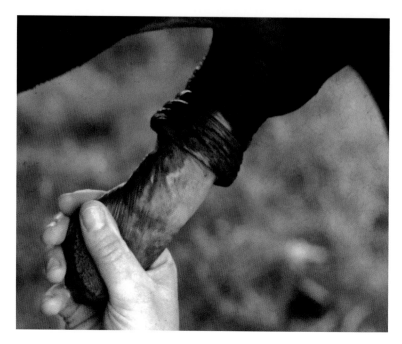

■ **Figure 91.2** Although not yet a laceration or erosion, the circular depression above the thumb in this image shows an indent left by a long-neglected, forgotten stallion ring. The young stallion began service, but the depression remained lifelong.
Image courtesy of C. L. Carleton.

 # SIGNALMENT/HISTORY

No age or breed predilection.

Risk Factors

Aggressive stallions/colts housed or handled in unsafe conditions are more likely to injure themselves and others.

 # CLINICAL FEATURES

Visual inspection generally reveals the laceration.

 # DIFFERENTIAL DIAGNOSIS

- Paraphimosis may be present, but it is often secondary to the laceration.
- Ulcerative lesions caused by neoplastic or parasitic diseases should not be considered lacerations for this discussion.

THERAPEUTICS

- Ensure urethral patency. Placement of a urinary catheter may be indicated.
- Cleanse and debride the wound as dictated by location and severity.
- Acute posttrauma lacerations can be sutured for first intention healing.
- Old or grossly contaminated lacerations may have to heal by second or third intention.
- Support the penis and prepuce with slings, hydrotherapy, and judicious exercise to prevent or eliminate extensive dependent edema.

Drug(s) of Choice

- NSAIDs including phenylbutazone (2–4 g/450 kg/day PO) or flunixin meglumine (1.1 mg/kg per day IV, IM, or PO) for patient comfort and to decrease inflammation. High initial dosages should be titrated to the lowest effective dose if more than 5 successive days of therapy are required.
- Systemic or local antibiotics for local infections and to prevent septicemia, if indicated.
- Emollient application to the penile surface as needed to prevent or address urine scalding, if indicated.

Precautions/Interactions

Phenothiazine tranquilizers should never be used in the intact male and used only with care in geldings.

Appropriate Health Care

- If retraction of the penis is not possible, hospitalization may be required for frequent evaluation and care of the exposed penis.
- If the penis can be maintained within the prepuce without support, less frequent evaluation may be appropriate.

Activity

Sexual stimulation is absolutely contraindicated until healing is complete.

COMMENTS

Possible Complications

- Urine leakage with extensive tissue necrosis is possible if the penile urethra has been lacerated.
- Wounds that cannot be treated surgically are usually those complicated by suppuration and cellulitis.

- Scar formation can result in phimosis, erectile dysfunction, impotence, or infertility.
- Hematomas generally arise from blood vessels superficial to the tunica albuginea. A hematoma that continues to enlarge is more likely attributable to a rent in the tunica albuginea, and closure of that defect is a priority.
- Paraphimosis is a common sequela to penile lacerations.
- Penile paralysis is possible as a result of the injury itself or secondary to paraphimosis.

Abbreviations

IM   intramuscular
IV   intravenous
NSAIDs   nonsteroidal anti-inflammatory drugs
PO   per os (by mouth)

See Also

- Breeding soundness examination, stallion
- Paraphimosis
- Penile paralysis
- Phimosis
- Semen collection, methods
- Semen evaluation, abnormal stallion

Suggested Reading

Ley WB, Slusher SH. 2007. Infertility and diseases of the reproductive tract of stallions. In: *Current Therapy in Large Animal Theriogenology*, 2nd ed. Youngquist RS, Threlfall WR (eds). St. Louis: Saunders Elsevier; 15–23.

Schumacher J, Varner DD. 2007. Surgical correction of abnormalities affecting the reproductive organs of stallions. In: *Current Therapy in Large Animal Theriogenology*, 2nd ed. Youngquist RS, Threlfall WR (eds). St. Louis: Saunders Elsevier; 23–36.

Schumacher J, Vaughan JT. 1988. Surgery of the penis and prepuce. *Vet Clin North Am: Equine Pract* 4: 443–449.

Vaughan JT. 1993. Penis and prepuce. In: *Equine Reproduction*. McKinnon AO, Voss JL (eds). Philadelphia: Lea & Febiger; 885–894.

Author: Carole C. Miller

chapter 92

Penile Paralysis

DEFINITION/OVERVIEW

Protracted extension of the penis in a flaccid state.

ETIOLOGY/PATHOPHYSIOLOGY

Injury to the sacral nerves, which innervate the penis or the retractor penis muscle, results in the inability to retract the penis into the prepuce.

Systems Affected

Reproductive

SIGNALMENT/HISTORY

Stallions (predominantly) or geldings of any age.

Risk Factors

- Chronic paraphimosis or priapism
- Exhaustion or starvation
- Spinal cord lesions

DIFFERENTIAL DIAGNOSIS

- Trauma: Direct penile trauma (Figs. 92.1 and 92.2), spinal cord injury, or disease. The presence of neurologic deficits other than the penile paralysis may link the penile problem (secondary) with primary spinal cord injury or disease.

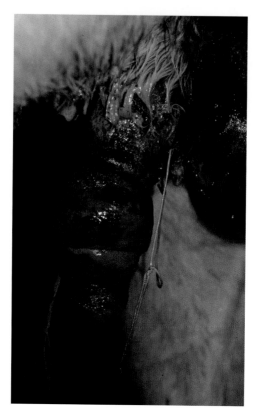

■ **Figure 92.1** Penile paralysis, pendant edema following a traumatic live cover, kick injury to the penis. Purse-string suture untied to allow the penis to drop for application of emollient. Stallion regained penile function within 14 days of the breeding accident.
Image courtesy of C. L. Carleton.

- Infectious disease: EHV-1, rabies, EIA, purpura hemorrhagica, or dourine (*Trypanosoma equiperdum*). A recent history of respiratory disease (affected horse or on its farm) may implicate EHV-1 as a possible cause.
- Drug-induced: Propiopromazine, acepromazine maleate, and reserpine have all been reported in the literature to contribute to penile paralysis (Fig. 92.3).
- Paraphimosis results in prolapse of the penis and prepuce, and dependent edema develops. The inability to retract the penis is generally due to the accumulated edema rather than true penile paralysis. However, penile paralysis can be a sequela to chronic, severe paraphimosis. Long-standing penile paralysis can present as paraphimosis due to the formation of extensive dependent edema.
- Priapism, a persistent erection with engorgement of the CCP, should not be confused with penile paralysis in which the penis is flaccid.

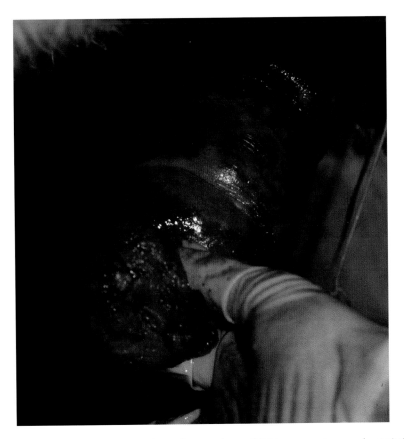

■ **Figure 92.2** Close-up of penis with pendant edema and superficial trauma and areas of excoriation. Image courtesy of C. L. Carleton.

DIAGNOSTICS

- *EHV-1:* Rising antibody titers from paired sera, collected at a 14- to 21-day interval; virus isolation from nasopharyngeal swabs in the acute stage of the disease.
- *EIA:* AGID or ELISA test (Coggins).
- *Dourine:* Identification of the causative agent in preputial or urethral exudates; serologic testing by CF. Note: This disease has been eradicated from North America and some areas of Europe.

THERAPEUTICS

- Replace the penis in the prepuce as soon as possible to prevent accumulation of dependent edema, drying of exposed surfaces, and traumatic injury. If replacement is impossible due to swelling, slings can be used to support the penis against the ventral abdominal wall (Fig. 92.4).

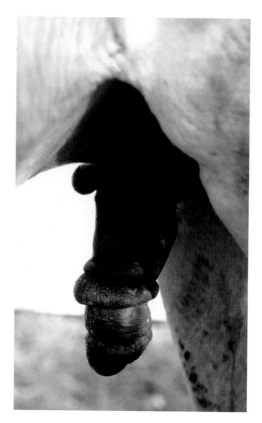

■ **Figure 92.3** Paraphimosis/paralysis following treatment with promazine tranquilizer. Image courtesy of C. L. Carleton.

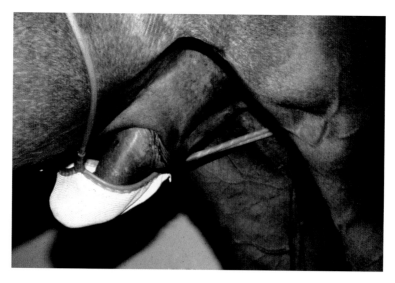

■ **Figure 92.4** Application of a web sling to minimize accumulation of edema with paraphimosis. Webbing allows urine to pass through and minimize urine scald of the penis.

- Lubricate the exposed mucosal surfaces with an emollient or antimicrobial ointment.

Drug(s) of Choice

Anti-inflammatory medication (phenylbutazone, 2–4 g/450 kg/day, PO) may be useful for patient comfort and to decrease inflammation.

Precautions/Interactions

Phenothiazine tranquilizers should be avoided.

Appropriate Health Care

Initial management is intensive, and frequent evaluation is of paramount importance. The stallion's ability to return and maintain the penis in the prepuce is a good prognostic indicator.

Surgical Considerations

In cases of chronic, unresponsive penile paralysis, surgical intervention, including penile amputation or penile retraction (Bolz technique), should be considered. Castration generally precedes these surgical techniques.

 COMMENTS

Possible Complications

- Libido often is maintained, but if erection is impossible, live cover will not be possible without human intervention and assistance.
- Some affected stallions can be trained to ejaculate into an AV or by an alternate system (e.g., application of hot compresses to the penis, semen collection into a bag [floor collection]).
- Possible secondary complications of paralysis:
  - Paraphimosis due to the accumulation of dependent edema.
  - Frostbite due to exposure.
  - Surface excoriations (i.e., ulcers, secondary bacterial contamination, and necrosis)

Abbreviations

AGID   agar gel immunodiffusion
AV   artificial vagina
CCP   corpus cavernosum penis
CF   complement fixation
EHV   equine herpes virus

EIA   equine infectious anemia
ELISA   enzyme-linked immunosorbent assay
PO   per os (by mouth)

See Also

- Behavior, evaluation, manipulation, stallion
- Breeding soundness examination, stallion
- Paraphimosis
- Priapism

Suggested Reading

Ley WB, Slusher SH. 2007. Infertility and diseases of the reproductive tract of stallions. In: *Current Therapy in Large Animal Theriogenology*, 2nd ed. Youngquist RS, Threlfall WR (eds). St. Louis: Saunders Elsevier; 15–23.

McDonnell SM, Turner RM, Love CC, et al. 2003. How to manage the stallion with a paralyzed penis for return to natural service or artificial insemination. Proc AAEP Available at www.ivis.org, Document No. P0642.1103.

Memon MA, Usenik EA, Varner DD, et al. 1988. Penile paralysis and paraphimosis associated with reserpine administration in a stallion. *Therio* 30: 411–419.

Vaughan JT. 1980. Surgery of the penis and prepuce. In: *Bovine and Equine Urogenital Surgery*. Walker DF, Vaughan JT (eds). Philadelphia: Lea & Febiger; 125–144.

Wheat JD. 1966. Penile paralysis in stallions given propiopromazine. *JAVMA* 148: 405–406.

Author: Carole C. Miller

chapter 93

Penile Vesicles, Erosions, and Tumors

DEFINITION/OVERVIEW

Any vesicular, ulcerative, or proliferative lesion associated with the penis or preputial folds.

ETIOLOGY/PATHOPHYSIOLOGY

- EHV-3, equine coital exanthema, is a relatively benign viral venereal disease of horses. The incubation period is typically 4 to 7 days. No proof of a nonclinically apparent carrier state exists. As with other herpes infections, virus recrudescence and formation of a new population of vesicles (infective stage) is associated with stress.
- Habronemiasis occurs when larvae of stomach nematodes are deposited on moist mucosal surfaces by stable flies. The larvae cause an influx of eosinophils to the affected tissues, resulting in granulomatous reactions and intense pruritus.
- Neoplasia: Appearance and progression vary with the type and size of neoplasia.

Systems Affected

- Reproductive
- Urinary
- Lymphatic
- Dermatologic

SIGNALMENT/HISTORY

Any age and breed can be affected.

Risk Factors

- Because EHV-3 is a venereal disease, natural breeding programs are more likely to have an outbreak than programs using AI. Similarly, unsanitary breeding practices can put the patients at greater risk.

- Unsanitary housing conditions or poor fly control can contribute to habronemiasis. It is more often seen in hot, humid locations in the spring or summer seasons.
- Gray horses are the most likely color pattern to present with melanoma. Most melanomas are typically found in aged animals.
- Lightly pigmented horses are more likely to have SCC, and geldings may be affected more often than stallions.
- Quarter horses are reportedly at higher risk for sarcoid development than other breeds.
- Young horses are more likely to present with papillomatous lesions.

Historical Findings

Most lesions are slow growing. Size, location, and presentation of the lesions vary. Dysuria or hematuria may be observed. Stallions may be unwilling to complete intromission; libido may be normal or diminished.

 CLINICAL FEATURES

- Lesions may be visible on the penis, prepuce, urethral process, or in the fossa glandis. Other mucocutaneous junctions may also be affected.
- Phimosis due to stricture formation, adhesions, or tumor proliferation can be observed.
- Paraphimosis due to secondary edema formation or mechanical impedance may be present.
- Hematuria or hemospermia may be present.
- Enlargement of local lymphatics or draining sinuses may be observed.

 DIFFERENTIAL DIAGNOSIS

- Viral infections: EHV-3. Typical presentation is multiple, circular, 1- to 2-mmm nodules that progress into vesicles and pustules and ultimately rupture to form ulcerations 5 to 10 mm in diameter on the penile/preputial mucosa (Figs. 93.1 and 93.2). Systemic involvement is rare, although lesions have been found on other mucocutaneous junctions in some cases.
- Parasites: Habronemiasis. Bollinger's granules, caseous masses in the exuberant granulation tissue, are diagnostic for habronemiasis. Lesions typically are extremely pruritic. Summer sores, the characteristic lesion, most often occur in the area of the urethral process or on the preputial ring (Figs. 93.3 and 93.4).
- Neoplasia: SCC, sarcoid, melanoma, papilloma, and hemangioma. Neoplastic lesions can be either ulcerative or proliferative. SCC is usually only locally invasive, although it can metastasize to regional lymph nodes and other body tissues. Biopsy should be used to confirm possible neoplasia (Fig. 93.5a and b).

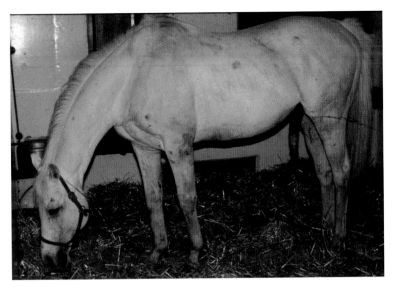

■ **Figure 93.1** Stallion presented by owner with complaint that since the previous week the stud had been standing for hours in his stall with his penis dropped. The stud could readily replace his penis into the prepuce when the owner startled the stud with an abrupt noise.
Image courtesy of C. L. Carleton.

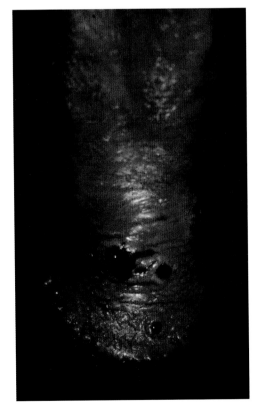

■ **Figure 93.2** Close up of active ulceration on the stallion's penis. Diagnosis: Equine herpesvirus type 3.
Image courtesy of C. L. Carleton.

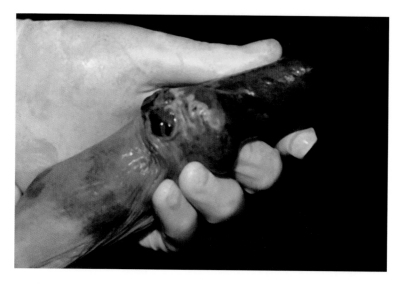

■ **Figure 93.3** *Habronema* lesion mid-shaft on a stallion's penis. He responded well and had complete resolution following treatment with ivermectin.
Image courtesy of C. L. Carleton.

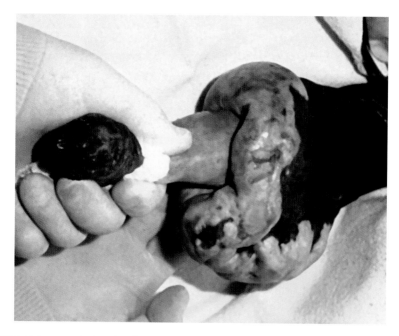

■ **Figure 93.4** *Habronema* lesion of stallion's prepuce.

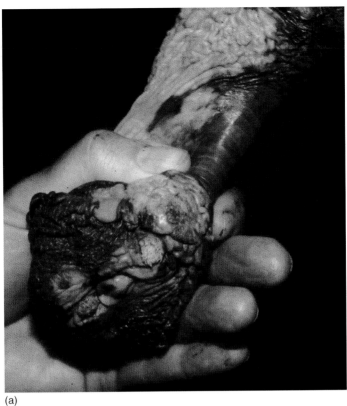

(a)

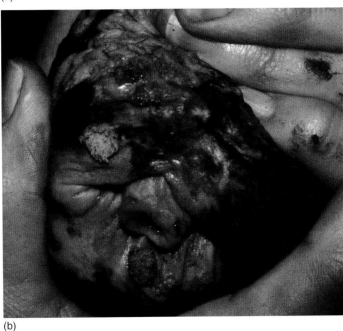

(b)

■ **Figure 93.5** *A,* Aged stallion presented with multiple lesions of his penis. *B,* Close up of glans penis. Histopath specimens collected from various glans penis lesions and results revealed the presence of *Habronema*, squamous cell carcinoma, sarcoid, and papillomatosis.
Images courtesy of C. L. Carleton.

- Trauma: Wounds, local irritants, and thermal injuries. Chronic traumatic lesions can mimic any other disease process. Diagnosis is established by history, exclusion, or response to therapy.
- Bacteria: Abscessation like that associated with bastard strangles.

DIAGNOSTICS

- EHV-3: Virus isolation from vesicular aspirates, rising antibody titers (paired sera collected at a 14- to 21-day interval) or the presence of intranuclear inclusion bodies on cytologic preparations may be diagnostic for EHV-3.
- Biopsy and histopathology can distinguish between the various tumor types and habronemiasis.

THERAPEUTICS

- Coital exanthema is a self-limiting disease with a course of disease of 3 to 5 weeks. The lesions can be quite uncomfortable, and secondary bacterial infections can occur. Daily cleansing and the application of emollient or antimicrobial ointments may be indicated for these reasons. Sexual rest while vesicles form, rupture, and heal prevents venereal transmission. After healing evidence of their presence remains in the form of irregular, scarred patches that may become confluent after repeated episodes (Figs. 93.6 and 93.7).
- Therapy for habronemiasis includes eradicating the infective larvae as well as controlling the local hypersensitivity reaction. Surgical resection of residual scar tissue may be necessary.
- Once diagnosed, tumors may be surgically excised or eliminated with cryosurgery, radiation therapy, hyperthermia, reefing, or phallectomy, dependent on their size, location, invasiveness, and type. Papillomas often regress spontaneously in 3 to 4 months. Topical or intralesional injections of chemotherapeutic agents have been used to address equine sarcoids and penile SCC.
- Chronic wounds should be cleansed, debrided, and closed, when possible. Local irritants (i.e., povidone iodine scrub) should be thoroughly rinsed off after application, if used.
- Streptococcal infections should be treated with systemic antibiotics.

Drug(s) of Choice

- *Habronema* larvae can be eradicated using ivermectin (0.2 mg/kg PO). Steroids have been used to diminish localized pruritic reactions (prednisone, 0.25–1.0 mg/kg PO, SID initially, then decreasing to the minimum effective dose).
- NSAIDs including phenylbutazone (2–4 g/450 kg/day PO) or flunixin meglumine (1 mg/kg/day IV, IM, or PO) are useful for symptomatic treatment of discomfort and to reduce local inflammation.

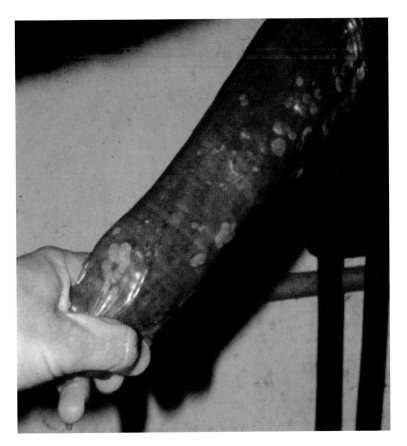

■ **Figure 93.6** Equine herpesvirus type 3 ulcerations that have recently healed; note gray scarred patches. Image courtesy of C. L. Carleton.

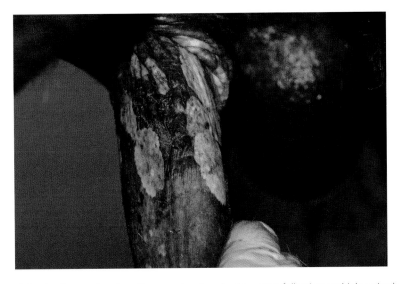

■ **Figure 93.7** Equine herpesvirus type 3, example of coalescing scars following multiple episodes of active equine herpesvirus type 3 (equine coital exanthema).
Image courtesy of C. L. Carleton.

- Systemic (Procaine penicillin G, 20,000–22,000 IU/kg IM, BID) or local (0.2% nitrofurazone ointment) antibiotics are used to treat primary or secondary bacterial infection.

Precautions/Interactions

- Nitrofurazone should not be used on horses intended for food.
- Chronic steroid use can result in iatrogenic Cushing's disease and may predispose the patient to developing laminitis due to systemic vasoconstrictive action.
- Phenothiazine tranquilizers should be used with caution, or not at all, due to the possibility of their causing priapism in intact stallions.

Alternative Drugs

- Trichlorfon (22 mg/kg diluted in 1–2 liters 0.9% NaCl, slow IV) has been used to eliminate *Habronema* larvae. There is risk of clinical organophosphate toxicity.
- Topical application of trichlorfon in 0.2% nitrofurazone (4.5 g trichlorfon in 4 ounces of 0.2% nitrofurazone) once daily to granulomatous lesions can be effective in the acute stage of habronemiasis.
- Autogenous vaccines have been suggested to deter the spread of papillomatosis within a herd.

Appropriate Health Care

The frequency of reevaluation depends on the inciting cause and severity of the lesion.

 COMMENTS

Possible Complications

- Chronic *Habronema* spp. infection involving the urethral process can result in peri-urethral fibrosis; if severe, it will necessitate amputation of the urethral process.
- Paraphimosis
- Phimosis
- Metastatic lesions in local lymph, lung, or other body tissues.
- Progression of squamous papillomatous lesions to SCC has been reported.
- Urethral blockage due to either the pathological condition or therapeutic intervention can occur; urethral patency should be closely monitored.
- Hemorrhage from penile lesions of any etiology may result in hemospermia and diminished ejaculate quality (Fig. 93.8).

Synonyms

- EHV-3
- Equine coital exanthema

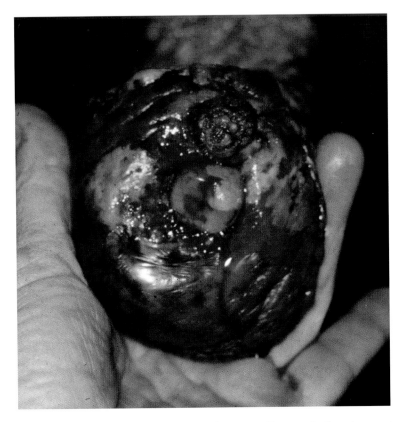

■ **Figure 93.8** Hemospermia. The act of the stallion serving a mare live or collection of semen in an artificial vagina led to bleeding from multiple sites with lesions.
Image courtesy of C. L. Carleton.

- Equine venereal balanitis
- Genital horse pox
- Habronemiasis
- Swamp cancer
- Genital bursatti
- Esponja
- Summer sores
- Warts

Abbreviations

AI	artificial insemination
BID	twice a day
EHV	equine herpesvirus
IM	intramuscular
IV	intravenous
NaCl	sodium chloride

NSAID   nonsteroidal anti-inflammatory drug
PO   per os (by mouth)
SCC   squamous cell carcinoma
SID   once a day

See Also

- Equine venereal diseases
- Paraphimosis
- Penile lacerations
- Phimosis

Suggested Reading

Couto MA, Hughes JP. 1993. Sexually transmitted (venereal) diseases of horses. In: *Equine Reproduction*. McKinnon AO, Voss JL (eds). Philadelphia: Lea & Febiger; 845–854.

May KA, Moll HD, Lucroy MD. 2002. Recognizing tumors of the equine external genitalia. *Compend Cont Educ Pract Vet* 24: 970–976.

Schumacher J, Varner DD. 2007. Surgical correction of abnormalities affecting the reproductive organs of stallions. In: *Current Therapy in Large Animal Theriogenology*, 2nd ed. Youngquist RS, Threlfall WR (eds). Philadelphia: WB Saunders; 23–36.

Vaughan JT. 1993. Penis and prepuce. In: *Equine Reproduction*. McKinnon AO, Voss JL (eds). Philadelphia: Lea & Febiger; 885–894.

Vaughan JT. 1980. Surgery of the penis and prepuce. In: *Bovine and Equine Urogenital Surgery*. Walker DF, Vaughan JT, (eds). Philadelphia: Lea & Febiger; 125–144.

Author: Carole C. Miller

chapter 94

Phimosis

DEFINITION/OVERVIEW

The inability to protrude the penis from the prepuce.

ETIOLOGY/PATHOPHYSIOLOGY

Constriction of either the external preputial orifice or the preputial ring can result in phimosis.

Systems Affected

Reproductive

SIGNALMENT/HISTORY

- Stallions or geldings of any age.
- Urination within the preputial cavity or dysuria is often reported.

Risk Factors

- Poor hygiene: accumulation of excessive smegma can lead to posthitis and subsequent phimosis from the formation of scar tissue.
- Coat/Skin color: light-colored skin is associated with an increased incidence of SCC. Gray horses are those most often diagnosed with melanomas. SCC and melanomas are more frequently diagnosed in middle-age to aged horses.
- Papillomas are more frequently diagnosed in young animals.

CLINICAL FEATURES

Visible or palpable thickening of the external preputial orifice or the preputial ring is noted. Excoriations due to urine scalding may be apparent.

DIFFERENTIAL DIAGNOSIS

Congenital

- Note: Phimosis during the first 30 days of life is normal due to fusion of the internal preputial lamina to the free portion of the penis.
- Stenosis of the preputial orifice
- Hermaphroditism
- Penile dysgenesis

Acquired

- Trauma: Breeding injury, postsurgical edema, or chronic posthitis.
- Neoplasia: Sarcoid, SCC, papilloma, melanoma, or hemangioma.
- Parasitism: Habronemiasis.
- Viral infections: EHV-3.

 DIAGNOSTICS

- Virus isolation using fluid from vesicular lesions, when present, may be diagnostic for EHV-3.
- Cytological evaluation or biopsy and histopathology may be useful to provide a definitive diagnosis for neoplastic, granulomatous, or herpesvirus lesions.

 THERAPEUTICS

If phimosis is due to:
- Postsurgical edema: hydrotherapy, massage, exercise, and diuretics are indicated. Cleansing and application of topical emollients or antibiotics may also be needed.
- Neoplastic or granulomatous lesions: surgical excision, cryosurgery, chemotherapy, or radiation as indicated by type, location, and size.
- A stricture of the external preputial orifice: surgical removal of a triangular section of the external preputial lamina.
- A stricture at the preputial ring: incise the internal preputial fold (preputiotomy). Circumcision (reefing) may be necessary to remove the constricting tissue in its entirety.

Drug(s) of Choice

- NSAIDs: including phenylbutazone (2–4 g/450 kg/day PO) or flunixin meglumine (1.1 mg/kg/day IV, IM, or PO) for symptomatic relief or to decrease inflammation.
- Systemic or local antibiotics: to treat local infections or prevent septicemia, if indicated.

- Diuretics: furosemide (1–2 mg/kg IV, every 6–12 hours) may be indicated in the acute phase to reduce edema.
- Specific topical or systemic treatments: for parasitic, fungal, or neoplastic conditions, as indicated by test results.

Precautions/Interactions

Phenothiazine tranquilizers should be avoided or used with caution (*see* Priapism).

Nursing Care

- Initially, daily evaluations: ensure that secondary posthitis, balanitis, balanoposthitis, urine scald, or penile or preputial excoriations are not complicating the phimosis.
- As the initial problem is effectively treated, less frequent examinations will be necessary.

 COMMENTS

Possible Complications

- Urination within the preputial cavity may cause inflammation of the epithelium, leading to a more extensive inflammation (e.g., posthitis, balanoposthitis) and scarring.
- Infertility or impotence can result if scarring becomes extensive.

Abbreviations

EHV	equine herpesvirus
IM	intramuscular
IV	intravenous
NSAIDs	nonsteroidal anti-inflammatory drugs
PO	per os (by mouth)
SCC	squamous cell carcinoma

See Also

- Paraphimosis
- Penile vesicles/erosions
- Venereal diseases

Suggested Reading

Blanchard TL, Varner DD, Schumacher J, et al. 2003. *Manual of Equine Reproduction*, 2nd ed. St. Louis: Mosby; 193–218.

Schumacher J, Varner DD. 2007. Surgical correction of abnormalities affecting the reproductive organs of stallions. In: *Current Therapy in Large Animal Theriogenology*, 2nd ed. Youngquist RS, Threlfall WR (eds). St. Louis: Saunders Elsevier; 23–36.

Schumacher J, Vaughan JT. 1988. Surgery of the penis and prepuce. *Vet Clin North Am Equine Practice* 4: 473–491.

Vaughan JT. 1980. Surgery of the penis and prepuce. In: *Bovine and Equine Urogenital Surgery*. Walker DF, Vaughan JT (eds). Philadelphia: Lea & Febiger; 125–144.

Author: Carole C. Miller

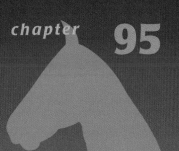

chapter 95

Priapism

DEFINITION/OVERVIEW

Persistent erection, with engorgement of the CCP, in the absence of sexual arousal.

ETIOLOGY/PATHOPHYSIOLOGY

- The smooth muscles of the arteries that supply, and the veins that drain, the CCP are under the control of the pudendal nerves. Parasympathetic stimulation of the pudendal nerves causes arterial dilation and venous constriction to and from the CCP to promote erection. Parasympathetic control also allows relaxation of the retractor penis muscles (causing penile prolapse) and the smooth muscle cells located in the walls of the CCP (allowing them to fill with blood).
- Detumescence is less well understood, but it is thought to be under sympathetic control. Adrenergic stimulation decreases arterial blood flow to the CCP and causes constriction of the smooth muscle cells lining the CCP. Agents or conditions that interfere with sympathetic stimulation are thought to directly or indirectly block detumescence.
- When detumescence fails, CO_2 tension in the CCP increases, causing increased blood viscosity and RBC sludging, and further occluding venous outflow from the CCP.
- Prolonged erection may then lead to secondary problems including paraphimosis or penile paralysis due to injury to the retractor penis muscles or the pudendal nerves proper.

Systems Affected

Reproductive

SIGNALMENT/HISTORY

- Predominantly seen in stallions, although geldings can be affected.
- It has been proposed that serum testosterone may contribute to the development of priapism.

- An alternative explanation may be that the lack of testosterone in geldings causes atrophy of the smooth muscles of the CCP, decreasing the size of the cavernous spaces available for filling with blood during the process of erection.

Risk Factors

- Most cases of priapism occur subsequent to administration of phenothiazine tranquilizer (including propiopromazine hydrochloride, chlorpromazine hydrochloride, and acepromazine maleate) to stallions.
- Avoid using this class of drugs in intact male equids.
- Rarely will these tranquilizers result in priapism in geldings.

CLINICAL FEATURES

The protruded, erect penis is usually evident. If the penis is only partially erect, the distended CCP can be detected by digital palpation.

DIFFERENTIAL DIAGNOSIS

- A history of phenothiazine tranquilizer administration to an intact stallion is significant.
- If there is evidence of debilitation, starvation, or systemic illness, these merit further investigation because they can contribute to the development of priapism.
- A complete neurologic examination is indicated to rule out spinal cord injury or disease as the inciting cause of priapism.
- Other causes that have been reported, but are rare, include general anesthesia, neoplasia, infectious diseases (i.e., purpura hemorrhagica), and postsurgical complication (e.g., castration).
- Paraphimosis is the prolapse of the penis and prepuce with extensive edema of those tissues. Paraphimosis may occur secondary to priapism, but paraphimosis may occur without a history of priapism.
- Penile paralysis is differentiated by a flaccid prolapsed penis, not erect or partially erect as is seen in priapism.

THERAPEUTICS

- As with paraphimosis, penile support in the form of slings, massage, application of emollient dressings to the penis and prepuce, and hydrotherapy are advocated to prevent the accumulation of edema and further penile injury.
- With the horse under anesthesia, manual compression of the erect penis and physically replacing it in the prepuce have been successful in some acute cases.
- Flushing the CCP with heparinized saline (10 units sodium heparin/mL 0.9% saline) using 12-gauge needles placed just proximal to the glans penis (ingress) and at the

level of the ischium (egress) has been used in cases of priapism unresponsive to cholinergic blocking or α-adrenergic agent administration.

- Surgical option: the creation of a vascular shunt between the CCP and the CSP has been successfully used in men and has been advocated for use in horses.
- Chronic cases that ultimately undergo detumescence, but leave the horse unable to retain his penis in the prepuce, may require surgery. Options are: circumcision (reefing), retraction (Bolz technique) to retain the penis within the prepuce, and in some cases, penile amputation.

Drug(s) of Choice

- A cholinergic blocker (benztropine mesylate, 8 mg, slow IV) has been used successfully to treat priapism caused by the administration of α-adrenergic blocking agents (e.g., phenothiazine tranquilizers). It should be administered during the acute phase.
- Injection of 10 mg of 1% phenylephrine HCl (an α-adrenergic agent) directly into the CCP during the acute phase has been advocated in cases unresponsive to cholinergic blocking agents.
- Superficial or deep laceration, secondary to exposure, may require topical or systemic antibiotics.
- Anti-inflammatory medication (phenylbutazone at 2–4 g/450 kg/day PO) is indicated if secondary paraphimosis or intractable inflammation exists.

Precautions/Interactions

- Phenothiazine tranquilizers are absolutely contraindicated.
- Benztropine mesylate and phenylephrine HCl should be avoided in patients with tachycardia or hypertension.

Alternative Drugs

Though not yet proven to be an effective treatment for equine priapism, the β-2 agonist clenbuterol has been suggested as an alternative drug (0.8–3.2 mg/kg PO).

Nursing Care

- Due to initial intensive patient management, hospitalization may be indicated to allow frequent reevaluation.
- Pain and discomfort are managed with physical therapy (e.g., massage, hydrotherapy, support) or pharmacologically with NSAIDs.
- Successful reduction of the erection and the stallion's ability to return his penis into the prepuce are considered good prognostic indicators.

 COMMENTS

Possible Complications

- Chronic priapism may cause inflammation of the pudendal nerve where it passes over the ischium. The pudendal nerve innervates the retractor penis muscle. Damage

to the pudendal nerve can cause malfunction of the retractor penis muscles, resulting in permanent penile paralysis.
- Secondary paraphimosis may develop as dependent edema accumulates.
- Impotence (inability to achieve an erection) can occur as a result of desensitization of the glans penis from nerve damage or fibrosis of the CCP.

Abbreviations

CCP	corpus cavernosum penis
CO_2	carbon dioxide
CSP	corpus spongiosum penis
HCl	hydrochloride
IV	intravenous
NSAIDs	nonsteroidal anti-inflammatory drugs
PO	per os (by mouth)
RBC	red blood cell

See Also

- Paraphimosis
- Penile paralysis

Suggested Reading

Blanchard TL, Schumacher J, Edwards JF, et al. 1991. Priapism in a stallion with generalized malignant melanoma. *JAVMA* 198: 1043–1044.

Blanchard TL, Varner DD, Schumacher J, et al. 2003. Surgery of the stallion reproductive tract. In: *Manual of Equine Reproduction*, 2nd ed. Blanchard TL, Varner DD, Schmacher J, et al.(eds). St. Louis: Mosby; 193–218.

Pauwels F, Schumacher J, Varner D. 2005. Priapism in horses. *Compend Contin Educ Pract Vet* 27: 311–315.

Pearson H, Weaver BMQ. 1978. Priapism after sedation, neuroleptanalgesia and anesthesia in the horse. *Eq Vet J* 10: 85–90.

Rochat MC. 2001. Priapism: A review. *Therio* 56: 713–722.

Schumaker J, Hardin DK. 1987. Surgical treatment of priapism in a stallion. *Vet Surg* 16: 193–196.

Schumacher J, Varner DD, Crabill MR, et al. 1999. The effect of a surgically created shunt between the corpus cavernosum penis and corpus spongiosum penis of stallions on erectile and ejaculatory function. *Vet Surg* 28: 21–24.

Schumacher J, Vaughan JT. 1988. Surgery of the penis and prepuce. *Vet Clin North Am, Equine Pract* 4: 473–491.

Author: Carole C. Miller

chapter 96

Reproductive Efficiency, Evaluation of Records

DEFINITION/OVERVIEW

- Reproductive records are important to establish measures of reproductive efficiency in horses, detect reproductive problems, and establish costs associated with reproduction.
- Recording systems vary depending on the extent of the evaluation. Reproductive efficiency can be estimated at the level of a state or country, stud farm, for a particular stallion, or in a particular clinic.
- Reproductive efficiency has three major components: stallion fertility, mare fertility, and personnel expertise (management).
- Data gathering (record keeping) is the cornerstone of all analyses no matter what statistical analysis and what the objectives of the analysis are.
- There are many problems using reproductive efficiency indices particularly when these calculations are done for the purpose of comparing stud farms or stallions.

SIGNALMENT/HISTORY

Requirements for Record Keeping

- To analyze reproductive efficiency, detailed reproductive records are necessary to develop common reproductive indices.
- Indices to determine the impact of some important factors such as stallion, stud farm, management procedure, breeding technique, mare fertility, and so on.
- The database can be as minimal or as detailed as desired.
- A detailed reproductive record should be kept for every mare and stallion.

Historical Findings

Mares

- All reproductive events should be recorded with appropriate date and time entries, including results of:
  - Foaling
  - Teasing records
  - U/S

- Breeding methods
- Stallion used
- Ovulation events
- Pregnancy diagnoses, results for each cycle bred.
- Abortion
- Health of each foal until weaned.

Stallions

- Reproductive events should include daily log of:
  - Natural (live) cover
  - Semen collection (date and time)
  - Identification and category of mare bred.
- When AI is used, breeding record should contain semen parameter data before shipping or freezing and at the time of insemination. Every ejaculate: motility, volume, and concentration. Monitor morphology at least on a monthly basis through each breeding season.
  - Interval from collection to insemination.
  - Interval from insemination to ovulation.
  - Identify person performing the insemination.

 ## CLINICAL FEATURES

For Everyday Simplified Overview

- Barn breeding charts
- Individual mare breeding season chart (Figs. 96.1a and b).
- These are valuable tools for a quick look at history and overall progress.

More Advanced Options

- Computerized spreadsheet or database, accessible/operated from desktop, laptop or Palm Pilot®.
- Advantage of generating daily stud farm breeding tasks, breeding history, and manipulation of data.
- Complete databases offer access to detailed individual history (mares and stallions), teasing, and TRP examination, including palpation data and results of pregnancy diagnoses.
- Can include image access (e.g., U/S, endometrial biopsy categories, and so on).
- Some databases and spreadsheets can be linked to powerful statistical packages.

Requirements for Record Analysis

For proper record analysis, it is important to observe a strict definition of the following parameters.

VETERINARY TEACHING HOSPITAL
WASHINGTON STATE UNIVERSITY

113376 Paulie the Palomino
WSU Teach Equine,
H:- W:(509)335-0711
Equine - Palomino
01/01/02 Fem Unknown

History: _4 year old maiden._
Bred 4/4/05 ovulated 4/5/05 Predicted due date **3/13/06** (342 days)
Vaccination current on all

Season: _2006_

Month	1	2	3	4	5	6	7	8	9	10	11	12	13	14	15	16	17	18	19	20	21	22	23	24	25	26	27	28	29	30	31
January																															
February							TRU TAU														Tx										
March					F											T-	T+	T+	TRU	TRU hCG	AI	OV									
April			PD⁺														PD⁻			TRU		TRU	TRU GnRH	AI	OV						
May								PD⁺Tx	P⁺	P⁺	P⁺	P⁺	P⁺	P⁺	P⁺	P⁺	P⁺	P⁺	P⁺	P⁺	P⁺PD⁺	Tx									
June																								PD⁺							
July																															
August																															
September																								TAU TRU							
October																															
November																															
December																															

Procedures/ Results Legend

AI = Artificial Insemination
F = Flush
Ov = Ovulation
PD = Pregnancy Diagnosis
PT = Parturition
T = Tease
TAU= Ultrasound (transabdominal)
TRU= Ultrasound (transrectal)
Tx = Treatment

Pharmaceutical Legend

GnRH = Gonadotropin releasing hormone
hCG = Chorionic Gonadotropin
O = Oxytocin
P+ = Progesterone
Pg = Prostaglandin F$_{2\alpha}$

(a)

Reproductive Exam Results

Date	Reason	L. Ovary	R. Ovary	Cervix	Uterus	Observation
2/7/06	Mammary development	–	–	Closed	normal pregnancy	Mammary edema - no secretion CUPT normal - Fetal HR = 80-90
2/21/06	Caslick's					Caslick's opened
3/8/06	Foaled					normal foaling & Placenta passed complete within 40 minutes
3/19/06	Pre-breeding exam	MSF	F35	± open	edema ++ small cysts	set up for frozen semen AI
3/20/06		MSF	F38	+ open	edema +++	hCG 2500IU, IM
3/21/06		MSF	F39 soft	+ open Relaxed	edema ++	AI, 3 hrs post hCG motility 45%
3/22/06		MSF	CH	± Relaxed	edema + no fluid	AI 24 hrs after ovulation -
4/05/06	Pregnancy diagnosis	F30	CL	tight	Toned vesicle 18 mm	Pregnant, Re-examine in 10-12 days
4/16/06	Pregnancy 25d.	F28	F30 CL	±	no tone, no edema	open - EED
4/20/06		F30	F26	±	·· ··	
4/22/06		F38	F35	+ Relaxed	edema ++	
4/23/06		F40	F38	± Relaxed	edema +++	GnRH (Deslorelin 1.5mg IM), 8 a.m.
4/24/06	Ovulation check					AI, frozen semen Progressive mot. 50% 5 P.m.
4/24/06	··	CH	CH	± Relaxed	edema ± no fluid	AI, frozen semen - Progressive mot. 60%
5/8/06	Pregnancy diagnosis 14d	CL	CL	Tight	Tone ++ 2 vesicles 20 mm - 18 mm	Crushed AV - 18mm Flunixin + Altrenogest for 10-12 days
5/10/06	Pregnancy	CL	CL	Tight	Tone + one vesicle 23mm	Pregnant keep on Altrenogest
5/21/06	Pregnancy Diag	CL	CL	Tight	Palpable vesicle tone	normal pregnancy, Heart beat seen check P₄
5/22/06	Caslick's					P₄ = 5.8 ng/mL. wean off Altrenogest Caslick's placed
6/24/06	Pregnancy 60 d.	CL MF	CL MF	Tight	pregnant	normal pregnancy
9/24/06	Preg evaluation	–	–	··	··	normal fetal activity, Transrectal Transabdominal start Pneumabort Ⓡ

(b)

■ **Figure 96.1** Individual mare season breeding records. *A,* Identification, history, and activity page. *B,* Examination results page.

Breeding Season

Should be precisely defined with specific dates:
- A stallion breeding season is the number of days between the first natural cover or collection until the date of last pregnancy diagnosis of the last mare bred in the season.
- For a mare the breeding season should be defined as the number of days from foaling or first teasing for nonfoaling mares until the pregnancy diagnosis of the last cycle of the season.

Types of Mares

Mares should be classified as foaling, maiden, or barren. This classification is important because it is related to mare fertility.
- *Foaling:* Mare that is to foal or has a foal at side during the breeding season. These mares are expected to have good fertility if no complications occurred during foaling or the postpartum period.
- *Maiden:* Mare that has never been bred prior to the current season. This group can be subdivided into three subgroups with decreasing order of fertility:
  - Young mares with no reproductive problems.
  - Young mares just retired from performance.
  - Older performance or pleasure mares (the *old maiden mare*).
- *Barren:* Mare that failed to become pregnant or lost a pregnancy in a previous season, entering current season open/non-pregnant. A subgroup is "barren by choice," which is a mare that foaled late in the prior season with the decision made to place her under lights and manage for early breeding the following season.

Pregnancy Status

Non-return to estrus has been used as the first indication of a possible pregnancy in the past.
- Today any serious equine breeding programs should include an early pregnancy diagnosis by U/S at 14 to 16 days post-ovulation.
- Two to three subsequent pregnancy examinations should be done to verify viability of the pregnancy and to confirm singleton versus twin.
- The last pregnancy diagnosis following a breeding season is generally done in autumn.

Cycle

A breeding cycle is defined as any opportunity the mare has to be bred again and get pregnant.

Maintenance of Reproductive Records

There are several means for data collection, manual to electronic.
- Most large farm will have some form of software for data collection and reproductive management.

- There are various software programs for keeping health and reproductive records appropriate to individual veterinary clinics.
- Mainframe data recording systems are available in countries where equine breeding is centralized at the level of National Stud Farms. This latter approach is also appropriate for the specialized, busy veterinary hospital.
- Regardless of the system used, data entry should be done promptly and verified for accuracy.
- Data systems should have built-in mechanisms to flag mares or stallions for specific actions (i.e., pregnancy diagnosis, factors indicating a decrease in fertility, and so on).

Reproductive Efficiency Measures

- Overall reproductive indices give an indication of the pregnancy rate and expected foal crop.
- A database should minimally allow calculation of the following common reproductive efficiency parameters: *Rates, Indices, Intervals,* and *Trends.*

Reproductive Rates

- Expressed in percentages of animals with the parameter of interest from the population of interest.
- The most common rates used in reproductive evaluation are:
  - *Seasonal Pregnancy Rate (SPR)*: the number of mares pregnant/number of mares bred in the season.
  - *Overall First cycle pregnancy rate* (OPR1): the number of mares pregnant on first cycle/number of mares bred in season.
  - *First cycle pregnancy rate for pregnant mares at the end of the breeding season* (PPRI) is the number of mares pregnant on first cycle/ number of mares pregnant in the season.
  - *Consecutive cycle pregnancy rates*: This is the pregnancy rate by cycle for mares bred several times in the breeding season (PPRII for all second-cycle breeding, PPRIII for all third-cycle breeding, etc.).
- For large populations of horses, these rates can be calculated separately for specific populations of mares:
  - PPR1 for maiden, foaling, and barren mares.
  - PPR1 for foal heat breeding.
- Other overall reproductive rates can be calculated and may yield valuable information on the reproductive efficiency of a population of horses, further serving to monitor and define reproductive performance, for example:
  - Double ovulation rate
  - Twinning rate
  - Early pregnancy loss, pregnancy rate
  - Abortion or fetal loss rate
  - Foaling rate
  - Endometritis event rate

- Dystocia rate
- Retained placenta rate
- Neonatal loss rate (foal losses from birth to weaning).

Reproductive Indices

Indices are important to determine the actual significance of a rate. For example, SPR alone does not address the time it took a mare to get pregnant. To increase the precision of analysis of reproductive performance, the following parameters are needed:
- Average number of cycles per pregnancy.
- Number of breedings per cycle. For efficient use of a stallion, this should be one breeding per cycle. For stallions with *large books*, good management requires that less than 10% of mares are bred more than once during a single estrus period. Increased number of matings (live, natural cover) or AI in one estrus period denotes an error in management of estrus and prediction of ovulation and leads to unnecessary overuse of a stallion.
- Number of breedings per cycle for pregnant mares.

Reproductive Intervals and Distributions

Because most reproductive parameters are calculated on a population basis, they lack precision in estimating the average weight of each factor. Distributions and intervals may provide strength in determining fertility trends.
- Distribution is plotted for:
  - Age of mares
  - Matings or AI dates
  - Pregnancy loss or abortion dates
  - Foaling dates
- The main intervals used for equine reproductive evaluation are:
  - Number of days from entry in the breeding shed to cover.
  - Number of days from entry in the breeding shed to pregnancy.
  - Number of days from foaling to foaling (for mares that have had a previous foal).
  - These intervals give an idea about reproductive efficiency but are also important to assess the cost of achieving a pregnancy.
  - Intervals are important for breeds that demand recording and reporting specific data (e.g., the official or a universal birth day for all foals [i.e., Thoroughbred breed]) or when advanced breeding techniques are used and their cost and efficacy are to be evaluated.
- Calculation of intervals between two specific reproductive events may be helpful for specific epidemiological data analyses. For example, analysis of reproductive loss should include not only rate of loss but also the interval from date of conception until date of pregnancy loss.

Trends

- Trend monitoring is an important factor in evaluation of reproductive efficiency in stud farms to determine seasonal effects as well as stallion fertility effects.

Date	Mare	-	-	-	-	-	-	-	-	-	-	-	-	-	0	+	+	+	+	+	+	+	+	+	+	+	+	+	+	+	+
3/1/07	M1															+															
3/2/07	M2														-																
3/2/07	M3															+															
3/2/07	M4																+														
3/4/07	M5																	+													
3/6/07	M6																		+												
3/6/07	M8																			+											
3/7/07	M9																				+										
3/7/07	M10																			+											
3/8/07	M11																				+										
3/8/07	M12																					+									
3/9/07	M13																						+								
3/10/07	M14																							+							
3/11/07	M15																						-								
3/11/07	M16																					-									
3/11/07	M17																				-										
3/13/07	M18																					+									
3/15/07	M19																				-										
3/15/07	M20																			-											
3/15/07	M21																		-												
3/15/07	M22																-														
3/18/07	M23																	+													
3/19/07	M24																-														

■ **Figure 96.2** Stallion Q-sum breeding analysis. Pregnancy diagnosis results are reported for all mares bred between March 1 and March 19. Plot shows good fertility from March 1 until the 11th, slowed by a poor trend thereafter as the stallion started being used heavily.

- Seasonal trends: Rates and indices listed previously can be calculated for specific months of the breeding season. Seasonal trend for pregnancy can also be expressed by a survival curve plot from the day mares enter the breeding shed until they are confirmed pregnant.
- Fertility trend for a stallion: Graphical illustration of fertility trends for a stallion can be illustrated with a Q-sum or pregnancy differential chart (Fig. 96.2).

Stallion Reproductive Efficiency

- Pregnancy rates listed previously are often used as a measure of stallion fertility or for the purpose of comparison between stallions. It is important to know the limitations of each type of indices.
- A stallion can achieve a low per cycle pregnancy rate but have an adequate cumulative season pregnancy rate. Factors that affect the overall reproductive efficiency of a stallion are:
  - Number of mares in each category of fertility.
  - Number of mares added to the stallion's *book* at the end on the breeding season, thus limiting the opportunities for them to become pregnant.
  - Number of mares that are switched from the "first stallion" to another stallion because they did not become pregnant.
  - Length of the breeding season.
  - Timing of the first pregnancy diagnosis.

- Season pregnancy rate can be misleading if the type of mares (e.g., aged, foaling, barren, or maiden) covered, and the extent of use of a stallion, are not taken into consideration.
- The fertility of a stallion may change over the season.
- When stallions are used in fresh cooled semen programs, sources of variation may include the interval from collection to breeding, mare management, and inseminator effect (difference).
- Pregnancy rate can also change during the season depending on the frequency of use or collection of the stallion.
- To alleviate some of these problems and more accurately analyze the pregnancy rate achieved by a stallion, evaluation/analysis should include:
  - Establishment of pregnancy rates and interval for each category of mare bred to a particular stallion.
  - First cycle pregnancy rate for pregnant mares should be used as the main rate to evaluate stallions (removes infertile mares from the pool).
  - Calculation of pregnancy rates should evaluate the effect of *frequency of use* of the stallion (specifically for live cover use). For this, pregnancy rate should be calculated for days when only one mare was bred versus one, two, or more.
  - Daily pregnancy rate: based on the number of mares bred each day and the pregnancy rate based on their *order of breeding* (daily pregnancy survival curve).
  - Pregnancy rate based on the *order of breeding* is relevant if the stallion live-covered multiple mares in 1 day.
  - Seasonal trends are demonstrated by pregnancy rate for each month.
  - Q-sum or pregnancy differential can be plotted on a daily basis to evaluate trends.

AI Program Efficiency

Stallion owners, stud farms, or veterinary clinics may benefit from evaluating the efficiency of an AI program. This can be done at three levels:

1. Semen production, at the time of collection or origin:
   a. Number of collections per season.
   b. Number of doses produced per season is equal to the number of collections less the number of ejaculates discarded for poor quality.
   c. Number of doses shipped or stored (frozen semen).
   d. Number of doses used per pregnancy.
2. AI success rate: pregnancy rates described previously can also be used for shipped or frozen semen.
   a. Overall pregnancy rate for cooled semen:
      i. Pregnancy rate with cooled shipped semen used at less than 24 hours.
      ii. Pregnancy rate with cooled shipped semen used 24 to 48 hours after collection.
      iii. Pregnancy rate with cooled shipped semen used more than 48 hours after collection.
      iv. Pregnancy rate by interval from AI to ovulation.
      v. Average number of doses used per cycle.

      vi. Average number of doses used per pregnancy.

      vii. Average number of cycles per pregnancy.

  b. Overall pregnancy rate with frozen semen:

      i.   Overall pregnancy rate.

      ii. Pregnancy rate by interval from AI to ovulation.

      iii. Average number of doses used per cycle.

      iv. Average number of doses used per pregnancy.

      v.   Average number of cycles per pregnancy.

3. Quality of semen at the user level:

  a. Quality of semen at destination (receiving end).

  b. Percentage of doses shipped but not used.

  c. Reasons given: poor or no motility, gross contamination, and so on.

ET Program Efficiency

Parameters used to evaluate success of an ET program include:

- Embryo recovery rate: percentage of times an embryo was collected from all collection attempts.
- Number of cycles flushed
- Average number of embryos per mare per season.
- Pregnancy rate after transfer
- Pregnancy loss rate
- Foaling rate
- Number of transfers per pregnancy

Reproductive Cost

- The only true measure of reproductive efficiency for the professional breeder is the differential between the value of a foal at sale and all costs incurred producing the foal until sale.
- A major portion of the cost of production is incurred by pregnancy, foaling, and management until weaning.
- Each aspect of the equine breeding program has an associated cost. The majority of costs are incurred with:
  - Stud fees
  - Boarding fees
  - Mare depreciation
  - Veterinary fees (including preventive drug cost and cost of management of a high-risk pregnancy).
  - Insurance fees

Abbreviations

AI   artificial insemination

ET   embryo transfer

OPR1   overall first cycle pregnancy rate

PPRI   first cycle pregnancy rate for pregnant mares at season's end
PPRII   consecutive cycle pregnancy rate, second cycle breeding
PPRIII   consecutive cycle pregnancy rate, third cycle breeding
SPR   seasonal pregnancy rate
TRP   transrectal palpation
U/S   ultrasound, ultrasonography

Suggested Reading

Love CC. 2003. The role of breeding record evaluation in the evaluation of the stallion for breeding soundness. *Proc Soc for Therio* 68–77.

Author: Ahmed Tibary

chapter 97

Semen, Chilled (for Transport)

DEFINITION/OVERVIEW

- "Chilled" semen is the term used for semen that is not frozen, but extended and cooled to a temperature above 0°C (most often 5°C), typically for transport to a distant facility for AI of a mare the day after the semen was collected.
- Cooled semen may also be maintained and used on farm, even when stallion and mares are residents, if the time between semen collection and AI is to be delayed.
- Chilled semen usually does not contain glycerol or other low molecular weight cryoprotectants (as are used in extenders for frozen semen).

ETIOLOGY/PATHOPHYSIOLOGY

Systems Affected

Reproductive

SIGNALMENT/HISTORY

- Common procedure used in breeds that accept the use of AI and shipped semen.
- Use of semen from a stallion (preferably of good fertility) if it has been determined to tolerate or survive extension, chilling, and transport to a distant location for AI of a mare(s).
- Semen used on site at a time frame longer than would survive on farm in the absence of extension and chilling.

CLINICAL FEATURES

Procedure

Semen collection and evaluation of the normal stallion:
- Semen is collected by AV.
- Gel fraction is removed:
  - By an in-line filter during collection.
  - By filtration or aspiration after collection.

- Evaluate motility of the raw semen.
- Measure (gel-free) semen volume.
- A small (1–5 mL) aliquot of raw semen (gel-free) is placed in a separate test tube for evaluation of concentration and sperm morphology.
- Measure sperm concentration of raw (gel-free) semen by hemocytometer or by spectrophotometric methods, if instrumentation is available.
- Semen is extended to a sperm concentration of 25 to 50 million sperm/mL or to a ratio of at least 3 to 4 volumes of extender per volume of raw semen.
- Evaluate motility of extended semen.
- Extended semen is packaged in plastic test tubes or plastic bags labeled with:
  - Stallion identification
  - Volume
  - Number of spermatozoa
  - Date packaged
- A data sheet is prepared for inclusion with the shipment, and semen is packed in a passive cooling system for gradual cooling to 5°C.
- In general, at least 1 billion spermatozoa are included in a package that will be considered a single AI dose; this will vary according to the stallion and success of transporting viable spermatozoa from that individual stallion.
- Target is for at least 500 million PMS available for AI.
- The volume of each AI dose can vary between 30 and 120 mL without affecting fertility:
  - AI of 170 mL (a large volume) was reported to have a high pregnancy rate.
  - May be that AI of a large volume could result in loss of extended semen via backflow through the cervix.
  - As long as sufficient numbers of PMS (more than 500 million) remain in the uterus after AI, fertility appears unaffected within range of volume limits reported here.

Variations in Procedure When Semen Does Not Transport Well

- Some stallion semen is sensitive to holding in an overly warm water bath or incubator following collection:
  - Motility can be diminished if the incubator or water bath warms the semen above 37°C.
  - Insulation, rather than incubation, is preferred to prevent cold shock.
  - Because equine semen is somewhat resistant to the detrimental effects of cooling between 37°C and 20°C, a slow decline in semen temperature while processing semen for shipment generally can be tolerated.
- Some stallion semen is sensitive to cooling:
  - Great care must be taken to extend the semen with a milk-based extender.
  - Insulate semen to cool it gradually, even if it is to be used for AI within 1 to 2 hours on farm, following collection.
- Some stallion semen is sensitive to incubation in seminal plasma:
  - With such semen and, in general when conditions permit the best possible practices, sperm motility and its survival are enhanced by removal of seminal plasma by centrifugation and resuspension in a milk-based extender.

- Centrifugation to remove seminal plasma generally results in a decreased tolerance to ambient temperature of semen.
  - To protect the semen from the effect of this cooling process, it is often necessary to dilute (extend) the semen in a milk-based extender prior to centrifugation.

Semen Extender, Components for Chilled Semen

- Usually a combination of glucose, milk, a buffer, and antibiotics.
  - Glucose for the bulk of the osmotic component to keep the solution isotonic.
  - Milk for cold-shock protection of the spermatozoa (may be by protecting the cell membrane from the detrimental effects of seminal plasma proteins; the definitive mechanism remains unclear).
  - Buffer is commonly sodium bicarbonate, to offset pH change caused by cellular respiration while the sample is in transit (CO_2 build-up).
  - Antibiotics to prevent a build-up of bacteria in stored semen. There is also some inevitable contamination of semen with microorganisms during semen collection.
- Egg yolk, a component to protect against cold-shock:
  - Mechanism is likely by neutralizing detrimental components of seminal plasma.
  - More commonly used in semen cryopreservation than in chilling of semen.
  - Tends to interfere with visual or photometric assessment of concentration, motility, and morphology, unless the extender has been centrifuged or clarified.
  - More difficult to package in a mix intended to be stored for long periods prior to use.
- Both milk and egg yolk are biological substances:
  - Quality may vary between batches.
  - Can be toxic if special steps are not taken during preparation.
- NFDSM causes the least complications in preparing chilled semen extenders, a generally safe form.
- Extenders containing only defined components of milk demonstrating beneficial qualities for storage of chilled semen:
  - Developed but not universally available.
- Antibiotics tested for use in equine semen extenders include:
  - Amikacin, gentamicin, streptomycin, potassium penicillin, sodium penicillin, ticarcillin/Timentin, polymyxin B, ceftiofur, combinations of penicillin and amikacin, and combinations of Timentin and clavulanic acid.
  - Gentamicin has demonstrated better efficacy than many of the other choices of antibiotics at eliminating bacterial growth from semen.
  - The combination of potassium penicillin and amikacin yielded better results than other antibiotics in maintaining motility of semen, also effective in suppressing bacterial growth.

Other Considerations for Chilled Semen Storage

Temperature

- Generally semen is transported and stored at 5°C until used.
  - When semen arrives, it can be transferred to a standard refrigerator set to 5°C if the storage limits of the container will be exceeded (the shipping box is incapable

of maintaining sample at desired temperature, 5°C, if more than 24 hours until it will be used).
  ▪ May prove that 15°C is superior to 5°C to maintain semen quality; however, transport containers maintaining semen at 15°C have not yet been designed for commercial use.

Cooling

▪ Equine spermatozoa are tolerant of cooling to 20°C.
▪ Cooling from 20°C down to 5°C is enhanced by a cooling rate of −0.1°C/minute.
  ▪ An even slower rate may be desirable.
▪ Containers for chilled shipment vary by type of insulation, type of frozen cold-pack, differences in design, insulating capacity, durability, volume of semen capable of being shipped (container capacity), and size/volume of the cold-pack in individual systems.
  ▪ All result in different rates of cooling, by system.

Volume

▪ Each transport container has an inherent capacity of extended semen that can be effectively cooled and stored in it.
▪ Often, when a stallion has produced an ejaculate with sufficient spermatozoa and only one mare is being inseminated from that ejaculate, two AI doses of 40 to 60 mL are prepared and shipped.
  ▪ Each contains 1 to 3 billion spermatozoa, extended to a concentration of 25 to 50 million/mL.
▪ Small volumes of highly concentrated fresh semen are capable of producing normal fertility in the mare.
  ▪ The larger AI volume inseminated with chilled, transported semen results from its dilution with semen extender.
  ▪ Concentration of extender to semen (a ratio) is intended to maintain motility for 24 to 48 hours.

Insemination of Chilled Transported Semen

Identification and Evaluation

▪ When the transport container arrives where AI will be performed, confirm the:
  ▪ Identity of the stallion.
  ▪ Labeling of the semen.
  ▪ Accompanying documents should be cross-checked (correct stallion for the mare).
▪ Prior to AI, a small aliquot of semen should be placed in a separate tube and checked for motility by examination under the microscope.
▪ Calculation of the number of PMS available for insemination should be performed (volume [mL] × concentration [M/mL] × percent progressively motile spermatozoa = millions of progressively motile sperm in the ejaculate [___ × 10⁶]).

Insemination

- If not prepackaged in an Air-Tite type syringe, semen is transferred to a syringe. (Do *not* use syringes with a rubber disk on the plunger).
- AI is performed trans-cervically with a mare AI pipet.
- Most semen/extender combinations do not require prewarming of the chilled sample before AI (semen extended in cream-gel may be semi-solid at 5°C).
- What to do with AI if multiple insemination doses are sent in the transport container?
  - Very often, two insemination doses will arrive in a chilled semen order.
  - Usually, each dose will be sufficient for an effective AI.
  - Calculation of PMS in each AI dose will confirm this.
  - Under most circumstances, a single dose inseminated on arrival is sufficient.
- Presupposes:
  - The stallion is normal and motility is well-maintained by the transport system
  - The mare is normal, ovulation will occur within 24 hours of insemination, and
  - PMS number is more than 500 million at the time of insemination.
- Options available are:
  - Inseminate one dose on the day of arrival.
  - Inseminate both doses on the day of arrival.
  - Inseminate one dose the day of arrival and the second dose the second day.
- Different studies of these options have not given identical results. What has been reported:
  - No difference between AI of both doses at 24 hours and,
  - AI of one dose at 24 and one at 48 hours.
  - One study showed a slight improvement in fertility with 24- and 48-hour inseminations.
- One possible conclusion might be that insemination of one or both doses on the day of arrival (at 24 hours postsemen collection) is generally sufficient but not always.
  - Mares and stallions differ, and circumstances differ (e.g., time of ovulation, intensity of uterine inflammatory response to AI, longevity of spermatozoa from different stallions and different ejaculates).
  - If the motility of the stallion's semen is known to decrease dramatically between 24 and 48 hours, insemination of both doses at 24 hours is indicated.

 COMMENTS

Client Education

- Semen from all stallions cannot successfully be extended, chilled, and transported.
- Individual variability and rates of success are to be expected.
- Success dependent also on stallion's sperm numbers and health (parameters: motility, concentration, morphology, and so on).

- Testing of ejaculate quality and its tolerance of chilling, including extension ratios, extender selection, and longevity (survival) of samples prior to anticipated time of shipment is highly recommended, well before any deadline to breed mares.

Possible Complications

- Semen from a subfertile stallion may not tolerate chilling and transport (poor semen quality).
- If initial testing fails to identify an extender or procedure compatible with a particular stallion, then shipment of chilled samples may not be possible.

Synonyms

- Cooled semen
- Liquid semen
- Extended semen
- Transported semen

Abbreviations

AI	artificial insemination
AV	artificial vagina
CO_2	carbon dioxide
NFDSM	nonfat dry skim milk
PMS	progressively motile spermatozoa

See Also

- Breeding soundness examination, stallion
- Semen collection, methods
- Semen collection, reproductive efficiency
- Semen collection, routine semen evaluation
- Semen cryopreservation
- Semen evaluation, abnormal stallion

Suggested Reading

Aurich C. 2005. Factors affecting the plasma membrane function of cooled-stored stallion spermatozoa. *Anim Reprod Sci* 89: 65–75.

Brinsco S, Varner DD, Blanchard TL. 2000. Transported equine semen. In: *Recent Advances in Equine Reproduction*. Ball BA (ed). Ithaca: IVIS. Document No. A0207.0400.

Varner DD, Scanlan CM, Thompson JA, et al. 1998. Bacteriology of preserved stallion semen and antibiotics in semen extenders. *Therio* 50: 559–573.

Author: Rolf E. Larsen

chapter 98

Semen Collection Techniques

DEFINITION/OVERVIEW

- The ideal method of semen collection is the one that yields an ejaculate as close as possible to the one the same stallion would deposit in the genital tract of a mare following a natural (live) cover.
- The choice of method of collection depends on several factors including:
  - Experience and training of the stallion.
  - Preference of the operator.
  - Preference of the stallion for specific collection conditions.
  - Health and soundness of the stallion.
- Several methods of semen collection have been devised for stallions. The main differences among methods are the:
  - Type of equipment used.
  - Presence or absence of a mount mare.
  - Presence or absence of copulation.
- Semen can also be obtained from the tail of the epididymis:
  - After castration
  - On death of terminally ill stallions.

ETIOLOGY/PATHOPHYSIOLOGY

- Ejaculation is a complex process involving several parameters related to behavioral, functional, and physical integrity.
- The normal ejaculatory process requires proper stimulation to obtain erection and to stimulate the stallion to obtain emission and ejaculation.
- Erection involves a series of reflexes primarily controlled by the parasympathetic system that result in engorgement of the CCP.
- Maximal erection is achieved with proper stimulation (i.e., pressure and temperature) during copulation.
- Ejaculation is the result of two types of contractions under sympathetic system control.
  - The first allows transport of semen from the tail of the epididymis to the pelvic urethra (emission).
  - The second is contraction of accessory sex glands and the urethra, and the forceful elimination of six to eight jets of semen, which comprise the ejaculate.

- Methods of semen collection are meant to mimic the stimulatory conditions provided by the mare's vagina during live cover (primarily pressure and temperature).
- Ideally, semen collection of the normal stallion should approximate the conditions of a "normal live cover," to encourage the stallion to exhibit normal behavior, including approach and copulation.
- Methods of semen collection vary depending on the objectives.
- Incapacitated stallions may require adoption of techniques that enhance stimulation of the erection and ejaculation process by:
  - Physical means: pressure on the glans penis, hot towels at the base of the penis.
  - Chemical means: to lower the threshold of erection and ejaculation.

Systems Affected

- Reproductive
- Multisystem

SIGNALMENT/HISTORY

- All stallions: routine semen evaluation or processing for use in AI.
- Stallions with different forms of incapacitating diseases or injuries, unable to cover naturally.
- Stallions with ejaculatory or erection disorders.
- All stallions should undergo a physical examination and be tested for venereal disease before collecting semen for the purpose of breeding or preservation.

Risk Factors

Stallions

- Older, debilitated stallion may require special techniques to successfully collect semen.

CLINICAL FEATURES

Techniques of Collection

Dismount Sample

- This technique consists of collecting and examining a few drops of the semen that dribble from the stallion after mating.
  - Routinely used to determine sperm motility and morphology for stallions with a large *book*, when AI is not allowed.
  - Goal is to gather information regarding semen quality without "wasting" an entire ejaculate.

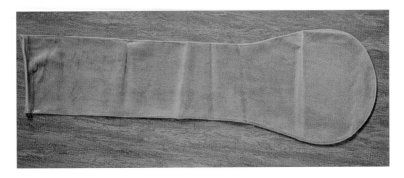

■ Figure 98.1 Condom used for semen collection in stallions.

- Main disadvantage: the sample is often not from the sperm-rich fraction and may not be representative of ejaculate quality.

Post-Coital Aspiration

- A more invasive technique.
- Consists of aspirating part of the ejaculate from the mare's vagina and uterus after natural (live) cover.
- Provides variable sample quality.
- Indicated for unruly or untrained stallions or when equipment for semen collection is unavailable (e.g., miniature horses).

Condom

- Seldom used nowadays because of problems with loss of erection, difficult intromission, and a high risk of loss of the condom after dismount (Fig. 98.1).
- Quality of rubber in the condom is important because some types of rubber may be sperm toxic.

Manual Stimulation

- May be indicated for stallions that cannot achieve a normal mount or small breeds (e.g., ponies, miniature horses). It has also been used to collect semen from zebras.
- Training of stallions to respond to manual stimulation is as easy as training for collection in an AV.
- The technique consists of stimulation of the stallion in the presence of an estrus mare until erection has been achieved.
  - A clean plastic bag is placed over the glans penis.
  - Ejaculation is obtained by exerting adequate pressure on the glans penis while either stroking the penile shaft using a warm towel or placing the warm towel at the base of the penis and applying pressure.
  - Ejaculation is generally obtained within a 10-minute stimulation period.
- Semen characteristics are similar to those of AV-collected ejaculates, with the exception of pH, which may be slightly lower with manual stimulation.

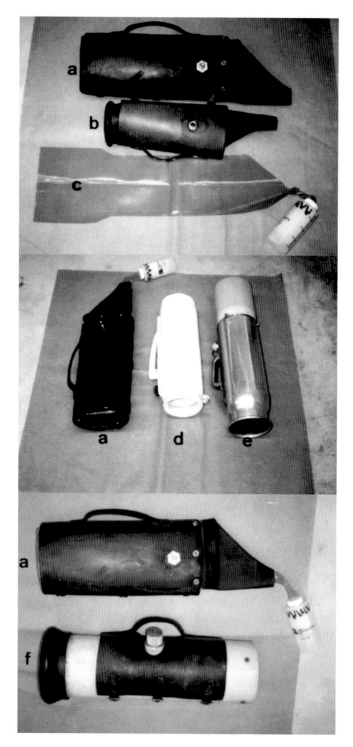

■ **Figure 98.2** Different models of artificial vaginas used for stallion semen collection: *A*, Missouri, large model; *B*, Missouri small (Pony) model; *C*, Inner liner for the Missouri model; *D*, French; *E*, known as the Japanese, the Nishikawa, or the Tokyo model; and *F*, Colorado.

AV

- The most often used technique for stallion semen collection.
- Most AVs are designed with double latex walls, filled with warm water to provide adequate temperature and pressure.
- There are several types of AVs (Fig, 98.2): Hannover, Missouri, Colorado, French.
    - They differ primarily by construction material, weight, and handling characteristics.
- Choice of equipment is determined by stallion and operator preference.
    - Missouri® model: most often used because of its light weight and ease of preparation (*see* Fig. 98.2). The coned-end of the latex can be cut off and used to collect semen fractions from its opened end (Fig. 98.3).
    - Colorado®/Lane-modified model: heavier, cumbersome, can also be used as an open-ended AV to collect a fractionated ejaculate (*see* Fig. 98.2).
    - The Hannover® AV model provides good stimulation of the glans penis because of its off-center proximal opening that provides increased pressure on the glans penis with each forward thrust.
- Most AV models are available in different sizes to accommodate different breeds of horses.
- AV components include an outer shell or liner, an inner liner, and a collection tube with or without an in-line filter in place (Fig. 98.4).

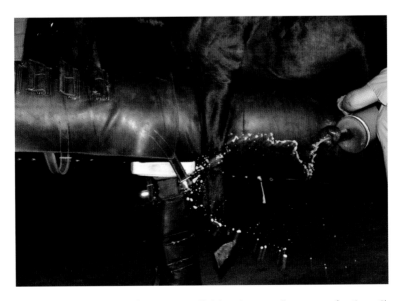

■ **Figure 98.3** Remodeled (cone cut-off) Missouri artificial vagina to collect semen fractions. Shown without individual cones and tubes to collect fractions.
Image courtesy D. D. Varner.

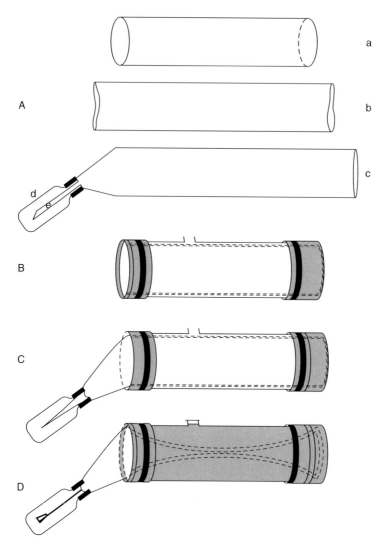

■ **Figure 98.4** Typical construction components of an artificial vagina: *A,* outer shell or tube; *B,* inner liner; *C,* disposable collection liner with collection tube and filter; *D,* collection bottle or bag, and *E,* in-line filter.

- Semen can be collected directly into the assembled system or by including a single-use plastic collection liner through its central lumen.
- Collection of semen without a plastic liner may expose semen to the harmful effect of rubber if the ejaculate is not delivered directly into the collection tube.
- The main factors in successful collection of semen using an AV are proper:
  - Preparation of the AV
  - Preparation and training of the stallion
  - Handling of the semen after collection

Preparation of the AV

- Three key parameters in AV preparation: temperature, pressure, and lubrication.
- The inside temperature of the AV should be approximately 45°C to 48°C at the time of collection.
- Pressure altered by fill volume is adjusted to allow penetration of the stallion's penis, with a snug fit that still allows comfortable thrusting within its lumen. Pressure at the level of the glans penis should be in the order of 100 to 240 mm Hg.
- Lubrication should be adequate to permit initial penetration of the penis. The type and volume of lubricant should be chosen carefully.
  - Most lubricants are water soluble and can mix with the ejaculate.
  - *Some lubricants* cause osmotic or pH changes that may be harmful to semen.
  - Priority-Care®, nonspermicidal, sterile gel has been shown to be the best choice. The volume of it used should be kept to a minimum.
  - Pre-seed®, a newly formulated lubricant, for use in equine AV preparation and for artificial insemination has been shown to give superior results (Fig. 98.5).
- Ideal parameters for AV preparation can vary significantly between stallions. Records of the preferred settings (i.e., temperature, pressure and lubrication) for each stallion ensure more reliable responses for stallions collected on a regular basis.

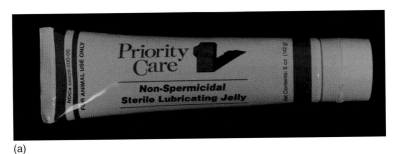

(a)

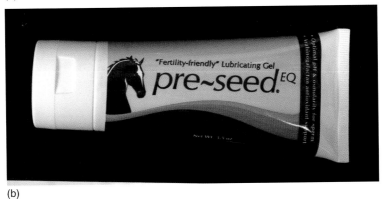

(b)

■ **Figure 98.5** Most commonly used lubricants for artificial vagina: *A,* Priority-Care® and *B,* Pre-seed®, a newly formulated lubricant for equine artificial vaginas and genital manipulations.

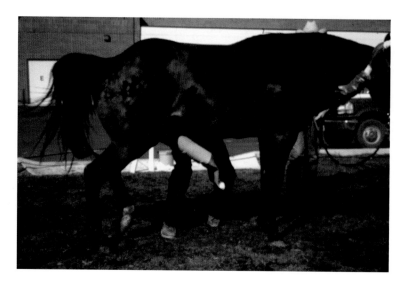

■ **Figure 98.6** Stallion collection on the ground (without mount).

Preparation and Training of the Stallion

- Most stallions readily accept semen collection in an AV, if they have already been trained to be handled for breeding.
- Stallion training for in-hand mating and stallion handler expertise are important parts to good semen collection.
- Semen collection area should be well designed to provide for the safety of the stallion and operators, as well as be in an environment conducive for the stallion to exhibit uninhibited mounting behavior.
- Collection of semen using an AV can be accomplished on a mount mare, a dummy (i.e., phantom), or *on the ground* (collection without mounting) (Fig. 98.6).
- Initial phases of stallion training are facilitated by the proximity of an estrus mare or an estrogen-treated ovariectomized mare.
- Most stallions will accept a dummy mare after only a few sessions of training in the presence of a tease mare.
- Advantages of phantom mare collections are safety, biosecurity (no contact with mares), and the ability to modify the height and inclination of the phantom to best suit the size of the stallion and accommodate health and physical conditions he may have.
- Dummy mounts are available commercially with some variations in construction. Sophisticated dummies such as Equidame® have a built-in port into which an AV can be inserted (for a hands-free collection), as well as a computerized system to collect semen fractions (Fig. 98.7).
- Stallions may prefer a particular model of AV, as well as a preferred temperature and pressure.

Proper Handling of AV

- The AV should be held at the approximate height and orientation of a mare's vulva and vagina.

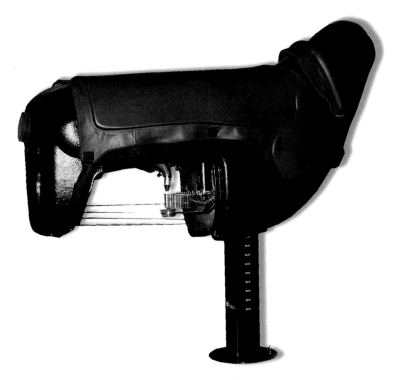

■ **Figuire 98.7** Equidame®: Computerized semen collection dummy.
Image courtersy Minitub®, Germany.

- Slightly deflect the stallion's glans penis and penile shaft toward the opening of the AV as he approaches the mare or phantom.
- Allow the stallion to move into the AV as he mounts and grips the mare/phantom with his forelimbs.
- The most common errors in handling the AV that may result in loss of erection or lack of ejaculation are:
  - Pushing the AV onto the penis rather than letting the stallion mount. This can result in an abnormal angle or cause discomfort for the stallion.
  - Grasping the penile shaft or glans penis too tightly.

Modification of Collection Conditions Using an AV

- Conditions for semen collection can be modified to accommodate specific medical or biological needs of a stallion. The most common modifications allow for collection of fractionated ejaculates or collection of the stallion *on the ground* (no mounting possible or desired).
- Fractionated ejaculates are desired to determine the anatomical origin of contaminants observed in an ejaculate (e.g., site of bleeding in cases of hemospermia, urine with urospermia, or to enable collection of only the sperm-rich fraction and eliminate the harmful effects of seminal plasma on preservation of semen).
- Fractionated ejaculates can be obtained by allowing the stallion to serve an open-ended AV.

- Separate jets of semen are collected into different collection tubes attached to a wide funnel.
- Technique requires an additional person or two to handle the collection tubes.
- Samples should be protected from light and change of temperature immediately after collection.
- This technique is not appropriate for field collections.
- A more thorough fractionation of the ejaculate is possible with the use of a computerized system such as the Equidame®.
- Standing (four-on-the-floor) collection is often required for stallions incapacitated by musculoskeletal injuries, chronic diseases, or that have undergone recent abdominal surgery (*see* Fig. 98.6).
  - The Missouri® AV is preferred for this technique.
  - AV temperature should be approximately 50°C at the time of collection. The AV is placed on the penis after proper stimulation of the stallion in the presence of an estrus mare.
  - Manual pressure on the glans penis should be provided during the stallion's thrusting movements. Ejaculation is usually obtained after five or six movements.
  - Up to 60% of stallions may respond to the first attempt. However, ejaculates may not be complete.

Electroejaculation

- This is not a routine technique and may be attempted only under general anesthesia.
- It has been used successfully in some debilitated stallions and wild equids.

Ex-Copula Ejaculation

- Pharmacological collection of semen is possible and may be indicated in stallions with erection or ejaculatory disorders (e.g., neurologic disease, penile paralysis, urospermia, retrograde ejaculation).
- The most common treatment combines the use of a tricyclic antidepressant (imipramine hydrochloride) and the α2-adrenergic agonist xylazine.
- Imipramine HCl is given orally 2 hours before administration of xylazine IV.
- Ejaculation occurs usually within 2 to 10 minutes after treatment, but it may range from 5 to 45 minutes.
- Response rates (successful ejaculation) are variable (10%–80%) and may be improved by titration of the dose of imipramine and xylazine for a particular stallion.
- Ejaculate quality is good. Some ejaculates will have a high sperm concentration due to a lack of adequate contributions from the accessory sex glands.

Post-Castration or Postmortem Semen Harvesting

- Semen can be harvested by flushing the tail of the epididymis after dissection following castration or postmortem collection of testes (Fig. 98.8).
- Collection of semen from the epididymis may be performed up to 24 hours if the testis is preserved at 5°C.

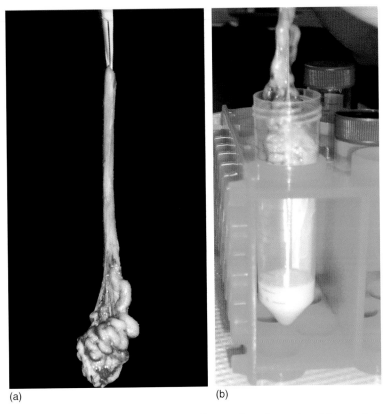

(a)   (b)

■ **Figure 98.8** Postmortem or postcastration collection of semen from the cauda epididymis: *A,* dissected cauda epididymis and ductus deferens; and *B,* direct flushing using Kenney's extender with 15% seminal plasma.

■ Semen processing for preservation and use for AI may need an initial phase of incubation with seminal plasma.

DIFFERENTIAL DIAGNOSIS

See Breeding Soundness Examination

DIAGNOSTICS

CBC/Biochemistry/Urinalysis

Dependent on the reason for semen collection.

Other Laboratory Tests

Microbiology may be required depending on the reason for semen collection.

Imaging

Videotaping and reviewing procedures used to collect semen may provide clues to the causes of a stallion's behavioral problems or difficulties resulting from stallion handling techniques.

 THERAPEUTICS

Drug(s) of Choice

- To enhance libido:
  - GnRH (50 μg) given SC 1 or 2 hours before collection.
  - Diazepam: 0.05 mg/kg by slow IV.
- To lower the ejaculatory threshold:
  - Imipramine HCl, 100 to 1000 mg orally 2 hours before collection
- To induce ejaculation ex-copula:
  - Imipramine HCl, 2.2 mg/kg orally 2 hours before xylazine
  - Xylazine: 0.66 mg/kg IV

 COMMENTS

Client Education

- Factors in semen collection that affect semen quality.
- Proper training and management of stallion.

Possible Complications

- Behavioral disorders
- Ejaculatory or erection disorders
- Musculoskeletal diseases
- Neurologic disorders

Abbreviations

AI	artificial insemination
AV	artificial vagina
CBC	complete blood count
CCP	corpus cavernosum penis
GnRH	gonadotropin releasing hormone
HCl	hydrochloride
IV	intravenous
SC	subcutaneous
Stallion's book	the number of mares contracted to be bred to a stallion in one breeding season

See Also

- Breeding soundness evaluation, stallion
- Behavior evaluation, stallion
- Ejaculatory disorders
- Sperm accumulation/stagnation

Suggested Reading

Foley BD, McDonnell SM. 1999. How to collect semen from stallions while they are standing on the ground. *Proc AAEP* 45: 142–145.

McDonnell SM. 2009. Stallion sexual behavior. In: *Equine Breeding Management and Artificial Insemination.* Samper JC (ed). Philadelphia: W. B. Saunders; 53–62.

Tibary A. 2006. Stallion reproductive behavior. In: *Current Therapy in Equine Reproduction.* Samper JC, Pycock JF, McKinnon AO (eds). St Louis: Saunders Elsevier; 174–184.

Author: Ahmed Tibary

chapter 99

Semen Evaluation, Routine

DEFINITION/OVERVIEW

- Refers to the most common examination techniques and tests performed on either freshly collected ejaculates or preserved semen (cooled shipped or frozen thawed) at the time of insemination.
- Should be performed by any veterinarian involved with equine theriogenology.
- It is important to observe the strict requirements of each test; use only high quality equipment and chemicals.
- The ejaculate or semen sample should be maintained in proper storage conditions during evaluation.
  - Errors in semen handling have deleterious effects on spermatozoa viability and test results.
  - Semen should be protected from temperature changes and toxic substances (e.g., water, chemicals) during all phases of the evaluation.
  - All equipment and supplies used must be maintained at 37°C.
- None of the routine sperm evaluation parameters taken individually are highly correlated with fertility.
- Minimum equipment and supplies for adequate semen evaluation (Table 99.1).

TABLE 99.1 Minimum Equipment and Supplies for Adequate Semen Evaluation.

- Artificial vagina with disposable liners and filter
- Nonspermicidal lubricant
- Heating plate
- Incubator or water bath
- Microscope with heating stage (preferably phase-contrast)
- Slides and cover slips
- Pasteur pipettes
- Precision pipettes for dilution
- Hemocytometer or calibrated sperm concentration determination
- pH paper or pH meter
- Eosin/Nigrosin stain
- Wright's stain or Diff Quick®
- Buffered formol saline
- Cooled semen extender
- Conical centrifuge tubes (50 mL)
- Commercial cooling containers
- Centrifuge

ETIOLOGY/PATHOPHYSIOLOGY

Multifactorial

- Factors affecting stallion semen parameters include:
  - Failure of normal physiological events (of the stallion).
  - Specific diseases (external impact).
  - Semen handling: techniques, conditions (i.e., iatrogenic).

Physiological Sources Causing Variation of Semen Parameters

- Age
- Season

Pathological Sources Resulting in Variation of Semen Parameters

- General health
- Testicular size and health
- Ejaculatory disorder (e.g., urospermia, hemospermia).
- Infection of the accessory sex glands

Systems Affected

Reproductive

SIGNALMENT/HISTORY

- Necessary for a stallion of any breed.
- An essential component of any BSE.
- Individual variation
- All stallions destined for breeding (live cover or AI).
- Stallion with visible abnormalities of the genital organs.
- Stallion with history of infertility or subfertility.
- Stallion recovering from a systemic illness.

CLINICAL FEATURES/DIAGNOSTIS

Physical and Chemical Characteristics

Volume (Fractions: Gel-free, Gel)

- Record the gel-free ejaculate volume (most equine AVs are equipped with a collection bottle or bag with a nylon or cotton mesh in-line filter).
- Precise determination of the volume can be obtained by using prewarmed (37°C) graduated cylinders. Specimen cups provide an estimated volume (much less accurate).

- Both the gel-free and gel portion of semen are measured. It is important to make sure that whole ejaculate is collected (confirm that all AV contents have been collected).
- Precise determination of ejaculate volume is necessary to determine the total sperm in an ejaculate.
- Physiological factors affecting ejaculate volume are:
  - Individual stallion variation
  - Breed
  - Age
  - Season
  - Rank of ejaculate (first, second, third in a day, or examination sequence within a set period of time).
- Pathological factors affecting ejaculate volume include:
  - Ejaculatory disorders
  - Urospermia
  - Hemospermia
- It is estimated that 10% to 15% of sperm cells are lost in the gel fraction.

General Appearance and Consistency

- The equine gel-free ejaculate is generally homogeneous and of a watery consistency.
- Turbidity increases with concentration (normal) or, with abnormal ejaculates (e.g., those with clumping, purulent material, or debris).
- Precipitates, or the presence of flocculent material, may be indicative of reproductive disorders (e.g., seminal vesiculitis, urethritis, or contamination).
- Viscosity is increased if the gel fraction has not been properly removed by filtration.
- Note the presence of debris is often due to smegma (i.e., poor preparation of the stallion, inadequate cleaning of the penis prior to collection).

Color

- The normal color of the equine ejaculate varies from grayish-white to white.
- Ejaculates contaminated with blood can range from light pink to a frank red (Figs. 99.1a and b).
- Old blood from the urethra may add a brownish or tan color to semen.
- With urospermia, the ejaculate may be amber or yellow (Fig. 99.2).
- With urospermia, the ejaculate will have a distinct urine odor.

pH

- Determine pH using pH meter or pH paper.
- Normal ejaculate should have a pH of 7.5 to 7.7
- pH increases suggest urine contamination or accessory sex gland infections.
- pH can decrease rapidly with metabolic activity in concentrated samples.

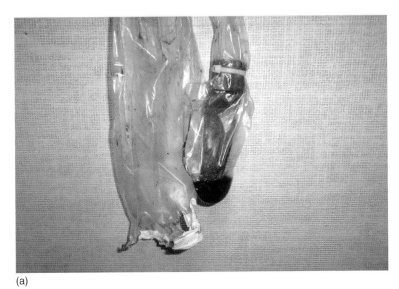

(a)

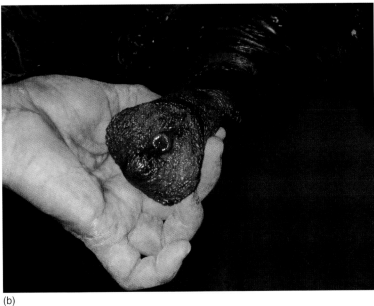

(b)

■ **Figure 99.1** Hemospermia: *A,* disposable liner showing bloody ejaculate; and *B,* blood dripping from the urethral orifice 5 minutes after semen collection.

Motility (Raw and Diluted)

- Evaluate both raw and extended semen samples, using a phase-contrast microscope with a heated stage.
- Semen should be maintained at body temperature. All slides, coverslips, pipets, and so on, in contact with the semen, should be prewarmed to prevent cold shock.
  - Motility of raw semen should be recorded immediately after collection because it can alter (diminish) quickly.

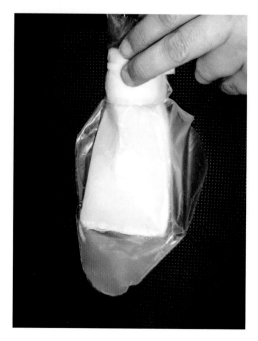

■ **Figure 99.2** Urospermia from a stallion with a neurological disorder.

- ■ Motility of at least 10 fields should be evaluated, at 200× and 400×
- ■ PM should be at least 60% in normal fresh ejaculates.
- ■ Both TM and PM should be estimated.
  - ■ Ideally, all fields examined should be recorded (videotape or digital file) as a permanent part of the medical record.
  - ■ TM is a record of the percentage of sperm cells showing *any type* of movement.
  - ■ PM is a record of the percentage of sperm cells with *forward* motility.
- ■ In most clinics, motility is estimated subjectively.
  - ■ CASA is becoming more common.
- ■ Sample preparation must be done carefully.
  - ■ *Raw semen motility*: a drop (10–20 μL) is placed on a prewarmed slide and covered with a coverslip, then observed at a power of 200× and 400×. A minimum of 5 to 10 fields should be examined to estimate motility.
  - ■ To estimate *motility of a diluted sample*: extend semen with a skim milk extender as is used to prepare fresh and cooled semen for breeding. The extension ratio should provide a final concentration of 25 to 50 million spermatozoa per mL.
- ■ General notations:
  - ■ Note the amount of sperm agglutination (clumping) present.
  - ■ Highly concentrated semen can give the illusion of increased motility.
  - ■ High rate of abnormal motility (backward or circular pattern) warrants evaluation of technique (cold shock) or abnormalities caused by the sperm's morphological defects in the ejaculate.

Live/Dead

- Differential stains for live and dead sperm cells are based on the ability of stains to diffuse through the plasma membrane of the dead spermatozoa.
  - Most common stain used is eosin/nigrosin, a supra-vital stain, to determine the percentage of live/dead, as well as for sperm morphology determination (Fig. 99.3).
  - Live sperm cells appear white; dead sperm cells appear varying shades of pink to red.
  - The relative percent of dead spermatozoa is determined after counting 100 sperm cells.
- The condition in which the sample is kept until staining and the physical and chemical proprieties of the stain may affect the percent of live/dead results.

Morphology

- Sperm morphology is the most important parameter in routine semen evaluation.
  - Can be determined on stained smears using various techniques. Most commonly used stain is eosin/nigrosin.
  - Morphology can also be determined under phase contrast of samples fixed in 10% PBS.
  - Sperm morphology assessment requires high power under oil (1000×).
- At least 100 sperm cells should be counted covering several fields. Counting 200 to 300 cells may be necessary to increase accuracy in some cases.
  - The frequency of normal cells and all types of abnormalities should be recorded (Fig. 99.4).

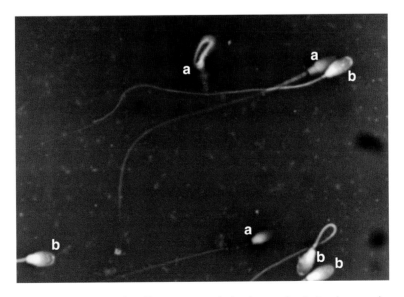

■ **Figure 99.3** Eosin/nigrosin stained stallion semen: eosin is taken up by *A,* Dead or membrane-damaged spermatozoa (i.e., pink to red color); and *B,* Live or membrane intact spermatozoa remain unstained.

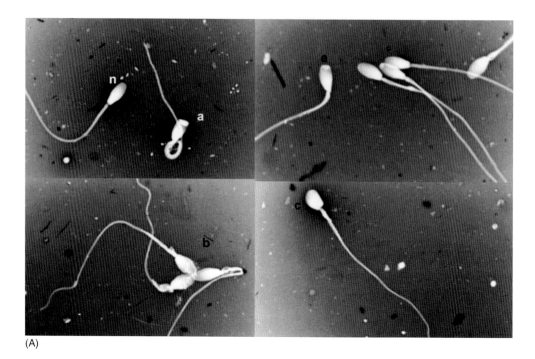

(A)

■ **Figure 99.4 A,** Selected abnormalities of the spermatozoa: (n) normal spermatozoa; (a) abnormal acrosome (knobbed); (b) head to head agglutination; (c) abnormal head shape. **B,** Mid-piece abnormalities: (a) normal spermatozoa; (b-c) thickened mid-piece; (d) mid-piece reflection; (e) coiled midpiece; (f) incomplete mid-piece; (g) distal droplet; and (h) proximal droplet. **C,** (a) distal mid-piece reflection; (b-d) coiled mid-piece and tail; and (e-f) bent tail.

- Abnormalities are generally grouped into major defects (related to infertility and thought to be due to abnormal spermatogenesis, of testicular origin) and minor defects (attributed to semen handling techniques, cold shock).
- Increased rate of abnormalities suggests testicular or epididymal disorders.
- If abnormalities exceed 40%, other (additional) examination techniques may be required.
- Stain quality (osmotic pressure, pH, purity) may affect results and needs to be checked regularly.

Concentration

- Sperm concentration is an important parameter for the determination of total sperm number in the ejaculate.
  - Used to detect sperm production or ejaculatory disorders.
  - Allows calculation of insemination doses.
- Concentration of the ejaculate can be determined manually with a hemocytometer or electronically using a Densimeter (modified spectrophotometer).
  - Sperm concentration using a hemocytometer on a diluted semen sample (1:100) is precise but tedious.

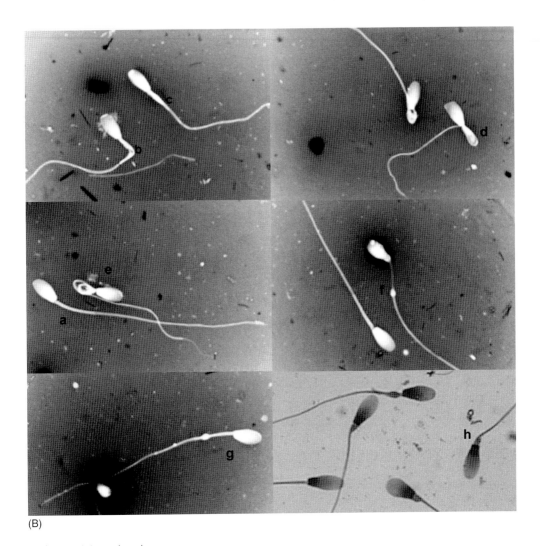

(B)

■ Figure 99.4 continued

- ■ Precise specimen preparation and dilution is important for accurate determination of concentration.
- ■ Numerous spectrophotometers or Densimeters for equine sperm concentration are available (Fig. 99.5). Errors in reading concentration occur if:
  - ■ The ejaculate deviates too much from the norm (too dilute or too concentrated), falling outside the reading sensitivity of the equipment.
  - ■ There is abnormal sample density, due to contamination by urine, blood, or smegma.
- ■ Record the number of spermatozoa per mL and the total number of sperm cells in the ejaculate (volume × concentration).
- ■ Total sperm number in the ejaculate can be affected by season, age, testicular size, and rank of ejaculation.

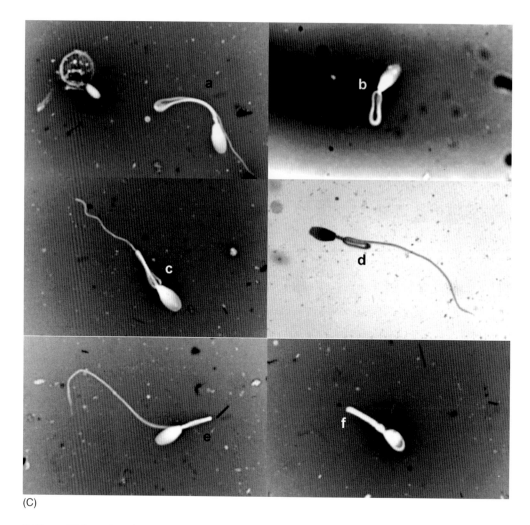

(C)

■ **Figure 99.4** continued

■ Reduced sperm number in the ejaculate can be due to testicular, epididymal, or ejaculatory disorders.

Longevity

■ This test estimates how long sperm can survive in the mare's reproductive tract and withstand the effect of cooling.
■ The test can be run on aliquots of extended semen incubated at room temperature (22°C) and at 5°C (chilled).
■ PM is estimated at 6, 12, 24, and 48 hours.

CBC/Biochemistry/Urinalysis

■ Records of baseline data should be determined for all stallions.
■ Indication for tests are based on physical findings and semen evaluation.

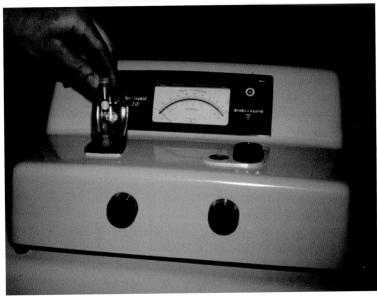

(a)

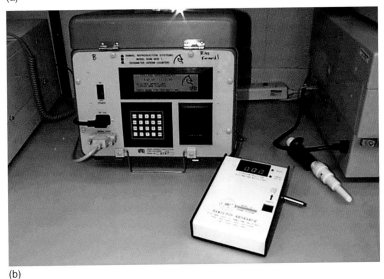

(b)

■ **Figure 99.5** Spectrophotometer used to determine equine semen concentration. *A*, Spectronic 20 by Bausch & Lomb; *B*, Densimeter by Animal Reproduction Systems; *C*, Accucell equine photometer by IMV; and *D*, SpermaCue by Minitube.

Other Laboratory Tests

Cytological Evaluation

- Stained smears using Giemsa, Wright's, Spermac, Diff-Quick®: to determine presence of WBCs and somatic cells such as germinal cells (spheroid) (Fig. 99.6).
- These stains also can help identify bacteria within semen.

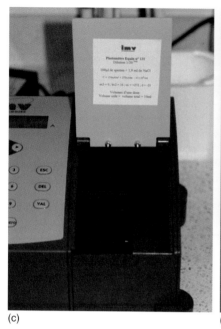

(c)

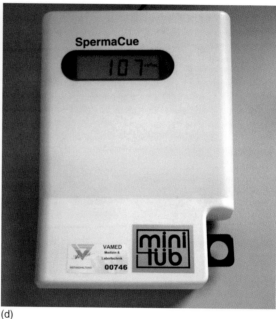

(d)

■ **Figure 99.5** continued

- Presence of round germinal cells suggests testicular degeneration (Fig. 99.7).

Bacteriological Evaluation

- Pre- and post-ejaculate urethral swabs are collected routinely during a stallion reproductive evaluation.
- Samples from semen should be also be submitted for bacteriological evaluation.

Other Biochemical Tests

- Semen samples should be saved and submitted for determination of creatinine or urea content, if urospermia is suspected.
- Seminal fluid from azoospermic ejaculates should be submitted for alkaline phosphatase:
  - To confirm or rule out an epididymal blockage.
  - Normal alkaline phosphatase level in a stallion ejaculate should be greater than 1000 IU/L.
  - Alkaline phosphatase level less than 100 IU/L suggests bilateral blockage.
  - Alkaline phosphatase levels between 100 and 1000 IU/L are difficult to interpret and the test should be repeated.

Pathologic Findings

See infertility and specific reproductive disorders by organ system.

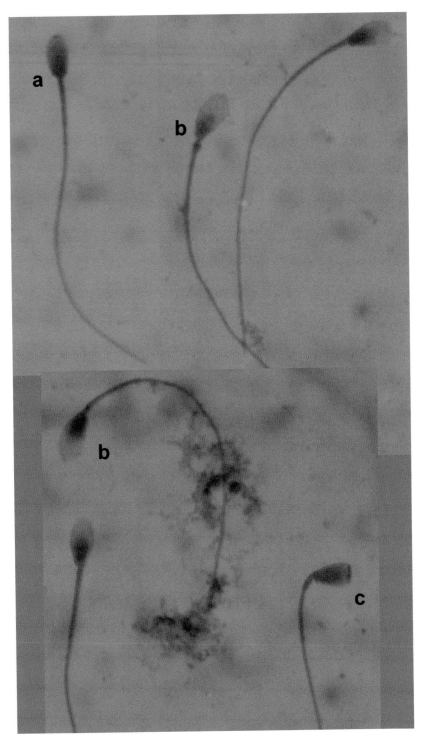

■ **Figure 99.6** Stallion semen smear stained with Spermac stain®. (a) normal head; (b) detached acrosome; and (c) knobbed acrosome.

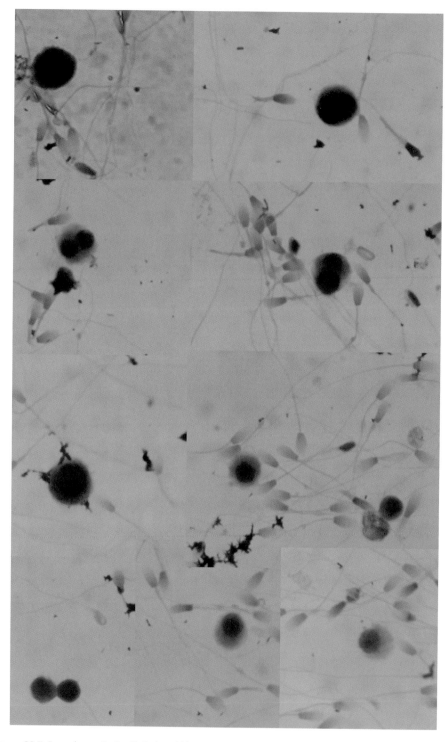

■ Figure 99.7 Round germinal cells (spheroids). Smears stained with DiffQuick®.

COMMENTS

Client Education

- Emphasize the importance of semen evaluation for stallions and of semen used for AI.
- Most breeders rely primarily (and often, solely) on motility, to make their breeding calculations. Reinforce to them that motility is a subjective test.
- Emphasize that these tests are not measures of fertility.

Abbreviations

AI   artificial insemination
AV   artificial vagina
BSE   breeding soundness examination
CASA   computer assisted semen analysis
CBC   complete blood count
PBS   phosphate buffered saline
PM   progressive motility (of spermatozoa)
TM   total motility (of spermatozoa)
WBC   white blood cells

See Also

- Breeding soundness examination, Stallion

Suggested Reading

Blanchard TL, Varner DD, Schumacher J, et al. 2003. Examination of the stallion for breeding soundness. In: *Manual of Equine Reproduction*, 2nd ed. Blanchard TL, Varner DD, Scumacher J, et al. (eds). Ithaca: IVIS; 143–164.

Kenney RM, Hurtgen J, Pierson R, et al. 1983. *Soc for Therio, Manual for Clinical Fertility Evaluation of the Stallion*, 1–100.

Author: Ahmed Tibary

chapter 100

Semen Cryopreservation, Managing the Freezing Ability of Stallion Semen

DEFINITION/OVERVIEW

- Post-thaw quality of cryopreserved stallion semen is highly variable.
- It is estimated that only 20% to 35% of all stallions will produce semen of consistently good freezing ability and post-thaw motility.
- Thirty percent to 60% of stallions have satisfactory freezability of semen (post-thaw motility that is greater than 30%).
- Twenty percent to 35% of stallions are described as "poor freezers."
- There are several reasons for the large variability of success in cryopreserving stallion semen.

ETIOLOGY/PATHOPHYSIOLOGY

- To manage the stallion with poor tolerance of semen cryopreservation, it is important to know the factors that may affect success.
- Cryopreservation damage to the spermatozoa involves several factors that may linked to the individual stallion (i.e., membrane stability, seminal plasma), interaction with extenders or behavior of the extender at low temperature.

Sources of Variation of Semen Cryopreservation Ability

- There are inherent differences among stallions in the ability of their semen to withstand the cooling/freezing/thawing cycle.
- These differences may be of genetic origin (i.e., cell membrane structure and function).
- Within the same stallion, semen freezability may change according to season, age, nutrition, and other unknown factors.
- Initial semen quality is an important factor in post-thaw quality and should be the first priority in managing a stallion with poor freezability.

Effect of Cryopreservation and Mechanisms of Cryo-Damage

- Spermatozoa are subjected to the effect of low temperature during the freezing and thawing process.

- During cryopreservation the spermatozoa undergoes several changes at the cell membrane and the intracellular level that affect both its metabolism and function.
- Prefreeze cooling and post-thaw warming cause rearrangement of the lipid and protein within the cell membrane; changing it from a liquid crystalline state to a gel state.
- In the absence of cryoprotection, cell death occurs primarily by damage to the cell membrane caused by ice formation or by the impact of the dramatically increased salt concentration on essential metabolic functions as free water *freezes out*. Note: this occurs not only during dehydration of cells but also as water molecules freeze leaving a higher and higher solute concentration.
- Semen freezing extenders are formulated to improve cell membrane stability and to reduce cryodamage by preventing intracellular water crystal formation and by changing the size and shape of ice crystals.
- Intracellular solute concentration effects are usually managed by adjusting the cooling and freezing rate.
- The best freezing rates should be slow enough to allow sufficient dehydration of the cell to avoid intracellular ice crystal formation, yet fast enough to avoid too long exposure to solute concentration.
- The effect of cryopreservation is different depending on membrane stability, type of cryoprotectant, and the freezing curve used.
- The effects observed during cryopreservation are also observed during the process of thawing and warming.
- Post-thaw changes in the cell membrane, as well as exposure to the hypotonic uterine environment, often cause spermatozoa to undergo capacitation-like changes that are detrimental to their survival.
- Factors involved in cryo-capacitation include the structure of the cell membrane, the type (penetrating versus non-penetrating), molecular weight, and concentration of the cryoprotectant.
- Individual differences in stallion semen cryopreservation may be explained by differences in cell membrane structure (amount of cholesterol), which determines their osmotic tolerance.
- This variety of mechanisms resulting in cryo-injury suggests that semen from different stallions may behave differently depending on the freezing and thawing methods tested.
- Therefore, adjustments of a freezing technique need to be made with attention given to the extender used (particularly the cryoprotectant selected), the cooling rate, equilibration time, and freezing and thawing rates.
- Post-thaw adjustments may have to be made to accommodate cryoprotectant removal, and timing of insemination with ovulation.

Systems Affected

- Reproductive
- Cellular level effects

Genetics

- Possible differences in seminal plasma biochemistry and cell membrane structure.
- Possible genetically determined ability of spermatozoa to withstand freezing/thawing.

Incidence/Prevalence

- Semen from about one third of all stallions will not withstand freezing.

Other Laboratory Tests

- Advanced techniques of sperm membrane evaluation
- Ejaculate motility

 THERAPEUTICS

Improving the Initial Semen Quality

- In nonsexually rested stallions post-thaw quality is best when semen is cryopreserved during the nonbreeding season (likelihood of their being more available and under less stress from the needs of their large book).
- In sexually rested stallions, extra-gonadal sperm reserves should be depleted by repeated collection before freezing (discard the first ejaculates, particularly in stallions that have a tendency for higher spermatozoal storage in their ampullae/epididymides).
- Appropriate semen collection frequency should be determined for a specific stallion. The intent is to collect semen of adequate concentration and as small a volume as possible.
- The main factors affecting initial semen quality, apart from the ability of the stallion, include the conditions surrounding semen collection (personnel, technique, protection of the ejaculate, cleanliness of the ejaculate, assessment of microbiological quality).
- In some stallions, semen quality may be improved by collection of a fractionated ejaculate or by collection directly into a suitable extender.

Dietary Supplementation

- Several dietary antioxidant supplements, such as ascorbic acid, tocopherol, selenium, L-carnitine, and folic acid have been tested with mixed results.
- Commercially available Nutriceutical products containing polyunsaturated fatty acid (ProSperm®) were shown to improve the quality of cooled semen.

Centrifugation

- Essential for removal of 80% to 95% of the seminal plasma before freezing.
- Essential for concentration of sperm from large volume ejaculates.

- Antioxidant properties of seminal plasma when added to extender may vary from one stallion to another.
- Improved semen quality may be obtained through the use of special centrifugation or filtration techniques in some stallions.
- The use of cushion techniques may allow greater centrifugation forces (g-force) to be used (1000 g for 20 minutes) to improve recovery of spermatozoa.

Extender Modifications (Proteins)

- Commercially available extenders vary primarily with regard to the type and concentration of cryoprotectants, egg yolk, and milk proteins.
- Newer, chemically defined media are being developed without the inclusion of complex biological substances such as milk or egg yolk.
- The species source of egg yolk (hen versus duck versus quail) has been shown to affect semen viability.
- The response attributable to egg yolk's inclusion may be due to the presence of progesterone and calcium, which are implicated in capacitation-like changes.
- Essential for concentration of sperm from ejaculates with very high volume.

Antioxidants and Cholesterol

- The lipid composition of sperm membranes influences the response of sperm to cooling and freezing.
- Antioxidant properties of seminal plasma and sperm cell membrane structure vary from one stallion to another.
- Addition of pyruvate to the extender has been shown to improve motility of frozen-thawed stallion sperm.
- Addition of cholesterol-loaded cyclodextrin to the extender seems to increase the cholesterol content of the sperm, thus improving membrane stability and preventing lipid loss and lipid/protein rearrangement within the sperm membrane during cooling.
- Increasing the cholesterol content may also improve osmotic tolerance and increase the permeability of the cryoprotectant.

Cryoprotectants

- Cryoprotectants are toxic to sperm under some conditions.
- Cryoprotectants induce cell volume changes that can harm the sperm. The choice of cryoprotectant used is critical for some stallions.
- Nonpenetrating cryoprotectants act purely as a solute, whereas penetrating cryoprotectants also act as a solvent.
- Glycerol is the most common cryoprotectant used in commercial extenders.
- The addition L-glutamine or proline (30–80 mM) allows the concentration of glycerol needed in the extender to be decreased or reduced.
- Dimethyl sulfoxide, ethylene glycol, methyl formamide, or dimethyl formamide have been shown to be superior to glycerol for some stallions.

- The temperature at which the cryoprotectant is used may affect post-thaw motility in some stallions.
- In most presently used techniques, semen is extended in the freezing extender at room temperature after centrifugation.

Cooling Rate

- Freezing techniques vary according to whether a cooling and equilibration phase at 5°C is necessary.
- Cooling of stallion spermatozoa from room temperature to 5°C is a critical step and may result in damage to the sperm's plasma membrane.
- Cooling rate may vary depending on the extender used and the stallion. It should be slow (between 0.05°C and 0.3°C/minute).
- Storage at 5°C may result in DNA fragmentation, so the length of the equilibration time is important.

Freezing Rate

- Optimal freezing rate ranges from 20°C to 100°C per minute.
- Freezing rate is primarily determined by the packaging type and volume.
- More advanced techniques, such as those incorporated into programmable freezers or directional freezing, may be necessary to precisely control the freezing process.
- These techniques control the initial crystal formation (seeding). Ice crystal propagation is controlled to optimize crystal morphology and homogenous cooling rate during the freezing process.

Thawing Rate and Cryoprotectant Removal

- Thawing rates are optimized for each packaging and freezing technique and should be observed carefully.
- Removal of the cryoprotectant after thawing may reduce cryo-capacitation and decrease cell injury when the sperm are placed in a hypotonic medium, but it is difficult to achieve reliably in practice.

Client Education

- Not all semen can successfully be frozen.
- A test freeze should employ a variety of techniques to find the best one for a stallion, but that can add significantly to expenses incurred.
- Freezing of stallion semen is best when accomplished during the stallion's years of peak reproductive capacity and not as a last resort or as an emergency procedure on illness or death of the stud.

See Also

- Artificial insemination, frozen semen
- Semen evaluation

- Semen cryopreservation
- Semen extenders

Suggested Reading

Clulow JR, Mansfield LJ, Morris LHA, et al. 2008. A comparison between freezing methods for the cryopreservation of stallion spermatozoa. *Anim Reprod Sci* 108: 298–308.

Loomis PR, Graham JK. 2008. Commercial semen freezing: Individual male variation in cryosurvival and the response of stallion sperm to customized freezing protocols. *Anim Reprod Sci* 105: 119–128.

Moore AI, Squires EL, Graham JK. 2005. Adding cholesterol to the stallion sperm plasma membrane improves cryosurvival. *Cryobiology* 51: 241–249.

Sieme H, Harrison RAP, Petrunkina AM. 2008. Cryobiological determinants of frozen semen quality with special reference to stallion. *Anim Reprod Sci* 107: 276–292.

Vidament M. 2005. French field results (1985–2005) on factors affecting fertility of frozen stallion semen. *Anim Reprod Sci* 89: 115–136.

Authors: Ahmed Tibary and Jacobo Rodriguez

Semen Evaluation, Abnormalities

chapter 101

DEFINITION/OVERVIEW

- Semen evaluation is an important part of the stallion BSE.
- Sperm production and quality are affected by internal and external factors.
- Abnormalities are not limited to morphology alone, and include alterations of volume, color, concentration, and motility.
- Abnormalities of semen quality may reflect events at various times or stages (e.g., spermatogenesis, sperm epididymal maturation, sperm storage in the epididymal tail or in the ampullae of the ductus deferens, at the time of ejaculation, or immediately after ejaculation).
- Abnormalities of the ejaculate may reflect specific reproductive tract diseases or a consequence of systemic disease processes.
- Sperm morphology varies widely among breeding stallions, but in general, fertile stallions have at least 50% morphologically normal spermatozoa.
- One means to determine a stallion's DSO is to collect two ejaculates 1 hour apart and then continue to collect a single ejaculate daily for 6 to 7 days.

ETIOLOGY/PATHOPHYSIOLOGY

Terms and Definitions of Abnormalities of Semen Quality

- Aspermia: absence of ejaculation
- Oligospermia: reduced semen volume
- Azoospermia: absence of spermatozoa in the ejaculate.
- Oligozoospermia: reduced sperm concentration and total sperm number.
- Asthenozoospermia: reduced spermatozoal motility in an ejaculate.
- Teratozoospermia: increased sperm abnormalities or presence of abnormal cellular components (round spermatid, medusa cells).
- Hemospermia: contamination of semen with blood.
- Pyospermia: contamination of semen with inflammatory cells or pus.
- Urospermia: contamination of semen with urine.

Physiological Factors Affecting Semen

- Age
  - Stallion fertility starts to decline on average by 15 years of age.

- Young stallions have lower sperm production and sperm quality. Semen quality and maximum sperm production are achieved around 4 years of age.
- Older stallions may have reduced sperm quality and sperm production.
- Seasonal changes are usually reflected by decreasing sperm motility, percentage of normal sperm morphology, and total sperm production.
- Individual variation exists among stallions with regard to total volume, gel volume, and the percentage of morphologically normal spermatozoa.
- The impact of season on semen quality varies significantly between individual stallions.
- Semen quality may be affected by the length of sexual inactivity. Normal fertile stallions have at least 50% morphologically normal sperm.

Environmental/External Factors Affecting Semen

- The main nongenital factors affecting semen quality in the stallion operate through reduction of normal spermatogenesis or alteration of sperm maturation and storage.
- Spermatogenesis and quality of extragonadal sperm reserves are affected by alterations in thermoregulation (e.g., excessive ambient temperature or fever, and rarely, frostbite [hypothermia]).
- Nutrition (primarily extreme loss of body condition or obesity) can affect semen production and quality.
- Iatrogenic/Management influences on semen quality may include inappropriate semen handling techniques, including but not limited to, those occurring during collection, evaluation, extension, exposure to excessive heat or cold, lubricant selection, exposure to disinfectants, sample contamination, and so on.

Behavioral Problems Affecting Semen

- Behavior-associated ejaculatory disorders may affect semen quality. Either incomplete or premature ejaculation may result in low semen volume and concentration.

Reproductive Pathologies Affecting Semen

- Diseases of the reproductive tract can affect semen quality in several ways.
- Trauma to the genital organs or inflammatory processes may affect semen concentration, motility, and morphology.
- Testicular degeneration, occluded ampullae, scrotal trauma, epididymitis, or orchitis may decrease the total number of spermatozoa in the ejaculate, its motility, and the percentage of morphologically normal spermatozoa.
  - The end result of infection or inflammation of the stallion's reproductive tract (primarily seminal vesiculitis) may be pyospermia.
  - External lesions of the penis, urethritis, seminal vesiculitis, or urethral rents may first become evident as hemospermia. Contamination of semen with blood causes a severe reduction in semen motility and viability.
- Neurologic disorders may be associated with urospermia because control of micturition can be compromised by neurologic deficits.

Systems Affected

Reproductive

SIGNALMENT/HISTORY/DIAGNOSTICS

Abnormalities of Color *(Macroscopic Evaluation)*

- A watery (pear juice color) diluted sample is indicative of oligozoospermia or azoospermia and is associated with ejaculatory disorders or severe testicular disease.
- A pinkish or red color is indicative of hemospermia and is associated with penile lesions (*Habronema*, squamous cell carcinoma), urethritis, urethral rents, or seminal vesiculitis (Figs. 101.1 and 101.2).
- A brownish color is indicative of old blood or contamination from the penis (inadequate cleaning of the penis prior to collection).
- A yellow color is indicative of urospermia and may be associated with problems of urinary bladder sphincter closure or secondary to neurologic disorders, viral infections (EHV-1), sorghum toxicity, or urolithiasis.
- A flocculent appearance to the ejaculate is indicative of pyospermia, often associated with infections of the accessory sex glands or a concentrated sample that may be associated with plugged ampullae.
- Semen normally is "odor neutral." If the sample has a urine-like smell, the impact or influence of urine can be diminished (diluted) by centrifugation. If the sample has a putrid odor, it should be discarded.

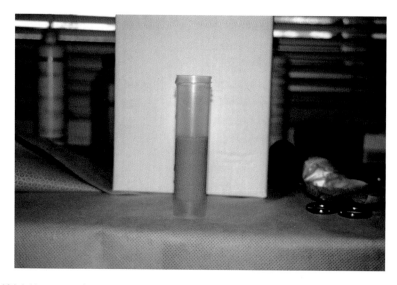

■ **Figure 101.1** Hemospermia, gross appearance.

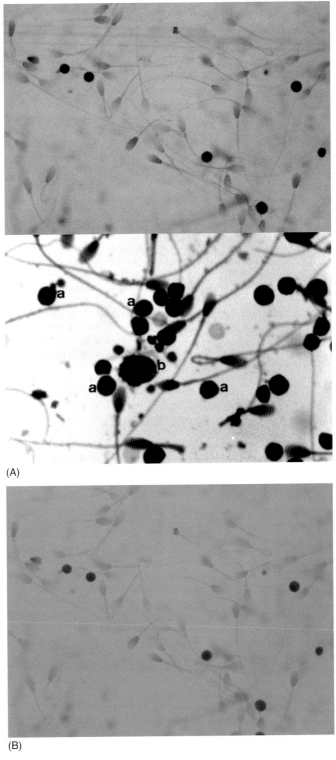

(A)

(B)

■ **Figure 101.2** *A,* Microscopic hemospermia (a) red blood cell and (b) white blood cell. *B,* Specimen, alternate staining.

Abnormalities of Volume (Total Semen Volume; Gel-Free Volume; Gel Volume)

- Excessive volume is often seen in stallions with high gel production (particularly with lengthy teasing) and in cases of urospermia.
- High ejaculate volume is affected by the time of the year (seasonal effect). Up to 50% of the ejaculate volume difference between the height of the breeding season and nonbreeding season is due to the volume of gel production.
- Draft horses and large breeds of donkeys ejaculate a larger volume.
- Ejaculate volume increases from 2 to 15 years of age and may also be affected by feed.
- Oligospermia with normal total sperm in the ejaculate is due to inadequate preparation of the stallion prior to collection or to the technique of semen collection (ex-copula ejaculation).
- Oligospermia combined with poor concentration and motility or the presence of WBCs could be associated with epididymitis, orchitis or testicular degeneration.
- Absence of ejaculation (aspermia or anejaculation) is primarily due to retrograde ejaculation or painful conditions during mounting.

Abnormalities of Motility *(Microscopic Evaluation)*

- Spermatozoal motility is positively correlated to the percent of morphologically normal spermatozoa.
- Decreased progressive motility is associated with an increase in some tail and mid-piece abnormalities.
- TM and PM are decreased by semen collection conditions and specific pathological process.
- Motility is severely reduced in cases of urospermia, pyospermia, hemospermia, plugged ampullae syndrome, and long periods of sexual rest in some stallions.
- Motility is severely reduced or completely absent (asthenospermia) if the ejaculate is contaminated with water, disinfectant or detergents.
- Asthenozoospermia may be observed as a syndrome in rare cases of "immotile cilia syndrome."
- Asthenozoospermia and sperm agglutination may be the result of the presence of anti-sperm antibodies.

Abnormalities of Concentration and Total Ejaculated Sperm (Sperm Concentration/mL; Total Number of Spermatozoa in the Ejaculate)

- Oligozoospermia is associated with testicular degeneration.
- Oligozoospermia and teratozoospermia may be the result of excessive use of anabolic steroids or progestogen treatment administered to modulate stallion behavior.
- Azoospermia is associated with severe bilateral testicular degeneration and atrophy, bilateral epididymal segmental aplasia, and severe bilateral spermastasis in the ampullae.
- Incomplete ejaculation (oligospermia).

- Very high concentration and an elevation of the total sperm number are features of spermastasis (plugged ampullae, aka sperm stagnation).
- Increased total sperm number in the second ejaculate taken 1 hour after the first is indicative of an ejaculatory disorder or poor semen collection technique (e.g., incomplete first ejaculation).

Abnormalities of Morphology

- A minimum of 100 spermatozoa (10 cells in 10 different fields) should be evaluated for evidence of morphological defects (*see* Fig. 99.3).
- Teratozoospermia is defined as:
  - More than 40% morphologically abnormal spermatozoa resulting in less than 1 billion normal spermatozoa per ejaculate.
  - More than 30% heads defects, greater than 25% proximal cytoplasmic droplets, or less than 40% normal sperm are problematic and reason for concern.
- Clinical observations show that a high incidence of a single abnormality may not be as critical to fertility as the presence of multiple abnormalities.
- Abnormalities in spermatozoal morphology have been classified as primary, secondary, or tertiary.
  - Primary abnormalities are considered to be associated with a defect in spermatogenesis.
  - Secondary abnormalities are created in the excurrent duct system.
  - Tertiary abnormalities develop in vitro as a result of improper semen collection and manipulation of semen.
- Abnormalities should reported in detail as follows:
  - Normal sperm
  - Abnormal acrosomal regions/heads (*see* Fig. 99.4a)
    - Detached
    - Rough
    - Knobbed
  - Heads defects
    - microcephalic (small, underdeveloped)
    - macrocephalic (large, giant)
    - pyriform
    - nuclear vacuoles (pouches or craters)
    - multiples heads
  - Proximal droplets
  - Distal droplets (Fig. 101.3)
  - Abnormal midpieces (*see* Fig. 99.4b)
    - Midpiece reflection (simple bent)
    - Segmental aplasia of the mitochondrial sheath
    - Fractured
    - Swollen (thick, pseudodroplet)
    - Roughed

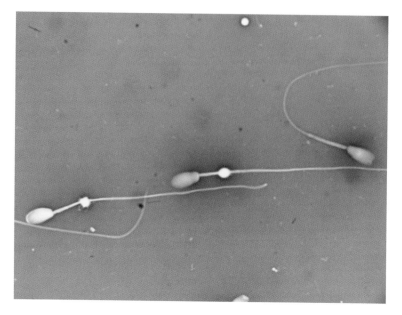

■ **Figure 101.3** Distal droplets.

  - ■ Swollen/roughed/broken
  - ■ Disrupted mitochondrial sheath
  - ■ Duplicate
  - ■ Stump tail
  - ■ Bent/coiled tails
- ■ Other cells (round germ cells, RBC, WBC, etc.).
- ■ Bent or coiled tails refer to those sperm in which the midpiece and the principal piece are bent or coiled, or the distal part of the principal piece is coiled (*see* Fig. 99.4c).
- ■ Some morphologic defects (cytoplasmic droplets, bent tails) seem to have a minor effect on fertility (*see* Fig. 101.3), whereas other defects (e.g., detached heads, abnormally shaped heads, an abnormally shaped midpiece, coiled tails, premature germ cells) have a greater impact on fertility.
- ■ Acrosomal abnormalities occurred more frequently in tandem with other sperm abnormalities, suggesting impaired spermatogenesis.
- ■ EM technique has increased the identification of some specific abnormalities of the sperm cell.
- ■ The SCSA has also been used to diagnose alterations in sperm chromatin stability due to disrupted spermatogenesis.
- ■ Sperm cytoplasmatic droplets are often the most prevalent defect in the ejaculate in young peripubertal stallions.
- ■ Knobbed acrosomes can be caused by environmental factors (e.g., increased testicular temperature, stress, toxins), but also could be of genetic origin (Fig. 101.4).
- ■ Increased abnormalities of spermatozoa are observed when thermoregulation of the testes is compromised (increased scrotal fat, scrotal edema, scrotal dermatitis,

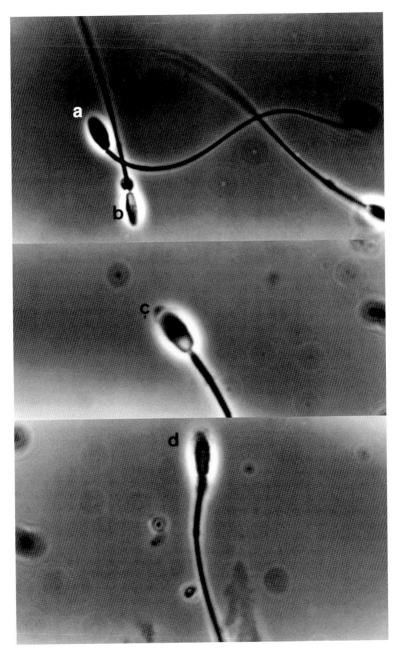

■ **Figure 101.4** Knobbed acrosome. (a) normal acrosome; (b) detached acrosome; (c) knobbed acrosome; and (d) swollen acrosome.

hydrocoele, hematocoele, pyocoele, trauma, orchitis, neoplasia, periorchitis and epididymitis, high ambient temperature, intense exercise, fever).
- Increased abnormalities of spermatozoa may be observed with prolonged stress and with the administration of exogenous hormones, such as progesterone or anabolic steroids.
- Increased free heads and midpiece defects are a characteristic of the first ejaculate after long periods of sexual rest and the sperm occluded ampullae syndrome (aka sperm stagnation).

Presence of Foreign Cells

- Stain with Giemsa or Diff Quick® (Fisher Scientific Co., LLC, Middletown, VA) to determine the presence of red cells, inflammatory cells, germinal cells (spheroids), and bacteria in semen (*see* Fig. 99.6).
- Round germ cells (Spheroids) are observed in peripubertal stallions and in early stages of testicular degeneration (Fig. 101.5).
- Spheroids and medusa cells are indicative of testicular degeneration.
- Presence of Sertoli cell containing degenerating germ cells is reported in stallions with irreversible testicular degeneration.
- More than six neutrophils per LPF are indicative of infection.

Abnormalities of pH

- Optimal pH 7.2 to 7.7.
- Low pH: associated with urospermia or pyospermia (Fig. 101.6).
- Abnormalities of pH are correlated with low motility and poor longevity.
- Spermatozoa are immobilized (no motility) by acidic conditions. Motility may be regained when the pH is corrected, but if spermatozoa were exposed to or placed in alkaline conditions, the immotility is irreversible.
- A high pH is correlated with low spermatozoa concentrations.

Centrifugation

- Centrifugation techniques are used to reconcentrate a high volume ejaculate or to select for highly motile or normal sperm.
- Centrifugation technique: in 40 to 60 mL conical tubes using specific cushion media.
- Semen is mixed with the centrifugation medium at a ratio of 1 to 1.
- Four hundred to 800 g-force for 10 to 20 minutes.
- Should be adapted for each stallion to ensure the best sperm recovery with the least damage caused by the centrifugation.

CBC/Biochemistry/Urinalysis

- See specific conditions.
- Creatinine levels greater than 2.0 mg/dL or a BUN level greater than 30 mg/dL is suggestive of urospermia.

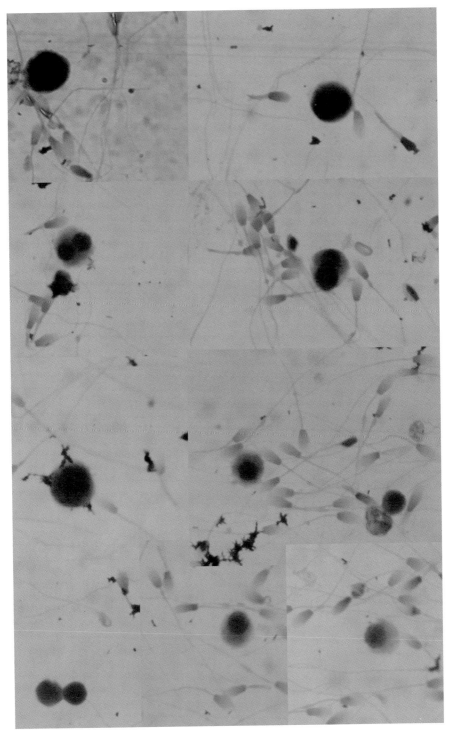

■ **Figure 101.5** Ejaculate from a stallion with testicular degeneration showing round spermatid (spheroids).

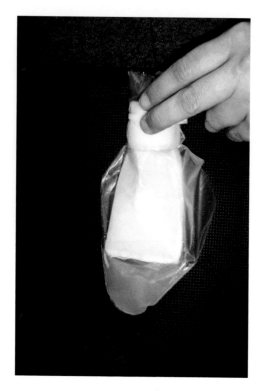

■ **Figure 101.6** Urospermia.

- The normal range of alkaline phosphatase in a stallion's seminal plasma is 1,640 to 48,700 IU/L.
- Alkaline phosphatase activity in the seminal plasma from a stallion with azoospermia is below 90 IU/L; a result of bilateral ampullar obstruction or epididymal blockage (Figs. 101.7 and 101.8).

Other Laboratory Tests

- Bacteriology
- See specific conditions

Imaging

- U/S of scrotal content and accessory sex glands
- See specific conditions

Other Diagnostic Procedures

- Urethroscopy
- Testicular biopsy

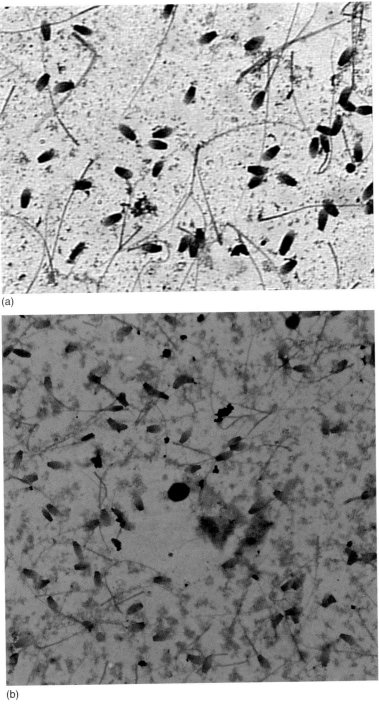

(a)

(b)

■ **Figure 101.7** *A-C,* High concentration of free heads from an ejaculate of a stallion with plugged ampullae syndrome.

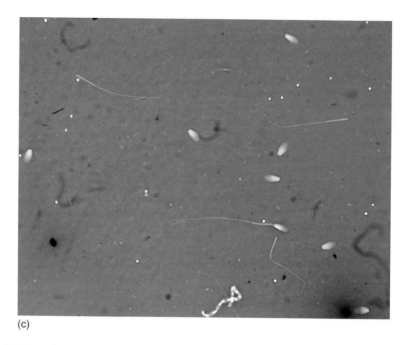

(c)

■ **Figure 101.7** continued

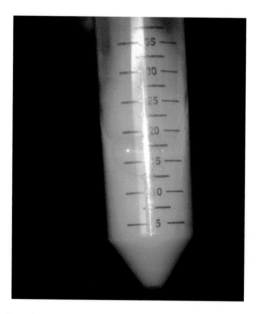

■ **Figure 101.8** Ejaculate of very high concentration (1.6 billion spermatozoa/mL) from a stallion with plugged ampullae.

COMMENTS

Age-Related Factors

- Puberty
- Senile changes

See Also

- BSE, stallion
- Semen collection, routine semen evaluation
- Semen collection, techniques
- Seminal vesiculitis
- Sperm accumulation/stagnation
- Behavior, ejaculatory disorders

Abbreviations

BSE breeding soundness examination
BUN blood urea nitrogen
CBC complete blood count
DSO daily sperm output
EHV equine herpesvirus
EM ejaculate motility
LPF low power field
PM progressive motility (of spermatozoa)
rcf radial centrifugation force
RBC red blood cell
SCSA sperm chromatin structure assay
TM total motility (of spermatozoa)
U/S ultrasound
WBC white blood cell

Suggested Reading

Brito LFC. 2007. Evaluation of stallion sperm morphology. *Clinical Techniques in Equine Practice* (6): 249–264.

Estrada AJ, Samper JC. 2006. Evaluation of raw semen. In: *Current Therapy in Equine Reproduction.* Samper JC, Pycock JF, Mc Kinnon AO (eds). St Louis: Saunders Elsevier; 253–257.

Tibary A, Rodriuez J, Samper JC. 2008. Microbiology and diseases of semen. In: *Equine Breeding Management and Artificial Insemination*, 2nd ed. Samper JC (ed). St Louis: Saunders Elsevier; 99–112.

Authors: Jacobo Rodriguez and Ahmed Tibary

chapter 102

Semen Extenders

DEFINITION/OVERVIEW

- Extenders are specially formulated solutions that prolong the viability of spermatozoa by:
  - Providing protection against temperature, pH, and osmotic changes.
  - Reducing contamination by the incorporation of antibiotics.
- Sugar molecules are often added to:
  - Balance the osmotic pressure.
  - Provide a substrate for spermatozoa metabolism.
- Semen extenders are generally grouped in two large categories:
  - Extenders for short-term preservation (shipped cooled semen).
  - Extenders for semen freezing.

ETIOLOGY/PATHOPHYSIOLOGY

Effect of Cooling on Semen

- Semen is usually shipped cooled at between 5°C and 8°C, however, some extenders have been formulated to allow shipment of semen at ambient temperature (INRA).
- Cooling causes various physical and chemical changes at the membrane level that may be deleterious to survival of the sperm cell and its function.
- Cooling induces a transition of sperm membrane from a liquid crystalline state to a gel state.
- Cold shock causes a loss of progressive motility (increase in circular or backward motion) and loss of fertilizing ability.
- Rapid cooling causes acrosomal damage and membrane changes with loss of intracellular components.
- Benefits of cooling:
  - Reduces metabolic activity of sperm cells.
  - Prevents peroxidation of membrane lipids.
  - Prevents changes in the pH.
- Extender components that prevent harmful effects on sperm caused by low temperature (cold shock):
  - Lipoprotein
  - Lipids
  - Lipophilic molecules
  - Sugars

TABLE 102.1 Composition of Extender for Fresh or Cooled Semen.

Tris egg yolk extender

Tris (g)	2.4	0.35	2.4
Glucose (g)	1.163	3.655	0.45
Citric acid (g)	1.326	0.151	1.25
Egg yolk (mL)	22.8	22.8	22.8
Glycerol	5.41	5.41	5.25
Distilled water (mL)	100	100	67.8
Sodium penicillin (UI)	50000	50000	6.99
Streptomycin (mg)	50	50	6.99
pH	7.0	7.0	298
Osmotic pressure (mOsm/kg)	340 to 360	340 to 360	

Gel-Cream extender

"Half and Half" cream* (mL)	88.7
Knox Gelatin** (g)	1.3
Deionized water (mL)	10.0
Antibiotic***	variable
pH	6.65
Osmotic pressure (mOsm/kg)	347

*Content: fat (11%), casein (2.8%), albumin (0.9%). Needs to be heated to 92°C–95°C for 4 minutes.

**Knox Gelatin®, Inc. Johnstown, New York. Dissolved in 10 mL of water then mixed with the cream.

***Added after cooling the cream-gelatin mix: Polymyxin B (1000 UI/mL) or Penicillin (1000 UI/mL) + Streptomycin (1 mg/mL) + Polymyxin (1000 UI/mL).

Kenny's skim milk*

Sanalac® powdered skim milk (g)	2.4
Glucose, monohydrate (g)	4.9
Na bicarbonate (solution 8.4%) (mL)	2.0
Gentamicin sulfate (mg)	100
Distilled water (mL)	92.01
pH	6.99
Osmotic pressure (mOsm/kg)	375

*Other variations of this extender exist; some do not contain Na bicarbonate. Some do not use any antibiotics and others use Ticarcillin/Timentin or Polymyxin or a combination Penicillin and Streptomycin.

Extender with heated UHT liquid milk (skim or half skimmed)

Skim or half skim milk (mL)	100
Polymixin B (UI/mL)	1000
pH	6.45–6.6
Osmotic pressure (mOsm/kg)	270–280

TABLE 102.2 Composition of INRA extenders.

INRA-82

Glucose, anhydrous (g)	25
Lactose, 1H$_2$O (g)	1.5
Raffinose, 5H$_2$O (g)	1.5
Citrate Na, 2 H$_2$O (g)	0.25
Citrate K, 1 H$_2$O (g)	0.41
Hepes (g)	4.76
Double distilled water QSP (mL)	500
Skim milk UHT (mL)	500
Gentamicin (sulfate) (mg)	50
Penicillin G (UI)	50,0000
pH	6.8
Osmotic pressure (mOsm/kg)	310

INRA-96 (Hank's salts with Glucose [67 mM] and lactose [126 mM])

CaCl$_2$ (g)	0.14
KCl (g)	0.4
KH$_2$PO$_4$ (g)	0.06
MgSO$_4$ 7 H$_2$O (g)	0.2
NaCl (g)	1.25
Na$_2$HPO$_4$, 12 H$_2$O (g)	0.118
NaHCO$_3$ (g)	0.35
HEPES (g)	4.76
Glucose (g)	13.21
Lactose (g)	45.39
Distilled water qsp (mL)	1000

- Phospholipids (low density lipoproteins) from egg yolk stabilize the sperm membrane.
- Additional protection of the sperm cell during cooling depends on:
  - Rate of cooling
  - Ability of a specific stallion's semen to withstand cooling.
- Extenders for cooled shipped semen can be subdivided in three groups:
  - Skim milk based extenders.
  - Egg yolk based extenders.
  - Sugar and salt based extenders (Tables 102.1, 102.2, and 102.3).
- Skim milk based extenders are the most commonly used in North America and are based on the original formulation of Kenney's extender.
  - Common components include skim milk, glucose, and sodium bicarbonate as a buffering agent.

TABLE 102.3 Lactose-EDTA-Egg Yolk Extender and Freezing Technique according to the East European Technique First Described by Naumenkov et Romenkova (1970).

Extender	
Lactose (g)	11
EDTA (g)	0.1
Na Citrate, 5.5 H$_2$O (g)	0.089
Na Bicarbonate (g)	0.008
Egg Yolk (g)	1.6
Glycerol (mL)	3.5
Penicillin (UI)	1,00,000
Dihydrostreptomycin (mg)	50
Distilled water (mL)	100
Dilution and centrifugation	No centrifugation needed if only sperm rich fraction is used. Dilution rate is 1:3 or 1:4 (semen-to-extender ratio) or to a concentration of 300 million spermatozoa per mL
Packaging	Aluminum tubes (20–25 mL)
Freezing	Slow cooling to 2°C–5°C in one (1) hour. Then freeze in liquid nitrogen vapors 2 to 4 cm above liquid nitrogen level for 7 to 9 minutes.
Thawing	Water bath at 40°C for 50 seconds

- The types of antibiotics added to these extenders vary.
- Some practitioners prefer the use of extenders without antibiotics. The most commonly used antibiotics are: potassium penicillin, amikacin sulfate, gentocin, and ticarcillin. Note: ticarcillin is still used in many countries, but is being replaced by timentin.
- Glycine egg yolk extenders are used primarily in some European countries (i.e., Holland and Germany).
  - Semen is centrifuged to remove seminal plasma before being resuspended in these extenders.
- INRA extender is a specially formulated extender for the short-term preservation of stallion semen that is particularly sensitive to temperature.
  - The use of INRA allows preservation of sperm viability and function up to 48 hours at temperatures between 12°C and 15°C.
  - This extender is based on Hank's salts, lactose, and phosphocaseinate (*see* Table 102.3).
- There are several other specialty extenders available in the literature but they remain in limited use.

Dilution of Semen for Cooled Storage

- Minimum extension for shipping chilled semen:
  - The ratio is 1:3 (one volume of semen to 3 volumes of extender).

- Dilution rate in skim milk based extenders should provide a final concentration of 25 to 50 million of motile spermatozoa per mL to prevent the deleterious effect of seminal plasma.
- Low concentration ejaculates should first be centrifuged to remove 80% to 95% of the seminal plasma and then resuspended appropriately with extender.

Effect of Freezing and Thawing on Semen

- Semen freezing presents greater challenges than those required to successfully cool and ship chilled semen.
  - Ice formation and concentration of salt solutes as cellular water freezes are deleterious to sperm viability and function and result in membrane injury and protein precipitation.
  - Similar challenges (detrimental effects) occur during thawing (i.e., a reversal of the process); water must successfully reenter the sperm cells at the time of thawing.
- The harmful effects of freezing and thawing can be reduced by using extenders and a freezing technique that reduces salt concentration and provides good cryoprotection of spermatozoa.

Freezing Extenders for Stallion Semen

- There are several techniques for freezing stallion semen.
- Most current techniques are two-step processes and use two different extenders.
  - The first extender is for centrifugation of semen and removal of seminal plasma.
  - The second extender is for resuspension of the centrifuged semen pellet in preparation for freezing.

Centrifugation Extender for Stallion Semen

- Seminal plasma has been shown to have deleterious effects on semen freezability and post-thaw fertility.
  - Stallion semen freezing requires an initial step of centrifugation to remove 90% to 95% of seminal plasma.
- Most techniques use as the centrifugation media, one of the extenders commonly used for shipped cooled semen. However, some techniques use unique, specially formulated, centrifugation extenders (Tables 102.4 through 102.9).
  - The dilution rate of semen for centrifugation is generally similar to those used for shipping cooled semen.
  - The purpose of the centrifugation extender is to maintain viability and provide a cushion to obtain a soft semen pellet after centrifugation.
  - Semen is centrifuged for 10 to 15 minutes at 400× to 800×g depending on the technique to be used.

Freezing Extenders

- Sperm pellets obtained by centrifugation are resuspended in the freezing extender.
- Freezing extenders vary according to methods.
  - Most contain skim milk, egg yolk, various sugars, electrolytes, and a cryoprotectant (*see* Tables 102.5 to 102.9).

TABLE 102.4 German Extender and Freezing Technique

Centrifugation Extender	
Glucose (g)	5.9985
Na Citrate, 2H$_2$O (g)	0.375
Na Bicarbonate (g)	0.120
EDTA (g)	0.37
Penicillin (UI)	50,000
Streptomycin (mg)	5,000
Distilled water (mL)	100

Freezing Extender	
Centrifugation extender (mL)	25
Egg yolk (mL)	20
Lactose (10%) (mL)	50
Orvus-es paste (mL)	0.5
Glycerol (mL)	5
Initial dilution and centrifugation	Dilution rate (semen-to-extender ratio) 1:1 to 1:4 Centrifugation: 650 × g for 15 minutes or 1000 × g for 5 minutes
Final dilution and packaging	Extend semen pellet to a concentration of 100 to 500 million spermatozoa/mL Package in 0.5-, 2.5-, or 4-mL straws
Freezing	Large straws: liquid nitrogen vapors for 20 minutes French straws: Liquid nitrogen vapors for 10 minutes
Thawing	Large straws: continuous agitation in a water bath at 50°C for 40 to 50 seconds French straws: 30 seconds in a 38°C water bath

- The most important difference between extenders is the type and concentration of cryoprotectants used.
- Some freezing techniques require the extended semen be cooled prior to freezing.
- Most stallion semen freezing extenders contain 2% to 2.5% egg yolk.
  - Higher concentrations of egg yolk seem to be harmful to stallion sperm cells.
  - Most extenders use chicken egg yolk.
  - Quail egg yolk is more suitable for freezing donkey semen.
- German extenders contain other substances known to stabilize the sperm membrane:
  - EDTA
  - Orvus-paste® (also known as Equex® STM Paste).

Cryoprotectants

- The primary cryoprotectant used in most extenders is glycerol.
  - Concentration of glycerol is generally kept at 2.5% to 3.5% of the final extender composition.

TABLE 102.5 Modified German Technique (Volkmann 1987).

Centrifugation Extender	
Glucose (g)	0.15
Na Citrate (2H$_2$O) (g)	0.2595
EDTA (g)	0.3699
Na Bicarbonate (g)	0.12
Polymixin B sulfate (UI)	1,000,000
Distilled water (mL)	100
Freezing Extender	
Lactose (11%) (g)	5.50
Centrifugation extender (mL)	50
Dialyzed egg-yolk (mL)*	21
Orvus-es Paste® (mL)	0.5
Glycerol (mL)	5
Initial dilution and Centrifugation	Semen is diluted to 1:3 to 1:4 ratio, placed on top of 0.25-mL layer of the hyperosmotic glucose solution. Centrifugation at 400 × g for 15 minutes at 20°C
Final dilution and packaging	Semen pellet is extended to achieve a concentration of 750 million spermatozoa/mL, packaged in 0.5-mL straws
Freezing	Computerized freezer or liquid nitrogen vapors
Thawing	6 seconds at 75°C then transfer to 37°C

*Egg yolk (150 mL) is dialyzed against deionized water (5–10 L). Water is changed every 8 to 12 hours.

TABLE 102.6 Freezing Extender according to the Japanese Technique (Nishikawa and Shinomyia 1972, Nishikawa 1975).

Centrifugation Extender	
Glucose (g)	5
Lactose (g)	0.3
Raffinose (g)	0.3
Na Citrate 5,5H$_2$O	0.15
Na$_2$HPO$_4$ (g)	0.05
Distilled water (mL)	100
Egg yolk (mL)	2.5
Penicillin (UI)	25,000
Streptomycin (µg)	25,000
Freezing Extender	
Centrifugation extender (mL)	90
Glycerol (mL)	10

TABLE 102.7 **Modified Japanese Freezing Extender (Palmer 1984, Magistrini et Vidament 1992).**

Centrifugation Extender	
Glucose (g)	5
Lactose (g)	0.3
Raffinose (g)	0.3
Na Citrate 5,5H$_2$O (g)	0.06
K Citrate (g)	0.082
Distilled water (mL)	100
Skim milk UHT (mL)	100
Egg yolk (mL)	4
Penicillin (UI)	200,000
Gentamicin (µg)	40,000
Freezing Extender	
Centrifugation extender (mL)	97.5
Glycerol (mL)	2.5
Initial dilution and Centrifugation	Dilution rate (semen-to-extender ratio) of 1:3 to 1:4 or to a concentration of 2.5 billion of spermatozoa in 45 mL. Slow cooling to 4°C in 1 hour. Centrifuge cooled at 600 × g for 10 minutes
Final dilution and packaging	Dilute pellet with freezing extender to a concentration of 100 million spermatozoa per mL. Equilibrate for 30 to 45 minutes. Package in 0.5-mL straws
Freezing	Liquid nitrogen vapors, held at 4 cm above liquid nitrogen level for 10 minutes
Thawing	Water bath at 37°C for 30 seconds

- Higher concentrations of glycerol have a negative effect on fertility.
- Glycerol may be harmful for semen from some stallions and contribute to capacitation-like changes upon thawing, and hypo-osmotic stress upon delivery (AI) into the uterus.
- Deleterious effects of glycerol are due to protein denaturation, alteration of microtubules, and alteration of the plasma membrane and glycocalyx.
- Glutamine (50 mM) improves cryopreservation of horse and donkey semen in the presence of glycerol.
  - Seems to act at the extra-cellular level, independent of glycerol.
- Other cryoprotectants such as alcohols (i.e., ethylene glycol) and amides (i.e., methyl formamide, dimethyl formamide, dimethyl acetamide) have proven to be less harmful and provide better post-thaw motility and fertility for some stallions.
  - Amides have the advantage of a lower molecular weight and greater water solubility and may induce less osmotic damage.

TABLE 102.8 Colorado Freezing Extender.	
Dried skim milk (g)	5.15
NaCL (mM)	18.5
KCl (mM)	5.0
KH_2PO_4 (mM)	0.6
$NaHCO_3$ (mM)	17.8
$MgSO_4$ (mM)	1.2
HEPES (mM)	5.0
$CaCl_2$, 2 H_2O (mM)	0.8
Fructose (mM)	42
Glucose (mM)	18.5
Na Pyruvate (mM)	0.6 mM
Na Lactate (mM)	6.55
BSA (mg) (mM)	160
Egg Yolk (%)	2
Glycerol (%)	3

- Amides are used in the freezing extender at concentrations of 2% to 3%, to improve post-thaw motility, cell integrity, and fertility in "poor freezing" stallions.
- Also available are new, specially formulated extenders containing cholesterol to adjust the phospholipid-to-cholesterol ratio.
  - May be helpful for some "poor freezing" stallions.

Freezing Process

- Semen should immediately be evaluated following collection. Record values for gel-free volume, initial motility, concentration, and morphology.
- Semen should be diluted with the appropriate extender to a concentration of 50 million spermatozoa per mL.
- Centrifugation is performed in aliquots of 40 mL of this diluted semen that has been placed into 50 mL conical tubes.
- The conical tubes are then centrifuged at 400 × g for 12 to15 minutes.
- The supernatant is discarded, but:
  - A quick evaluation of the supernatant (pipet a drop of the supernatant onto a warmed slide, coverslip it, and observe at 400×) provides an additional gauge of the adequacy of the centrifugation protocol used.
  - If the sperm pellet is too soft, or the supernatant laden with high numbers of spermatozoa, the subsequent centrifugation time or g-force can be appropriately increased.
  - If the pellet is too hard and is re-suspended only with great difficulty and the supernatant is void of motile sperm, the centrifugation protocol may be adjusted downward (less time or g-force) for processing subsequent ejaculates.

TABLE 102.9 **Burns Technique (Burns 1992).**		
Centrifugation Extender		
Sucrose (g)		5
Glucose (g)		3
Bovine Serum Albumin (g)		1.5
Ticarcillin (mg)		100
Distilled water (mL)		100
pH		6.8
Osmotic pressure (mOsm/kg)		350
Freezing Extender		
Powdered skim milk (g)	2.4	
Glucose (g)	4.9	
Clarified egg yolk (mL)*	8	
Ticarcillin (mg)	100	
Glycerol (% volume)	3.5	
Distilled water (mL) qsp	100	
Initial dilution and centrifugation	One part of semen to two parts of centrifugation extender Centrifuge at 350 × g for 5 minutes	
Final dilution and packaging	Dilute semen pellet (after centrifugation) to a concentration of 100 million spermatozoa per mL Package in 5-mL straws	
Freezing	Freeze in liquid nitrogen vapor, 4 cm above liquid nitrogen level for 15 minutes	
Thawing	Continuous agitation in 52°C water bath for 52 seconds	

*Egg yolk is clarified by centrifugation in centrifugation extender (equal volume, 25 mL) at 10,000 × g for 15 minutes.

- The semen pellet is re-suspended in freezing media to obtain the desired concentration:
  - Four hundred to 1,600 million spermatozoa per mL for freezing in 0.5-mL straws.
  - Two hundred million/mL for freezing in 5.0-mL straws.
- The use of some freezing extenders (i.e., French extenders) requires slow cooling of semen to 5°C for 2 hours prior to packaging (filling straws) and freezing.
  - This can be accomplished with an extended sample being suspended (protected from water contamination, but partially submerged) within a water bath to provide a measured, cooling rate.
  - Equitainers®, used for preparation of chilled semen for shipping, can also be used to achieve the same end.
- After packaging (generally in 0.5-, 2.0-, or 5.0-mL straws), semen is frozen in liquid nitrogen vapor.
  - Computerized freezers are available in which the straws are held at a specific distance above liquid nitrogen level (3–6 cm) to achieve the appropriate cooling/freezing rate.

- Straws can also be frozen in vapor, positioned on a rack in a container 2 to 3 cm above liquid nitrogen. Thick-walled Styrofoam boxes can serve this purpose well (lower equipment budget, but good results can be achieved).
- In both systems, straws are plunged into liquid nitrogen after 15 minutes.
- Straws are then placed into goblets; goblets onto canes; and the canes transferred into canisters of a properly maintained liquid nitrogen tank.

System Affected

Reproductive

 # DIAGNOSTICS

Other Laboratory Tests

- Semen quality should be determined before addition of extenders.
- Microbiological quality of semen and extenders should be determined as part of quality control and to choose the antibiotic to be added to an extender.
- Quality of ingredients in extenders should be verified.
- Physical and chemical properties of extenders (i.e., pH, osmotic pressure) should be determined periodically, or if problems have been encountered in preserving semen.

 # THERAPEUTICS

Drug(s) of Choice

- Choice of antibiotic in the extender is determined by several factors:
  - Bacteria found to be present in a stallion's ejaculate.
  - The culture and sensitivity of the organisms, including assessment of potential pathogens versus contaminants.
  - The effect of specific antibiotics on semen viability.
- Polymixin B sulfate has been shown to reduce sperm motility after storage at 5°C.
- Amikacin sulfate, ticarcillin (or Timentin) or the combination of amikacin sulfate and potassium penicillin G are the preferred antibiotics for cooled shipped semen.
- Overuse of antibiotics in semen extenders is believed to be responsible for the increase in fungal endometritis.

 # COMMENTS

Possible Complications

Adverse reactions may occur when breeding mares with semen diluted using some extenders.

Expected Course and Prognosis

The ability of stallion semen to withstand cooling and freezing depends on several factors:

- Individual stallion and ejaculate
- Cooling and freezing protocol used
- Freezing media and particularly the interaction between the individual stallion's semen and the cryoprotectant used.
- Semen should be test frozen with different methods to determine the best protocol for a particular stallion.

Abbreviations

AI   artificial insemination
EDTA ethylenediaminetetraacetic acid
INRA Institut National de la Recherche Agronomique

See Also

- Artificial insemination
- Breed soundness examination, stallion
- Semen evaluation, fertile stallion
- Semen evaluation, infertile stallion

Suggested Reading

Alvarenga MA, Papa FO, Landim-Alvarenga FC, et al. 2005. Amides as cryoprotectants for freezing stallion semen: A review. *Anim Reprod Sci* 89: 105–113.

Khlifaoui M, Battut I, Bruyas JF, et al. 2005. Effects of glutamine on post-thaw motility of stallion spermatozoa: an approach of the mechanism of action at spermatozoa level. *Therio* 63: 138–149.

Moore AI, Squires EL, Graham JK. 2005. Effect of seminal plasma on the cryopreservation of equine semen. *Therio* 63: 2372–2381.

Samper JC, Morris CA. 1998. Current methods for stallion semen cryopreservation: A survey. *Therio* 49: 895–903.

Samper JC. 2000. Artificial insemination. In: *Equine Breeding Management and Artificial Insemination.* Samper JC (ed). Philadelphia: W. B. Saunders; 109–132.

Squires EL, Keith SL, Graham JK. 2004. Evaluation of alternative cryoprotectants for preserving stallion spermatozoa. *Therio* 62: 1056–1065.

Thomas AD, Meyers SA, Ball BA. 2006. Capacitation-like changes in equine spermatozoa following cryopreservation. *Therio* 65: 1531–1550.

Tibary A, Anouassi A, Sghiri A, et al. 2005. Insémination artificielle chez les équides. In: *Reproduction Equine III, Biotechnologies appliqué.* Tibary A, Bakkoury M (eds). Rabat, Morocco: Actes Edition; 9–155.

Author: Ahmed Tibary

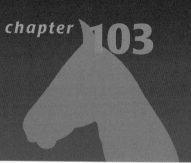

Semen, Frozen, Artificial Insemination

DEFINITION/OVERVIEW

- Frozen semen is the term used for semen that has been diluted in special extender (usually with low molecular weight cryoprotectants such as glycerol), frozen to LN2 temperature, and maintained at that temperature until being thawed for AI.
- AI with frozen semen is used less commonly in the horse than natural cover, AI with fresh semen, and AI with chilled transported semen:
  - Reasons for this are expense and,
  - Expectation of lower pregnancy rates than with the previously mentioned options.
- Other terms used: Cryopreserved semen.

ETIOLOGY/PATHOPHYSIOLOGY

Systems Affected

Reproductive

CLINICAL FEATURES

Procedure for Preparation of Frozen Semen

Semen Collection and Evaluation of the Normal Stallion

- Semen collection and evaluation is performed as for preparation for AI with fresh or chilled semen.
- Minimum standards of motility and total spermatozoa in the ejaculate are typically higher than those used for AI with fresh or chilled semen.
  - When these threshold standards are not exceeded, the ejaculate should not be frozen and used for AI with frozen semen.

Semen Packaging

- Semen has been frozen:
  - In plastic straws that vary in size from 0.25 mL up to 5 mL.
  - In pellets of extended semen frozen directly on dry ice that are subsequently placed in plastic tubes

- In various plastic, glass, and metal containers.
  - The most typical containers are 0.5-mL straws and 5-mL straws.
- When semen is frozen in 0.5-mL straws, it is often necessary to inseminate the contents of more than one straw to bring total sperm numbers up to an acceptable complete AI dose.

Semen Freezing

- Spermatozoa are usually concentrated by centrifugation before freezing; this is usually done immediately after dilution in a milk-based extender; centrifuged semen will often be held or processed at room temperature after this procedure.
- Semen is resuspended after centrifugation in semen freezing extender or in an interim solution; final concentration of spermatozoa will be between 200 and 400 million/mL.
- Extended semen may be cooled to 5°C before freezing and held for up to 18 hours, but immediate freezing is sometimes also done.
- Glycerol is added to the semen either after cooling or immediately on dilution with the final freezing extender.
- Semen is loaded in straws or other types of packages after the glycerolated extender has been added and final concentration has been reached.
- Straws are frozen in a programmable freezer or on a rack suspended above the surface of LN2 (freezing occurs while straws are held in the vapor above the LN2).
  - One technique used with 0.5-mL straws in the programmable freezer is cooling at −10°C/min until −15°C is reached and then at −15°C/min until −120°C is reached.
- After straws have reached −120°C they are submerged (plunged) in LN2 and placed in goblets and canes if necessary (necessary with 0.5-mL straws) and transferred to a LN2 tank.
- A test straw is evaluated for post-thaw motility; other viability tests may be performed.

Variations in Procedure and General Considerations

- Centrifugation is less harmful to spermatozoa (motility and fertility) if done at lower speed (400 to 800 g) rather than at faster speeds (greater than 1000 g) and at room temperature (22°C–25°C) rather than at 5°C.
- Semen can be extended and cooled to 5°C and stored for up to 18 hours while maintaining adequate motility and fertility after freezing, but it is more typical for semen to be frozen without cooling to 5°C, or after only 1 to 2 hours of cooling to 5°C.
  - Longer storage before freezing would only be used when semen must be shipped from the farm where it was collected to the semen preservation facility.
- Extenders for freezing semen usually contain egg yolk and may contain both egg yolk and skim milk; the bulk of the osmotic component is made up of sugars (i.e., glucose, fructose, lactose, sucrose, and sometimes more complex sugars), and often a buffer is added, although yolk and milk also act as buffers.

- Many different components are added to equine semen extender in an attempt to improve post-thaw motility and fertility:
  - Equex (sodium triethanolamine lauryl sulfate, a detergent that interacts with yolk and improves yolk/spermatozoa interactions).
  - EDTA
  - Sodium citrate (a buffer that also helps to clarify the yolk)
  - And a variety of other inorganic and organic buffers.
- pH of semen extender is usually titrated to 6.8 to 7.4 because the addition of yolk and milk can often move pH away from this physiological range.
- Antibiotics are added for control of bacterial growth during processing and to reduce the risk of transmitting a pathogen during AI.
- Glycerol is the most common low molecular weight cryoprotectant added to equine semen extenders:
  - It is toxic and attempts to reduce its concentration and detrimental effects are made by freezing semen at 2% to 3.5% final concentration and by adding glycerol after cooling and incubation at 5°C.
  - However, experimenting with addition of glycerol earlier or later in the preparation of frozen semen sometimes gives conflicting results (one study suggested that adding glycerol at 22°C was preferable to adding it after cooling to 5°C).
- The addition of low molecular weight cryoprotectants other than glycerol has been attempted with some success, but the long history of glycerol use tends to inhibit radical changes in this part of the freezing procedure.
  - Cryoprotectants that may have promise include ethylene glycol (antifreeze), methyl formamide, and dimethyl formamide.

Variations in Procedure When a Stallion Produces Semen That Does Not Freeze Well

- Some stallions are known as poor "coolers" and poor "freezers."
  - This may be a result of obvious problems such as abnormal morphology, low sperm output, poor initial motility, and sensitivity to normal handling procedures.
  - In some cases, this can be mitigated by selecting and freezing only ejaculates that meet threshold standards.
  - In other cases the ejaculate may appear normal until post-thaw evaluation and fertility results reveal substandard results.
- Stallions extremely sensitive to incubation or cooling in seminal plasma can be collected directly into prewarmed milk-based semen extender and have centrifugation take place immediately to remove seminal plasma.
- Experiments with nonglycerol cryoprotectants have as one objective finding less toxic low molecular weight products to use on semen sensitive to the toxic effects of glycerol.
- Combinations of milk and egg yolk may be beneficial in extenders for stallions producing semen that freezes poorly in extenders containing only one or the other.
- Experimenting with cooling rate and incubation time before freezing may identify a protocol that works better than standard techniques.

Other Considerations in Frozen Semen Storage

Maintaining Temperature at −196°C (LN2 temperature)

- Frozen semen must be kept in LN2 until it is thawed for AI. There are ultra-cold freezers that operate by standard refrigeration technology that are capable of holding semen at less than −100°C but these are rarely used for holding frozen semen.
- When semen is checked for identification by lifting the canister into the neck of the LN2 tank the operator must keep the semen well down inside the neck (at or below the frost line) and minimize the time spent with the semen outside the main bulk of the tank's interior.
  - The temperature in the neck can rise above −40°C and that will damage the frozen semen.

Transport to the Site of AI

- Frozen semen is often transported via package service, air freight, bus, or train in nitrogen vapor tanks designed for this purpose.
  - Depending on the amount of LN2 needed to charge such tanks, their holding time at −196°C can range from 1 to 3 weeks.
  - When a vapor tank is first being charged, a minimum of 48 hours is usually needed to fully saturate the liner. Serial additions of LN2 are required over 2 days. Continue additions until some LN2 remains in the bottom of the central canister 6 to 8 hours after the final addition; it ensures it will hold at the safe temperature for semen maintenance during transport and during the holding period if straws are not transferred to a LN2 tank.
  - It is important for the veterinarian on the mare end of frozen semen AI to maintain a standard LN2 tank into which the transported semen will be transferred upon arrival.
- All LN2 tanks must be maintained in an upright position to function normally; transport vapor tanks are designed to maintain proper temperature for a matter of days, even if there is a spill or the tank tips.
  - Allowing the vapor tank to be transported or stored on its side or upside-down will degrade its performance.

Microorganisms Preserved in Frozen Semen

- Bacteria and viruses shed in semen are well-preserved by the freezing process used with semen.
  - Stallions shedding EAV must be identified. The risks of storing semen from such a stallion should be passed on to the owners of mares interested in using the frozen semen.
- Insemination will inevitably set up an inflammatory reaction in the uterus of the mare; addition of pathogens to this normal reaction may result in uterine infection rather than normal inflammation.

Insemination of Frozen Semen

Identification and Evaluation

- When frozen semen arrives, the identification of the semen and stallion should be confirmed by documents that accompany the shipment and the label on the frozen semen itself.
- Total numbers of spermatozoa available for insemination should be calculated:
  - If there are 10 straws with 200 million spermatozoa per straw, there are 2 billion spermatozoa available.
  - This would be sufficient for five inseminations of 400 million spermatozoa or two inseminations of 1 billion cells.
  - The semen processor should designate how many cells and how many straws constitute one AI dose.

Thawing and Insemination

- The mare should be prepared for insemination and all equipment organized before thaw.
- The equivalent of one AI dose should be thawed as per the instructions of the processor; this may be a two-step procedure with two water baths.
  - The default procedure, when no detailed instructions are available, is to thaw in a 37°C water bath for 30 seconds if using 0.5-mL straws, and for 2 minutes if larger straws. Gently agitate (move) the straws through the water bath during thawing to ensure a more even and rapid thaw.
- If the package is designed in a way that is not water tight, the operator should not let water come into direct contact with the frozen semen.
- Broken straws or broken containers should be discarded.
- If a single 0.5-mL straw represents a complete AI dose, specialized straw pipets to deliver the contents of the straw can be used; with greater volumes or multiple straws, the semen can be thawed and transferred to a plastic test tube and aspirated into an AI pipette or two-piece syringe.
- The semen is inseminated into the body of the uterus by passing an AI pipette through the cervix and expressing the complete volume of the AI dose through the pipette using the syringe.
- DHI technique using intra-uterine endoscopy to deliver the semen dose onto the ostium (uterotubal junction) of the uterine horn on the side of ovulation, can conserve the number of straws/spermatozoa needed to achieve pregnancy.
  - DHI, a low-dose AI technique.
  - May be of particular interest when using semen from stallions that have died or when semen is available in limited supply or at great expense.

Fertility of Frozen Semen

- Pregnancy rates with frozen semen have been variously reported at 51% for first cycle bred and 75% for the season (876 mares); 46% per cycle and 64% foaling rate/year (more than 1000 mares).

- Pregnancy rates for mares recognized as problem mares are lower when inseminated with frozen semen than when inseminated with fresh semen (37% versus 59%).
- Adequate numbers of spermatozoa must be available for multiple inseminations per cycle and for multiple cycles, if potential foaling rates of 60% to 75% are to be realized.
- Optimum results with frozen semen demand frequent U/S examination of the mare's ovaries and at least one insemination of a full dose of semen within the 24-hour period that spans 12 hours before and 12 hours after ovulation.
  - Unless U/S examinations can be performed two to four times per day, AI within this 24-hour period may demand multiple inseminations within one cycle.

 COMMENTS

Abbreviations

AI	artificial insemination
DHI	deep horn insemination
EAV	equine arteritis virus
EDTA	ethylenediaminetetraacetic acid
LN2	liquid nitrogen
U/S	ultrasound, ultrasonography

See Also

- Artificial insemination
- Semen collection, routine evaluation
- Semen, cryopreservation, managing freezability
- Semen evaluation, abnormalities

Suggested Reading

Backman T, Bruemmer JE, Graham JK, et al. 2004. Pregnancy rates of mares inseminated with semen cooled for 18 hours and then frozen. *J Anim Sci* 82: 690–694.

Moore AI, Squires EL, Graham JK. 2005. Effect of seminal plasma on the cryopreservation of equine spermatozoa. *Therio* 63: 2372–2381.

Vidament M. 2005. French field results (1985–2005) on factors affecting fertility of frozen stallion semen. *Anim Reprod Sci* 89: 115–136.

Author: Rolf E. Larsen

chapter 104

Seminal Vesiculitis

DEFINITION/OVERVIEW

- Inflammation/infection of the seminal vesicles resulting in specific changes in seminal characteristics and subfertility or infertility.

ETIOLOGY/PATHOPHYSIOLOGY

- Colonization of the seminal vesicle (can be unilateral or bilateral) by an infectious agent disrupts its secretory function.
- The inflamed seminal vesicle becomes enlarged and painful.
- Impaired secretory function of the seminal vesicle affects semen quality and viability.
- Presence of WBC, frank blood, inflammatory products, and infectious organisms compromises sperm cell function and leads to infertility.
- Transmission of infectious organisms to mares at breeding results in endometritis and infertility.

Systems Affected

Reproductive

SIGNALMENT/HISTORY

Historical Findings

- Stallion usually presents for infertility
- Reluctance to breed
- Relatively uncommon
- Poor semen quality: poor motility, sperm agglutination
- Hemospermia or pyospermia
- Mares bred to affected stallion return to estrus or develop endometritis

CLINICAL FEATURES

Physical Examination Findings

- Symptoms vary depending on duration.
- Chronic cases do not show outward clinical signs.
- Acute cases may show pain during ejaculation or TRP.
- Dysuria or abnormal stance during micturition.
- Anorexia and colic have been reported but are rare.
- Septic bacterial infections may be ascendant or hematogenous.
- Reported isolates include *Pseudomonas aeruginosa, Klebsiella pneumoniae, Streptococcus* spp., *Staphylococcus* spp., *Proteus vulgaris, Brucella abortus,* and *Acinetobacter calcoaceticus.*

DIFFERENTIAL DIAGNOSIS

- Other causes of hemospermia: urethritis, urethral defects (rents).
- Other causes of leukospermia: epididymitis, ampullitis (rare), or urethritis.

DIAGNOSTICS

CBC/Biochemistry/Urinalysis

- CBC and biochemistry are unremarkable, unless complications develop.
- Urinalysis may show increased WBC and RBC.

Other Laboratory Tests

- Semen evaluation shows microscopic or macroscopic hemospermia (ejaculate color dirty pink to brownish), poor motility, increased sperm clumping, increased percentage of detached heads.
- Cytology: Giemsa, Modified Wrights, DiffQuick® or Gram-stained semen smears show PMNs and bacteria.
- Bacteriology of semen, samples taken directly from the seminal vesicle gland by endoscopy or by fractioned semen collection.
- Collection of seminal vesicle gland secretions may be obtained by transrectal massage following sexual stimulation of the stallion.

Imaging

Per Rectum U/S of the Seminal Vesicles

- Two- to threefold increase in vesicle size.
- Change in their echogenicity and increased thickness of the wall.
- Increased echogenicity and flocculent material in the gland.

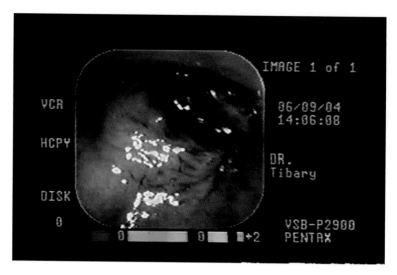

■ Figure 104.1 Inflamed *colliculus seminalis* in a stallion with seminal vesiculitis.

Fibroscopy or Video-Endoscopy

- Inflammation of the colliculus seminalis.
- Direct visualization of the seminal vesicle lumen and aspiration of its contents is possible with a small diameter (9-mm) flexible endoscope. Contents may be muco-purulent or hemorrhagic (Figs. 104.1 and 104.2).

THERAPEUTICS

Drug(s) of Choice

- Antimicrobial selection is based on culture and sensitivity.
- Combination of local instillation (amikacin sulfate for 2 days) and systemic treatment with antimicrobials (trimethoprim/sulfadiazine for 8 days) has been successful in some cases.
- Lavage and systemic treatment with gentamicin (800 mg BID, IV) and amoxicillin (5 g, BID).
- Enrofloxacin has been shown to reach the seminal vesicle in sufficient concentration after parenteral administration.

Appropriate Health Care

- Obtain sample for cytology and culture and sensitivity from fractionated ejaculate or directly by endoscopy.
- NSAIDs may be helpful in acute painful cases.
- Systemic antimicrobials are not efficacious; they do *not* reach the gland at sufficient concentration.

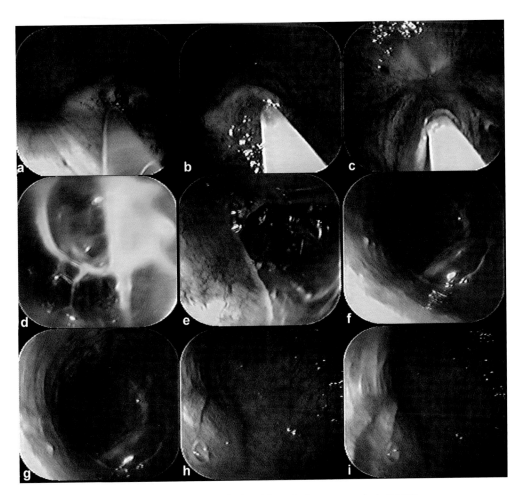

■ **Figure 104.2** Endoscopic lavage of the seminal vesicle, note its mucopurulent content.

- Best treatment approach:
  - Endoscopic lavage and local antimicrobial infusion into the lumen of the gland (*see* Fig. 104.2).
- Direct collection of semen into an antibiotic-containing extender may be helpful in the management of some cases.
- Breeding with MCT (infusion of antibiotic-containing extender before breeding) and uterine lavage after breeding when AI is not allowed by a particular breed registry.
- Refractory cases may require collection of semen directly into an antibiotic-containing extender (preplaced in the AVs collection bag/bottle).

Surgical Considerations

- Vesiculectomy has been described but may lead to complications (e.g., loss of ejaculatory function).

COMMENTS

Client Education

- Strict hygienic measures during natural breeding
- Recommend regular BSE of a stallion

Patient Monitoring

- Monitor semen quality

Prevention/Avoidance

- Meticulous breeding hygiene

Possible Complications

- Infertility
- Ampullitis, epididymitis

Expected Course and Prognosis

- Fair to guarded for fertility

Synonyms

- Seminal vesicle adenitis
- Vesicular gland adenitis

Abbreviations

AI	artificial insemination
AV	artificial vagina
BID	twice a day
BSE	breeding soundness examination
CBC	complete blood count
IV	intravenous
MCT	minimum contamination technique
NSAID	nonsteroidal anti-inflammatory drug
PMN	polymorphonuclear cell
RBC	red blood cell
TRP	transrectal palpation
U/S	ultrasound, ultrasonography
WBC	white blood cell

See Also

- BSE, Stallion
- Sperm accumulation/stagnation

Suggested Reading

Freestone JF, Paccamonti DL, Eilts BE, et al. 1993. Seminal vesiculitis as a cause of signs of colic in a stallion. *JAVMA* 203: 556–557.

Malmgrem L, Sussemilch BI. 1992. Ultrasonography as a diagnostic-tool in a stallion with seminal vesiculitis. A case report. *Therio* 37: 935–938.

Varner DD, Schumacker J, Blanchard TL, et al. 1991. Diseases of the accessory genital glands. In: *Diseases and Management of Breeding Stallions*. DD Varner (ed). Goleta, CA: American Veterinary Publications; 257–263.

Author: Ahmed Tibary

chapter 105

Sperm Accumulation/Stagnation

DEFINITION/OVERVIEW

- Accumulation of sperm in the ampullae of the ductus (vas) deferens is one kind of ejaculatory dysfunction.
- Characterized by low sperm concentration ejaculates or a high concentration of abnormal sperm and poor motility.

ETIOLOGY/PATHOPHYSIOLOGY

- The ampullae are the caudal dilations of the ductus deferens as it approaches the ejaculatory duct (pelvic urethra).
  - Length 20 to 25 cm.
  - Width in the mature stallion 2 to 3 cm.
  - They function as a sperm reservoir and also have a secretory function (branched tubulo-alveolar glands).
  - The reservoir of sperm is emitted at the time of ejaculation by the contraction of the tunica muscularis, comprised of an inner circular layer and an outer longitudinal layer of smooth muscle.
- Accumulation of sperm and glandular secretion in the ampullar crypts results in inspissation of the gland contents and distension of its glandular portion.
- Increased glandular inspissation results in blockage of sperm flow.
- Etiology: unknown

Systems Affected

Reproductive

SIGNALMENT/HISTORY

- Stallions of all ages (2–30 years of age) and breeds.
- Uncommon, incidence estimated at 1% to 2%.

Historical Findings

- History of subfertility
- Oligozoospermia or azoospermia
- High rate of detached sperm heads
- High sperm concentration with poor motility
- Sperm clumping or agglutination (Fig. 105.1)

 ## CLINCAL FEATURES

Physical Examination Findings

- General physical examination is unremarkable.
- TRP reveals enlarged ampullae.
  - Ampullar diameter is often greater than 3 cm and may reach 10 cm.
  - May be unilateral or bilateral.

 ## DIFFERENTIAL DIAGNOSIS

- Other causes of oligozoospermia or azoospermia:
  - Severe testicular degeneration or atrophy.
  - Epididymal diseases: epididymitis, epididymal occlusion, or segmental aplasia.
- Other causes of poor motility and hemospermia (seminal vesiculitis).
- Other causes of teratospermia: epididymitis or orchitis.
- Other causes of ejaculatory dysfunction.

 ## DIAGNOSTICS

CBC/Biochemistry/Urinalysis

- CBC and biochemistry are unremarkable.
- Urinalysis unremarkable.

Other Laboratory Tests

- Ejaculate may be thick (creamy appearance) and flocculent (*see* Figs. 105.1a and 105.1b).
- Semen evaluation typically reveals oligospermia, oligozoospermia, azoospermia, or very high concentration (total sperm numbers in the ejaculate are excessively high or they present an inconsistent pattern), poor motility, increased clumping of the sperm, or detached heads.
- Cytology: Giemsa, Modified Wright's, DiffQuick® or Gram-stain semen smears.
- PMNs occasionally seen.
- Hemospermia and tags of tissue may be present in the ejaculate after treatment by massage or oxytocin.

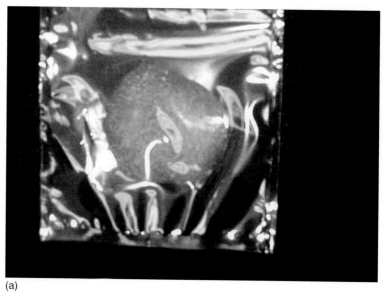

(a)

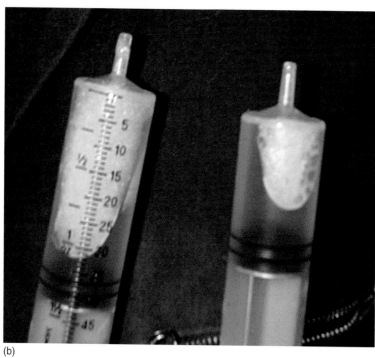

(b)

■ **Fig 105.1** *A, B,* Thick viscous ejaculate obtained from a stallion with plugged ampullae; samples were collected after oxytocin and transrectal massage therapy.

Imaging

Transrectal U/S of ampullae:

- U/S of the ampullae may aid the diagnosis if obvious ampullar changes are present.
- Enlargement of ampullar diameter and length.
- Change in the echogenicity of content; increased thickness of the wall of the ampullae.
- Presence of echodense areas or foci corresponding to inspissated or clumps of sperm.
- A "plug" (dead agglutinated sperm plus epithelial cells from the ampullae) may be visible caudal to the area of maximal accumulation of sperm. If present, it will appear hyperechoic with U/S.

 ## THERAPEUTICS

Drug(s) of Choice

- Oxytocin (20 IU, IV) to increase smooth muscle contraction.
- $PGF_2\alpha$ (0.01 mg/kg, IM) to increase smooth muscle contraction.

Appropriate Health Care

- Transrectal manual massage of the ampullae to dislodge the occlusion prior to semen collection.
- Administration of $PGF_2\alpha$ after massage may help to eliminate clumps of semen.
- Oxytocin (20 IU, IV) immediately prior to semen collection or transrectal massage (ampullae are composed of smooth muscle, stimulate contractions).
- Serial daily semen collections until semen parameters are within normal limits. This may take 5 to 21 days depending on severity.
- Semen collection several times (two to four times) per day may be necessary.
- Chronically affected stallions may require regular collections year-round to remain unoccluded or to lessen the degree of blockage between collections.

Nursing Care

Daily collection through the period of breeding season to prevent accumulation and reoccurrence.

 ## COMMENTS

Patient Monitoring

- Monitor semen quality

Prevention/Avoidance

- Maintain stallion on a regular semen collection schedule.
- Check ampullae by TRP.
- Check semen quality at the beginning of the breeding season or after a period of sexual inactivity.

Possible Complications

- Infertility
- Development of antisperm antibodies due to erosion of the epithelial lining of the ampullae.

Expected Course and Prognosis

- Good

Synonyms

- Plugged ampullae syndrome
- Occluded ampullae
- Spermastasis in the ampullae
- Sperm accumulation syndrome
- Sperm accumulators (name designation of affected stallion)

Abbreviations

CBC   complete blood count
IM   intramuscular
IV   intravenous
PMN   polymorphonuclear cells
TRP   transrectal palpation
U/S   ultrasound, ultrasonography

See Also

- Abnormal scrotal size
- Abnormal testicular size
- Breeding soundness examination, stallion
- Testicular degeneration

Suggested Reading

Love CC, Riera FL, Oristaglio RM, et al. 1992. Sperm occluded (plugged) ampullae in the stallion. *Proc Soc Therio* 117–125.

Author: Ahmed Tibary

chapter 106

Spermatogenesis and Factors Affecting Sperm Production

 DEFINITION/OVERVIEW

- *Spermatogenesis* occurs in testicular seminiferous tubules (Fig. 106.1) and is the process of:
  - Mitotic proliferation of spermatogonia.
  - Meiotic divisions of primary (first meiotic division) and secondary spermatocytes (second meiotic division) to form spermatids.
  - Maturation of spermatids into spermatozoa capable of motility and fertilization.
  - In the horse, this sequence takes approximately 55 to 57 days.
- *Spermiogenesis* is the portion of spermatogenesis that involves the maturation of round spermatids into spermatozoa.
- *Epididymal maturation* or passage of sperm through the epididymis is thought to be necessary in many animals, including the horse, for spermatozoa to achieve normal motility and fertilizing ability.
  - Passage through the epididymis takes approximately 9 days in the horse.

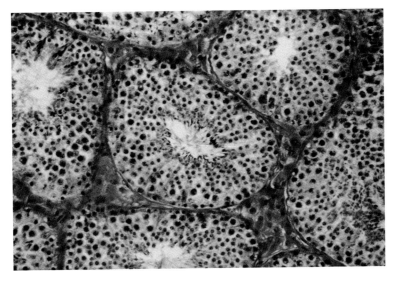

■ Figure 106.1 Normal seminiferous tubules in an equine testis. Image courtesy of Charles Love.

ETIOLOGY/PATHOPHYSIOLOGY

Spermatogenesis is a major component of normal reproductive physiology in the stallion.

Endocrine Considerations

- Testosterone tissue concentrations in the testis seem to be positively associated with spermatogenic activity.
  - Tissue concentrations of testosterone are related to blood concentrations.
  - It is difficult to assess testosterone activity in the testis or circulating levels with a single blood sample.
- Modulation of spermatogenesis involves LH, FSH, GnRH, testosterone, estrogen, inhibin, and other paracrine/autocrine factors not yet completely characterized.

Seasonal Patterns

- Some studies report a higher testicular concentration of testosterone in stallions during the breeding season.
- There are seasonal variations in sperm production and output.
- Sperm production during the winter (short-daylight months) may be half of the level observed during months of maximum photoperiod.
- Normal stallions produce spermatozoa year-round and are potentially fertile year-round.
  - Sperm motility and percent normal morphology vary little throughout the year.

Age-Related Factors

- At puberty, testis weight is positively correlated with:
  - Potential DSO, based on histologic evaluation of seminiferous tubules.
  - Quantitative measures of spermatogenesis.
- In 1- to 3-year-old horses, spermatogenic efficiency does not reach normal adult levels of 14 to 18 million spermatozoa per gram of testicular tissue per day until the individual testis weight reaches 70 to 80 g, or a combined testicular volume of 133 to 152 mL (or cm³).
  - Some 3-year-old stallions may reach this testicular volume without producing sufficient spermatozoa to rank them as *satisfactory* during a BSE.
  - From puberty on, sperm production may continue to increase for years. Some studies have found sperm production continues to increase past 12 years of age. Full maturity of the stallion with regard to sperm production is often considered to be 6 years.
- Intratesticular testosterone (testosterone produced per gram of testicular tissue) increases with age and is related to sperm production.
  - Differences in intratesticular testosterone between stallions may explain differences in sperm production.
- In general:
  - Testicular size increases with age.
  - Sperm production and sperm output increase with testicular size.

Causes of or pathophysiological mechanisms associated with arrested or disrupted spermatogenesis include the following.

Congenital

- Testicular hypoplasia due to hypogonadotropic hypogonadism:
  - Abnormally low GnRH, LH, and FSH result in low testosterone.
  - Probably rare
- Primary testicular degeneration:
  - Unknown if this is part of a congenital lesion or is acquired.
- Chromosomal anomalies such as XXY.
- Intersex conditions
- Cryptorchidism

Acquired

- Although relatively rare, testicular neoplasia can occur in stallions (Fig. 106.2).
- Testicular heating due to infection, fever, environment, and scrotal insulation.
  - Heating could result from a hydrocele, ventral edema, inflammation, and trauma.
- Testicular degeneration (Fig. 106.3) associated with testicular metabolic changes is incompletely characterized at present, but it might be associated with either of the following:
  - Anabolic steroid treatment, or treatment with steroids or medications with steroid-like effects (i.e., androgens, estrogens, or progestins) administered for behavioral or medical conditions can interfere with normal endocrine feedback loops resulting in decreased GnRH and LH.
  - Interference with normal metabolism by nutritional deficiencies, or exposure to one or more of many toxic substances (Table 106.1), some of which target specific populations of sperm precursors. Diagnosis is challenging and few cases have been specifically documented in the stallion.

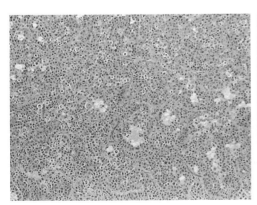 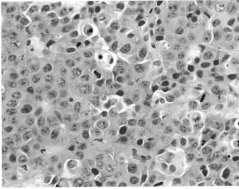

■ **Figure 106.2** An equine seminoma.
Images courtesy of Charles Love.

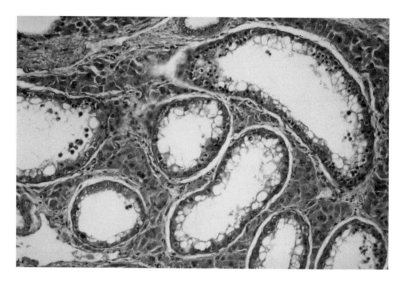

■ **Figure 106.3** Severe degeneration of seminiferous tubules with some germ cell precursors still present.

SIGNALMENT/HISTORY

Risk Factors

Azoospermia and Oligospermia

- Exposure to toxicants (*see* Table 106.1)
- Metabolic disorders
- Testicular heating
- Trauma
- Neoplasia
- Inflammation

Historical Findings

One or more of the following:
- Possibly abnormal sexual behavior or changes in sexual behavior.
- Alterations in appearance or size of the testes.
- Decreased sperm numbers in ejaculates.
- Changes in sperm motility or morphology.
- Decreased conception or foaling rates.

CLINICAL FEATURES

- Azoospermia or the absence of spermatozoa.
- Oligospermia or oligozoospermia indicating that few spermatozoa are present

TABLE 106.1 Toxicants and Physiological Factors That Adversely Affect Spermatogenesis.

Toxicant/Factor	Potential Adverse Effect(s) on Stallions*
Antimicrobials	
Metronidazole	High doses: ↓ sperm number and ↑ abnormal morphology
Tetracycline	Very high doses: ↓ sperm number; ↓ sperm capacitation; testis atrophy
Trimethoprim	One-month course: ↓ sperm numbers by 7% to 88%
Exogenous Hormones	
Androgens	↓ Sperm number; testicular degeneration
Anabolic steroids	↓ Sperm number, motility and normal morphology
Estrogens	↓ Sperm number; behavioral feminization
Progestins	↓ Sperm number and normal morphology; ↓ aggression
Antihistamines	
Chlorpheniramine	In vitro experiments: ↓ sperm motility
Gastrointestinal Tract Drugs	
Cimetidine	↓ Sperm number
Anti-inflammatory Medications	
Phenylbutazone	Inhibition of sperm acrosome reaction; unknown effect on fertility
Prednisone	↓ sperm number and motility; ↓ testosterone
Insecticides	
Pyrethrins	In vitro: 40% to 60% ↓ in testosterone binding to androgen receptor
Heavy Metals	
Lead	↓ Testosterone; ↓ sperm number; ↓ fertilization rates
Physiologic Factors	
Stress	↓ Sperm motility
Fever (hyperthermia)	Damaged sperm chromatin and quality

*Note:

These potential toxicants (many of them are medications commonly used in equine practice) and physiologic factors have adversely affected spermatogenesis in one or several animal species (including horses in some instances).

It is assumed that high enough or long enough exposures to any of these could potentially have similar effects in stallions, despite few or no reported cases.

Depending on the stage of sexual development at the time of exposure, adverse effects can vary in their severity and reversibility.

Adapted with permission from Ellington JE, Wilker CE. 2006. In: *Small Animal Toxicology*, 2nd ed. Peterson ME, Talcott PA (eds). St. Louis: Elsevier Saunders.

- Small testes
- Abnormally large testes, especially with neoplasia or following trauma (Fig. 106.4).
- Softening or increased firmness of the testes.
- Possibly altered sexual behavior.
- Poor semen characteristics:
  - Reduced motility
  - Increased morphological defects (Fig. 106.5).
  - Reduced total sperm numbers per ejaculate or DSO.

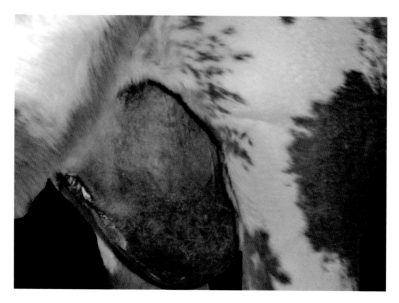

■ **Figure 106.4** Testicular enlargement that can be seen in conjunction with either neoplasia or trauma. Image courtesy of Charles Love.

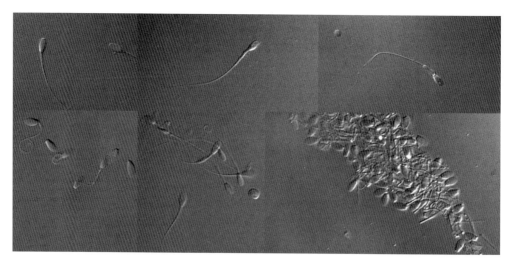

■ **Figure 106.5** Various abnormalities are shown in individual sperm in the top row. Images of multiple sperm with different types of abnormalities, including sperm clumping (bottom right), are shown in the bottom row. Images (top and bottom center and bottom right) courtesy of Charles Love and courtesy (bottom left) of Peter Sutovsky.

 DIFFERENTIAL DIAGNOSIS

- Refer to Causes and Age-Related Factors.
- Failure to ejaculate
- Abnormal ejaculation

- Blockage of the excurrent duct system
- Behavioral disturbances

DIAGNOSTICS

Assessment of Overall Health and Well-Being

- Complete physical examination
- CBC with differential, as well as serum biochemical data to determine inflammatory or stress leukocyte response, as well as other organ system involvement

Semen Evaluation

- Evaluate a set of two ejaculates collected at a 1-hour intervals.
  - The minimum sample size to assess fertility or sperm production ability.
  - Evaluate sperm numbers, motility (total and progressive) and morphology.
  - Sperm numbers and motility can be assessed manually or by use of instrumentation, such as spectrophotometers (sperm concentration) and CASA systems for both sperm concentration, motility (including velocity and direction), and morphology.
  - DIC or phase contrast microscopy are much superior to normal bright-field light microscopy for evaluating sperm motility and morphology.
- DSO arrived at by collecting daily until sperm numbers stabilize.
- Rule out:
  - Bilateral blockage of the excurrent duct system.
  - Ejaculatory disturbances.
  - Behavioral abnormalities that cause failure of normal ejaculation.
- If the cause of azoospermia or, especially, oligospermia is thought to be transient in nature, it is advisable to reevaluate the stallion's semen in at least 60 days (duration of spermatogenesis) after cessation of the insult or disease thought to be causing the problem, to check for improvement. Depending on what aspects of spermatogenesis are affected, the period of recovery might be as long as 60 to 70 days (the duration of spermatogenesis and epididymal maturation and transport).

U/S Imaging

- Assess testicular dimensions and volume and presence of fluid within space between the parietal and visceral vaginal tunics.
- Assess testicular texture and presence of abnormal masses in testis or epididymis.
- Evaluate ampullae if blockage or sperm accumulation is suspected.

Other Diagnostic Procedures

- Measurement of serum/plasma concentrations of FSH, LH, estrogen, inhibin, and testosterone.
  - Daily blood samples for 3 days recommended by some laboratories.
- GnRH stimulation test:
  - Single dose of 25 µg GnRH given IV at 9 AM.

- Blood collected at pre-GnRH treatment and at 30-minute intervals (i.e., 0, 30, 60, 90, and 120 minutes).
- Serum/plasma assayed for LH and testosterone.
- Triple pulse GnRH stimulation test (given in nonbreeding season):
  - Three intravenous doses of 5 µg of GnRH given 1 hour apart.
  - Samples taken 1 hour before and 6 hours after GnRH administration.
  - Assayed for LH
- hCG stimulation test
  - Give 10,000 units hCG IV.
  - Collect blood samples 1 hour before and 6, 24, and either 48 or 72 hours after hCG. Those final samples are now recommended because occasional delayed increases in testosterone have been reported.
  - Assay for testosterone and estrogen.
- Testicular biopsy:
  - Three tissue samples recommended.
  - One biopsy sample fixed in Bouin's fluid or modified Davidson's solution for histopathological evaluation (*see* Figs. 106.2 and 106.3).
  - Two tissue samples placed in PBS and snap-frozen for assay of paracrine/autocrine factors.
- Flow cytometric procedures such as the SCSA or SUTI:
  - Detect alterations in sperm integrity (Fig. 106.6).
  - May be available in some specialized university or research settings.

Pathological Findings

Azoospermia or Absence of Spermatozoa in the Ejaculate

- Absence of germ cells in the seminiferous tubules (rare).
- Arrested spermatogenesis.
- Bilateral blockage of the epididymis or ductus deferens.
- Typically, stallions with congenital absence of spermatogenesis or arrested spermatogenesis will have smaller testes than normal.

Oligospermia or Fewer Spermatozoa in the Ejaculate than Considered Normal

- Small testicular volume with reduced sperm-producing tissue.
- Congenital malformations.
- Testicular degeneration/disruption of spermatogenesis due to toxicants (specific sperm precursors can be targeted), metabolic disorders, or testicular heating (*see* Fig. 106.3).
- Trauma
- Neoplasia (*see* Fig. 106.2).
- Inflammation of the testes or epididymides.
- Partial blockage of the duct system.
- Typically, stallions with chronic oligospermia due to reduced testicular production of spermatozoa will have smaller than normal testes.

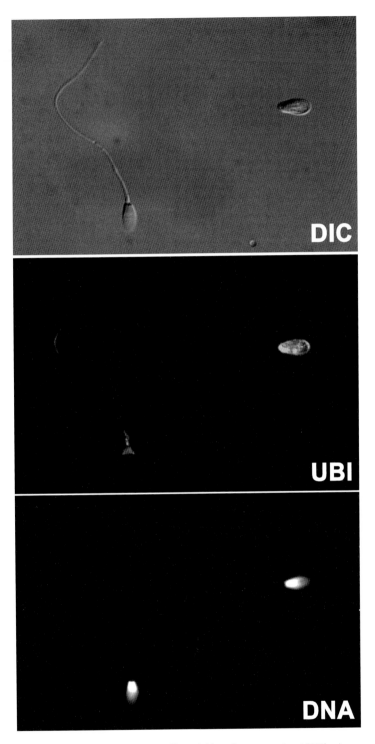

■ **Figure 106.6** Two spermatozoa are shown by differential interference contrast (DIC) microscopy and by fluorescent staining for either ubiquitin (UBI) or DNA. Abnormal sperm are *tagged* with ubiquitin, and the amount of sperm ubiquitination can be assessed using sperm ubiquitin tag immunoassay.
Image courtesy of Peter Sutovsky.

Poor Fertility Following Cryopreservation or Cooling

- The sperm's ability to tolerate these special procedures varies with stallion.
- The causes of increased susceptibility of some stallion's sperm to damage during cryopreservation or cooling are best described as idiopathic.
  - Subtle disruptions in spermatogenesis may not have been identified and cannot be ruled out.
  - Further diagnostics might be indicated.

 # THERAPEUTICS

- Resolve underlying disease condition, if it can be identified.
- Hemi-castration may be indicated if one testis in a valuable breeding animal has been affected by trauma, inflammation, infection, or neoplasia.
- Treatments of infertility due to abnormal spermatogenesis are speculative at best, if the etiology and underlying pathological process remain unidentified.
- If the cause of azoospermia, or especially, oligospermia, is thought to be transient in nature, it is advisable to reevaluate the stallion's semen in at least 60 days (duration of spermatogenesis) after cessation of the insult or disease thought to be causing the problem, to check for improvement.

Nursing Care

- May be indicated in instances of systemic disease or hemi-castration.

Diet

- Stallions should be fed a diet with proper levels of energy, protein, vitamins, and minerals, unless contraindicated by concurrent disease.
- There is recent evidence to suggest that supplementation of stallions with omega-3 and omega-6 fatty acids, as well as their precursors (e.g., docosahexaenoic acid or DHA) can improve some sperm parameters when semen from supplemented stallions is cooled or frozen.

Activity

- Stallions need exercise in a stress-free environment.
- Reproductive function of some stallions is transiently impaired while they are actively involved in competition.

Surgical Considerations

- Hemi-castration may be indicated if one testis in a valuable breeding animal has been affected by trauma, inflammation, infection, or neoplasia.

COMMENTS

Client Education

- An understanding of the length of the spermatogenic cycle and the need for patience are critical.
- Depending on what aspects of spermatogenesis are affected, the period of recovery might be as long as 60 to 70 days (the duration of spermatogenesis and epididymal maturation and transport).

Patient Monitoring

- Semen evaluation following treatment or resolution of underlying condition.
- Minimum recheck interval or BSE of an injured or affected stallion is approximately 2 months from date of recovery (e.g., body temperature has returned to normal post-fever, recovery from frostbite affecting the scrotum or hemi-castration of a testis affected by trauma, inflammation, infection, or neoplasia.

Prevention/Avoidance

- Control fever in instances when stallions become ill or following vaccination.
- Manage minor scrotal edema and underlying etiology.
- Do not administer anabolic steroids or progestins to stallions that currently are or will eventually be used for breeding.
- Use caution in the administration of medications or dietary supplements to stallions that currently are or will eventually be used for breeding.
- Although somewhat controversial, if possible, avoid excessive exposure of breeding stallions to endophyte infected fescue, especially during the breeding season.

Synonyms/Disease Conditions Closely Related to Azoospermia and Oligospermia

- Infertility
- Oligozoospermia
- Shooting blanks
- Sterility
- Subfertility

Abbreviations

BSE	breeding soundness examination
CASA	computer-assisted sperm analysis
CBC	complete blood count
DIC	differential interference contrast
DSO	daily sperm output
FSH	follicle-stimulating hormone

GnRH   gonadotrophin-releasing hormone
hCG   human chorionic gonadotrophin
IV   intravenous
LH   luteinizing hormone
PBS   phosphate-buffered saline
SCSA   sperm chromatin structure assay
SUTI   sperm ubiquitin tag immunoassay
U/S   ultrasound, ultrasonography

See Also

- Abnormal scrotal size
- Abnormal testicular size
- Anatomy review, stallion
- Castration, routine and Henderson technique
- Cryptorchidism
- Disorders of sexual development
- Inguinal hernias
- Semen, chilling of
- Semen evaluation, abnormal
- Semen evaluation, normal
- Semen extenders
- Semen, freezing/cryopreservation
- Seminal vesiculitis
- Sperm accumulation/stagnation
- Testicular biopsy

Suggested Reading

Brinsko SP, Varner DD, Love CC, et al. 2005. Effect of feeding DHA-enriched nuticeutical on the quality of fresh, cooled and frozen stallion semen. *Therio* 63: 1519–1527.

Card C. 2005. Cellular associations and the differential spermiogram: Making sense of stallion spermatozoal morphology. *Therio* 64: 558–567.

Proc 4th International Symposium on Stallion Reproduction, Hannover, Germany, October 2005. *Anim Reprod Sci* 89(1–4): 1–321.

Robinson NE (ed.). 2003. *Current Therapy in Equine Medicine 5*. Philadelphia: Saunders.

Roser J. 2001. Endocrine diagnostics for stallion infertility. In: *Recent Advances in Equine Reproduction*. Ball BA (ed). Ithaca: IVIS.

Samper JC, Pycock JF, McKinnon AO (eds). 2007. *Current Therapy in Equine Reproduction*. St. Louis: Elsevier-Saunders.

Youngquist RS, Threlfall WR (eds). 2007. *Current Therapy in Large Animal Theriogenology*, 2nd ed. St. Louis: Elsevier-Saunders.

Authors: Rolf E. Larsen and Tim J. Evans

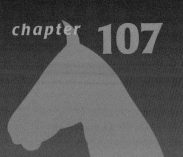

chapter 107

Testicular Biopsy

DEFINITION/OVERVIEW

A testicular biopsy is the surgical collection of a suitable size and quality sample of testicular tissue for histopathologic examination.

ETIOLOGY/PATHOPHYSIOLOGY

- Testicular biopsy is a method of evaluating fertility disorders in the male.
- May be used in combination with semen evaluation to aid in the diagnosis and classification of stallions suffering varying degrees of testicular failure.
- Of particular use as a diagnostic test in veterinary medicine because the economic practicality of hormone assays is limited.

Systems Affected

Reproductive

SIGNALMENT/HISTORY

- It was first recommended to use testicular biopsy to diagnose cases of obstructive versus nonobstructive aspermia, to classify oligozoospermia, and to aid in determining treatment and prognosis.
- Testicular biopsy can help determine many disorders, including but not limited to germinal cell aplasia, germinal cell arrest, hypogonadotropic eunuchoidism, hypospermatogenesis, Klinefelter's syndrome, and hypogonadotropism.
- Testicular biopsy can also help discriminate between inflammatory and noninflammatory disorders, as well as neoplasms.

Risk Factors

- Injuries or illnesses may predispose the stallion to testicular damage.
- If a stallion's fertility has been compromised, depending on the results of a BSE and outcomes of additional less invasive testing, testicular biopsy may be indicated.

Historical Findings

- Inherited conditions that affect the testes are usually evident earlier in life prior to the onset of breeding.
- Otherwise, results of the BSE may indicate the appropriateness, need, or particular indications for a testicular biopsy.

CLINICAL FEATURES

- Decreased/decreasing conception rates.
- Alteration in testicular size.
- Testes that are larger or smaller than normal.
- Indicators on a BSE that biopsy is indicated.
- Palpable changes in the consistency or shape of the testes as detected during a thorough scrotal evaluation.
- Less commonly, lesions identified on U/S, the origin of which cannot otherwise be explained, may be biopsied.

DIFFERENTIAL DIAGNOSIS

Testicular biopsy is an effective means to distinguish between degenerative, inflammatory, and neoplastic findings.

DIAGNOSTICS

- The preferred biopsy technique is the split needle method. The procedure is performed with the stallion standing and sedated. The sedative is chosen by the clinician/surgeon.
- The scrotum is surgically scrubbed with cotton, water, and chlorhexidine or Betadine surgical scrub (Fig. 107.1).
- Local anesthesia of the skin is sufficient. The area to be infiltrated with a bleb of local anesthetic lies at the cranial aspect of the testis, ventral to (below) the caput epididymis (epididymal head).
  - Puncture of the tunic is painless because there normally are no sensory neural pain fibers between the dermal layer and the tunica albuginea.
  - Care must be taken not to enter into the rete testes with the split needle near the anterior aspect of the testes.
  - Removal of the testicular tissue isolated in the biopsy instrument is also relatively painless because of the lack of innervation in the testes.
- Only the scrotal skin is incised with a guarded tip of a scalpel blade.
  - Gently raise up a small pinch of tissue directly over the bleb containing the local anesthetic and nick the skin full-thickness at that site.

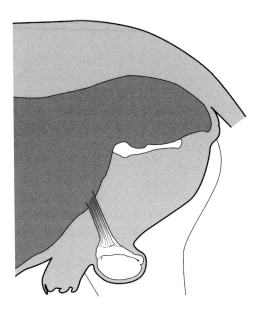

■ **Figure 107.1** Position of the testis in the scrotum.

- The split needle is pushed gently through the incised area, through the tunic albuginea and into the testicular tissue (Figs. 107.2, 107.3, and 107.4).
  - The split needle causes minimal testicular trauma.
  - The testicular sample is held over the container with fixative and gently teased free of the needle's chamber. This is a critical step. It is essential to avoid inducing tissue changes to the small (but nonetheless representative) sample.
  - Although 10% BNF may be used, it is preferable to use Bouin's fixative. Bouin's is particularly useful in defining nuclear tissue detail (e.g., rapidly dividing nuclei of cells; testes, tumors/neoplasms).
- The scrotal incision is closed with an appropriate suture or covered with a wound protective dressing and not sutured.
- No antibiotics are necessary after this procedure.
- This procedure will provide tissue samples of approximately 1.0 mm in diameter and between 2.0 to 6.0 mm in length.

Pathological Findings

- Based on histopathology of the testicular biopsies.
- Results of testicular histopathology from biopsies have included:
  - Maturation arrest, hypospermatogenic tubules, tubular generation, coagulation necroses, interstitial fibrosis, fibrosis of the tunics, neutrophilic inflammation, neutrophilic lymphocytic inflammation, giant cells, tubular degeneration, absence of Leydig cells, arterial thrombi, interstitial hemorrhage, mineralization of tubules, spermatocele and hyperplastic tubules.

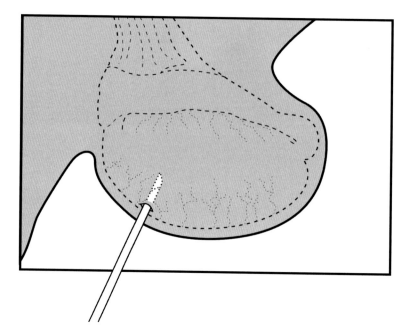

■ **Figure 107.2** Insertion of the split needle biopsy instrument through the tunic into the testis.

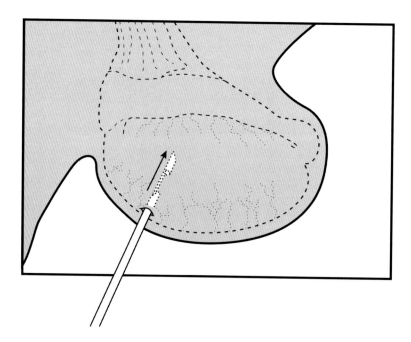

■ **Figure 107.3** Advancing the inner portion of the split needle deeper into the testis.

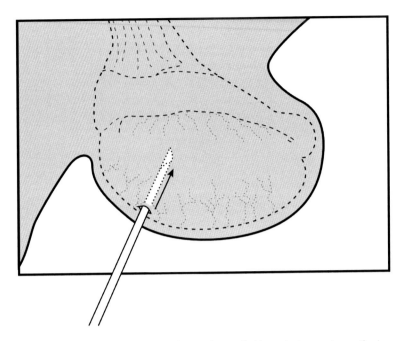

■ **Figure 107.4** Insertion of the outer portion of the split needle biopsy instrument over the inner portion.

 THERAPEUTICS

Drug(s) of Choice

- The local anesthetic is to be placed in or under the skin only. It is important to avoid injecting any of the local anesthetic into the testicular tissue; these agents have very irritant properties.
- Suggested medications for the stages of this procedure:
  - Xylazine: 0.75 to 1.2 mg/kg (0.3–0.5 mg/lb) body weight; dormosedan: 20 to 40 µgm/kg (1–1.5 mL/400 kg) body weight, IV.
  - Lidocaine or Carbocaine (2%): 2 to 3 mL per skin incision site.

Appropriate Health Care

Following the procedure, pay attention to the stallion for any evidence of scrotal swelling or rear limb discomfort. Although I have seen no complications following any biopsies collected with the split needle biopsy method, the potential exists.

Activity

There are no activity restrictions needed following this procedure.

Surgical Considerations

- Contraindicated: Incisional biopsies are frequently associated with adhesions of the testis to scrotum, as well as reduction of testicular size following this technique.
- In all instances, incisional biopsy induced more lesions and more severe lesions than did the split needle biopsy technique.

 COMMENTS

Client Education

Clients should know that additional diagnostic tests are available for delineating causes of subfertility or infertility.

Patient Monitoring

Observation of the scrotum for swelling for the first 3 days is indicated.

Prevention/Avoidance

- Regarding the incisional biopsy technique:
  - It is more invasive; larger pieces of testicular stroma protruding through a surface incision are excised.
  - Adhesions of the testis to scrotum and reduction of testicular size are frequently observed following incisional biopsies.
  - Therefore, this technique is not recommended.
- Proper surgical preparation is important to prevent introducing infection into the testis.
- Entry into the testis with the split thickness needed, as described, facilitates a safer entry into the testis, helps avoid blood vessels surrounding the testes, and thus avoids the probability of hemorrhage.
- Handle biopsy tissue carefully during transfer to the fixative.

Possible Complications

- The most frequently reported complication is hemorrhage from the testicular vessels into the scrotum.
- Hematoma is seen between testicular tissue and the tunics, or between the tunics and scrotum (most common). This is usually due to vigorous manipulation of the testicle.
- Testicular biopsy must be performed gently, without excess tension or torsion on the testicle, the spermatic cord, or the vasculature to the testicle.
- In most cases during split needle biopsy, if hemorrhage is present it can be controlled by exerting gentle pressure with a sterile sponge on the site for 1 to 2 minutes. If pressure is applied until it is certain that bleeding has stopped (has been properly controlled), hematoma rarely results.

Expected Course and Prognosis

Prognosis depends on the histopathologic findings of the testicular biopsy.

Abbreviations

BNF   buffered-neutral formalin
BSE   breeding soundness examination
IV   intravenous
U/S   ultrasound, ultrasonography

See Also

- Abnormal scrotal enlargement
- Abnormal testicular size
- Anatomy review, reproductive, stallion
- BSE, stallion
- Disorders of sexual development
- Reproductive efficiency, measures of
- Spermatogenesis and factors affecting sperm production
- Teratoma

Suggested Reading

Threlfall WR, Lopate C. 1993. Testicular biopsy. In: *Equine Reproduction.* McKinnon AO, Voss JL (eds). Ames, IA: Wiley Blackwell; 943–949.
Threlfall WR, Lopate C. 1987. Testicular Biopsy. *Proc Soc Therio* 65–73.

Author: Walter R. Threlfall

chapter 108

Vaccination Protocols, Stallion

DEFINITION/OVERVIEW

Before vaccinating the stallion, certain considerations need to be addressed:
- The stallion's vaccination status, geographical location, his likelihood of being transported and moved off-farm (showing, breeding, production sale, and so on), the client's budgetary constraints, morbidity/mortality associated with individual diseases for which vaccines are available, and the efficacy of different vaccine products.
- Timing a stallion's vaccinations tends to less complicated than those for mares.
- Scheduling annual vaccinations is determined by season or incidence of endemic disease.

ETIOLOGY/PATHOPHYSIOLOGY

Systems Affected

- Hemic
- Lymphatic
- Immune

SIGNALMENT/HISTORY

Risk Factors

- Do not give tetanus antitoxin to stallions because there is an increased risk of developing serum hepatitis (Theiler's Disease).
- When an injury occurs, if it has been more than 6 months because his prior tetanus protection, the stallion should be administered a booster injection of tetanus toxoid and placed on appropriate antibiotics.

CLINICAL FEATURES

All North American stallions should be vaccinated against: tetanus, EEE, WEE, WNV, and rabies where it is endemic. These vaccines are considered core due to their demonstrated efficacy, safety, and low risk of side effects. In unvaccinated individuals, these diseases usually result in death. In addition, rabies is a zoonotic disease.

- Unvaccinated stallions, or stallions with an unknown vaccinal history, will require an initial series of vaccinations similar to the recommendations for foals.

  Diseases are included in order of their importance, morbidity/mortality/frequency of exposure or relationship to equine health:

Tetanus

- The stallion requires an annual vaccination. As tetanus has a worldwide distribution, all individuals should be administered this vaccine.

EEE/WEE

- Annual vaccination is required.
- If insects are present year-round, semi-annual vaccination may be necessary.

VEE

- Recommendations for VEE mirror those for EEE/WEE in areas where it is present or outbreaks have been reported.
- Present in Mexico and South and Central America; therefore, equids residing in the southern United States are potentially at greater risk for exposure.

WNV

- The protocol employed is dependent on the product chosen. Currently four products are marketed for protection against WNV.
  1. Inactivated vaccine: The timelines for vaccination mirror those for the encephalitides. If starting a vaccination series in an unvaccinated stallion, optimal protection is not achieved until 3 to 4 weeks after the booster has been administered.
  2. Canary pox vaccine: Vaccination follows the protocol for EEE/WEE. If starting a series in an unvaccinated stallion, some protection is achieved after the initial vaccination with optimal protection after administration of the booster vaccine.
  3. Flavivirus chimera vaccine: Vaccination follows the protocol for EEE/WEE. In the unvaccinated stallion, one vaccination provides protection. In an unvaccinated stallion during the vector season, this is the vaccine of choice.
  4. DNA vaccine: This vaccine uses purified DNA plasmids to stimulate an immune response. Annual vaccination provides a 12-month duration of immunity. In unvaccinated stallions, an initial vaccine is given with a booster vaccination administered 4 weeks later, followed by annual vaccination. Not currently being marketed.
- Annual vaccination may be administered using any of the aforementioned products without concern for the product used the previous year.

Rabies

- The stallion needs to receive an annual vaccination.
- Because rabies is zoonotic and fatal, all horses in or traveling to endemic areas should be protected.

Herpes/Rhinopneumonitis

- EHV-1 and EHV-4
- Most often results in respiratory disease, rather than its neurologic form (EHV-1).
- Herpes viruses persist and can recrudesce during periods of stress (e.g., transport, introduction of new horses, and so on).
- Recommendations for vaccination will vary depending upon potential risk factors for the stallion, such as travel, natural cover, and so on.
- Efficacy of the vaccine is no better than 80% (i.e., vaccinated animals may still develop disease).
- No vaccine protects against the neurologic form of EHV-1. Older animals may be at greater risk of developing neurologic Herpes.
- Pneumabort-K may infrequently cause muscle swelling and soreness post-vaccination. If a horse has reacted at a prior vaccination period, selection of an alternate killed product or a MLV for foals and stallions may be appropriate.

Influenza

- The stallion should be administered an annual vaccination prior to the breeding season.
- There are two types of vaccine, an inactivated form and an intranasal MLV.
  - Many companies market an inactivated vaccine. Calvenza® (Boehringer-Ingelheim) is an inactivated product that can be used either IM or intranasally.
  - A MLV vaccine is also available and is called Flu-avert® (Intervet).

Strangles

- Vaccination for Strangles should only be considered for stallions when there is a high likelihood for exposure, such as large breeding farms.
- There are two types of vaccine, an inactivated form (cell wall preparation, Strepguard) and an intranasal MLV (Pinnacle).

Botulism, If Endemic

- Stallions are vaccinated annually. If the stallion has never been vaccinated, he will need a series of three vaccinations administered at monthly intervals.
- Although multiple toxins exist, the vaccine only contains the B-toxin, which is predominant in the southeast and west coast.

PHF

- The current vaccine contains only one strain of *Neorickettsia risticii*. Multiple inactivated, whole cell vaccines of this strain exist.
- However, of the more than 14 strains of *N. risticii*, the vaccine is not protective against these other strains.
- Booster vaccines are typically given every 3 to 4 months during the vector season.

EVA

- Venereal disease (predominately), respiratory (secondary incidence).
- Eighty percent of Standardbred horses have seroconverted by the time they are adults. Exposure is presumed to occur during early months at training stables (nasal transmission) or on-farm. Other breeds have a much lower percentage of sero-conversion.
- Approximately 30% of stud colts exposed at a young age become shedders of EAV in their semen, for variable periods of time. The majority will be short-term, a few months or less. A smaller number will become life-long shedders of EAV.
- EAV can persist in frozen semen.
- A MLV vaccine (Arvac®) is produced by Pfizer Animal Health.
- If a stallion is intended for export, vaccine administration may be contraindicated as some countries prohibit entry of horses with a titer against EAV. Dependent on the country, stable or falling titers (minimum 3-week testing interval) will be acceptable; other countries require there be no (negative) titer. It is important to review the requirements of countries to which a horse might be transported prior to vaccination.
- Vaccination of stallions may be appropriate, but only if prior evaluation has been done, to include serum titer and confirmation of no shedding in his semen (viral isolation).
- Annual vaccination for previously vaccinated stallions. Vaccinations should be more than 4 weeks prior to the onset of the equine breeding season. Vaccinated stallions should be isolated (for 1 month) from nonvaccinated or sero-positive horses, especially pregnant broodmares.
- A cause of respiratory disease in young horses.

 DIAGNOSTICS

Strangles or WNV: may test for high titer before electing to vaccinate.

 THERAPEUTICS

Precautions/Interactions

Strangles: the development of purpura hemorrhagica is possible either from disease or of vaccine origin.

Appropriate Health Care

If a stallion reacts to a certain vaccine, first assess the risk of disease/complications versus the benefit of the vaccine. If vaccination is deemed necessary, initially, select a different company's vaccine because the adjuvant will be different. If the stallion still reacts to the vaccine and the vaccine is a combination product, vaccinate the stallion with the individual component vaccines. In addition, premedicating the stallion with flunixin meglumine may be warranted.

COMMENTS

Client Education

- Because muscle soreness may occur post-vaccination, do not vaccinate within 7 to 10 days of showing.
- Also, to reduce the risk of the stallion developing multiple sore muscles, limit the number of vaccines given at one time to no more than two or three products and give any subsequent vaccines at least 1 week later.

Possible Complications

- Abscessation at injection site.
- Clostridial myositis has been reported post-vaccination.

Abbreviations

EEE	eastern equine encephalitis
EHV	equine herpes virus
EAV	equine arteritis virus
EVA	equine viral arteritis
IM	intramuscular
MLV	modified live virus
PHF	Potomac Horse Fever
VEE	Venezuelan equine encephalitis
WEE	western equine encephalitis
WNV	West Nile Virus

See Also

May refer to specific diseases against which vaccinations are to be protective.

Suggested Reading

AAEP Vaccination Guidelines, revised 2008. www.aaep.org/vaccination_guidelines.htm.

Foote CE, Love DN, Gilkerson JR, et al. 2004. Detection of EHV-1 and EHV-4 DNA in unweaned Thoroughbred foals from vaccinated mares on a large stud farm. Eq Vet J 36: 341–345.

Holyoak GR, Balasuriya UB, Broaddus CC, et al. 2008. Equine viral arteritis: current status and prevention. Therio 70(3): 403–414.

www.boehringer-ingelheim.com/corporate/products/animal_health_horse_01.htm.

www.intervet.ca/products/flu_avert__i_n__vaccine/020_product_details.asp.

http://merial.com.

http://pfizer.com/products/animal_health/animal_health.jsp.

Author: Judith V. Marteniuk

Fetal/Neonatal

Acute Renal Failure

chapter **109**

DEFINITION/OVERVIEW

Acute renal failure is defined as a relatively rapid loss of renal function due to damage to the kidneys. As a result, nitrogenous (i.e., urea, creatinine) and non-nitrogenous waste products accumulate. The occurrence of metabolic disturbances, electrolyte abnormalities and fluid balance problems depends on the severity and duration of the renal dysfunction. Urine production may be decreased (oliguria) or stop entirely (anuria).

ETIOLOGY/PATHOPHYSIOLOGY

Acute renal failure may be subdivided into three categories depending on the cause: pre-renal, renal, and post-renal.

- *Prerenal* disease is the result of changes in the blood supply to the kidney. This is the result of a decrease in circulating blood volume, decrease in renal perfusion pressure, sepsis, or thrombosis of the renal vasculature.
- *Renal* causes of acute failure depend on damage to the kidney itself. This may be iatrogenic from the administration of nephrotoxic drugs. Environmental toxins, myoglobin, hemoglobin, neoplasia, and glomerulonephritis can also diminish renal function.
- *Postrenal* causes of acute failure are the result of obstruction of the urinary tract distal to the kidney. Urolithiasis, pharmacological agents preventing bladder emptying, and a blocked urinary catheter are the most likely causes.

Systems Affected

- Cardiovascular: edematous conditions may result from fluid overload. Electrolyte derangements (hyperkalemia) may affect heart rhythm.
- Endocrine/Metabolic: metabolic acidosis due to hypovolemia is likely.
- Hemic/Lymphatic/Immune: peripheral edema is likely due to fluid overload.
- Musculoskeletal: muscle fasciculations may be present.
- Nervous: altered cell membrane potentials increase excitability and lower the threshold to depolarization (hyperkalemia, acidosis).
- Renal/Urologic: decreased urine volume.
- Respiratory: increased respiratory rate and effort due to respiratory compensation of metabolic acidosis.

SIGNALMENT/HISTORY

Risk Factors

- Decreased renal perfusion: hypovolemia and hypotension as a result of blood or fluid loss.
- Dehydration: hypovolemia due to inadequate fluid intake or excessive losses.
- Perinatal asphyxia: hypoxia and ischemia may result in loss of vasomotor tone of renal vasculature.
- Sepsis: nephritis from dissemination of bacteremia, poor vasomotor tone.
- Nephrotoxic disease: intravascular hemolysis, or myositis.
- Iatrogenic: nephrotoxic drug administration: aminoglycosides, NSAIDs.

Historical Findings

- Decreased or absent urine production
- Peripheral edema
- Weakness
- Apparent colic
- Weakness
- Depression
- Seizure activity

CLINICAL FEATURES

- Peripheral edema
- Uremic breath
- Elevated heart and respiratory rate
- Oliguria progressing to anuria
- Neurological disturbances: in advanced cases, blindness, head-pressing, and seizure activity may occur.

DIFFERENTIAL DIAGNOSIS

- Gastrointestinal disease: peripheral edema due to protein loss and lack of urine due to dehydration from excessive fluid losses. Production of high volume watery feces.
- Inadequate fluid intake: monitor mare milk production.
- Inadequate food intake: foals drink to meet energy, not fluid, requirements. Assess caloric intake and blood glucose levels.
- Uroperitoneum: presence of a large volume of peritoneal fluid, gross abdominal distension.

DIAGNOSTICS

- Confirm oliguria or anuria: average urine output for healthy neonate is 6 mL/kg per hour. In addition to decreased renal function, consider uroperitoneum and decreased fluid intake.
- Monitor USG: affected foals are unable to concentrate urine and will maintain within the isothenuric range (1.008–1.015) in the face of varying fluid loads.
- U/S of the kidneys: consider size, echogenicity, clarity of the corticomedullary junction, renal pelvis dilation, and the presence of any perirenal edema. Loss of normal echogenicity, dilation of the renal pelvis, and perirenal edema are of concern.
- Electrolyte disturbances: hyponatremia, hypochloremia, hyperkalemia, hypocalcemia, hyperphosphatemia.
- Elevated BUN, creatinine.
- Lack of urine production in response to fluid load, onset of peripheral edema.
- Urinalysis: renal tubular damage as indicated by tubular casts and increased tubular enzymes (γGT).

Pathological Findings

Histological evidence of renal tubular necrosis, fibrosis, and inflammation of the renal parenchyma.

 THERAPEUTICS

- Address concurrent disease: fluid loss and sepsis.
- Discontinue and avoid further usage of potentially nephrotoxic drugs.
- Combat hypotension/hypovolemia: intravenous crystalloids, colloids, pressor agents.
- Avoid over-hydration: monitor fluid balance.
- Increase urine output: mannitol 0.50 to 1 g/kg IV, furosemide 1 mg/kg IV (usage of loop diuretics is controversial), dopamine (controversial), dobutamine.
- Manage hyponatremia: renal wasting may be occurring if tubular function is compromised. Avoid fluid overload. Restrict hypotonic fluid intake. Administer hypertonic saline if refractory.
- Manage hyperkalemia: intravenous dextrose (transport into cells) and bicarbonate (address acidosis).
- Manage azotemia: intravenous fluids to establish a diuresis.
- Manage neurological disorders: seizures.
- If refractory, peritoneal dialysis is indicated to combat hyperkalemia and azotemia. Peritoneal dialysis is technically difficult due to requirements for sterility. Omental plugging of dialysis catheter can occur.

Precautions/Interactions

Avoid nephrotoxic drugs.

COMMENTS

Client Education

- Acute renal failure may not respond to aggressive treatment.
- Irreversible renal changes may lead to progressive loss of renal function over time and precipitate renal failure.

Patient Monitoring

- Assess BUN, creatinine, and electrolyte levels.
- Monitor fluid intake and urine production.
- Monitor USG.

Prevention/Avoidance

Care with nephrotoxic agents in hemodynamically compromised neonates.

Expected Course and Prognosis

Approximately 50% eventually recover

Synonyms

Renal failure

Abbreviations

γGT   γ glutamyl transaminopeptidase
BUN   blood urea nitrogen
IV   intravenous
NSAID   nonsteroidal anti-inflammatory drug
U/S   ultrasound, ultrasonography
USG   urine specific gravity

Suggested Reading

Brewer BD. 1980. The urogenital system, Section 2: Renal diease. In: *Equine Clinical Neonatology.* Koterba AM, Drummond WH, Kosch PC (eds). Philadelphia: Lea & Febiger; 446–458.

Author: Peter R. Morresey

chapter 110

Angular Limb Deformities

 DEFINITION/OVERVIEW

Disorders of the musculoskeletal system may be associated with congenital malformations, intrauterine sepsis, abnormal length of gestation, small for gestational age foals, and twinning. Trauma at delivery, neonatal bacterial sepsis, and postnatal injury can lead to additional musculoskeletal problems. Limb deformities can involve angular, flexural, and rotational deviations.

- Angular limb deformities are defined as deviations in the frontal plane, with the name dependent on the joint acting as the pivot point.
- Flexural deformities occur in a plane perpendicular to the frontal plane.
- Rotational deviations are commonly seen concurrent with angular deformities and occur along the long axis of the limb.
- Discussion will be limited to angular deformities. These are further described as varus (distal limb is medial to the affected joint) or valgus (distal limb is lateral to the affected joint) (Fig. 110.1).

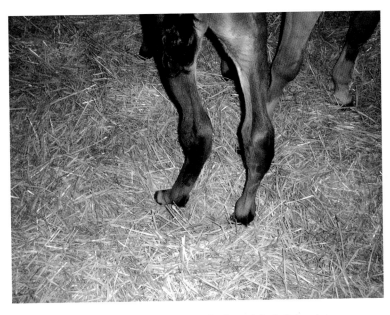

■ **Figure 110.1** Angular limb deformities. Left limb tarsal valgus; right limb tarsal varus.

ETIOLOGY/PATHOPHYSIOLOGY

- Laxity of periarticular supporting tissue
- Cuboidal bones: incomplete ossification or trauma
- Physeal deviations: trauma
- Uneven longitudinal growth along the metaphysis and epiphysis.

Systems Affected

- Musculoskeletal: development of appropriate musculature of affected limbs is affected.
- Skin/Exocrine: interference of limbs during ambulation can cause superficial trauma.

SIGNALMENT/HISTORY

Carpal valgus is the most commonly reported syndrome.

Risk Factors

- Abnormal *in utero* positioning
- Prematurity: incomplete ossification of the cuboidal bones.
- Gestational insults: infectious, nutritional (copper deficiency, caloric restriction).
- Postnatal physeal injury: premature asymmetrical closure of the physis.
- Abnormal weight-bearing: contralateral limb injury leads to overloading of the affected limb.

Historical Findings

Abnormal angulation of the distal limb.

CLINICAL FEATURES

- Apparent lameness or limb interference.
- Valgus: predominantly carpal, tarsal. Carpal valgus (2–5 degrees) appears normal for the early neonate.
- Varus: fetlock is most often affected.
- Abnormal hoof wear: hoof wall on convex aspect of deviation becomes abnormally abraded.

DIAGNOSTICS

- Examine on a flat, level surface.
- Examine weekly until 1 month of age, then monthly until weaning.

- Standing examination: flex limbs to determine ligamentous laxity. Stand in-line with limb.
- Walking examination: determine contribution of ligamentous laxity to appearance of deviation.
- Radiographs: determine degree of angulation, level of deviation (joint, physis of long bone), and degree of cuboidal bone ossification. Assess joint for arthritis. Assess physis for uneven width. Assess shape of cuboidal bones.

Pathological Findings

Malalignment along the long axis of the affected limb. Bony or ligamentous pathology may be present.

 # THERAPEUTICS

Drug(s) of Choice

Analgesics: to stimulate bone growth, remove excessive weight bearing on affected limb if being used to spare contralateral limb.

Diet

Nutritional management: ensure appropriate growth rate and mineral intake.

Activity

Controlled exercise. Avoid overloading affected limbs.

Surgical Considerations

- Physeal origin: minor cases self-correct.
  - Trim hoof to balance compressive forces: release excessive compressive force from concave side of limb (lateral hoof for valgus, medial hoof for varus).
  - Hoof extensions: apply to medial wall for valgus, lateral wall for varus deformities. Useful when no improvement seen in 2 to 3 weeks with more conservative management.
  - Surgical intervention: for more severe cases. Periosteal elevation (on concave aspect) stimulates metaphyseal growth and avoids over-correction. Transphyseal bridging (on convex aspect) slows physeal growth on the convex aspect of the limb allowing concave limb aspect to even up.
- Delayed ossification of cuboidal bones.
  - Strict stall rest
  - Limb splinting/external support: tubular cast to provide rigid support until endochondral ossification completed.
  - Serial radiographs appropriate to monitor ossification and response to treatment.

COMMENTS

Client Education

Carpal valgus is most common, but all angular deformities are regularly reported. Multiple joints are often affected.

Possible Complications

Pressure sores with external supporting bandages and casts.

Expected Course and Prognosis

Mildly affected cases may spontaneously resolve with corrective hoof trimming. External support and surgical correction of most cases is successful.

Synonyms

Knock knees (bilateral carpal valgus)

Suggested Reading

Hardy J, Latimer F. 2003. Orthopedic disorders in the neonatal foal. *Clin Tech Eq Pract* 2: 96–119.

McIlwraith CW. 2002. Diseases of joints, tendons, ligaments and related structures. In: *Lameness in Horses*, 5th ed. Stashak TS, Adams OR (eds). Baltimore: Lippincott Williams & Wilkins; 459–644.

Trumble TN. 2005. Orthopedic disorders in neonatal foals. *Vet Clin North Am Equine Pract* 21: 357–385.

Author: Peter R. Morresey

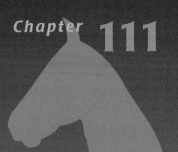
Botulism

DEFINITION/OVERVIEW

A generalized flaccid paralysis caused by the exotoxin of *Clostridium botulinum*. The condition is considered endemic in the eastern United States but has sporadic occurrence elsewhere. Diagnosis is aided by eliminating other causes of neurologic disease.

ETIOLOGY/PATHOPHYSIOLOGY

Blockage of acetylcholine release at neuromuscular junctions results from the presence of *Clostridium botulinum* toxin (eight different toxins). Associated in adults with a suspicion of spoiled feed ingestion. In the neonate, gastric ulceration is considered the most common predisposing factor. This allows germination of *Cl. botulinum* spores in devitalized tissue, with production and local absorption of toxin. Soil contamination of wounds with anaerobic conditions also allows spore germination.

Systems Affected

- Musculoskeletal: muscle wasting through disuse
- Neuromuscular: ascending flaccid paralysis
- Respiratory: death by respiratory failure

SIGNALMENT/HISTORY

Risk Factors

- Foal from unvaccinated mare
- Ingestion of preformed toxin. Less common in foals.
- Gastrointestinal colonization permitted by presence of gastric ulceration (toxoinfectious botulism). Most common in foals.
- Spores germinate in abscess or devitalized tissue where anaerobic conditions prevail (wound botulism). Less common in foals.

Historical Findings

Sudden onset of weakness.

 ## CLINICAL FEATURES

- Generalized weakness
- Fasciculations of the antigravity muscles
- Dysphagia: milk discharge from nose and mouth following suckling
- Ptosis
- Recumbency
- Respiratory paralysis
- Death

 ## DIFFERENTIAL DIAGNOSIS

- HIE
- PAS
- Sepsis

 ## DIAGNOSTICS

- Characteristic clinical signs: weakness to tongue pull, weak resistance to manipulation of eyelids.
- Toxin or spores: assay feed material or affected animal's feces.

Pathological Findings

No pathognomonic lesions for this condition. Diagnosis by exclusion.

 ## THERAPEUTICS

- Antitoxin: monovalent, polyvalent
- Antimicrobials with anaerobic spectrum: penicillins, metronidazole
- Supportive therapy: nutrition, fluids, electrolytes
- Management of recumbent horse: decubital ulcers, myopathy, corneal ulceration.
- Mechanical ventilation: in severe cases with respiratory paralysis.

Drug(s) of Choice

- Monovalent (type B) or polyvalent antitoxin: expensive and most beneficial if used when foals first display suggestive signs.

- Penicillin: 50,000 units/kg (K: IV, every 6 hours; procaine: IM, every 12 hours).
- Metronidazole: 25 mg/kg, PO, every 12 hours.

Precautions/Interactions

Avoid drugs that may potentiate respiratory depression: sedatives and aminoglycosides.

Alternative Drugs

- Cephalosporins: ceftiofur 5 to 10 mg/kg IV, every 12 to 24 hours, 2 mg/kg IM, every 12 hours.
- Trimethoprim-sulfa: 25 to 30 mg/kg, PO, every 12 hours.

Nursing Care

Management of recumbent animal to avoid decubital ulceration.

Diet

Parenteral or assisted enteral feeding (indwelling nasogastric tube) likely required.

 COMMENTS

Client Education

Prolonged treatment may be required. Response to appropriate therapy may be delayed.

Patient Monitoring

Monitor return of muscle strength.

Prevention/Avoidance

Vaccination of pregnant mare in late gestation aids in production of colostral antibodies.

Possible Complications

Decubital ulceration, inhalation pneumonia, recumbency, and death.

Expected Course and Prognosis

Response fair with early treatment and in those cases where the site of intoxication can be eliminated (manage gastric ulceration, treatment of infected anaerobic focus). Poor outcome expected with cases that are advanced at time of presentation.

Synonyms

Shaker foal

Abbreviations

HIE hypoxic ischemic encephalopathy
IM intramuscular
IV intravenous
PAS perinatal asphyxia syndrome
PO per os (by mouth)

See Also

- Meningitis
- Neonatal evaluation

Suggested Reading

Green SL, Mayhew IG. 1980. Neurologic disorders. In: *Equine Clinical Neonatology*. Koterba AM, Drummond WH, Kosch PC (eds). Philadelphia: Lea & Febiger; 496–530.
MacKay RJ. 2005. Neurologic disorders of neonatal foals. *Vet Clin North Am Equine Pract* 2: 387–406.
Wilkins PA, Palmer JE. 2003. Botulism in foals less than 6 months of age: 30 cases (1989–2002). *J Vet Intern Med* 17: 702–707.

Author: Peter R. Morresey

Chapter 112

Cardiovascular Congenital Anomalies

DEFINITION/OVERVIEW

Congenital cardiovascular lesions are rare, as opposed to murmurs, which are common in neonatal foals. These murmurs tend to be predominantly physiologic in nature. Congenital lesions should be considered when a cardiac murmur, signs of CHF, or cyanosis are present in the neonate. Lesions present may include valvular abnormalities, abnormal vessels, or shunting of blood across the atrial or ventricular septum.

ETIOLOGY/PATHOPHYSIOLOGY

Developmental anomalies are likely genetic in origin; however, exposure to unknown environmental toxins or infectious agents may also have a role.

Systems Affected

- Musculoskeletal: wasting of musculature due to poor perfusion.
- Renal/Urologic: renal function compromised due to insufficient perfusion.
- Respiratory: increased pulmonary pressures, pulmonary edema with cardiac failure.

SIGNALMENT/HISTORY

Congenital cardiac malformations have no known inciting cause and are considered evenly distributed across all groups. However, a large retrospective study showed an overrepresentation of purebred or half-bred Arabian foals.

Risk Factors

- Genetic component unknown
- Unknown *in utero* stress, exposure, toxic insult, or nutritional deficiency. Such a factor may be dependent on developmental (gestational) time of exposure for its effect.

Historical Findings

Signs in affected foals range from inapparent to severe exercise intolerance and labored breathing.

CLINICAL FEATURES

Dependent on severity of the lesion and potential for blood shunting: desaturation of arterial blood and cyanosis due to venous admixture.

- Left to right shunt (where systemic pressures exceed pulmonary): ASD, VSD, persistent PDA. Where significant shunting occurs, exercise intolerance, pulmonary edema, tachypnea, respiratory distress, and ventral edema may be evident.
- Right to left shunt (where pulmonary pressures exceed systemic): pulmonary pathology, tricuspid atresia (shunts right to left through VSD and ASD, respectively). May be present with complex abnormalities such as Tetralogy of Fallot. Hypoxemia develops with variable clinical signs evident. Growth is generally poor in affected individuals.

DIFFERENTIAL DIAGNOSIS

- Infectious causes of cardiac compromise: pericarditis, vegetative endocarditis, and valvular endocarditis.
- Thoracic trauma
- Hypovolemia: ongoing hemorrhage, hypoplastic bone marrow.
- Respiratory disease

DIAGNOSTICS

- Auscultation:
  - Left to right shunt: systolic murmur. Most commonly murmur of PDA (continuous, machinery) that can occur up to 4 days before closure in the normal foal.
  - Right to left shunt: systolic murmur. Indicates raised pulmonary circulation pressure and septal defect to allow passage of blood.
  - Valvular lesion: detect by auscultation over the representative area.
- Echocardiography:
  - Allows detection of ventricular dilation, imaging of septal (atrial, ventricular) defects, regurgitant jets, valvular incompetence, vegetative lesions (valvular, mural) and ruptured chorda tendineae.
  - Abnormal anatomy characteristic of more complex anomalies can be detected.
- Radiography
  - Detect cardiomegaly
  - Assess pulmonary vessels or associated pulmonary changes.
- ECG
  - Rhythm disturbances

Pathological Findings

Characteristic anatomical abnormalities of the particular congenital anomaly.

TABLE 112.1 Cardiac Drugs in Common Usage *(Consult specialist text for more complete listing.)*
Antimicrobials
■ K-penicillin 50,000 units/kg IV every 6 hours
■ Ceftiofur 5 to 10 mg/kg IV every 6 to 12 hours
■ Amikacin 25 mg/kg IV every 24 hours
■ Metronidazole 25 mg/kg PO every 12 hours, 15 mg/kg IV every 8 hours.
■ Enrofloxacin 5 mg/kg IV every 24 hours. Care with duration of therapy (5–7 days) and body weight estimation during dose calculations. Discontinue at first sign of synovitis.
Systemic anti-inflammatories
■ Flunixin 1 mg/kg PO, IV every 12 hours
■ Ketoprofen 2 mg/kg IV every 12 to 24 hours
Miscellaneous
■ Furosemide 1 mg/kg IV or IM every 12 hours

IM, intramuscular; IV, intravenous; PO, per os (by mouth).

THERAPEUTICS

Serial examination is necessary to monitor progression of all cardiac anomalies.

- Volume overload, CHF, edema: diuretics, ACE-inhibitors.
- VSD: often an uncomplicated, asymptomatic incidental finding. No treatment may be necessary. More severely affected cases display atrial fibrillation, pulmonary edema, and CHF.
- ASD: uncommon in foals. Exercise (increasing systemic pressure) decreases blood flow across the defect. Small isolated defects may not require treatment. Large defects or those with concurrent anatomical anomalies carry a poor prognosis.
  - PDA: May be secondary to pulmonary pathology (increases right circulation pressure) therefore manage pulmonary disease, if possible. Evaluate for concurrent cardiac pathology. Manage volume overload and CHF.
- Tricuspid atresia: poor prognosis.
- Valvular lesions: manage volume overload resulting from regurgitation.
- Complex congenital anomaly: no treatment possible, therefore, manage secondary heart failure or euthanasia is indicated.

Drug(s) of Choice

See Table 112.1.

Surgical Considerations

Affected animal may be a poor anesthetic risk due to depressed cardiac output, abnormal blood pressure, or deficient blood oxygenation.

COMMENTS

Client Education

Congenital lesions may lead to progressive decline in cardiac function and seriously limit athletic performance. However, many are clinically silent and of no risk to the long-term well-being of the horse.

Patient Monitoring

Regular echocardiography is advisable to monitor any progression of cardiac lesions.

Possible Complications

- Pulmonary edema
- Poor exercise tolerance
- Ill thrift
- Sudden death

Expected Course and Prognosis

- May be clinically in apparent and require no treatment.
- Mildly affected animals may improve with treatment (lifelong treatment may be necessary). Exercise tolerance may be reduced.
- Severely affected animals respond poorly to treatment and are debilitated.

Abbreviations

ACE   angiotensin-converting enzyme
ASD   atrial septal defect
CHF   congestive heart failure
ECG   electrocardiogram
PDA   patent ductus arteriosus
VSD   ventricular septal defect

See Also

- Congenital disorders
- Fetal evaluation
- Neonatal evaluation

Suggested Reading

Bonagura JD, Reef VB. 2004. Disorders of the cardiovascular system. In: *Equine Internal Medicine*. Reed SM, Bayly WM, Sellon DC (eds). St. Louis: Saunders; 355–460.

Lombard CW. 1980. Cardiovascular diseases. In: *Equine Clinical Neonatology*. Koterba AM, Drummond WH, Kosch PC (eds). Philadelphia: Lea & Febiger; 240–261.

Marr CE (ed). 1999. *Cardiology of the Horse*. London: Saunders.

Author: Peter R. Morresey

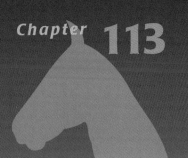

Chapter 113

Cataracts

DEFINITION/OVERVIEW

Opacities of the lens or lens capsule. May be in association with other ocular abnormalities.

Ocular conditions in the foal often go undiagnosed because examination is not commonly performed unless for insurance or sale purposes.

When compared to the adult horse, a number of differences are noted in the foal:

- The pupil is relatively round (contrast to ovoid adult pupil).
- Prominent Y sutures of the lens capsule are present and should not be confused with cataract formation.

ETIOLOGY/PATHOPHYSIOLOGY

- Both congenital and acquired causes
- Heritable: Belgian, Morgan, Quarterhorse, and Thoroughbred
- Traumatic: leakage of lens protein
- In utero insult
- Post-inflammation

Systems Affected

- Nervous: visual impairment
- Skin/Exocrine: cutaneous trauma due to misadventure

SIGNALMENT/HISTORY

Less affected cases are often an incidental finding during routine examination.

Risk Factors

- Genetics
- Ocular insult

Historical Findings

Visual deficiencies in cases that have extensive cataracts.

CLINICAL FEATURES

- Unilateral or bilateral lens opacity; may involve surface of lens or lens itself.
- Visual disturbances may be present.

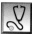

DIFFERENTIAL DIAGNOSIS

- Corneal disease
- Aqueous flare
- Hypopyon

DIAGNOSTICS

- History: occurrence of ocular abnormalities in siblings and other close relatives.
- Assess eyes for concurrent abnormalities.
- PLR and blink evaluation: foal should have appropriate PLR and blink with a bright light shining in the eye.
- Pupillary dilation: retinal examination for abnormalities

Pathological Findings

Characteristic finding of lens opacity

THERAPEUTICS

Surgical Considerations

- Phacoemulsification: young foals (less than 6 months of age) are the best surgical candidates.
- Preoperative evaluation: electroretinography, ocular U/S

COMMENTS

Prevention/Avoidance

Ophthalmological screening of breeding stock

Possible Complications

May have heritable component

Expected Course and Prognosis

Visual disturbances can be compensated for if minor; however, the presence of extensive cataracts or concurrent ocular abnormalities are problematic.

Abbreviations

PLR   pupillary light response
U/S   ultrasound, ultrasonography

Suggested Reading

Gelatt KN. 2000. Equine ophthalmology. In: *Essentials of Veterinary Ophthalmology*. Gelatt KN (ed). Philadelphia: Lippincott Williams & Wilkins; 337–376.

Turner AG. 2004. Ocular conditions of neonatal foals. Vet *Clin North Am Equine Pract* 20: 429–440.

Whitley RD. 1990. Neonatal equine ophthalmology. In: *Equine Clinical Neonatology*, vol. 1. Koterba AM, Drummond WH, Kosch PC (eds). Philadelphia: Lea & Febiger; 531–557.

Author: Peter R. Morresey

Coloboma of the Eyelid

Chapter 114

DEFINITION/OVERVIEW

Ocular conditions in the foal often go undiagnosed because examination is not commonly performed unless for insurance or sale purposes.
- A defect in the eyelid margin. Considered an agenesis because it is a full-thickness defect.
- Similar agenesis can occur in the iris and ciliary body (iris or ciliary body coloboma) resulting in lens abnormalities. Refer to listed texts for further information.

ETIOLOGY/PATHOPHYSIOLOGY

Systems Affected

Ophthalmic: visual disturbances and corneal disease possible.

SIGNALMENT/HISTORY

Congenital lesion

Risk Factors

Unknown

Historical Findings

Epiphora, conjunctivitis, and corneal opacity (keratitis).

CLINICAL FEATURES

- Variable: short full-thickness lesions may appear as a notch in the eyelid margin. Larger defects occur.

- Predominantly lower eyelid
- Corneal ulceration and pigmentation with larger, chronic lesions.

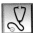 **DIFFERENTIAL DIAGNOSIS**

Trauma

 DIAGNOSTICS

Clinical signs are characteristic.

Pathological Findings

Characteristic eyelid defects

 THERAPEUTICS

Appropriate Health Care

Manage concurrent corneal pathology: ulceration and keratitis.

Surgical Considerations

- Minor cases require no treatment.
- Remove local hair contacting cornea.
- Larger defects: surgical repair

 COMMENTS

Expected Course and Prognosis

Chronic conjunctival and corneal pathology without treatment. Surgical intervention likely curative.

See Also

- Corneal ulceration
- Conjunctivitis

Suggested Reading

Gelatt KN. 2000. Equine ophthalmology. In: *Essentials of Veterinary Ophthalmology*. Gelatt KN (ed). Philadelphia: Lippincott Williams & Wilkins.

Turner AG. 2004. Ocular conditions of neonatal foals. *Vet Clin North Am Equine Pract* 20: 429–440.

Whitley RD. 1990. Neonatal equine ophthalmology. In: *Equine Clinical Neonatology*, vol. 1. Koterba AM, Drummond WH, Kosch PC (eds). Philadelphia: Lea & Febiger; 531–557.

Author: Peter R. Morresey

Chapter 115

Congenital Disorders in Foals

DEFINITION/OVERVIEW

Congenital disorders result from defects in growth or from *in utero* damage to a developing fetus. These disorders are highly variable in their causation and the resulting abnormalities. Significance of the deviation from the expected developmental outcome is dependent on the interaction between the disorder and the extrauterine environment. Unfortunately, those of a genetic basis or those of a severe nature are not often amenable to treatment.

ETIOLOGY/PATHOPHYSIOLOGY

Congenital abnormalities have a number of causes:
- Genetic abnormalities: heritable conditions.
- Chromosomal abnormalities: disrupted cell division or gene translocation.
- Errors of development: disruption to appropriate cellular and tissue growth from exogenous factors.
- Compromises to the intrauterine environment: inflammatory or degenerative changes leading to fetal deprivation.

Systems Affected

- Cardiovascular: Septal defects, persistence of fetal circulation, vascular anomalies, and multiple cardiac anomalies.
- Endocrine/Metabolic: *In utero* deprivation can alter responsiveness to insulin later in life and thyroid abnormalities (e.g, hypothyroidism, goiter, hyperplasia).
- Gastrointestinal: Segmental aplasia, stenosis, aganglionosis (Lethal White Foal), and cleft palate.
- Hemic/Lymphatic/Immune: Severe Combined Immunodeficiency, hemophilia A (Factor VIII deficiency), and IgM deficiency.
- Hepatobiliary: Hyperammonemia of Morgan foals.
- Musculoskeletal: Skeletal malformations, patellar abnormalities, angular limb deformities, agenesis or duplication of the digits, tendon laxity/contracture, muscle storage diseases, HYPP, and occipito-atlantal-axial malformation.

- Nervous: Hydrocephalus, cerebellar hypoplasia, idiopathic epilepsy.
- Ophthalmic: Alterations in the eyelids, microphthalmia, cataracts, and the orbit.
- Renal/Urologic: Ectopic ureter, ruptured bladder, urachal defects, renal agenesis, and polycystic kidneys.
- Reproductive: Intersex conditions, aneuploidy (Turner's syndrome).
- Respiratory: Choanal atresia.
- Skin/Exocrine: HERDA (also known as Hyperelastosis cutis), epitheliogenesis imperfecta, papillomatosis, and umbilical hernia.
- Multiple: Lavender Foal Syndrome.

SIGNALMENT/HISTORY

Present at birth or apparent soon after. Predilections dependent on disorder.

Risk Factors

Genetics, *in utero* stress, and unknown environmental or infectious agents acting as teratogens.

Historical Findings

Physical or physiological deviation of neonate from that expected.

CLINICAL FEATURES

- Cardiovascular: ill thrift, exercise intolerance, and persistent cardiac murmur. With vascular ring anomalies, esophageal obstruction may be evident.
- Endocrine/Metabolic: weakness, low plasma thyroid levels, and musculoskeletal abnormalities.
- Gastrointestinal: structural anomaly of gastrointestinal tract (cleft palate), fecal production abnormal or absent, and abdominal distension and pain.
- Hemic/Lymphatic/Immune: tendency to bleed, immunoglobulin deficiency, chronic illness, and ill thrift that may progress to death.
- Hepatobiliary: Morgan weanlings within 2 to 3 weeks of weaning develop persistent hyperammonemia, ill thrift, and central neurological dysfunction.
- Musculoskeletal: characteristic limb abnormalities (i.e., angular deviations, tendon contracture or laxity, digital absence or duplication), vertebral malformations may result in neurological deficits, and muscle storage diseases become apparent with age.
- Nervous: cerebral abnormalities may lead to abnormal behavior/mentation and seizures. Cerebellar abnormalities lead to uncoordinated movements and tremors. Spinal cord abnormalities lead to unilateral or bilateral weakness and proprioceptive deficits.
- Ophthalmic: characteristic anatomical abnormalities of eyelids (i.e., entropion, ectropion, coloboma), globe (microphthalmia), lens (cataracts), or malformation of the orbit (may be associated with other facial bone deformities).

- Renal/Urologic: anuria (renal developmental abnormalities or *in utero* hypoxia/ischemia, may have concurrent peripheral edema), stranguria (ruptured bladder, may be associated with abdominal distension, pain, electrolyte abnormalities and neurological signs if longstanding), urinary incontinence (ectopic ureter), and patent urachus.
- Reproductive: ambiguous external genitalia. Infertility from gonadal abnormalities or agenesis of the tubular genital tract will not be apparent until later in life.
- Respiratory: dyspnea and cyanosis in the absence of pulmonary pathology.
- Skin/Exocrine: characteristic abnormalities of the skin (detachment of epidermis from deeper layers, HERDA). Multiple papillomas may be acquired *in utero*.
- Multiple: Lavender Foal Syndrome: Arabians only, coat color dilution (may have lightened tips of hair), gray-lavender coat color. Weak and unable to stand, will progress to seizures and death. No known test or cure.

Pathological Findings

Characteristic for lesion.

THERAPEUTICS

See individual condition.

Surgical Considerations

See individual condition.

COMMENTS

Client Education

Heritable factors may contribute to abnormality. Consider genetic testing (if available) of affected animal or parent stock.

Possible Complications

Diminished growth, function, and survivability of affected offspring.

Expected Course and Prognosis

Dependent on type and severity of congenital lesion.

Abbreviations

HERDA   hereditary equine regional dermal asthenia
HYPP   hyperkalemic periodic paralysis
IgM   immunoglobulin M

See Also

- Fetal evaluation
- Neonatal evaluation
- Disorders of the cardiovascular system
- Disorders of the gastrointestinal system
- Disorders of the musculoskeletal system
- Disorders of the neurological system
- Disorders of the ophthalmic system
- Disorders of the respiratory system
- Disorders of sexual development system
- Disorders of the urinary system

Suggested Reading

Finno CJ, Spier SJ, Valberg SJ. 2009. Equine diseases caused by known genetic mutations. *Vet J* 179(3): 336–347.

Lester GD. 2005. Maturity of the neonatal foal. *Vet Clin North Am Equine Pract* 2: 333–355.

Page P, Parker R, Harper C, et al. 2006. Clinical, clinicopathologic, postmortem examination findings and familial history of 3 Arabians with lavender foal syndrome. *J Vet Intern Med* 6: 1491–1494.

Reef VB. 1985. Cardiovascular disease in the equine neonate. *Vet Clin North Am Equine Pract* 1: 117–129.

Saperstein G. 2002. Congenital defects and hereditary disorders in the horse. In: *Large Animal Internal Medicine*. Smith BP (ed). St. Louis: Mosby; 1556–1588.

Author: Peter R. Morresey

Chapter 116

Conjunctivitis

DEFINITION/OVERVIEW

Ocular conditions in the foal often go undiagnosed because examination is not commonly performed unless for insurance or sale purposes.

When compared to the adult horse, a number of differences are noted in the foal:

- The menace response is not present until approximately 2 weeks of age; however, it may develop at any time prior to that.
- Comparatively low tear production
- Corneal sensitivity to stimulation is low, predisposing to traumatic lesions.

Conjunctivitis is inflammation of the conjunctival membranes.

ETIOLOGY/PATHOPHYSIOLOGY

May be the result of direct irritation, blockage of the nasolacrimal duct system, bacterial infection, or a manifestation of systemic disease.

Systems Affected

- Ophthalmic: blepharospasm may obstruct vision.
- Skin/Exocrine: regional tear staining and skin irritation in severe cases.

SIGNALMENT/HISTORY

Risk Factors

- Primary cases due to environmental irritants
- Secondary to other ocular pathology
- Secondary to systemic disease: sepsis, pneumonia (i.e., bacterial, viral)

Historical Findings

Epiphora, reddened eye, and swelling of conjunctiva.

CLINICAL FEATURES

Early signs include serous discharge, hyperemia, and chemosis. Discharge may progress to mucopurulent in chronic cases with secondary bacterial involvement.

DIFFERENTIAL DIAGNOSIS

- Conjunctival foreign body
- Systemic disease: bacterial, viral, or immune mediated.

DIAGNOSTICS

Clinical Signs

- Culture and sensitivity of conjunctival swabs
- Conjunctival scrapings: cytology may show causative agent to be bacterial or viral (intranuclear inclusions) and local cellular response. WBC (eosinophils) where allergic reaction is predominant.
- Assess tear film: check adequacy of production
- Assess nasolacrimal duct patency
- Assess corneal health: ulceration
- Assess intraocular health: uveitis
- Assess palpebral function: decreased blinking leads to chronic drying
- Examine conjunctival sacs for foreign bodies.

THERAPEUTICS

- Flush conjunctival sacs where irritant bodies present: normal saline.
- Flush nasolacrimal duct if blockage suspected: fluorescein dye transport from conjunctival sac to nasolacrimal opening at nares.
- Topical antimicrobials: broad spectrum where conjunctivitis is secondary to another condition. Select based on sensitivity in primary cases.
- Topical anti-inflammatories: care with corticosteroids; rule out ulcer presence.
- Topical antifungals: when indicated
- Topical antivirals: when indicated
- Cycloplegics: relieve ciliary body spasm markedly reducing pain.
- Systemic anti-inflammatories: intraocular inflammation and pain reduction.

Drug(s) of Choice

See Table 116.1.

TABLE 116.1 Ophthalmic Drugs in Common Usage *(Consult specialist text for more complete listing.)*
Topical Antimicrobials
Chloramphenicol 1% every 4 to 8 hours broad spectrum, good ocular penetration.
Gentamicin: 0.3% solution every 2 to 6 hours, 0.3% ointment every 2 to 6 hours.
Neomycin-bacitracin-polymyxin B: every 2 to 6 hours
Tobramycin: 0.3% solution every 2 to 6 hours, 0.3% ointment every 4 to 8 hours. Useful with resistant organisms.
Topical Anti-inflammatories
Topical corticosteroids: prednisolone acetate 1%, dexamethasone 0.1% every 4 to 24 hours. Ensure corneal ulceration is not present. Treatment frequency is dependent on severity of disease. Subconjunctival corticosteroids may be useful if topical application is impractical.
Topical NSAID: flurbiprofen 0.03% every 8 to 12 hours.
Topical Antifungals
Miconazole 1%, natamycin 5% every 2 to 4 hours. Systemic fluconazole 4 mg/kg PO every 24 hours or Itraconazole 3 mg/kg every 12 hours, indicated if local vascularization of the ulcer is present or corneal infiltration is deep.
Topical Antivirals
Trifluridine 1% every 2 to 6 hours
Idoxuridine 0.1% solution every 2 hours
Cycloplegics
Atropine 1% topically every 6 to 24 hours until pupillary dilation, then maintain every 12 to 24 hours.
Systemic Anti-inflammatories
Flunixin 1 mg/kg PO, IV every 12 hours
Phenylbutazone 2 to 4 mg/kg PO every 12 to 24 hours
Anti-collagenase
Serum: autologous serum every 2 to 4 hours
EDTA: 0.05% every 2 to 4 hours
Acetylcysteine 5% every 2 to 4 hours
EDTA, ethylene diamine tetra acetic acid; IV, intravenous; NSAID, nonsteroidal anti-inflammatory drug; PO, per os (by mouth).

 COMMENTS

Client Education

Maintain animal in environment with minimal irritants.

Patient Monitoring

Assess corneal health regularly.

Possible Complications

Chronic low tear production and blockage of nasolacrimal system may occur.

Expected Course and Prognosis

Good response to treatment is expected unless conjunctivitis is secondary to physical irritation or underlying systemic disease.

Abbreviations

WBC   white blood cell

Suggested Reading

Gelatt KN. 2000. Equine ophthalmology. In: *Essentials of Veterinary Ophthalmology*. Gelatt KN (ed). Philadelphia: Lippincott Williams & Wilkins; 337–376.

Turner AG. 2004. Ocular conditions of neonatal foals. *Vet Clin North Am Equine Pract* 20: 429–440.

Whitley RD. 1990. Neonatal equine ophthalmology. In: *Equine Clinical Neonatology*, vol. 1. Koterba AM, Drummond WH, Kosch PC (eds). Philadelphia: Lea & Febiger; 531–557.

Author: Peter R. Morresey

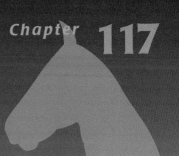

Chapter 117

Corneal Ulceration

DEFINITION/OVERVIEW

Disruption and erosion of the corneal epithelium, basement membrane, and stroma. May progress to an extent that rupture of the globe may even occur.

Ocular conditions in the foal often go undiagnosed because examination is not commonly performed unless for insurance or sale purposes.

When compared to the adult horse, a number of differences are noted in the foal:

- The menace response is not present until approximately 2 weeks of age; however, it may develop at any time prior to that.
- Comparatively low tear production
- Corneal sensitivity to stimulation is low, predisposing to traumatic lesions.

ETIOLOGY/PATHOPHYSIOLOGY

Superficial ulceration may involve only the corneal epithelium and basement membrane. This is usually the result of mechanical trauma to the cornea. Secondary bacterial infection increases severity and discomfort associated with ulceration. Deeper ulcers may progress to involve the full depth of the corneal stroma.

Systems Affected

- Nervous: visual deficiencies from corneal opacity or blepharospasm.

SIGNALMENT/HISTORY

Risk Factors

- Trauma
- Concurrent debilitating disease
- Foreign bodies
- Entropion
- Facial nerve paralysis: lack of blinking

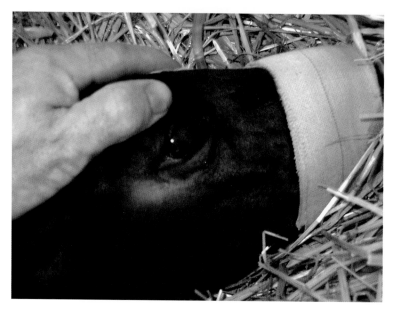

■ **Figure 117.1** Corneal edema and conjunctivitis in devitalized foal.

Historical Findings

Epiphora, blepharospasm, or sensitivity to light

 CLINICAL FEATURES

- Acute ulcer is painful, a chronic ulcer less so
- Epiphora
- Blepharospasm
- Corneal edema, clouding (Fig. 117.1).
- Corneal neovascularization: limbal vessels or corneal vessels.

 DIFFERENTIAL DIAGNOSIS

- Corneal foreign body
- Conjunctivitis
- Trauma
- Uveitis

DIAGNOSTICS

- Ocular examination: light source, assess cornea, pupil, iris, and eyelids.
- Examine for foreign body.
- Flush nasolacrimal duct to ensure patency.
- Assess ulcer margins: be concerned if margins are raised, or if corneal discoloration is evident (necrosis). If a descemetocele is present (as an ulcer), it is a surgical emergency.
- Fluorescein dye uptake determines stromal involvement.
- Culture: bacterial or fungal
- Cytology: corneal scrapings; bacteria or fungal hyphae.

THERAPEUTICS

Treatment is dependent on severity of the ulceration. Uveitis is a likely concurrent condition.

- Superficial, epithelial disruption:
  - Topical antimicrobials
  - Atropine: diminish ciliary body spasm and pain.
  - Systemic NSAID
- Infected:
  - Topical antimicrobials
  - Topical antifungals (if indicated)
  - Systemic NSAID
  - Local clearing of ulcer debris.
  - Atropine: pupillary dilation, decrease ciliary muscle spasm, and pain.
- Melting:
  - Emergency treatment required.
  - Medical treatment as previously mentioned.
  - Surgical intervention: corneal graft, conjunctival flap, or tarsorraphy.
- It is important to detect and aggressively treat fungal involvement. Loss of vision or enucleation is reported in half of all eyes with fungal infection.
- Collagenolysis: prevent with topical autologous serum, 0.05% EDTA, acetylcysteine 5%.

Drug(s) of Choice

See Table 116.1.

Appropriate Health Care

Strict adherence to the recommended treatment schedule

Nursing Care

Discourage and prevent self-trauma to affected eye.

Surgical Considerations

Intervention in cases of deep or melting ulcers (e.g., corneal graft, conjunctival flap, tarsorrhaphy).

 COMMENTS

Client Education

May result in loss of vision or globe despite aggressive management.

Patient Monitoring

Repeated ocular examinations to monitor progress

Possible Complications

Loss of visual field or globe

Expected Course and Prognosis

Superficial ulcers usually respond well if not allowed to progress to deeper corneal defect. Deep or melting ulcers may easily progress to descemetocele and rupture of the globe.

Abbreviations

EDTA   ethylene diamine tetra acetic acid
NSAID   nonsteroidal anti-inflammatory drug

See Also

- Uveitis

Suggested Reading

Gelatt KN. 2000. Equine ophthalmology. In: *Essentials of Veterinary Ophthalmology.* Gelatt KN (ed). Philadelphia: Lippincott Williams & Wilkins; 337–376.

Turner AG. 2004. Ocular conditions of neonatal foals. *Vet Clin North Am Equine Pract* 20: 429–440.

Whitley RD. 1990. Neonatal equine ophthalmology. In: *Equine Clinical Neonatology*, vol. 1. Koterba AM, Drummond WH, Kosch PC (eds). Philadelphia: Lea & Febiger; 531–557.

Author: Peter R. Morresey

Chapter 118

Delayed Ossification of the Cuboidal Bones

DEFINITION/OVERVIEW

Disorders of the musculoskeletal system may be associated with congenital malformations, intrauterine sepsis, abnormal length of gestation, small for gestational age foals, and twinning.

Growth or ossification of the cartilaginous template of the cuboidal bones is delayed. Early and aggressive management of this condition is necessary to allow the normal ossification process to proceed without the development of permanent deformities resulting from crushing of cuboidal bones.

ETIOLOGY/PATHOPHYSIOLOGY

Deprivation *in utero* or premature delivery

Systems Affected

Musculoskeletal: valgus or varus deformity of either carpus or tarsus.

SIGNALMENT/HISTORY

Risk Factors

- Prematurity, dysmaturity
- Congenital hyperplastic goiter

Historical Findings

Visual deformity of joints

CLINICAL FEATURES

- Angular limb deformity: level of carpus, tarsus.
- Hyperextension of carpus, tarsus.

DIFFERENTIAL DIAGNOSIS

- Limb fracture: involving joint or cuboidal bones.
- Periarticular soft tissue laxity

DIAGNOSTICS

Clinical Signs

- Radiography: lack of ossification, deformity of cuboidal bones. Serial studies to monitor progress.

Pathological Findings

Misshapen cuboidal bones. Ossification may be incomplete.

THERAPEUTICS

Nursing Care

Splinting or casting of affected limbs

Diet

Assess nutrition

Activity

- Strict stall rest: allow endochondral ossification to proceed.
- Controlled exercise

Surgical Considerations

Application of rigid external support while endochondral ossification proceeds.

COMMENTS

Client Education

Athletic function likely compromised in affected neonates.

Patient Monitoring

Serial radiographs to assess cuboidal bone ossification and shape.

Possible Complications

Degenerative joint disease. Angular or flexural limb deformity.

Expected Course and Prognosis

Prognosis is guarded with all but mildly affected cases, subject to early and aggressive treatment.

See Also

Angular limb deformities

Suggested Reading

Hardy J, Latimer F. 2003. Orthopedic disorders in the neonatal foal. *Clinical Techniques in Equine Practice* 2: 96–119.

McIlwraith CW. 2002. Diseases of joints, tendons, ligaments and related structures. In: *Lameness in Horses*, 5th ed. Stashak TS, Adams OR (eds). Philadelphia: Lippincott Williams & Wilkins; 459–644.

Trumble TN. 2005. Orthopedic disorders in neonatal foals. *Vet Clin North Am Equine Pract* 21: 357–385.

Author: Peter R. Morresey

Chapter 119

Diarrhea (Bacterial): *Clostridium difficile*

DEFINITION/OVERVIEW

Diarrhea due to intestinal tract infection with *Clostridium difficile*.

ETIOLOGY/PATHOPHYSIOLOGY

Infection with *Cl. difficile* is by the fecal-oral route. Spores persist in the environment for extended periods but overcome gastric acidity and resume vegetative growth in the gut. Pathogenic strains produce toxins A (enterotoxin) and B (cytotoxin), and these toxins act synergistically to produce inflammation, fluid secretion, and mucosal disruption.

Systems Affected

Hemic/Lymphatic/Immune: sepsis

SIGNALMENT/HISTORY

May cause rapid progression from colic to diarrhea and subsequently death within the first few days of life. Antimicrobial usage can predispose to infection and disease.

Risk Factors

- Disruption of normal colonic flora: naïve gut, antimicrobial usage.
- Overgrowth of gut with pathogenic, toxin producing strain.

Historical Findings

Profuse fetid diarrhea, dehydration, and depression.

CLINICAL FEATURES

- Fever initially, hypothermia when advanced
- Diarrhea: mild to severe colitis

- Dehydration
- Colic: secondary to colonic distension
- Anorexia
- Metabolic acidosis
- Electrolyte derangements: hyponatremia
- Hypoproteinemia

 DIFFERENTIAL DIAGNOSIS

- Bacterial diarrhea
- Nutritional changes
- Parasites: *Cryptosporidium, Giardia* spp.

 DIAGNOSTICS

- Clinical signs
- Fecal toxin recovery: refrigerate sample until analysis

Pathological Findings

Severe colitis

 THERAPEUTICS

- Discontinue previous antimicrobial therapy where possible; however, inflammation of the gastrointestinal mucosal barrier allows bacterial translocation and dissemination in neonatal foal.
- Specific anticlostridial antimicrobials: metronidazole.
- Supportive therapy
- Correct fluid and electrolyte disturbances
- Hyperimmune plasma

Drug(s) of Choice

See Table 119.1.

Appropriate Health Care

Maintain fluid and electrolyte balance.

Diet

Parenteral nutrition advantageous

TABLE 119.1 Gastrointestinal Drugs in Common Usage (Consult specialist text for more complete listing.)

Antimicrobials

- Metronidazole: 25 mg/kg PO every 12 hours, 15 mg/kg IV every 8 hours.
- Enrofloxacin: 5 mg/kg IV every 24 hours. Care with duration of therapy (5–7 days) and body weight estimation during dose calculations. Discontinue at first sign of synovitis.
- Ceftiofur: 5 to 10 mg/kg IV every 6 to 12 hours
- Oxytetracycline: 10 mg/kg IV every 24 hours
- Impenem: 10 mg/kg IV every 6 to 12 hours
- Systemic Anti-inflammatories
- Flunixin: 1 mg/kg PO, IV every 12 hours
- Ketoprofen: 2 mg/kg IV every 12 to 24 hours

Anti-ulcer (H$_2$ Blockers and Proton Pump Inhibitors)

- Cimetidine: 6.6 mg/kg IV every 6 to 8 hours, 20 mg/kg PO every 8 hours
- Ranitidine: 2 mg/kg IV every 8 hours, 6.6 mg/kg PO every 8 hours
- Omeprazole: 4 mg/kg PO every 24 hours

Gastrointestinal Protectants

- Sucralfate: 20 mg/kg PO every 6 to 8 hours

Miscellaneous

- N-butylscopolammonium bromide: 0.3 mg/kg IV. Will accelerate heart rate post-infusion.
- Bethanechol: 0.07 mg/kg SC every 8 hours
- Polymyxin B: 6000 units/kg IV in 1-L fluids every 8 hours. Care with duration of therapy and monitor renal values closely.
- Acetylcysteine enema: 8 g in 200 mL water (add 20 g sodium bicarbonate)

IV, intravenous; PO, per os (by mouth); SC, subcutaneous.

 COMMENTS

Client Education

Highly contagious. Outbreaks may occur on farms with a maternal component to disease transmission suspected.

Prevention/Avoidance

Adequate colostrum ingestion. Good hygiene practices.

Possible Complications

Sepsis

Expected Course and Prognosis

Severely affected cases of rapid onset are challenging to treat. Early and aggressive treatment required.

See Also

- Bacterial diarrhea

Suggested Reading

Bueschel D, Walker R, Woods L, et al. 1998. Enterotoxigenic Clostridium perfringens type A necrotic enteritis in a foal. *JAVMA* 213: 1305–1307, 1280.

Byars TD. 2002. Diarrhea in foals. In: *Manual of Equine Gastroenterology*. Mair T, Divers T, Duscharme N (eds). Philadelphia: W. B. Saunders; 493–495.

East LM, Dargatz DA, Traub-Dargatz JL, et al. 2000. Foaling-management practices associated with the occurrence of enterocolitis attributed to Clostridium perfringens infection in the equine neonate. *Prev Vet Med* 46: 61–74.

Wilson JH, Cudd TA. 1980. Common gastrointestinal diseases. In: *Equine Clinical Neonatology*. Koterba AM, Drummond WH, Kosch PC (eds). Philadelphia: Lea & Febiger; 412–430.

Author: Peter R. Morresey

Diarrhea (Bacterial): *Clostridium perfringens*

Chapter 120

DEFINITION/OVERVIEW

Widespread soil and alimentary tract inhabitant. Five types (A through E) based on production of four toxins: α, β, ϵ, and ι. Enterotoxin is produced in an alkaline environment.

ETIOLOGY/PATHOPHYSIOLOGY

Enterotoxins produce hemorrhagic necrosis of the gut wall. Bacterial overgrowth is favored by antimicrobial usage and age-related susceptibilities (naïve neonatal gut).

Systems Affected

- Hemic/Lymphatic/Immune: sepsis

SIGNALMENT/HISTORY

May cause rapid progression from colic to diarrhea and subsequently death within the first few days of life. Older foals present with severe hemorrhagic diarrhea and depression.

Risk Factors

Disruption of normal colonic flora: antimicrobial usage, diet change, and concurrent infection.

Historical Findings

Sudden onset of debilitating diarrhea. Hemorrhagic nature may not be noted.

CLINICAL FEATURES

- Fever initially, progressing to hypothermia when disease is advanced
- Diarrhea: profuse, often hemorrhagic

- Dehydration: rapid onset of profound dehydration is possible
- Depression
- Anorexia
- Abdominal distension: secondary to colonic distension
- Colic: due to inflammation of intestinal wall and gross distension
- Peritonitis: bacterial translocation across the devitalized gut wall

 ## DIFFERENTIAL DIAGNOSIS

Bacterial diarrhea: Salmonellosis

 ## DIAGNOSTICS

- Hematology: leukopenia, left shift, and toxicity
- Clinical chemistry: hypoproteinemia, acidosis, hypoglycemia, and azotemia.
- U/S: ileus, gastric distension, colonic distension, and peritoneal fluid.
- Toxin identification: feces (refrigerate until tested)
- Microbiology: Gram stain or culture of organisms in feces

Pathological Findings

Hemorrhagic gastroenteritis

 ## THERAPUETICS

- Supportive therapy
- Anticlostridial antimicrobials: metronidazole.
- Empiric antimicrobial coverage: susceptible to bacteremia with the loss of mucosal integrity
- Anti-inflammatories, analgesics
- Intravenous fluids and electrolytes: correct deficits and replace losses
- Hyperimmune plasma
- Parenteral nutrition: enteral nutrition may not be able to be digested and adds to osmotic diarrheal component of disease

Drug(s) of Choice

See Table 119.1.

Appropriate Health Care

Maintain fluid and electrolyte balance.

Diet

Parenteral nutrition advantageous

 COMMENTS

Client Education

Highly contagious. Outbreaks may occur on farms with a maternal component to disease transmission suspected.

Prevention/Avoidance

Adequate colostrum ingestion. Good hygiene practices.

Possible Complications

Sepsis

Expected Course and Prognosis

Severely affected cases of rapid onset are challenging to treat. Early and aggressive treatment is required.

Abbreviations

U/S   ultrasound, ultrasonography

See Also

- Bacterial diarrhea

Suggested Reading

Bueschel D, Walker R, Woods L, et al. 1998. Enterotoxigenic Clostridium perfringens type A necrotic enteritis in a foal. *JAVMA* 213: 1305–1307, 1280.

Byars TD. 2002. Diarrhea in foals. In: *Manual of Equine Gastroenterology*. Mair T, Divers T, Duscharme N (eds). Philadelphia: W. B. Saunders; 493–495.

East LM, Dargatz DA, Traub-Dargatz JL, et al. 2000. Foaling-management practices associated with the occurrence of enterocolitis attributed to Clostridium perfringens infection in the equine neonate. *Prev Vet Med* 46: 61–74.

Wilson JH, Cudd TA. 1980. Common gastrointestinal diseases. In: *Equine Clinical Neonatology*. Koterba AM, Drummond WH, Kosch PC (eds). Philadelphia: Lea & Febiger; 412–430.

Author: Peter R. Morresey

Chapter 121

Diarrhea (Bacterial): *Salmonella*

DEFINITION/OVERVIEW

Salmonella is a gram-negative bacteria that is a common pathogen of the equine gastro-intestinal tract. A number of types are described; however, Group B is the most commonly associated with disease. Clinical episodes of Salmonellosis may occur in outbreaks and be a recurrent problem on some farms.

ETIOLOGY/PATHOPHYSIOLOGY

- Between 1% and 2% of the equine population are considered to shed *Salmonella* in their feces at any one time. These horses act as a reservoir of infection for other horses. Virulence of the organism varies widely between strains, with host factors greatly affecting susceptibility to infection and disease. Environmental stressors (especially heat), disturbances in normal gastrointestinal health (i.e., altered motility, pH, altered feeding, loss of commensal flora), and iatrogenic factors (i.e., antimicrobial usage, transport, herding, surgical procedures) have all been associated with the onset of disease.
- Once mucosal invasion has occurred, *Salmonella* organisms have the ability to survive and disseminate within the phagocytic cells. Although spread is limited to the intestinal tract and mesentery in adults, neonatal foals may experience bacteremia, multifocal septic foci, and sepsis.

Systems Affected

- Hemic/Lymphatic/Immune: sepsis
- Musculoskeletal: septic arthritis and osteomyelitis are possible.
- Ophthalmic: hypopyon
- Renal/Urologic: prerenal azotemia from dehydration, however, renal disease is reported.
- Respiratory: pneumonia

SIGNALMENT/HISTORY

May cause acute enterocolitis with rapid progression from colic signs to death from sepsis. Severe profuse watery diarrhea and depression are characteristic findings. Blood and fibrin may be found in feces as may mucosal casts (sloughed intestinal mucosa). Multi-organ failure may follow.

Risk Factors

Disruption of normal colonic flora, physiological and social stressors, antimicrobial usage, dietary change, and concurrent infection.

Historical Findings

Sudden onset of debilitating malodorous diarrhea. Hemorrhagic nature may not be noted.

 # CLINICAL FEATURES

- Fever initially, progressing to hypothermia when disease is advanced.
- Diarrhea: profuse, voluminous, malodorous, and sometimes hemorrhagic.
- Dehydration: rapid onset of profound dehydration is possible.
- Depression
- Anorexia
- Abdominal distension: secondary to colonic distension.
- Colic: due to inflammation of intestinal wall and gross distension.
- Peritonitis: bacterial translocation across devitalized gut wall.
- Disseminated foci of infection: septic arthritis, osteomyelitis.
- Thrombosis

 # DIFFERENTIAL DIAGNOSIS

- Bacterial diarrhea
- Sepsis

 # DIAGNOSTICS

- Hematology: leukopenia, left shift, and toxicity.
- Clinical chemistry: hypoproteinemia, acidosis, hypoglycemia, azotemia, electrolyte derangements (e.g., hyponatremia, hypokalemia, hypochloremia, hypocalcemia).

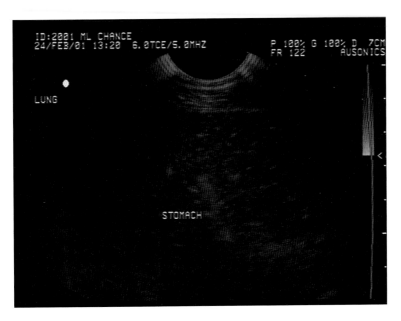

■ **Figure 121.1** Enlarged stomach visible with ultrasound over the left midthoracic area.

- U/S: ileus, gastric distension (Fig. 121.1), colonic distension, and peritoneal fluid.
- Microbiology: Culture of organisms in feces (5 daily cultures), however sensitivity may only be 30% to 50%. Blood culture if sepsis is suspected.
- PCR: single sample to detect organism is useful in early stages; sensitivity of the test is high.

Pathological Findings

Hemorrhagic gastroenteritis

 THERAPEUTICS

- Intravenous fluids and electrolytes: correct deficits and replace losses.
- Specific antimicrobial usage with known efficacy for *Salmonella*: foals are especially susceptible to bacteremia with loss of mucosal integrity.
- Anti-inflammatories and analgesics.
- Hyperimmune plasma
- Supportive therapy
- Parenteral nutrition: enteral nutrition may not be able to be digested and adds to osmotic diarrheal component of disease.

Drug(s) of Choice

- Dependent on isolate sensitivity (variable): enrofloxacin, third generation cephalosporin, oxytetracycline, imipenem.
- See Table 119.1.

Appropriate Health Care

Maintain fluid and electrolyte balance.

Diet

Parenteral nutrition advantageous

Surgical Considerations

Secondary septic orthopedic foci require early and aggressive management to preserve athletic potential.

 COMMENTS

Client Education

Highly contagious. Outbreaks may occur on farms with carrier animals suspected as the source. If new introductions have occurred, screen for shedding.

Prevention/Avoidance

Adequate colostrum ingestion. Good hygiene practices.

Possible Complications

- Sepsis
- Orthopedic: degenerative joint disease and pathological fracture.
- Chronic protein losing enteropathy/malabsorptive syndrome.
- Renal failure
- Infarction: peripheral or splanchnic vessels.
- Pulmonary aspergillosis

Expected Course and Prognosis

Severely affected cases are challenging to treat with poor prognosis. Early and aggressive treatment required to preserve life and athletic potential.

Synonyms

Salmonellosis

Abbreviations

PCR   polymerase chain reaction
U/S   ultrasound, ultrasonography

See Also

- Bacterial diarrhea

Suggested Reading

Byars TD. 2002. Diarrhea in foals. In: *Manual of Equine Gastroenterology*. Mair T, Divers T, Ducsharme N (eds). Philadelphia: W. B. Saunders; 493–495.
Wilson JH, Cudd TA. 1980. Common gastrointestinal diseases. In: *Equine Clinical Neonatology*. Koterba AM, Drummond WH, Kosch PC (eds). Philadelphia: Lea & Febiger; 412–430.

Author: Peter R. Morresey

Chapter 122

Diarrhea (Viral): Rotavirus

DEFINITION/OVERVIEW

An infectious disease characterized by profuse diarrhea, fever, depression, and inappetance. It can affect older foals but is more common in neonatal or young foals. Diarrhea usually lasts 4 to 7 days, although it can persist for weeks. Shedding may continue for up to 10 days post-diarrhea.

ETIOLOGY/PATHOPHYSIOLOGY

Rotavirus destroys the enterocytes on the tips of the villi in the small intestine. Subsequent villus atrophy and intestinal crypt proliferation leads to malabsorption and increased secretion.

Systems Affected

- Hemic/Lymphatic/Immune: secondary bacterial infections are common
- Musculoskeletal: muscle wasting
- Respiratory: secondary pneumonia possible

SIGNALMENT/HISTORY

Suckling foals are most at risk. Neonates are immunologically naïve and the most susceptible. Foals up to 6 months of age can be infected, but the disease is predominantly seen at less than 3 months of age.

Risk Factors

Crowding and other social stresses may lead to increased viral shedding.

Historical Findings

Depression and anorexia progressing to watery diarrhea.

CLINICAL FEATURES

- Diarrhea: loss of intestinal brush border epithelium and enzymes within it (lactase) leads to lactose intolerance. Lactose enters the colon allowing bacterial overgrowth; fermentation occurs releasing osmotically active substances and osmotic diarrhea results.
- Abdominal distension: severe colonic distension due to ileus, gas production, and loss of fluid into the lumen.
- Fever
- Depression
- Loss of body condition

 # DIFFERENTIAL DIAGNOSIS

- Foal heat diarrhea (unknown etiology, likely nutritional and maturation changes).
- Bacterial diarrhea
- Nutritional changes
- Parasites: *Cryptosporidium*, *Giardia* spp.

 # DIAGNOSTICS

- U/S: distended colon
- Fecal virus: EM, ELISA, latex agglutination (Rotazyme®)

Pathological Findings

Colitis, dehydration, and emaciation

 # THERAPEUTICS

- Supportive
- Intravenous fluids and electrolytes: correct deficits and replace ongoing losses.
- Hyperimmune plasma
- Empiric: antimicrobials (controversial although neonates are susceptible to bacteremia), anti-ulcer, anti-diarrheals.
- Prevention: mare vaccination pre-foaling

Drug(s) of Choice

See Table 119.1.

Appropriate Health Care

Lactase: 100 units/kg PO every 8 hours

Nursing Care

Maintain appropriate fluid and electrolyte balance.

Diet

Oral feeding may have to be discontinued to avoid distension and colic. Loss of lactase enzyme in the brush border may lead to transient lactose intolerance.

Surgical Considerations

Not a surgical condition; however, severe colonic distension may necessitate surgical decompression in cases of intractable pain.

 COMMENTS

Client Education

Disease is highly contagious. Virus may be shed up to 10 days following apparent recovery and is known to persist up to 9 months in the environment.

Prevention/Avoidance

- Vaccination of pregnant mares
- Adequate colostral protection
- Phenolic disinfectants: bleach, chlorhexidine, and quaternary compounds do not appear to be effective.

Possible Complications

Weight loss, poor growth rate, and general ill thrift may persist for some time following recovery from diarrhea.

Expected Course and Prognosis

Older and less severely affected foals have a shorter duration of disease and faster recovery.

Abbreviations

EM   electron microscopy
ELISA   enzyme-linked immunosorbant assay
PO   per os (by mouth)
U/S   ultrasound, ultrasonography

See Also

- Bacterial diarrhea

Suggested Reading

Byars TD. 2002. Diarrhea in foals. In: *Manual of Equine Gastroenterology*. Mair T, Divers T, Duscharme N (eds). Philadelphia: W. B. Saunders; 493–495.

East LM, Dargatz DA, Traub-Dargatz JL, et al. 2000. Foaling-management practices associated with the occurrence of enterocolitis attributed to Clostridium perfringens infection in the equine neonate. *Prev Vet Med* 46: 61–74.

Wilson JH, Cudd TA. 1980. Common gastrointestinal diseases. In: *Equine Clinical Neonatology*. Koterba AM, Drummond WH, Kosch PC (eds). Philadelphia: Lea & Febiger; 412–430.

Author: Peter R. Morresey

Chapter 123

Disorders of Sexual Development

DEFINITION/OVERVIEW

- Sexual differentiation occurs sequentially at three levels: genetic, gonadal, and phenotypic. Errors at any level lead to varying degrees of genital ambiguity and aberrant reproductive function.
- Affected animals are known as intersexes or as particular classes of hermaphrodites: true hermaphrodites or pseudohermaphrodites, with the latter further subdivided into male and female.

ETIOLOGY/PATHOPHYSIOLOGY

- Genetic sex is established at fertilization.
- Gonadal sex is controlled by genetic sex determination.
- Phenotypic sex is governed by gonadal function and target-organ sensitivity.

Disorders of Genetic Sex

- *Sex chromosomes abnormalities*: result from an abnormal number (aneuploidy) or abnormal structure (i.e., deletion, duplication/insertion, reciprocal exchange, fusion, inversion) of the chromosomes.
- *Chimera*: an individual with coexisting, genetically distinct cell populations admixed *in utero* from different genetic sources.
- *Mosaic*: an individual with coexisting, genetically distinct cell populations caused by errors in chromosomal segregation during cell division of a single genetic source.
- Normality of genetic sex development depends on normality of sex chromosomal pairings during gametogenesis and fertilization. Spontaneous errors during cell division affecting gonadal development may occur early during embryonic life.
- The SRY gene initiates testicular development.
  - If present, the animal develops testicular tissue regardless of the number of X chromosomes present.

- 63,XO: the most common abnormality noted and considered similar to Turner's syndrome in humans.
  - Also known as ovarian dysgenesis.
  - Affected horses are small in stature and are phenotypic females.
- 65,XXY: similar to Klinefelter's syndrome in humans. Phenotypic males with hypoplastic testes and normal to hypoplastic genitalia.
- Numerous possible sex chromosome combinations (mixoploidies) are reported.

Disorders of Gonadal Sex

- Sex reversal syndromes: gonadal and genetic sex may disagree. This can result from autosomal recessive genes or translocation of the TDF to the X chromosomes.
- XY with no testes: considered to be an XY female. Female phenotype with hypoplastic ovary/streak gonad, acyclic, and sterile.
- XX with varying degrees of testicular development: an extreme form is the XX male, otherwise a true hermaphrodite is considered to result.
- True hermaphrodite with ovotestes: these horses have ambiguous genitalia and are named by their genetic makeup, either XX or XY.

Disorders of Phenotypic Sex

- Genetic and gonadal sex agree, but ambiguous external genitalia is present.
- Phenotypic sex development involves differentiation of tubular genitalia (mesonephric and paramesonephric ducts) and external genitalia under direction of the gonad.
- Degree of masculinization of external genitalia relates to the proportion of testicular tissue on the intersex gonad.
- Male reproductive tract formation is dependent on the gonad producing testosterone (Leydig cells) and Müllerian-inhibitory substance (Sertoli cells) at the appropriate time during gestation.
- Target tissue (duct system) must have cytosolic receptors for testosterone and enzyme 5α-reductase to produce dihydrotestosterone, the androgen responsible for tubular and external genitalia differentiation.
- Hypospadia: urethra opens ventrally on penis.
- Epispadia: urethra opens dorsally on penis.
- Pseudohermaphrodite: named by the gonadal tissue present: male (testes), female (ovary).
- Testicular feminization: genetic/gonadal male but external genitalia female due to target-organ insensitivity to dihydrotestosterone.

Systems Affected

- *Renal/Urologic*: anatomical abnormalities of distal urinary tract may lead to urine stasis and ascending infections.
- *Reproductive*: retention of normal reproductive tract secretions may lead to septic foci.

SIGNALMENT/HISTORY

- Genetic basis possible due to abnormal chromosomal number or gene translocation from sex chromosome to autosome.
- Familial basis due to chromosomal abnormalities possible.

Risk Factors

- Congenital: heritable (from pre-existing) or spontaneous (due to cell division abnormalities).
- Genetic abnormalities: zygote fusion during embryogenesis leading to chimerism. Placental admixture not reported in equines (compare to ruminant species).
- Exogenous: steroid hormone use during pregnancy: Progestins and androgens reported to masculinize females. Estrogens and antiandrogens can feminize males.

Historical Findings

- Abnormal external genitalia
- Lack of appropriate behavior: cyclicity, mating.
- Infertility

CLINICAL FEATURES

Abnormal sexual differentiation presents as a congenital disorder (present at birth). However, normal external genitalia may be present, delaying detection of problems until the affected individual enters a breeding program.

Reproductive Performance

- Failure to display appropriate reproductive behavior with opposite sex or attraction to same sex.
- Infertility/sterility

Physical Examination Findings

External

- Female: normal or hypoplastic vulva, presence of an enlarged clitoris or os clitoris. Purulent vulvar discharge due to retention of secretions by segmental anomalies of the tubular tract.
- Male: penis and prepuce may be normal or hypoplastic. Testes can appear scrotal or cryptorchid. Penile urethral abnormalities include hypospadia and epispadia (abnormal position of urinary orifice, closure of urethra).

Internal

- Abnormal gonadal position (cryptorchid), form (hypoplastic, fibrous) or type (ovotestis).
- Aberrant ductal derivatives: aplasia, hypoplasia or cysts associated with the tubular genitalia.

DIFFERENTIAL DIAGNOSIS

Phenotypically Normal

- *Female*: infectious infertility (endometritis), noninfectious infertility (endometrial degeneration).
- *Male*: infectious infertility (venereal diseases), noninfectious infertility (testicular hypoplasia or degeneration).

Aberrant Behavior

- Female: granulosa-theca cell tumor.
- Male: estrogen secreting tumor (Sertoli cell tumor).

DIAGNOSTICS

CBC/Biochemistry/Urinalysis: Unremarkable, unless cystitis or infection results from aberrant genital structure.

Hormonal Assays

- Testosterone: hCG challenge: collect baseline serum sample then administer 3000 IU hCG. Collect blood samples at 3 and 24 hours, and the final at 48 to 72 hours (a few horses will exhibit a delayed rise in serum testosterone levels). An increase in testosterone indicates testicular tissue is present, more specifically a functional Leydig cell population.
- Estrone Sulfate: Its source in the male is the Sertoli cells of the testicles. Couple its measurement with testosterone (hCG challenge as above) to improve diagnostic accuracy.

Immunology

- Test for 5α-reductase or cytosolic receptor.
- Use labial skin only, as receptors are site specific.

Karyotyping

- Culture of peripheral blood leukocytes and examination of metaphase chromosome spreads to identify sex chromosomes. Collect whole blood in heparin or ACD and send samples unrefrigerated by rapid courier. Cultures require 48 to 72 hours.

PCR

- Detection of SRY. Uses whole blood in EDTA.

Imaging

- U/S, coupled with TRP, in the female or of the scrotal content in the stallion.
- Visualize mass lesions (neoplastic) or cysts (segmental aplasia with fluid dilations).

Pathological Findings

Disorders are categorized by histopathology of the gonad, morphology of the tubular genitalia (duct derivatives), the accessory glands (male), and appearance of the external genitalia (increased anogenital distance, vulvar folds, blind-ended vagina).

 THERAPEUTICS

Treatment is not always required.
- Management: to avoid aberrant sexual behavior where indicated.
- Surgical correction of genital abnormalities if they are leading to secondary complications.

Appropriate Health Care

Not applicable, unless resulting pathology or physical/behavioral problems develop that require gonadectomy or hysterectomy to modify behavior.

Activity

Removal from breeding programs

Surgical Considerations

Correction of genital tract abnormalities if secondary complications arise (e.g., persistent urinary tract infections).

COMMENTS

Client Education

Remove from breeding programs. If a genetic basis is suspected, screen the parent stock.

Patient Monitoring

Only if physical or behavioral complications develop

Prevention/Avoidance

Remove carrier animals from the breeding population: gonadectomy.

Possible Complications

If not detected early, pyometra, cystitis, hematuria, or gonadal neoplasia (intra- abdominal testis) may result.

Expected Course and Prognosis

Uneventful condition if secondary complications do not occur. Prognosis for life good, for reproduction poor.

Synonyms

- Hermaphrodite
- Intersex
- Klinefelter's syndrome: trisomy
- Mesonephric: Wolffian
- Paramesonephric: Müllerian
- Pseudohermaphrodite
- Turner's syndrome: monosomy X

Abbreviations

ACD	acid citrate dextrose
CBC	complete blood count
EDTA	ethylene diamine tetraacetic acid
hCG	human chorionic gonadotropin
PCR	polymerase chain reaction
SRY	sex-determining region of the Y chromosome
TDF	testis-determining factor
TRP	transrectal palpation
U/S	ultrasound, ultrasonography

Suggested Reading

Bowling AT, Hughes JP. 1993. Cytogenetic abnormalities. In: *Equine Reproduction*. McKinnon AO, Voss JL (eds). Philadelphia: Lea & Febiger; 258–265.

Halnan CR. 1985. Equine cytogenetics: role in equine veterinary practice. *Equine Vet J* 17: 173–177.

Meyers-Wallen VN. 1997. Normal sexual development and intersex conditions in domestic animals. In: *Proc Reprod Path Symp*. Sponsored by the ACT/SFT. Hastings, Nebraska; 18–28.

Meyers-Wallen VN, Hurtgen J, Schlafer D, et al. 1997. Sry XX true hermaphroditism in a Pasofino horse. *Equine Vet J* 29: 404–408.

Milliken JE, Paccamonti DL, Shoemaker S, et al. 1995. XX male pseudohermaphroditism in a horse. *JAVMA* 207: 77–79.

Author: Peter R. Morresey

Chapter 124

Entropion

DEFINITION/OVERVIEW

Ocular conditions in the foal often go undiagnosed because examination is not commonly performed unless for insurance or sale purposes.

When compared to the adult horse, a number of differences are noted in the foal:

- The menace response is not present until approximately 2 weeks of age; however, it may develop at any time prior to that.
- Comparatively low tear production
- Corneal sensitivity to stimulation is low, predisposing to traumatic lesions. Inward rolling of the eyelid margin causing corneal irritation from cutaneous contact.

ETIOLOGY/PATHOPHYSIOLOGY

An inherited primary defect in Thoroughbreds; however, secondary causes are more common. Secondary causes include enophthalmos from weight loss or dehydration, spastic entropion resulting from ocular inflammation, and conformational problems.

Systems Affected

Ophthalmic: corneal abrasion, keratitis, and ulceration. Epiphora and blepharospasm result.

SIGNALMENT/HISTORY

May be congenital or acquired secondary to systemic illness, ocular inflammation, or regional trauma.

Risk Factors

- Prematurity
- Dehydration, weight loss: eyelid contacts cornea
- Recumbency, general debilitation

- Blepharospasm from ocular pathology and inflammation
- Corneal ulceration: corneal pain with spastic contraction of *obicularis oculi*
- Microphthalmos

Historical Findings

Epiphora, enophthalmos

 CLINICAL FEATURES

- Epiphora
- Secondary keratitis and corneal ulceration may develop due to abrasion of cornea from hair.
- Lower lid more commonly affected.

 DIFFERENTIAL DIAGNOSTICS

- Trauma
- Conjunctivitis and chemosis

 DIAGNOSTICS

- Topical analgesics relieve spasm and allow assessment of eyelid position and corneal inspection. Do not use therapeutically because continued usage is detrimental to the corneal epithelium.

 THERAPEUTICS

- Dependent on cause
- Restore hydration and nutrition of systemically ill patients
- Manage secondary ulceration, if present

Drug(s) of Choice

- Lubricating ophthalmic ointment

Nursing Care

Minor cases may resolve with periodic *rolling out* of affected lower eyelid and application of ophthalmic lubricants.

Surgical Considerations

Suture: mattress sutures to evert lower eyelid. Assess when eyelid muscular spasm has resolved. Ectropion may result following repair. Sutures may remain in place for 7 to 21 days. Apply topical antimicrobial or lubricating treatments to affected eye as required.

 # COMMENTS

Client Education

Repeated procedures may be necessary to achieve resolution.

Expected Course and Prognosis

Complete resolution is expected with timely repair. Secondary ulceration and keratitis may prolong therapy time.

Suggested Reading

Gelatt KN. 2000. Equine ophthalmology. In: *Essentials of Veterinary Ophthalmology*. Gelatt KN (ed). Philadelphia: Lippincott Williams & Wilkins; 337–376.
Turner AG. 2004. Ocular conditions of neonatal foals. Vet *Clin North Am Equine Pract* 20: 429–440.
Whitley RD. 1990. Neonatal equine ophthalmology. In: *Equine Clinical Neonatology*, vol. 1. Koterba AM, Drummond WH, Kosch PC (eds). Philadelphia: Lea & Febiger; 531–557.

Author: Peter R. Morresey

Chapter 125

Fetal Evaluation

DEFINITION/OVERVIEW

- Despite advances in neonatal intensive care, perinatal death is still a major cause of foal mortality.
- Assessment of feto-placental well-being during the later stages of pregnancy aims to identify mares at risk of an abnormal pregnancy or delivery, identifying them for closer supervision during the periparturient period.
- Fetal evaluation may also allow earlier detection, treatment, and possibly prevention of neonatal morbidity and mortality.

ETIOLOGY/PATHOPHYSIOLOGY

- Maternal history: illness during gestation can result in *in utero* fetal deprivation. A previous delivery of a compromised neonate is also a risk factor for the current pregnancy.
- Prolonged gestation: may indicate fetal deprivation.
- Placental pathology: placentitis leads to placental thickening or premature separation.

Systems Affected

- Cardiovascular
- Endocrine/Metabolic
- Gastrointestinal
- Hemic/Lymphatic/Immune
- Hepatobiliary
- Musculoskeletal
- Nervous
- Neuromuscular
- Ophthalmic
- Renal/Urologic
- Reproductive
- Respiratory
- Skin/Exocrine

SIGNALMENT/HISTORY

- History of previous pregnancy failure or compromise.
- Systemic illness noted during the current gestation.

Risk Factors

- Placentitis
- Placental dysfunction/insufficiency other than from placentitis: microcotyledonary development is poorest in aged multiparous mares; degenerative endometrial changes.
- Aged primiparous mares have markedly decreased microcotyledon density compared to young multiparous mares.

Historical Findings

- Premature udder development
- Premature lactation
- Vaginal discharge
- Sudden increase of abdominal volume
- Surgery

DIAGNOSTICS

Mare

Fetal compromise is difficult to detect with a routine physical examination of the mare.

Clinical Examination

- Due to the size of the fetus and dam, a physical evaluation of the entire conceptus during the later stages of gestation is difficult.
- Examination per rectum: volume of fetal fluids, uterine size, and presence of fetus.
- Excessive volume of fetal fluids in cases of hydrops allantois or hydrops amnion (Fig. 125.1).
- Decreased fetal fluids may indicate a dead fetus.
- Uterine tone may vary during late pregnancy due to periods of myometrial activity.
- Fetal movements are variably present during a *per rectum* examination. Fetal activity alternates with periods of quiescence in late pregnancy.
- A speculum or manual examination *per vaginum* is of greatest use when purulent or sero-sanguineous discharge is present.
- Abdominal palpation is unreliable, provides little information unless active fetal movements are felt.

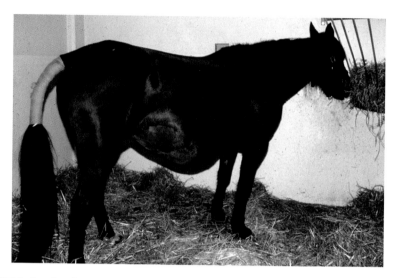

■ **Figure 125.1** Grossly enlarged late gestational mare affected by hydrops allantois. A viable fetus was delivered from this mare.
Image courtesy of C. L. Carleton.

U/S Evaluation

- Monitoring of the fetus and placenta is useful for mares near term considered at risk of abortion.
- Evaluation of the late gestation fetus includes the fetal HR, activity, size, position, and aspects of the utero-placental unit. Identification of fetuses, later born compromised or even dead, is possible. A favorable evaluation does not guarantee a positive outcome.
- Transrectal and transabdominal evaluation of the equine fetus near term is difficult because of its large size, ventral position in the abdomen, and the limited depth of penetration of commonly available ultrasound equipment.

Fetus

HR

- Fetal HR of normal fetuses declines gradually as parturition approaches. There is a huge variation in values, even within an individual's serial examinations.
- Short periods of tachycardia are common; considered normal, especially if concurrent with fetal movements.
- Persistent tachycardia is a concerning sign and may indicate fetal or placental infection, maternal illness, or fetal compromise.

Breathing

- Observed when diaphragm is visualized.
- Noted from 8 months gestation to term.

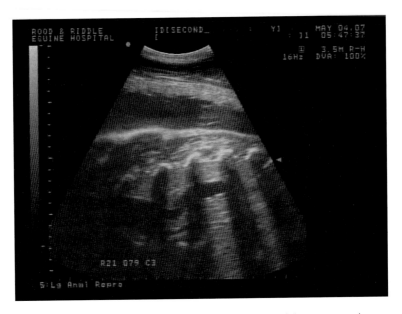

■ **Figure 125.2** Transabdominal ultrasonography showing fetal heart and the great vessels.

Activity

- A reflection of fetal CNS function.
- Late gestation fetal movements range from limb flexion and extension, to generalized, coordinated activities.
- Simple fetal movements are present regularly from day 90 onward.
- Complex movements are normal in the last 3 months of gestation.
- Inactivity observed in fetuses of all ages; more common late in gestation.
- Prolonged inactivity or hyperactivity is suggestive of fetal distress.

Size

- U/S measurement of fetal body structures: crown-rump length, biparietal diameter of the cranium, aortic diameter, and the dimensions of the eyeball (Fig. 125.2).
- Fetal aortic diameter is significantly correlated with neonatal foal weight, girth, and hip height in normal pregnancies.
- Aortic diameter can serve as an indicator of unfavorable intrauterine conditions.
- Significant relationship between fetal orbital size and gestational age, to estimate fetal growth trend.

Presentation

- Frequent changes in fetal presentation have been observed in studies investigating the mobility of the equine fetus.

- Variability of fetal presentation decreases with advancing gestational age. From day 270 to term, presentation is anterior, occasionally transverse. Equal likelihood of anterior or posterior presentation during the first 5 months of gestation.
- Fetus in posterior presentation in the last 2 month of gestation is unusual.

Placenta

Placental Membranes and Fluid

- Utero-placental thickness: CTUP is measured at the level of the cervical-placental junction during a transrectal examination or at a place where no fetal parts are in contact with the placenta, if it is performed transabdominally.
- Premature or exaggerated increases in CTUP, or where placental separation is detected, suggests placentitis.
- Fetal fluid volume: if excessive, suggests hydrops; decreased amount, suggests fetal compromise.
- Fetal fluid content: Anechoic fluid, during late gestation debris is present in amniotic fluid.
- Considerable debris detected in the fetal fluids on several occasions may indicate placental pathology or fetal demise.
- In known cases of placentitis, changes in the echogenicity of the fetal fluids often has not been observed.

Other

Hormonal/Biochemical Maternal Values

- Declining concentrations of estrogens before day 280 are related to fetal compromise.
- Some mares show no decrease in estrogen concentrations before aborting.
- Progesterone, various other progestagens and their metabolites, differ between normal and abnormal pregnancies; however, no clear link exists between maternal progestagens and pregnancy maintenance.
- Mares with placentitis had increased concentrations of either P5 and P4 and several metabolites, suggesting increased fetal production of P5 and P4 and increased metabolism in the utero-placental tissues in response to chronic stress.
- Mares with other placental pathology had raised P4 concentrations, while 5α-DHP and 3β-5P were low possibly due to reduced placental function.

Fetal ECG

- Fetal ECG is useful for noninvasive, long-term monitoring of HR and rhythm.

Abbreviations

CNS   central nervous system
CTUP   combined thickness of the uterus and placenta
ECG   electrocardiogram

HR heart rate
P4 progesterone
P5 pregnenolone
U/S ultrasound, ultrasonography

See Also

- Placental basics
- Placentitis
- Placental insufficiency
- Neonatal evaluation

Suggested Reading

Allen WR, Wilsher S, Turnbull C, et al. 2002. Influence of maternal size on placental, fetal and post-natal growth in the horse. I. Development in utero. *Reproduction* 123: 445–453.

Bucca S, Fogarty U, Collins A, et al. 2005. Assessment of feto-placental well-being in the mare from mid-gestation to term: transrectal and transabdominal ultrasonographic features. *Therio* 64: 542–557.

Giles RC, Donahue JM, Hong CB, et al. 1993. Causes of abortion, stillbirth, and perinatal death in horses: 3,527 cases (1986–1991). *JAVMA* 203: 1170–1175.

Reef VB, Vaala WE, Worth LT, et al. 1996. Ultrasonographic assessment of fetal well-being during late gestation: development of an equine biophysical profile. *Eq Vet J* 28: 200–208.

Renaudin C, Troedsson M, Gillis C, et al. 1997. Ultrasonographic evaluation of the equine placenta by transrectal and transabdominal approach in the normal pregnant mare. *Therio* 47: 559–573.

Rossdale P. 2004. The maladjusted foal: Influences of intrauterine growth retardation and birth trauma. *Proc AAEP* (Denver, CO); 75–126.

Vaala WE, Sertich PL. 1994. Management strategies for mares at risk for periparturient complications. *Vet Clin North Am Equine Pract* 10: 237–265.

Wilsher S, Allen WR. 2003. The effects of maternal age and parity on placental and fetal development in the mare. *Eq Vet J* 35: 476–483.

Author: Peter R. Morresey

chapter 126

Fetal Gender Determination, Equine

DEFINITION/OVERVIEW

- Fetal gender determination by transrectal and transabdominal U/S.
- *Early gestation*: 57 to 80 days gestation (ideal time 60–70 days), transrectal U/S.
- *Mid- to advanced gestation*: 100 to 260 days gestation, by transrectal or transabdominal U/S examination.

ETIOLOGY/PATHOPHYSIOLOGY

Systems Affected

Reproductive

SIGNALMENT/HISTORY

- Either technique can both be applied to most equine breeds.
- Transabdominal approach is more appropriate for very small breeds.

DIAGNOSTICS

- Early gestation technique:
  - To identify the GT and its location (Fig. 126.1).
  - GT: precursor of the clitoris in the female fetus and the penis in the male fetus (Figs. 126.2 and 126.3).
  - *Advantages*: early diagnosis (57–80 days), solely by transrectal U/S examination.
  - *Disadvantages*:
    - ninety-seven percent reliability for colt fetus.
    - small fetal size and high fetal mobility.
    - only one diagnostic parameter, the GT.
- Mid- to advanced gestation technique:
  - To identify: primary sex organs; perineal contour; anatomical structure of gonads.
    - *Advantages*: 100% reliability; wide diagnostic window (100–260 days); three to four diagnostic parameters to confirm diagnosis.

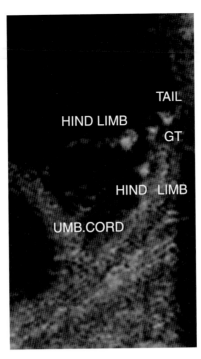

■ **Figure 126.1** A 63-day filly fetus. Oblique plane. Genital tubercle close to tail. Caudal left of sonogram; cranial right of sonogram.

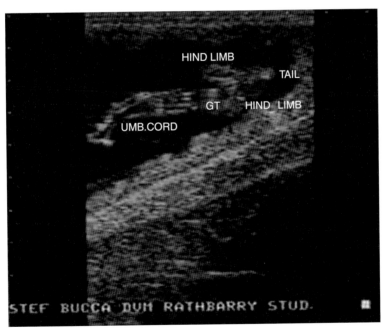

■ **Figure 126.2** A 65-day male fetus. Genital tubercle close to umbilical root. Caudal left of sonogram; cranial right of sonogram.

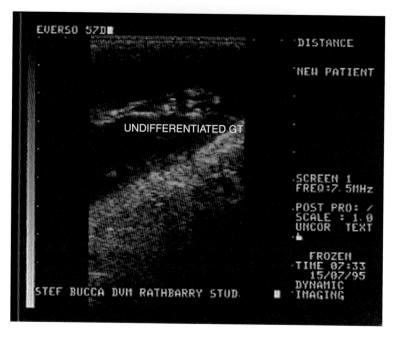

■ **Figure 126.3** A 55-day fetus. Frontal plane. Undifferentiated genital tubercle lying between thighs. Caudal left of sonogram; cranial right of sonogram.

- *Disadvantages*: U/S equipment with increased scanning depth may be required for transabdominal imaging.

Imaging

U/S

- GT appears like a hyperechoic equals sign (=).
- GT location: close to the tail in a female fetus versus close to the root of the umbilicus in the male fetus
- *Fetal gonads*:
  - *Female*: oval-shaped; distinct cortex and medulla (Fig. 126.4).
  - *Male*: oval-shaped; uniformly echodense; hyperechoic central line visible on long axis (Fig. 126.5).
- *Additional female fetus characteristics*:
  - *Mammary gland*: triangular or trapezoidal hyperechoic area, uniformly echodense (Figs. 126.6 and 126.7).
  - *Nipples*: two large hyperechodense dots emerging from the ventral border of the mammary gland (*see* Figs. 126.6 and 126.7).
  - *Clitoris*: hyperechoic structure, bulging out of the buttocks, just below the anus (Figs. 126.8, 126.9, and 126.10).
  - *Vulva*: labiae and commissure may be visualized between anus and clitoris (*see* Figs. 126.8 and 126.11).
  - *Female perineum*: no other structures below clitoris.

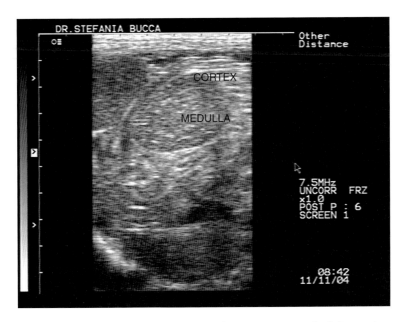

■ **Figure 126.4** A 130-day filly fetus. Posterior presentation. Features: gonad: distinct cortex and medulla. Caudal left of sonogram; cranial right of sonogram.

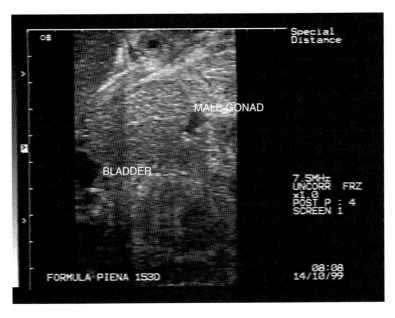

■ **Figure 126.5** A 150-day male fetus. Posterior presentation. Features: gonad: uniformly echogenic; distinct hyperechoic central line. Caudal left of sonogram; cranial right of sonogram.

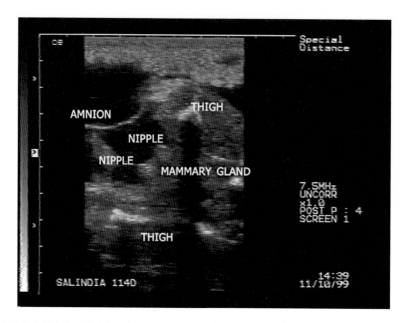

■ **Figure 126.6** A 114-day filly fetus. Transverse presentation; ventro-caudal position. Features: mammary gland and nipples. Caudal left of sonogram; cranial right of sonogram.

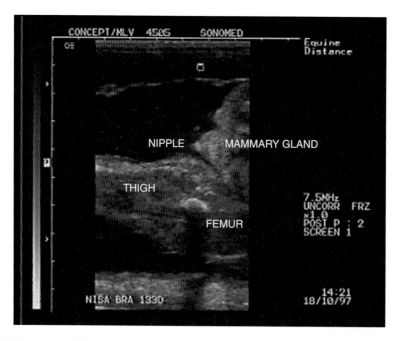

■ **Figure 126.7** A 133-day filly fetus. Transverse presentation; ventro-caudal position. Features: mammary gland and nipple. Caudal left of sonogram; cranial right of sonogram.

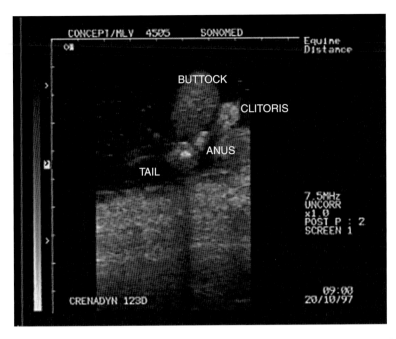

■ **Figure 126.8** A 123-day filly fetus. Transverse presentation; dorso-caudal position. Features: clitoris, vulva, anus and tail. Caudal left of sonogram; cranial right of sonogram.

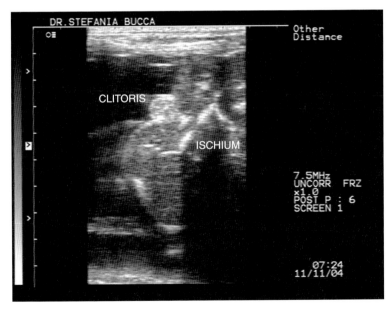

■ **Figure 126.9** A 180-day filly fetus. Posterior presentation. Features: clitoris. Caudal left of sonogram; cranial right of sonogram.

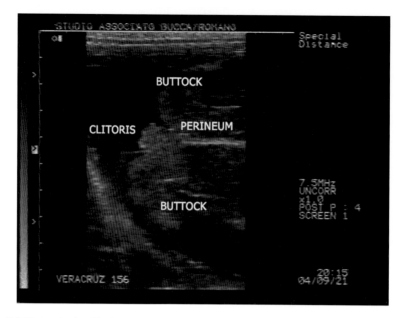

■ **Figure 126.10** A 156-day filly fetus. Posterior presentation. Features: clitoris and perineum. Caudal left of sonogram; cranial right of sonogram.

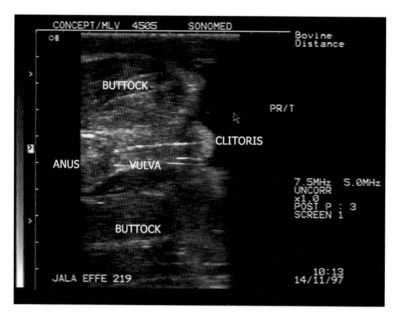

■ **Figure 126.11** A 219-day filly fetus. Transverse presentation; dorso-caudal position. Features: clitoris, vulva and anus. Caudal left of sonogram; cranial right of sonogram.

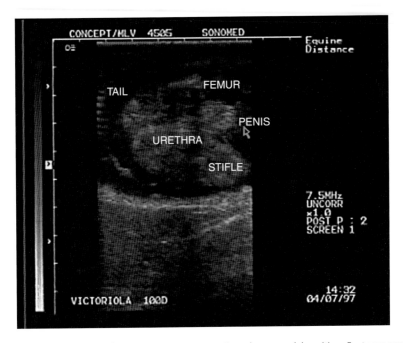

■ **Figure 126.12** A 100-day male fetus. Transverse presentation; dorso-caudal position. Features: prepuce/penis and urethra. Caudal left of sonogram; cranial right of sonogram.

- *Additional male fetus characteristics*:
  - *Male perineum*: can visualize the urethra.
  - *Penis*: just caudal to the root of the umbilical cord, may be encased within the prepuce, fully extended or occasionally erect (Figs. 126.12, 126.13, 126.14, and 126.15).
  - *Urethra*: visualized as a double line in longitudinal section and as a hyperechoic small circle in cross-section (Fig. 126.16).
  - *Scrotum*: the scrotal compartments appear as two symmetrical, oval, less echo-dense areas (Figs. 126.17 and 126.18).

Other Diagnostic Procedures

Early Gestation

- Equipment options:
  - U/S: B-mode, real-time scanners.
  - Transrectal transducer: linear-array, 5 to 8 MHz.
- Scan fetus in cross-sectional and frontal planes.
- GT is identified:
  - Assess its distance from the tail and the umbilical root on the frontal plane.
- Diagnosis is confirmed on cross-section.

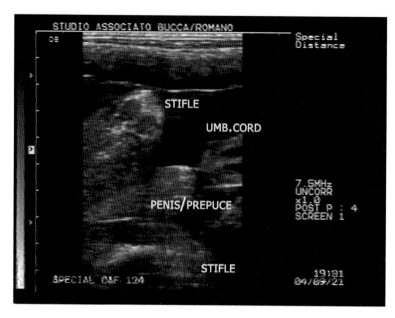

■ **Figure 126.13** A 124-day male fetus. Transverse presentation; dorso-caudal position. Features: prepuce/penis. Caudal left of sonogram; cranial right of sonogram.

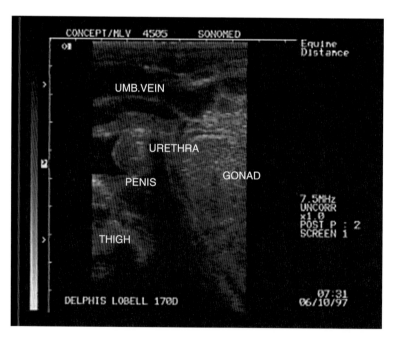

■ **Figure 126.14** A 170-day male fetus. Posterior presentation. Features: cross-section of erected penis showing the urethra. Caudal left of sonogram; cranial right of sonogram.

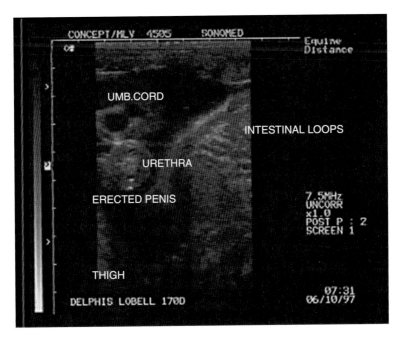

■ **Figure 126.15** A 170-day male fetus. Posterior presentation. Features: umbilical cord and cross-section of erected penis showing the urethra. Caudal left of sonogram; cranial right of sonogram.

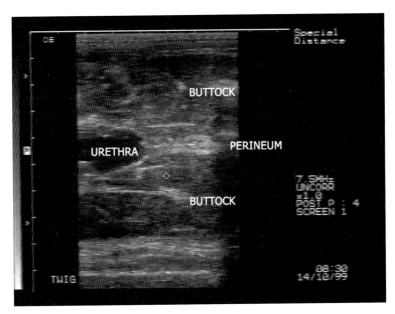

■ **Figure 126.16** A 160-day male fetus. Posterior presentation; ventro-caudal position. Features: perineum and urethra in longitudinal and cross-sections. Caudal left of sonogram; cranial right of sonogram.

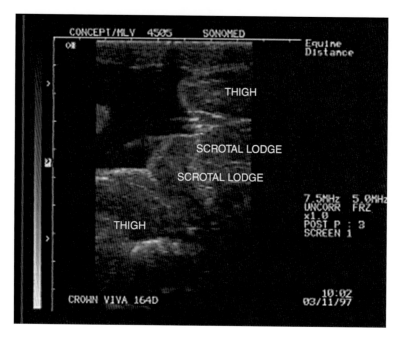

■ **Figure 126.17** A 150-day male fetus. Posterior presentation. Features: scrotum and scrotal compartments. Caudal left of sonogram; cranial right of sonogram.

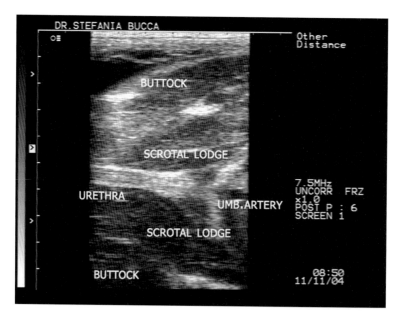

■ **Figure 126.18** A 185-day male fetus. Posterior presentation. Features: urethra and scrotal compartments. Caudal left of sonogram; cranial right of sonogram.

Mid- to Advanced Gestation

- Equipment:
  - U/S: B-mode, real-time scanners.
  - Transrectal transducer: linear-array, 5 to 8 MHz.
  - Transabdominal approach: sector or convex-array transducer, 2.5 to 5.0 MHz frequency.
- Locate fetus, scan in both longitudinal and cross-sectional planes.
- Assess fetal presentation and position.
- Evaluate fetal gonads by scanning caudal portion of the fetal abdomen, hindquarters, and buttocks.

Typical Characteristics Imaged at Different Stages of Gestation

- 55 to 60 days: small fetus
  - GT difficult to identify, may not have fully migrated (*see* Fig. 126.3).
  - Transducer: transrectal, 5 to 8 MHz, linear array.
- Sixty to 70 days: ideal time for early diagnosis (*see* Figs. 126.1 and 126.2).
  - GT: distinct and fully migrated.
  - Transducer: transrectal, 5 to 8 MHz, linear array.
- Seventy to 80 days: fetus slightly more difficult to reach (near to or descending over pelvic brim).
  - Transducer: transrectal, 5 to 8 MHz, linear array.
- Eighty to 100 days: difficult to access fetus, by either transrectal or transabdominal examination.
- One hundred to 150 days: fetus accessible transrectally.
  - Difficult to adequately visualize fetal details by transabdominal scan prior to 150 days gestation.
  - Transrectal U/S diagnosis possible most of the time despite presentation.
  - Anticipate frequent changes of presentation during course of a single examination.
  - Gonads are fully developed.
  - Transducer: transrectal, 5 to 8 MHz, linear array.
- One hundred fifty to 210 days:
  - Transrectal diagnosis possible with fetuses in posterior and transverse presentation;
  - Fetus fully accessible by transabdominal U/S approach;
  - Transducer:
    - 5 to 8 MHz linear, linear array transducer.
    - 3.5 to 5 MHz convex or sector scan transducer for transabdominal.
- Two hundred ten to 260 days: diagnosis by transabdominal U/S.
  - Gender may be determined transrectally if fetuses are in posterior presentation.
  - Transducer:
    - 5 to 8 MHz linear array.
    - 2.5 to 5 MHz convex or sector scan transducer.

Synonyms

Fetal sexing

Abbreviations

GT   genital tubercle
U/S   ultrasound, ultrasonography

See Also

- Fetal Monitoring
- Assessment of feto-placental well-being

Suggested Reading

Bucca S. 2005. Equine fetal gender determination from mid- to advanced gestation by ultrasound. *Proc SFT* 568–571.

Curran SS, Ginther OJ. 1989. Diagnosis of equine fetal sex by location of the genital tubercle. *J Eq Vet Sci* 9: 77.

Holden RD. 2000. Fetal sex determination in the mare between 55 and 150 days gestation. *Proc AAEP* 321–324.

Renaudin CD, Gillis CL, Tarantal AF. 1997. Transabdominal combined with transrectal ultra-sonographic determination of equine fetal gender during mid-gestation. *Proc AAEP* 252–255.

Authors: Stefania Bucca and Andrea Carli

Fetal Stress, Distress, and Viability

DEFINITION/OVERVIEW

- Fetal stress, distress, and viability are parameters, often found in conjunction with *high-risk pregnancies* and impaired placental function, that indicate less-than-ideal conditions for fetal survival.
- Fetal stress is a normal physiological response to potentially life-threatening situations.
- If these life-threatening circumstances are not addressed quickly enough, fetal stress progresses to distress, which is a pathophysiological condition leading to fetal demise or delivery of a severely compromised foal.

ETIOLOGY/PATHOPHYSIOLOGY

The specific conditions that lead to concern regarding fetal stress, distress, or viability often involve maternal disease or compromised placental function and include the following:

Etiology

Pre-existing Maternal Disease

- Equine Cushing's-like disease
- Laminitis
- Chronic, moderate to severe endometrial inflammation, endometrial periglandular fibrosis, or endometrial cysts leading to impaired placental function.

Gestational Maternal Conditions

- Malnutrition
- Colic
- Endotoxemia
- Hyperlipemia
- Prepubic tendon rupture
- Uterine torsion
- Dystocia
- Ovarian granulosa cell tumor

947

- Laminitis
- Musculoskeletal disease
- Exposure to ergopeptine alkaloids in endophyte-infected fescue or ergotized grasses or grains
- Exposure to other xenobiotics
- Exposure to abortigenic infections, especially EHV, and bacterial contaminants on ETC setae

Placental Conditions

- Placentitis
- Placental insufficiency
- Umbilical cord torsion or torsion of the amnion
- Placental separation
- Hydrops of fetal membranes
- MRLS

Fetal Conditions

- Twins (often resulting in placental insufficiency for one or both twins).
- Fetal abnormalities, such as hydrocephalus.
- Delayed fetal development for gestational age; IUGR.
- Fetal trauma

Pathophysiology

Depending on the specific cause, the pathophysiological mechanisms for fetal stress, distress, and viability can involve one or more of the following:
- Maternal systemic disease; placental infection, insufficiency, torsion, or separation; and fetal abnormalities, all of which impede efficient fetal gas exchange and nutrient transfer.
- The fetus initially responds physiologically (i.e., stress) to these alterations in oxygenation and nutrient supply and might initiate the cascade of events leading to parturition.
- If the impaired oxygenation or nutritional compromise are not resolved quickly that the fetus can respond physiologically in an adequate manner, its pathophysiologic response (i.e., distress) to these alterations in oxygenation and nutrient supply (e.g., passing and aspirating meconium pre- or perinatally, decreased respiratory movements, or irregular heartbeat), potentially leads to fetal compromise and death.
- In some cases, acute fetal stress may cause premature birth of a nonviable foal.
- In other cases, fetal stress progressing to distress results in fetal death or the delivery of a severely compromised foal.

Systems Affected

- Maternal: Reproductive and other organ systems, depending on the nature of the maternal disease.
- Fetal: All organ systems.

SIGNALMENT/HISTORY

Risk Factors

- May be nonspecific
- Thoroughbreds, Standardbreds, draft mares, and related breeds predisposed to twinning
- Mares more than 15 years of age
- American Miniature Horse mares
- Same as those listed previously under Etiology/Pathophysiology.

Pre-existing Maternal Disease

- Equine Cushing's-like disease.
- Laminitis
- Chronic, moderate to severe endometrial inflammation, endometrial periglandular fibrosis, or endometrial cysts, leading to impaired placental function.

Gestational Maternal Conditions

- Malnutrition
- Colic
- Endotoxemia
- Hyperlipemia
- Prepubic tendon rupture
- Uterine torsion
- Dystocia
- Ovarian granulosa cell tumor
- Laminitis
- Musculoskeletal disease
- Exposure to ergopeptine alkaloids in endophyte-infected fescue or ergotized grasses or grains.
- Exposure to other xenobiotics.
- Exposure to abortigenic infections, especially EHV and bacterial contaminants on ETC setae.

Placental Conditions

- Placentitis
- Placental insufficiency
- Umbilical cord torsion or torsion of the amnion
- Placental separation
- Hydrops of fetal membranes
- MRLS

Fetal Conditions

- Twins (often resulting in placental insufficiency for one or both twins).
- Fetal abnormalities, such as hydrocephalus.

- Delayed fetal development for gestational age; IUGR.
- Fetal trauma

Historical Findings

One or more of the following:
- Maternal disease during gestation, such as colic, hyperlipidemia, prepubic tendon rupture, uterine torsion, and so on.
- Mucoid, hemorrhagic, serosanguineous, or purulent vulvar discharge.
- Premature udder development and dripping of milk.
- Previous examination indicating placentitis or fetal compromise.
- Previous abortion, high-risk pregnancy, or dystocia.
- History of delivering a small, dysmature, septicemic, or congenitally malformed foal.
- Pre-existing maternal disease at conception, such as laminitis, equine Cushing's-like disease, endometrial inflammation, fibrosis, or cysts.
- Previous exposure to endophyte-infected fescue or ergotized grasses or grains.
- Previous exposure to abortigenic or teratogenic xenobiotics or infections.

 CLINICAL FEATURES

Maternal and Placental Signs

- Anorexia, fever, or other signs of concurrent, systemic disease.
- Abdominal discomfort
- Mucoid, mucopurulent, hemorrhagic, serosanguineous, or purulent vulvar discharge.
- Premature udder development and dripping of milk (except in cases of fescue toxicosis where there is little or no udder development).
- Premature placental separation (*red bag*).
- Placentitis, placental separation, or hydrops of fetal membranes by transrectal or transabdominal U/S.
- Excessive swelling along the ventral midline and evidence of body wall weakening or rupture by palpation or transabdominal U/S (Fig. 127.1).
- Excessive abdominal distention.
- Alterations in maternal circulating levels of progestins (progestagens), estrogens, or relaxin, reflecting changes in fetal well-being or placental function.

Fetal Signs

- The sole clinical sign of fetal stress or distress might be the premature delivery of a live or dead foal or the late delivery of a severely compromised foal, unable to stand and suckle (Fig. 127.2).
- Fetal hyperactivity or inactivity (concurrent with maternal or placental abnormalities) may suggest a less-than-ideal fetal environment or fetal compromise.
- Can be assessed by visual inspection (external) or by TRP (internal) of the mare.

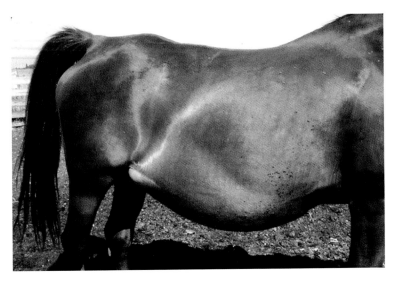

■ **Figure 127.1** The mare shown has severe ventral edema, which, as well as being an early indicator of body wall tears, also has the potential to additionally weaken the ventral abdominal wall. The severity of ventral edema in this mare warrants further examination or monitoring of the condition and signals the need to consider potential adverse effects on fetal well-being.
Image courtesy of D. Volkmann.

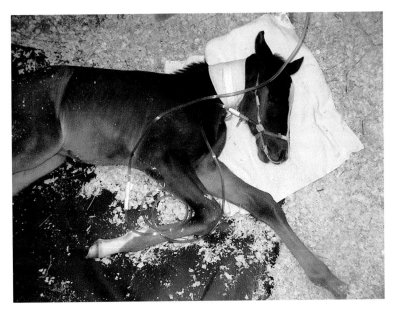

■ **Figure 127.2** The only clinical sign to indicate fetal stress or distress might be the delivery of a severely compromised foal. Its dam had been exposed to ergopeptine alkaloids during the last 30 days of gestation. This foal was unable to stand and suckle on its own and was eventually euthanized.
Image courtesy of B. Ramanathan.

- Alterations in parameters assessed using transrectal or transabdominal U/S (see Diagnostics).

DIFFERENTIAL DIAGNOSIS

Normal, uncomplicated, pregnancy with an active, normal fetus as assessed by TRP, transrectal or transabdominal U/S, or various laboratory tests.

DIAGNOSTICS

Maternal Assessment

- Complete physical examination.
- CBC with differential, as well as serum biochemical data, to determine inflammatory or stress leukocyte response, as well as other organ system involvement.
- ELISA or RIA analyses for maternal progesterone may be useful at less than 80 days of gestation (normal levels vary from greater than 1 to greater than 4 ng/mL, depending on the reference laboratory). At more than 100 days of gestation, RIA detects both progesterone (very low if more than 150 days) and cross-reacting 5α-pregnanes of utero-fetoplacental origin. Acceptable levels of 5α-pregnanes vary with stage of gestation and the laboratory used. Decreased maternal 5α-pregnane concentrations during late gestation are associated with fescue toxicosis and ergotism and are reflected in RIA analyses for progestins.
- Maternal estrogen concentrations can reflect fetal estrogen production and viability, especially conjugated estrogens (e.g., estrone sulfate).
- Decreased maternal relaxin concentration is thought to be associated with abnormal placental function.
- Decreased maternal prolactin secretion during late gestation is associated with fescue toxicosis and ergotism.
- There are anecdotal reports of lower T_3/T_4 levels in mares with history of conception failure, EED, high-risk pregnancies, or abortion. The significance of low T_4 levels is unknown and somewhat controversial.
- Feed or environmental analyses might be indicated for specific xenobiotics, ergopeptine alkaloids, phytoestrogens, heavy metals, or fescue endophyte (*Neotyphodium coenophialum*).

Fetal Assessment

- Transrectal and transabdominal U/S can be useful in diagnosing twins, assessing fetal stress, distress, or viability, monitoring fetal development, evaluating placental health and diagnosing other gestational abnormalities (e.g., hydrops of fetal membranes).
- In predisposed individuals (i.e., barren, older mares, or mares with history of high-risk pregnancy, placentitis, abortion, EED, conception failure, or endometritis), transrectal or transabdominal U/S should be performed on a routine basis during the entire pregnancy to assess fetal stress and viability.

- Confirmation of pregnancy and diagnosis of twins should be performed any time serious, maternal disease occurs or surgical intervention is considered for a mare bred within the last 11 months.
- Twin pregnancy can be confirmed by identifying two fetuses (easier by transrectal U/S when gestational age is less than 90 days) or ruled out by the presence of a nonpregnant uterine horn (by transabdominal U/S) during late gestation.
- Fetal stress, distress, or viability can best be determined by transabdominal U/S during late gestation. View the fetus in both active and resting states for at least 30 minutes. Make not of abnormal fetal presentation and position.
- Abnormally high FHR after activity (greater than 100 bpm), or more than a 40 bpm difference between resting and active rates reflects fetal stress, rather than distress.
- Abnormal fetal heart rhythm by echocardiography may occur immediately before, during, or after foaling and might indicate distress from acute hypoxia.
- Abnormally low resting FHR is less than 60 bpm or less than 50 bpm after day 330 of gestation.
- Bradycardia and absence of heart rate variation with activity indicate CNS depression, probably from acute hypoxia.
- Persistent bradycardia correlates well with poor prognosis for survival.
- Absence of fetal heartbeat is a reliable sign of fetal death.
- Absence of fetal breathing movements correlates well with fetal distress.
- Alterations in fetal fluid amounts.
- Increased amounts of amniotic fluid reflect hydrops amnion (*hydramnios*); low amounts indicate fetal distress and longstanding, chronic hypoxia.
- Sudden changes in the echogenicity of the amniotic fluid in late gestation can indicate meconium expulsion and fetal distress.
- Increased echogenicity of the allantoic fluid more than 44 days prior to the anticipated foaling date may reflect fetal distress; floating particulate matter normally gets gradually larger 10 to 36 days prior to foaling. Sudden increases in the echogenicity of the allantoic fluid can be indicative of fetal or placental abnormalities.
- The mean vertical distance of the allantoic fluid in uncomplicated pregnancies from less than 300 days to term is generally 1.9 ± 0.9 cm.
- Fetal ECG has been used to detect twins and to assess fetal viability and distress, but largely has been replaced by transabdominal U/S with ECG capabilities.
- While a higher-risk technique in horses than in humans, U/S-guided amniocentesis or allantocentesis and analysis of the collected fluids might become a future means to assess fetal karyotype, pulmonary maturity, and to measure fetal proteins.
  - Samples might reveal bacteria, meconium, or inflammatory cells.
- Since the 2001 outbreak, MRLS research is underway to develop fetal catheterization techniques and other methods of prepartum evaluation.

Pathological Findings

- Evidence of villous atrophy or hypoplasia on the chorionic surface of the fetal membranes (Fig. 127.3).
- Thickening and edema of the chorioallantois or allantochorion (*see* Fig. 127.3).

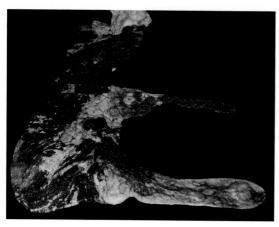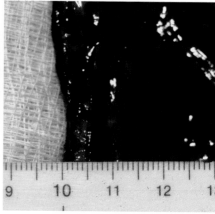

■ **Figure 127.3** Areas of severe villous atrophy or hypoplasia of the chorion, corresponding to the anatomical location of large maternal endometrial cysts shown on the left. A thickened and edematous section of chorioallantois/allantochorion, linked with maternal exposure to endophyte-infected fescue, is shown on the right.
Images courtesy of D. Volkmann (left image) and C. L. Carleton (right image).

- An endometrial biopsy can demonstrate the presence of moderate to severe, chronic endometritis, endometrial periglandular fibrosis with decreased normal glandular architecture, or lymphatic lacunae (see EED).

    # THERAPEUTICS

Drug(s) of Choice

See recommendations for specific conditions, such as dystocia, fescue toxicosis, high-risk pregnancy, induction of parturition, prepubic tendon rupture, RFM, hydrops, and so on.

Appropriate Health Care

Monitoring/managing fetal stress/distress, including the prolonged examination times required for complete serial transabdominal fetal assessments, is best performed at a facility prepared to manage high-risk pregnancies, especially if distress is severe and parturition (induction or C-section) is imminent.

- Early diagnosis of at-risk pregnancies is essential for successful treatment. The impact of maternal disease on fetal and placental health cannot be underestimated.
- Foal survival is improved with maternal body wall tears, when circumstances allow conservative management, without induction of parturition or elective C-section.
- With prolonged fetal stress or distress, maintenance of pregnancy (while attempting to treat the cause of fetal compromise) must be balanced with the need to induce

parturition (with or without C-section), if that becomes necessary to stabilize the mare's health.

- Parturition requires close supervision in cases of fetal stress and distress. The neonatal foal will very likely require intensive treatment.
- Individual circumstances and their sequelae will require consideration to determine nature and timing of treatment.
- Physical examination findings.
- CBC and biochemistry profile results.
- Stage of gestation.
- Nature of maternal disease.
- Hydrops of fetal membranes.
- Evidence of fetal stress, distress, or impending fetal demise.
- Maternal health risks or impending maternal demise.
- Occurrence of complications such as dystocia or RFM, FPT in the foal, or fetal dysmaturity, with or without septicemia.
- Financial considerations; relative value of mare and foal.
- Refer to individual topics for treatment recommendations.

Nursing Care

- Depending on the nature of the maternal disease, fetal distress, and the necessity for surgical intervention, intensive nursing care might very well be required for the neonatal foal and mare.
- Special attention should be given to the possibility of FPT in the neonate, which would require that the foal receive a plasma transfusion.

Diet

- Feed the mare an adequate, late-gestational diet with proper levels of energy, protein, vitamins, and minerals, unless contraindicated by concurrent maternal disease.

Activity

- For most cases, exercise will be somewhat limited and supervised.
- Body wall tears, prepubic tendon rupture, laminitis, or fetal hydrops may necessitate severe restrictions, or complete elimination of exercise.

Surgical Considerations

- C-section may be indicated when vaginal delivery is not possible or in dystocias not amenable to resolution by vaginal manipulation alone.
- Surgical intervention might be indicated for future repair of anatomical defects predisposing mares to endometritis and placentitis.
- Depending on the specific circumstances, certain future diagnostic and therapeutic procedures might also involve some surgical interventions in the mare or the foal.

COMMENTS

Client Education

- Clients should be aware that early diagnosis is essential for fetal survival.
- Predisposing conditions compromising fetal well-being must be corrected or managed for a successful outcome.
- Induction of parturition and C-section are not without risk to the mare and foal.

Patient Monitoring

- Mare and fetus need frequent monitoring until pregnancy either reaches term or is lost prematurely.
- Specific monitoring depends on the therapy undertaken, nature of the maternal or fetal disease, and complications that develop.
- Mares should be carefully monitored for premature or inadequate udder development.
- Within 24 hours of delivery, the foal should be assessed and, if necessary, appropriately treated for FPT.
- Vaginal speculum examination and uterine cytology and culture (as indicated) can be performed 7 to 10 days postpartum, or sooner, depending on the circumstances.
- Endometrial biopsy may be indicated as part of the postpartum examination as a prognostic tool for future reproduction.
- Appropriate therapeutic steps should be taken based on these findings.

Prevention/Avoidance

- Early recognition of at-risk mares and potential high-risk pregnancies.
- Correction of perineal conformation to prevent placentitis.
- Management of pre-existing endometritis before breeding.
- Early monitoring of mares with a history of fetal stress, distress, or viability concerns.
- Complete breeding records, especially for recognition of double ovulations, early diagnosis of twins (less than 25 days of pregnancy; ideally, days 14–15) and selective embryonic or fetal reduction.
- Careful monitoring of pregnant mares for vaginal discharge and premature mammary secretion.
- Removal of pregnant mares from fescue pasture or ergotized grasses or grains during last trimester (minimum of 30 days prepartum).
- Use ET procedures with mares predisposed to EED or high-risk pregnancies.
- Avoid breeding or using ET procedures in mares that have produced multiple stressed, distressed, or dead foals due to congenital and potentially inheritable conditions.
- Prudent use of medications in pregnant mares.

- Avoid exposure to known toxicants.
- Management of ETCs for prevention of MRLS.

Possible Complications

- Abortion, dystocia, RFM, endometritis, metritis, laminitis, septicemia, reproductive tract trauma, or impaired fertility that will all affect the mare's well-being and reproductive value.
- Fetal stress or distress.
- Fetal death
- Stillbirth
- Neonatal death
- Neonatal foals from at-risk pregnancies have potentially been compromised during gestation and are more likely to be dysmature, septicemic, and subject to FPT or angular limb deformities than foals from normal pregnancies.

Expected Course and Prognosis

- The ability to prevent and treat the conditions leading to fetal stress or distress have improved dramatically over the last twenty years. However, the successful management of at-risk pregnancies requires rigorous monitoring of the mare, fetus, and neonatal foal. The goal is to address treatable health concerns as soon as possible during the pregnancy and to avoid or minimize challenges to maternal, fetal, and placental health.
- If the predisposing conditions can be treated or managed, pregnancies in which fetal stress has been diagnosed have a guarded prognosis for successful completion.
- If there is evidence of fetal stress progressing to distress and the distress continues in the face of treatment for the predisposing conditions, fetal viability and maternal health become major concerns. The prognosis for successful completion of gestation under these circumstances is guarded to poor.

Synonyms/Closely Related Conditions

- Abortions, spontaneous infectious and noninfectious
- High-risk pregnancy
- Placental insufficiency
- Twins

Abbreviations

BPM   beats per minute
CBC   complete blood count
CNS   central nervous system
ECG   electrocardiogram
EED   early embryonic death
EHV   equine herpesvirus

ELISA   enzyme-linked immunosorbent assay
ET   embryo transfer
ETC   Eastern tent caterpillar
FHR   fetal heart rate
FPT   failure of passive transfer
IUGR   intrauterine growth retardation
MRLS   mare reproductive loss syndrome
RIA   radioimmunoassay
RFM   retained fetal membranes, retained placenta
T_3 triiodothyronine
T_4 thyroxine
TRP   transrectal palpation
U/S   ultrasound, ultrasonography

See Also

- Abortion, spontaneous, infectious or noninfectious
- Dystocia
- EED
- Endometrial biopsy
- Endometritis
- ET
- High-risk pregnancy, neonate
- High-risk pregnancy
- Hydrops amnion/allantois
- Induction of parturition
- Placental insufficiency
- Placentitis
- Twins

Suggested Reading

Christensen BW, Troedsson MH, Murchie TA, et al. 2006. Management of a hydrops amnion in a mare resulting in birth of a live foal. *JAVMA* 228 (8): 1228–1233.

Koterba AM, Drummond WH, Kosch PC. 1990. *Equine Clinical Neonatology*. Philadelphia: Lea & Febiger.

Madigan JE. 1997. *Manual of Equine Neonatal Medicine*, 3rd ed. Woodland, CA: Live Oak.

Robinson NE (ed). 2003. *Current Therapy in Equine Medicine 5*. Philadelphia: Saunders.

Ross J, Palmer JE, Wilkins PA. 2008. Body wall tears during late pregnancy in mares: 13 cases (1995–2006). *JAVMA* 232(2): 257–261.

Youngquist RS, Threlfall WR (eds). 2007. *Current Therapy in Large Animal Theriogenology*, 2nd ed. St. Louis: Elsevier-Saunders.

Author: Tim J. Evans

chapter 128

Flexor Contracture and Tendon Laxity

DEFINITION/OVERVIEW

Disorders of the musculoskeletal system may be associated with congenital malformations, intrauterine sepsis, abnormal length of gestation, small for gestational age foals, and twinning. Trauma at delivery, neonatal bacterial sepsis, and postnatal injury can lead to additional musculoskeletal problems.

Mildly contracted or flaccid tendons are a common presentation in newborn foals.

ETIOLOGY/PATHOPHYSIOLOGY

- Tendon contracture: uterine malposition is incriminated; however, this is unlikely a common cause due to frequent repositioning of the fetus. Unknown gestational insults (teratogens), goiter, and genetic factors alone or in combination are also possible causes.
- Tendon laxity: associated with birth of premature or dysmature foals, or concurrent systemic illness. Other signs of systemic weakness are present. Severity varies greatly.

Systems Affected

- Musculoskeletal: rupture of affected or apposing tendons possible. Muscle wasting as a result of disuse of affected limb or general debility.
- Skin/Exocrine: superficial skin trauma due to misadventure.

SIGNALMENT/HISTORY

Risk Factors

- Tendon contracture (flexural deformities): intrauterine malposition, insult, or secondary to bony malformation.
- Tendon laxity (resulting in hyperextension): prematurity or dysmaturity, catabolism in the postnatal period.

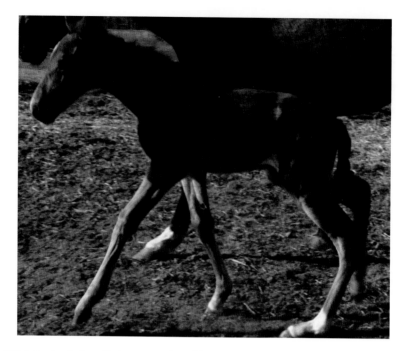

■ **Figure 128.1** Tendon laxity with hyperextension of joint.
Image courtesy of C. L. Carleton.

Historical Findings

Hyperextended or hyperflexed joint, usually fetlock or carpus (Fig. 128.1).

 CLINICAL FEATURES

- Contracture
  - Multiple joints in same limb.
  - Carpus, fetlock, tarsus, proximal interphalangeal joints are most often affected.
- Standing may be difficult.
- Laxity
  - General lack of muscle tone.
  - Fetlocks: most commonly affected, especially in the hind limbs.
  - Hyperextension of pastern: weight-bearing on heel bulbs, toe loses contact with ground (Fig. 128.2).

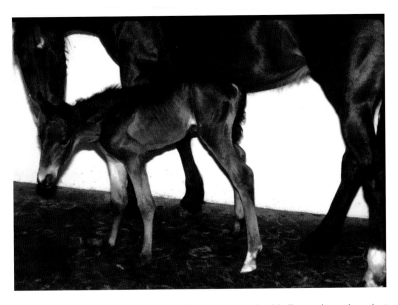

■ **Figure 128.2** Tendon laxity of severe degree, weight-bearing on heel bulbs, and toes have lost contact with ground.
Image courtesy of C. L. Carleton.

DIFFERENTIAL DIAGNOSIS

- Tendon rupture
- Trauma: sesamoid fracture, cuboidal bone collapse
- Congenital abnormality

DIAGNOSTICS

- Contracture: palpate affected limb when extended to ascertain the affected flexor tendons.
- Laxity: characteristic clinical presentation. Assess for injury or illness if condition develops outside the early postnatal period. Assess neurological status of neonate.
- Radiographs: no bony abnormalities. Alignment of bones may be abnormal with hyperextension of the joint.

Pathological Findings

Abnormal length of tendons relative to bony structures. May have secondary articular malformation or degeneration.

THERAPEUTICS

- Physical support applied to limb
- Corrective trimming/shoeing
- Analgesia when required

Drug(s) of Choice

- Flunixin meglumine: 1 mg/kg, IV, every 12 hours
- Ketoprofen: 2 mg/kg, IV, every 12–24 hours

Surgical Considerations

- Contracture
  - Standing and ambulating foal: spontaneous correction in mild cases.
  - Splinting: physically stretch contracted tendons.
  - Controlled exercise: encourage weight-bearing.
  - Analgesia: relieve discomfort of soft tissue or causative condition (e.g., physitis) allowing more appropriate weight-bearing.
  - Alternative Drug, Oxytetracycline: 50 mg/kg IV: controversial mechanism. Establish diuresis with intravenous fluids at time of administration. Nephrotoxic drug potential in dehydrated animals. In addition, a breakdown metabolite present in aged preparations (anhydroepitetracycline) is a known renal toxin.
  - Desmotomy: check ligament(s).
- Laxity
  - Spontaneous correction if mildly affected.
  - Manage concurrent disease: if present to reverse catabolism.
  - Corrective trimming: lower heel to eliminate the "rocker motion" and restore a flat weight-bearing surface. Do not trim the toe.
  - Corrective shoeing: heel extensions to restore appropriate sole placement.
  - Protect volar aspect of limb and treat soft-tissue trauma.
  - Avoid supportive bandaging: this delays strengthening of the affected muscles and can worsen laxity.

COMMENTS

Client Education

Multiple treatments may be required in severely affected cases.

Possible Complications

- Secondary trauma to fetlock periarticular tissue if contact occurs with the ground.
- Common digital extensor rupture can occur with flexor contracture.

Expected Course and Prognosis

Progressive improvement with time.

Abbreviations

IV   intravenous

See Also

- Angular limb deformities

Suggested Reading

Hardy J, Latimer F. 2003. Orthopedic disorders in the neonatal foal. *Clin Tech Eq Pract* 2: 96–119.

McIlwraith CW. 2002. Diseases of joints, tendons, ligaments and related structures. In: *Lameness in Horses*, 5th ed. Stashak TS, Adams OR (eds). Baltimore: Lippincott Williams & Wilkins; 459–644.

Trumble TN. 2005. Orthopedic disorders in neonatal foals. *Vet Clin North Am Equine Pract* 21: 357–385.

Author: Peter R. Morresey

chapter 129

Foal Nutrition

DEFINITION/OVERVIEW

Nutrition of neonatal foals is critical to their survival.

- The need for colostrum in the first 12 hours of life is well recognized, but little research has been done on optimal nutrition after that first critical period.
- The nursing foal obtains 80% to 100% of its nutrition from its dam in the first month or so; however, it starts sampling feed as early as 1 week, and if the feeds available (i.e., that which is being fed to the mare) are not balanced for growth, problems can occur.
- Major nutrient concerns are protein, calcium, phosphorus, and other minerals (magnesium, copper, selenium) to support muscular and skeletal growth.
- Excess protein (16%–20% in ration) does *not* cause problems per se, but over-feeding calories, especially in the form of high carbohydrate concentrate feeds, can lead to DOD, in foals genetically predisposed. Protein deficits will result in stunting and poor body condition.

Phases of Nutrient Concerns

Neonatal (First 24 Hours)

- Critical issue is the provision of colostrum (10%–15% BW divided into three to four feedings) if a mare is agalactic or rejects her foal.
- It is important not to introduce any other oral supplements before feeding the colostrum. There is evidence that this may cause premature "closure" of the GI wall that then prevents absorption of intact colostral antibodies.

First 1 to 2 Months

- Mare's milk provides more than 80% of the nutrients needed.
- The mare's ration will affect her milk mineral content but not the volume produced to any great extent.
- White muscle disease (caused by inadequate selenium intake) in some regions.

2 to 3 Months to Weaning

- Although the mare's milk can provide adequate nutrients for survival and some growth, supplemental feeds are increasingly important for steady growth during this phase.

- If feeds specifically formulated for growth are not provided, it is critical that the forages and feeds provided to the mares contain adequate nutrients for growth because the foals will increase their intakes of the solid feeds.

ETIOLOGY/PATHOPHYSIOLOGY

- Inadequate protein intake (less than 14% in the total ration) will cause reduced skeletal growth.
- Inadequate or grossly imbalanced minerals will cause improper mineralization of osteochondral matrices, leading to epiphysitis, angular and flexural deformities, and osteochondrosis desiccans.
- There is some evidence that hyperinsulinemia, due either to feeding high carbohydrate feeds or genetically linked insulin resistance, may affect growth hormone secretion and bone mineralization too.
- Genetics

Mare

- Some mares are better "milkers" than others, and it is difficult, if not impossible to affect overall milk quantity without totally starving the dam.

Foal

- Genetic predisposition to DOD is well documented in many breeds.
- There is increasing evidence that relative insulin resistance (high insulin responses to glucose challenges with or without hyperglycemia) may be a factor in the appearance of OCD lesions.
- Rapid growth rates have been selected for in some breeds and are associated with increased incidence of growth related problems, however merely slowing the rate of growth by depriving the foal of adequate energy and protein will not improve bone quality or density.

Incidence/Prevalence

- Over 40% of Hanoverians and Standardbreds in separate studies were reported to have evidence of DOD in the first 2 years of life.
- Prevalence of OCD lesions that required surgical correction in a survey of Thoroughbred breeding farms ranged from 0% to over 50%.

SIGNALMENT/HISTORY

- Foals from birth to weaning at 4 to 6 months.
- Improper nutrition will result in:
  - Poor body and hair coat condition.

- Slow growth rates, stunting.
- DOD: Epiphysitis, flexure and angular limb deformities, OCD.
- Causes
  - Excess calories (exceeding 125% of NRC recommendations), especially if provided predominantly by high carbohydrate feeds, excess phosphorus, zinc and potentially other trace minerals, or heavy metals that may interfere with calcium metabolism.
  - Deficit of protein, calcium, phosphorus, copper, selenium, or zinc.

Risk Factors

- Genetic predisposition.
- Feeding over 50% of ration as high carbohydrate feeds that lack adequate minerals.

 DIFFERENTIAL DIAGNOSIS

- Poor body and hair coat condition: clinical illness, intestinal parasitism.
- Slow growth rates, stunting: clinical illness, intestinal parasitism.
- DOD: Epiphysitis, flexure and angular limb deformities, OCD: inadequate or excessive exercise, genetics, poor hoof trimming.

 DIAGNOSTICS

- Ration analysis

 CBC/BIOCHEMISTRY/URINALYSIS

- Use to rule out clinical infection/illness, toxicities.
- Blood concentrations of most nutrients do *not* reflect intake or dietary adequacy, especially with respect to calcium, phosphorus, magnesium, potassium, and vitamins such as A and E.

Other Laboratory Tests

- If a nutrient imbalance is suspected, get the feed (i.e., hay, pasture, concentrates) analyzed to determine actual intake.
- Analysis of the mare's milk may reveal gross mineral imbalances but normal ranges are not well established.

Imaging

- Radiographs may be useful in determining the presence or absence of true epiphysitis or OCD.

- Many foals, especially warmblood breeds, have naturally large physes that can be misdiagnosed visually as epiphysitis.
- OCD lesions apparent at less than 12 months of age often disappear without surgery or major dietary manipulation.

 ## THERAPEUTICS

Diet

Neonatal (First 24 to 36 Hours)

- Ten percent to 15% BW colostrums in first 12 to 24 hours, either by bottle or naso-gastric intubation if foal is unwilling or unable to nurse adequately from the mare.
- Nothing else should be administered per os during this period.

Zero to 2 Months

- Ten percent to 15% BW in mare's milk or milk replacer, preferably divided into at least six feedings, per day.
- Foals normally nurse at least once per hour during the first month of life.
- Free choice (1%–2% BW) of good quality forage (hay or pasture).
- Mare should be fed concentrates that are formulated for growth/lactation with higher than maintenance concentrations of protein, calcium, phosphorus and trace minerals.

Two to 6 Months

- Free choice (1.0%–2.0% BW) good quality forage (hay or pasture) and 0.5% to 1.5% BW concentrate formulated for growth that complements the forage being fed. Actual amounts fed will depend on breed and body condition score. Nutrient concentration of concentrates will be dictated by forage nutrient content. Examples:
  - If only grass or grass hay is the base forage, the concentrate should provide greater than 14% protein, more than 0.7% calcium and more than 0.45% phosphorus.
  - If alfalfa (Lucerne) is the base forage, the concentrate can contain 12% to 14% protein, 0.6% to 0.8% calcium and 0.45% to 0.65 % phosphorus.
- Warmblood, draft, and draft-cross foals do well on lesser amounts of concentrate (with higher mineral concentrations); approximately 80 to 90% of what is recommended by the NRC.
- Light horse breeds such as Thoroughbreds may require higher concentrate intakes to sustain adequate growth and body condition.
- The mares should be fed the same concentrates as their foals.
- Salt (sodium chloride) and water should be available free choice.

Activity

- No restrictions
- Best if kept lean and fit.

Surgical Considerations

- Because some OCD lesions that are apparent radiographically at younger than 1 year of age will resolve spontaneously, it may be prudent not to advise surgical correction in foals that are less than 6 months of age unless there are clinical signs of joint effusion and lameness.

 COMMENTS

Client Education

- Disregard most of what is on the internet and most lay magazines.

Prevention/Avoidance

Avoid:
- Obesity
- Excessive weight loss
- Inadequate calcium, phosphorus, copper, and selenium intake.
- Excessive grain, especially sweet feeds.

Possible Interactions

- Excess selenium will interfere with copper absorption/utilization and vice versa.
- Excess zinc will interfere with calcium metabolism.
- Excessive grain will predispose to obesity and insulin resistance.

Patient Monitoring

- Body Condition
- Limbs assessed weekly or biweekly.
- Foal weights can also be monitored with a walk-across scale.

Abbreviations

BW	body weight
CBC	complete blood count
DOD	development orthopedic disease
GI	gastrointestinal
NRC	National Research Council
OCD	osteochondrosis desiccans

See Also

- Nutrition of the mare
- Nutrition of the stallion

Suggested Reading

Black A, Ralston SL, Shapses SA, et al. 1997. Skeletal development in weanling horses in response to high dietary energy and exercise. *J Anim Sci* 75: 170.

Kronfeld DS, Meacham TN, Donoghue S. 1990. Dietary aspects of developmental orthopedic disease in young horses. *Vet Clinics of North Am Eq Prac* 6: 451–465.

Lewis LD. 1996. *Feeding and Care of the Horse*, 2nd ed. Philadelphia: Lippincott Williams & Wilkins.

National Research Council. 2007. *Nutrient Requirements for Horses*, 8th ed. Washington, DC: National Academy Press.

Ralston SL. 2004. Hyperinsulinemia and glucose intolerance. In: *Equine Internal Medicine*, 2nd ed. Reed S, Bayly W, Sellon D (eds). St. Louis: Elsevier; 1599–1603.

Ralston SL. 1997. Diagnosis of nutritional problems in horses. www.rcre.rutgers.edu/pubs/publication.asp?pid=FS894.

Ralston SL. 1998. Feeding the rapidly growing foal. www.rcre.rutgers.edu/pubs/publication.asp?pid=FS895.

Rich GA, Breuer LH. 2002. Recent developments in equine nutrition with farm and clinic implications. *Proc AAEP*, Orlando; 48: 24–40.

Ropp JK, Raub RH, Minton JE. 2003. The effect of dietary energy source on serum concentration of insulin-like growth factor-I, growth hormone, insulin, glucose, and fat metabolites in weanling horses. *J Anim Sci* 81: 1581–1589

Vervuert I, Coenen M, Borchers A, et al. 2003. Growth rates and the incidence of osteochondrotic lesions in Hanoverian warmblood foals. *Proc 18th Equine Nutrition and Physiology Symp*, East Lansing, MI; 18: 113–114.

Author: Sarah L. Ralston

chapter 130

Foal Vaccination Protocols

DEFINITION/OVERVIEW

Before vaccinating the foal, certain considerations need to be addressed:

- The dam's vaccination status, the foal's age, geographical location, its likelihood of being transported and moved off-farm (i.e., showing, moving, production sale, and so on), client's budgetary constraints, morbidity/mortality associated with individual diseases for which vaccines are available, and the efficacy of different vaccine products.
- To ensure adequate immunity within the first year of life, foals will normally receive a series of vaccinations. In general, for foals of unvaccinated dams, vaccination programs will be instituted at an earlier age than those of dam's with a known and adequate vaccination program.

ETIOLOGY/PATHOPHYSIOLOGY

Systems Affected

Hemic/Lymphatic/Immune

SIGNALMENT/HISTORY

Risk Factors

Avoid intramuscular injections in the nursing foal's neck because they may result in soreness and an inability to nurse.

CLINICAL FEATURES

All North American foals should be vaccinated against: tetanus, EEE, WEE, WNV, and rabies where it is endemic. These vaccines are considered core due to their demonstrated efficacy, safety, and low risk of side-effects. In unvaccinated individuals, these diseases usually result in death. In addition, rabies is a zoonotic disease.

Diseases included are in order of their importance, based on morbidity, mortality, frequency of exposure, or relationship to equine health:

Tetanus

- If the dam has been vaccinated, the series for the foal is started at 4 to 6 months of age with a booster vaccination administered approximately 4 weeks later. The subsequent booster vaccination is administered at 1 year of age and repeated annually.
- If the dam has not been vaccinated or her vaccination history is unknown, the foal's vaccinations may begin as early as 1 month of age, and repeated twice at 4-week intervals, with a booster administered at one year of age, and then annually.

EEE/WEE

- If the dam has been vaccinated, the foal's series is started at 4 to 6 months of age with a booster vaccination approximately 4 weeks later. It is next given at 1 year of age prior to the appearance of insect vectors. Annual vaccination is required. However, if insects are present year-round, vaccination may be necessary twice a year.
- If the dam has not been vaccinated or her vaccination history is unknown, or in areas where vectors are present year-round, vaccination may begin as early as 3 to 4 months of age and repeated twice at 4-week intervals. Following a booster vaccine at one year of age, it is then administered annually or semi-annually.

VEE

- Recommendations for VEE mirror those for EEE/WEE in areas where it is present or outbreaks have been reported.
- Present in Mexico and South and Central America, therefore equids residing in the southern United States are potentially at greater risk for exposure.

WNV

- The protocol employed is dependent on the product chosen. Currently four products are marketed for protection against WNV.
  1. Inactivated vaccine: the vaccination series begins at 4 to 6 months of age when the dam has been vaccinated previously. The timelines for vaccination mirror those for the encephalitides. For the foal of the unvaccinated dam, vaccination begins at 3 to 4 months of age. Vaccinal protection is not optimal until 3 to 4 weeks following administration of the booster vaccination.
  2. Canary pox vaccine: Regardless of the dam's vaccination status, the foal's initial vaccination is *not* given until 5 to 6 months of age. Vaccination boosters then follow the protocol for EEE/WEE.
  3. Flavivirus chimera vaccine: Initial vaccination is given at 5 to 6 months of age. The subsequent booster is administered at 1 year of age prior to the appearance of vectors.
  4. DNA vaccine: This vaccine uses purified DNA plasmids to stimulate an immune response. Initial vaccination is administered at 5 to 6 months of age with a booster

vaccination 4 weeks later, followed by an annual vaccination. The DNA vaccine provides a 12-month duration of immunity. Not currently being marketed.

■ Annual vaccination may be administered using any of the aforementioned products without concern for the product used the previous year.

Rabies

■ If the dam has been vaccinated, the series is started at 6 months of age with a booster approximately 4 weeks later. A booster vaccination is administered at 1 year of age and then repeated annually.

■ If the dam has not been vaccinated or her vaccinal history is unknown, vaccination begins at 3 to 4 months of age. It is repeated once 4-weeks later. A booster vaccine is administered at 1 year of age, and then annually.

■ Because rabies is zoonotic and fatal, all horses in or traveling to endemic areas should be protected.

Herpes/Rhinopneumonitis

■ EHV-1 and EHV-4: Most often results in respiratory disease in foals rather than its neurologic form.

■ EHV-4: Vaccination of the foal does not provide adequate protection since vaccination is *not* started prior to 4 to 6 months of age. EHV-4 can be transmitted between the dam and foal as early as the first 2 weeks of the foal's life. EHV-1 transmission between the mare and her foal occurs later.

■ Herpes viruses persist and can recrudesce during periods of stress (e.g., weaning, transport, show, introduction of new horses, and so on).

■ Two types of vaccine are available, killed and MLV. The protocol for vaccination for either is similar, beginning at 4 to 6 months of age, with a booster vaccination administered approximately 4 weeks later. In the face of exposure, revaccination may be done at a 6-month interval. Efficacy of the vaccine is no better than 80% (i.e., vaccinated animals may still develop disease).

■ Pneumabort-K may infrequently cause muscle swelling and soreness post-vaccination. If a horse has reacted at a prior vaccination period, selection of an alternate killed product or a MLV for foals and stallions may be appropriate.

Influenza

■ Maternal antibody, if present, can blunt the foal's response to vaccination. The initial vaccination is therefore not administered prior to 6 months of age.

■ There are two types of vaccine, an inactivated form and an intranasal MLV. Administration of the inactivated vaccine follows a protocol similar to that for tetanus. With the intranasal MLV vaccine, the initial dose is given at 6 to 7 months of age and the booster at 12 months of age.

■ Many companies market an inactivated vaccine. Calvenza® (Boehringer-Ingelheim) is an inactivated product that can be used either IM or intranasally.

■ A MLV vaccine is also available and is called Flu-avert® (Intervet).

Strangles

- Vaccination of foals against Strangles should only be considered when/where there is a high likelihood for exposure.
- There are two types of vaccine, an inactivated form (cell wall derivative, Strepguard) and an intranasal MLV (Pinnacle). The inactivated vaccine follows a protocol similar to that for protection against tetanus. For the intranasal MLV vaccine, the initial dose is given at 6 to 7 months of age and the booster at 12 months of age.

Botulism (*Clostridium botulinum*), If Endemic

- Foals may be vaccinated as early as 2 weeks of age if at high risk, as maternal antibodies do not interfere with vaccination protection.
- Otherwise, vaccination begins at 2 to 3 months of age with two boosters, administered 4 weeks apart (a series of three).
- Although multiple toxins exist, the vaccine only contains the B-toxin, which is predominant in the southeast and west coast.

PHF

- The current vaccine contains only one strain of *Neorickettsia risticii*. Multiple inactivated, whole cell vaccines of this strain exist.
- However, of the more than 14 strains of *N. risticii*, the vaccine is not protective against these other strains.
- If the vaccine is given, the first dose should be administered at 5 months of age with the booster administered 4 weeks later.

EVA

- MLV (Arvac®) produced by Pfizer Animal Health.
- If used in male foals, the colt should be serotyped/blood tested prior to vaccination to establish his negative status to EVA prior to vaccination. Because maternal antibodies may persist for up to 6 months, testing of the colt should not be performed prior to that time.
- Colts are vaccinated with a single dose at 6 to 12 months of age.

DIAGNOSTICS

Strangles or WNV: may test for high titer before electing to vaccinate.

THERAPEUTICS

Precautions/Interactions

Strangles: the development of purpura hemorrhagica is possible from either disease or of vaccine origin.

COMMENTS

Rotavirus: there is no product available for vaccination of foals.

Client Education

Since muscle soreness may occur post-vaccination, do not vaccinate within 7 to 10 days of showing. Also, to reduce the risk of the foal developing multiple sore muscles, limit the number of vaccines given at one time to no more than two or three products. Administer any subsequent vaccines at least 1 week later.

Possible Complications

- Abscessation at injection site.
- Clostridial myositis has been reported post-vaccination.

Abbreviations

EEE   eastern equine encephalitis
EHV   equine herpes virus
EVA   equine viral arteritis
IM   intramuscular
MLV   modified live virus
PHF   Potomac Horse Fever
VEE   Venezuelan equine encephalitis
WEE   western equine encephalitis
WNV   West Nile Virus

See Also

- May refer to specific diseases against which vaccinations are to be protective.

Suggested Reading

AAEP Vaccination Guidelines, revised 2008. www.aaep.org/vaccination_guidelines.htm.
Foote CE, Love DN, Gilkerson JR, et al. 2004. Detection of EHV-1 and EHV-4 DNA in unweaned Thoroughbred foals from vaccinated mares on a large stud farm. *Eq Vet J* 36: 341–345.
Holyoak GR, Balasuriya UB, Broaddus CC, et al. 2008. Equine viral arteritis: current status and prevention. *Therio* 70(3)403–414.
www.boehringer-ingelheim.com/corporate/products/animal_health_horse_01.htm.
http://merial.com.
http://pfizer.com/products/animal_health/animal_health.jsp.
www.intervet.ca/products/flu_avert__i_n__vaccine/020_product_details.asp.

Author: Judith V. Marteniuk

chapter 131

Gastric Ulceration

DEFINITION/OVERVIEW

- Some degree of gastric ulceration is a common finding in the neonatal foal, with prevalence estimated between 25% and 50%. The majority of cases are asymptomatic, with disease usually advanced by the time clinical signs become apparent.
- Subclinical duodenal ulceration is uncommon, with lesions in the proximal duodenum ranging from diffuse inflammation to focal bleeding ulcers.
- Advanced duodenal ulceration can lead to an acute onset of gastric emptying dysfunction, duodenal perforation with resultant peritonitis, adhesion formation, duodenal stricture, ascending cholangitis, and hepatitis.
- Ulcer disease can also worsen in the face of apparent clinical improvement.

ETIOLOGY/PATHOPHYSIOLOGY

Hydrochloric acid is continuously secreted. Gastric pH of the foal can become very acidic, with ulcers being secondary to prolonged periods of not eating or nursing, exercise, or delayed gastric emptying (concurrent illness).

Systems Affected

- Gastrointestinal: intestinal stricture, perforation and peritonitis can result from severe ulcer disease.
- Hemic/Lymphatic/Immune: sepsis

SIGNALMENT/HISTORY

Affected foals often have a concurrent debilitating illness. This leads to reduced gastric mucosal blood flow and diminished protection from acid erosion. Physiologic and social stresses also impair mucosal defenses.

Risk Factors

- Decreased nursing and feeding: increased gastric acidity causes lesions in both the gastric squamous and glandular mucosa.
- NSAID usage

Historical Findings

Onset of salivation, teeth grinding and colic signs

CLINICAL FEATURES

- Colic: foals may seek and remain in dorsal recumbency.
- Bruxism, ptyalism: gastroesophageal reflux secondary to severe gastroduodenal ulceration causes a functional or anatomic gastric outflow obstruction.
- Anorexia
- Diarrhea
- Weight loss
- Death: gastroduodenal perforation with onset of septic peritonitis.

DIFFERENTIAL DIAGNOSIS

- Enterocolitis: abdominal distension or colic
- Intestinal accident: volvulus or intussusception
- Oral pathology: foreign body or trauma leading to hypersalivation.
- Esophageal obstruction: spontaneous reflux

DIAGNOSTICS

- Fever
- Hematology: anemia, leukopenia, or leukocytosis
- Chemistry: hyperfibrinogenemia. May have reflux cholangiohepatitis.
- Abdominal U/S: gastric and duodenal dilation. Thickened duodenal wall. Peritonitis resulting from perforation.
- Contrast radiography (barium swallow): delayed gastric emptying or duodenal stricture.
- Fecal examination: occult blood
- Paracentesis: peritonitis
- Endoscopy: definitive diagnosis. Visualization of gastric and esophageal ulceration (if reflux is present).

Pathological Findings

Ulceration of gastric mucosa, esophagus, and duodenum. Physical evidence of duodenal stricture and peritonitis.

THERAPEUTICS

- Diminish gastric acid secretion: H_2 receptor antagonists or proton-pump blockers.
- Oral protectants: sucralfate binds ulcerated glandular mucosa, inhibits pepsin, enhances gastric mucosal barrier, and enhances mucosal blood flow.
- Oral antacids: aluminum hydroxide, magnesium hydroxide.
- Enhance gastric emptying if it is delayed: bethanechol.
- Parenteral nutrition and fluids: when gastric outflow obstruction leads to gastric dilation and abdominal discomfort. May be successful in allowing resolution of stricture if it is of short duration and stomach exhibits a partial ability to empty.

Drug(s) of Choice

See Table 119.1.

Appropriate Health Care

Withhold feed and water in cases of suspected outflow obstruction.

Diet

Provide parenteral nutrition during periods of fasting where possible.

Surgical Considerations

Gastrojejunostomy: where outflow obstruction is unresponsive to medical therapy or obstruction is complete at the time of presentation. A considerable amount of pre- and postsurgical management is required. Parenteral nutrition is essential to rest the gastrointestinal system because food and water need to be withheld for a prolonged period.

COMMENTS

Client Education

- Gastric ulceration can be widespread and is sometimes a clinically silent disease.
- Ulceration may progress rapidly to a life-threatening condition secondary to ulcer perforation.

Prevention/Avoidance

Avoidance of stressful situations. Consider concurrent antacid treatment along with all treatments for primary disease processes.

Expected Course and Prognosis

Mild cases respond rapidly and completely to control of acid production. Advanced cases require prolonged and aggressive therapy. Stricture formation is a serious event that may necessitate surgery or euthanasia.

Abbreviations

NSAID   nonsteroidal anti-inflammatory drug.
U/S   ultrasound, ultrasonography

Suggested Reading

Wilson JH, Cudd TA. 1980. Common gastrointestinal diseases. In: *Equine Clinical Neonatology*. Koterba AM, Drummond WH, Kosch PC (eds). Philadelphia: Lea & Febiger; 412–430.

Author: Peter R. Morresey

chapter 132

Hypoxic Ischemic Encephalopathy

DEFINITION/OVERVIEW

A multitude of factors lead to and perpetuate neuronal cell damage from ischemia and hypoxia. The common manifestation of these factors is HIE. Alternative name used by many internists is PAS because it is a multi-systemic syndrome.

ETIOLOGY/PATHOPHYSIOLOGY

Neonatal hypoxic-ischemic brain injury is the product of many biochemical cascades and events.

- Cerebral ischemia: from systemic hypoxemia depressing myocardial performance. Reduced cerebral blood flow decreases delivery of oxygen and energy substrates to the brain causing a combined hypoxic-ischemic insult. Anaerobic metabolism depletes the brain's stores of glucose and high energy phosphates. Glutamate uptake is impaired resulting in accumulation and overstimulation of receptors (excitotoxicity). Reperfusion and reoxygenation injury also occurs.
- Free radical production: the neonatal brain is highly susceptible to free radical-mediated injury. Multiple enzyme systems and antioxidants scavenge these in the healthy individual. During reperfusion following ischemia, oxygen-derived free radical production is overwhelming.
- Neurotransmitter release: regardless of the inciting cause, neural injury results in increased release of neurotransmitters and inflammatory mediators, with apoptosis and electrolyte derangements occurring.
- Maternal infection: shown to be strongly associated with neonatal brain injury. Intrauterine infection may injure the brain indirectly via the induction of sepsis and poor perfusion, or directly by the production of inflammatory mediators that devitalize neurons.
- Intracranial hemorrhage: shown associated with neurological compromise and found more frequently in premature foals, in foals born dead, and in foals born following assisted delivery, compared to normal foals and those delivered without intervention.

Systems Affected

- Gastrointestinal: motility and mucosal integrity of the intestinal tract is compromised. Diarrhea and sepsis can result from intestinal bacterial overgrowth, with possible toxin absorption and profound fluid and electrolyte losses.
- Renal/Urologic: hypoxic and ischemic insult to renal function leads to electrolyte and fluid balance derangements.
- Cardiovascular: hypoxic insult to the myocardium can occur concurrently with the cerebral damage, leading to decreased cerebral perfusion.
- Respiratory: aberrant pulmonary function can result from insult to the central respiratory centers. This can lead to abnormal gas exchange via decreased ventilation efforts, allowing retention of carbon dioxide. Central depression and abnormal blood acid-base balance ensue.

SIGNALMENT/HISTORY

Pregnancy or maternal health usually known to have been compromised, however HIE can occur without prior warning. Events at delivery can precipitate problems.

Risk Factors

- Placental disease: placentitis or placental edema
- Placental insufficiency: maternal disease, endometrial degeneration, or IUGR.
- Premature placental separation: placentitis, usually ascending at the cervix.
- Dystocia: prolonged delivery or physical trauma

Historical Findings

Abnormal placental appearance. Sudden onset of neonatal foal depression and neurological dysfunction.

CLINICAL FEATURES

- Signs of neurological dysfunction may be present at birth or develop within the first 2 days of life.
- Initially, behavior changes such as loss of affinity for mare, depression, and wandering may be all that is apparent (Fig. 132.1).
- Loss of suckle reflex may develop (Fig. 132.2).
- Later, seizure activity, beginning as focal muscle fasciculations and progressing to overt generalized seizures, may occur.
- If seizures are not observed, the presence of unexplained physical trauma may be noted (Fig. 132.3). Concurrent vital organ dysfunction may be detected on routine examination.

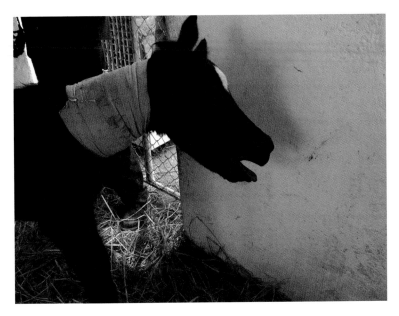

■ **Figure 132.1** Loss of affinity for the mare can be a subtle sign of neonatal neurological dysfunction. Image courtesy of Dr. B. Ramanathan.

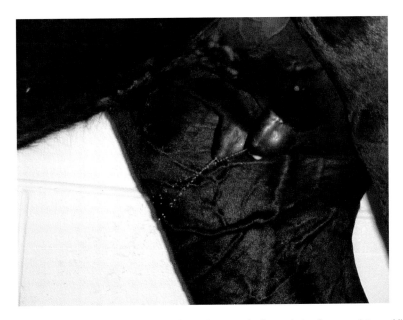

■ **Figure 132.2** Spontaneous expulsion of milk from the mare indicates lack of appropriate suckling activity by the foal.

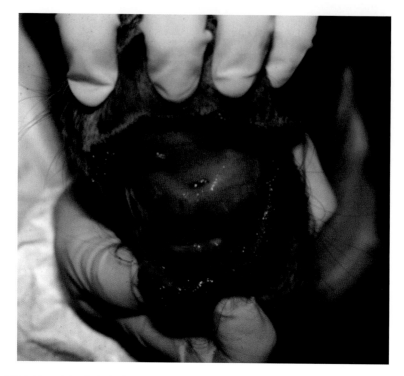

■ **Figure 132.3** Unexplained physical trauma may be the only indication of unobserved seizure activity.

DIFFERENTIAL DIAGNOSIS

- Sepsis: hematological signs of infection. Fever or hypothermia may occur. May progress to meningitis.
- Head trauma: palpable skull damage or superficial lacerations and contusions.
- Malnutrition: lack of urine production, diminished weight gain, or spontaneous lactation by mare.

DIAGNOSTICS

- History: birthing or gestational related trauma.
- Clinical signs: deranged neurological function and overt seizure activity.
- Concurrent major organ system dysfunction: renal (acute renal failure, oliguria/anuria) and gastrointestinal (diarrhea, intestinal ileus, abdominal distension).

Pathological Findings

Possibility of cerebral hemorrhage. Histological evidence of neuronal cell death.

THERAPEUTICS

- Control seizure activity and normalize cerebral function: diazepam, phenobarbital, or thiamine.
- Control cerebral edema and inflammation: DMSO, mannitol, or NSAID.
- Control NMDA receptor activation: magnesium sulfate.
- Control oxidative damage: DMSO or antioxidants.
- Prevent sepsis: administer broad spectrum antimicrobials. Normalize immunoglobulin levels by plasma transfusion.
- Manage concurrent disease: renal, respiratory, or gastrointestinal.
- Supportive therapies: nutritional adequacy and monitor fluid and electrolyte balance.

Drug(s) of Choice

Seizure Control and Metabolic Support

- Diazepam: 0.05 to 0.4 mg/kg, IV. Short-acting control.
- Phenobarbital: 5 to 25 mg/kg, IV over 30 minutes followed by 2–4 mg/kg PO every 12 hours. Long-acting control.
- Thiamine: 10 mg/kg, IV every 24 hours. Cerebral metabolic support.

Control Cerebral Edema and Inflammation

- Hypertonic saline: 7 ml/kg, IV as 7.5% solution.
- Mannitol: 1 mg/kg, IV as 20% solution.
- Flunixin: 1.1 mg/kg, IV, every 12 hours, PO every 24 hours.

Control Oxidative Damage

- Vitamin C: 100 mg/kg, IV, every 24 hours.
- Vitamin E: 20 IU/kg, SC, every 24 hours.
- Dimethyl sulfoxide: 1 g/kg, IV, every 12 hours as 10% solution.

Precautions/Interactions

Be careful with potentially nephrotoxic drugs in patients with renal compromise.

Appropriate Health Care

Monitor closely for and control seizure activity.

Nursing Care

Decubital ulcers are common with recumbent neonates.

Diet

Ensure adequate caloric intake while avoiding aspiration of feed.

Activity

Maintain in environment with minimal stimulus if seizure activity present.

Surgical Considerations

Avoid unnecessary procedures and care with depth of sedation.

 COMMENTS

Client Education

Recovery of appropriate mentation may be delayed.

Patient Monitoring

Assess neurological function regularly.

Prevention/Avoidance

Maintain maternal health. Ensure problem/high-risk foal deliveries are monitored.

Possible Complications

Decreased growth. Secondary infections in areas of cutaneous trauma from recumbency. Prolonged periods of intermittent seizure activity if presenting signs indicate severe hypoxic insult.

Expected Course and Prognosis

Mild hypoxic insult, early presentation, and aggressive management of cases will most likely allow complete recovery with minimal to no short term deficits. Severe hypoxic insult or cases presented later in the clinical course of the condition less likely to fully recover in a reasonable time frame. Central depression leads to decreased feeding activity, loss of body condition and increased susceptibility to secondary or opportunistic infections.

Synonyms

- Dummy foal
- Neonatal maladjustment
- Perinatal asphyxia syndrome

Abbreviations

DMSO   dimethyl sulfoxide
HIE   hypoxic ischemic encephalopathy
IV   intravenous

IUGR   intrauterine growth retardation
NMDA   N-methyl D-aspartate
NSAID   nonsteroidal anti-inflammatory drug
PAS   perinatal asphyxia syndrome
PO   per os (by mouth)
SC   subcutaneous

Suggested Reading

Green SL, Mayhew IG. 1980. Neurologic disorders. In: *Equine Clinical Neonatology*. Koterba AM, Drummond WH, Kosch PC (eds). Philadelphia: Lea & Febiger; 496–530.

MacKay RJ. 2005. Neurologic disorders of neonatal foals. *Vet Clin North Am Equine Pract* 2: 387–406.

Author: Peter R. Morresey

Chapter 133

Idiopathic Tachypnea

DEFINITION/OVERVIEW

A transient elevation in respiratory rate of unknown etiology. Diagnosis depends on the elimination of the possibility of organic disease.

ETIOLOGY/PATHOPHYSIOLOGY

Idiopathic tachypnea is thought to result from immature thermoregulatory mechanisms in certain foal breeds.

Systems Affected

Endocrine/Metabolic: increased rectal temperature

SIGNALMENT/HISTORY

Risk Factors

- Breed. idiopathic or transient tachypnea has been observed primarily in Clydesdale, Thoroughbred, and Arabian foals.
- Environmental conditions are usually warm and humid around the time of onset; however, this condition is thought to result from immature or dysfunctional thermoregulatory mechanisms.

Historical Findings

Sudden onset of increased respiratory rate.

CLINICAL FEATURES

- Increased respiratory rate and rectal temperature
- Onset reported within a few days of birth and tachypnea may continue for several weeks.
- Normal blood gas analysis

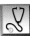

DIFFERENTIAL DIAGNOSIS

- Infectious respiratory disease
- Aspiration pneumonia
- Pain from orthopedic problems
- Pain from thoracic wall trauma (e.g., rib fractures or contusions).
- Diaphragmatic hernia
- Structural abnormalities of the upper respiratory tract

DIAGNOSTICS

Rule out infectious causes of respiratory disease:
- Hematology: lack of inflammatory leukogram makes infectious cause less likely.
- Auscultation: absence of abnormal pulmonary air sounds.
- Thoracic U/S: detect pleural fluid, pulmonary consolidation or fractured ribs.
- Thoracic radiography: pulmonary parenchymal inflammation or consolidation, fractured ribs

Rule out respiratory compensation for a metabolic acidosis.

Pathological Findings

Characteristic histological changes have not been described.

THERAPEUTICS

- Treatment involves modifying the foal's environment to avoid heat and humidity.
- Topical treatment to encourage heat dissipation: body clipping or cool water or alcohol baths.
- Broad-spectrum antimicrobial drugs are recommended until infectious pneumonia can be ruled out.

Drug(s) of Choice

As prescribed for bacterial pneumonia until it has been ruled out

Precautions/Interactions

Avoid drugs that may cause hyperthermia: macrolides.

Appropriate Health Care

Provide cool, low humidity environment.

COMMENTS

Expected Course and Prognosis

- Spontaneous recovery is expected.
- Response to antipyretics is poor.

Abbreviations

U/S   ultrasound, ultrasonography

Suggested Reading

Bedenice D, Heuwieser W, Brawer R, et al. 2003. Clinical and prognostic significance of radiographic pattern, distribution, and severity of thoracic radiographic changes in neonatal foals. *J Vet Intern Med* 17: 876–886.

Wilkins PA. 2003. Lower respiratory problems of the neonate. *Vet Clin North Am Equine Pract* 19: 19–33.

Author: Peter R. Morresey

Chapter 134

Lethal White Syndrome

DEFINITION/OVERVIEW

Intestinal aganglionosis. Lethal white foals are characterized by an unpigmented hair coat and light blue irises. Histologically, they lack myenteric ganglia in terminal portions of the ileum, cecum, and colon. This is a congenital, heritable condition for which there is no treatment.

ETIOLOGY/PATHOPHYSIOLOGY

Overo horses are defined as having white coloration on the abdomen that extends toward, but does not cross, the dorsal midline between the withers and tail. Extensive white markings are usually present on the head. An inherited defect of the endothelin receptor gene (the Ile118Lys EDNRB mutation) is responsible for the syndrome. In homozygotes, lethal white syndrome occurs. However, in heterozygotes the desirable frame overo phenotype usually is present.

Systems Affected

Gastrointestinal: obstruction of the intestinal tract, abdominal distension, and pain.

SIGNALMENT/HISTORY

Mostly white coat color, light blue irises, and pigmented retinas.

Risk Factors

- Autosomal recessive gene: foal of two overo Paint parents.
- Carriers: tobiano, solid colored horses with overo color patterns in their ancestors.
- Equal frequency in both males and females.

Historical Findings

Non-passage of meconium or persistent abdominal discomfort.

CLINICAL FEATURES

- Normal at birth; stand, suckle mare appropriately
- Do not pass meconium.
- Colic develops within the first 12 hours, progressively worsens.
- Abdominal distension
- Fecal staining may be present at the anus.

 DIFFERENTIAL DIAGNOSIS

- Meconium retention: not all foals born solid white from suspect breedings will be affected. Therefore, provide treatment in the first instance until diagnosis is confirmed.
- Atresia of the intestinal tract

 DIAGNOSTICS

- Signalment
- Overo parentage
- Compatible clinical signs and onset
- U/S: small intestinal distention
- Radiography: small intestinal distention
- Genetic testing: DNA mutation. Whole blood and hair samples with roots (plucked mane, tail hairs). Detect carriers, non-carriers, and affected animals. Submit to University of California, Davis or University of Minnesota veterinary schools diagnostic laboratory.

Pathological Findings

Necropsy findings of colonic meconium impaction or contraction of the small colon.

 THERAPEUTICS

- No treatment, grave prognosis
- Euthanasia: recommended; will die naturally within 2 to 3 days.

Surgical Considerations

None

COMMENTS

Client Education

Genetic counseling regarding at-risk overo-overo matings

Prevention/Avoidance

Avoid susceptible breedings.

Expected Course and Prognosis

Affected foals develop intractable abdominal distension and pain. Euthanasia is indicated.

Abbreviations

U/S   ultrasound, ultrasonography

See Also

- Meconium impaction
- Intestinal accident

Suggested Reading

Santschi EM, Vrotsos PD, Purdy AK, et al. 2001. Incidence of the endothelin receptor B mutation that causes lethal white foal syndrome in white-patterned horses. *AJVR* 62: 97–103.

Wilson JH, Cudd TA. 1980. *Common gastrointestinal diseases. In: Equine Clinical Neonatology.* Koterba AM, Drummond WH, Kosch PC (eds). Philadelphia: Lea & Febiger; 412–430.

Author: Peter R. Morresey

Chapter 135

Meconium Aspiration

DEFINITION/OVERVIEW

Aspiration of meconium by the fetus can occur during any time of *in utero* stress or during respiratory efforts at the time of parturition. This will result in inflammatory and consolidating pulmonary disease that decreases compliance of the lungs themselves. Respiratory failure can result from fatigue.

ETIOLOGY/PATHOPHYSIOLOGY

- MAS has been identified as an important cause of neonatal morbidity and mortality. The free fatty acids in aspirated meconium displace surfactant, resulting in additional atelectasis and decreased lung compliance.
- Proteolytic digestive enzymes are active. In the lungs, meconium inhibits phagocytosis allowing bacterial overgrowth.
- Meconium also induces chemical pneumonitis accompanied by alveolar collapse and edema. Type II alveolar cells produce less surfactant, causing an increase in alveolar surface tension and a decrease in compliance. The resulting atelectasis leads to pulmonary vascular constriction, hypoperfusion, and lung tissue ischemia.
- Sloughed epithelium, protein, edema, and hyaline membrane formation further contribute to respiratory distress. Dysplasia of the respiratory epithelium results. Pneumothorax, pneumomediastinum, or interstitial emphysema from labored respiratory effort can result in severe cases.

Systems Affected

- Cardiovascular: persistent pulmonary hypertension may result from the increased cardiac workload to perfuse consolidated lung.

SIGNALMENT/HISTORY

Clinical signs become apparent in the early neonatal period, although suspicion of meconium aspiration is raised by the presence of meconium-staining of the fetal membranes or gross discoloration of the fetal fluids. Overt meconium staining over the body, meconium discharge from the nares, and elevated respiratory rate and effort are highly suggestive in the neonate.

Risk Factors

- Acute pre- or intrapartum asphyxiation: dystocia, prolonged delivery, or premature placental separation.
- Fetal distress leading to passage of meconium *in utero*: indicated by a persistently elevated or highly variable fetal heart rate may result from maternal illness or hemodynamic compromise.

Historical Findings

Gross meconium staining of fetus, nasal discharge, and increased respiratory effort.

 # CLINICAL FEATURES

- Range from mild to severe: may result in perinatal death, especially if allowed to progress.
- Increased respiratory effort and rate, may lead to physical exhaustion.
- Respiratory distress: lower airway obstruction, inadequate blood gas exchange.
- Secondary bacterial pneumonia

 # DIFFERENTIAL DIAGNOSIS

- Infectious causes of pneumonia: bacterial, viral
- Trauma: fractured ribs or diaphragmatic hernia or rupture
- Idiopathic tachypnea
- Congenital cardiovascular anomaly: shunting and admixture of deoxygenated blood

 # DIAGNOSTICS

- History: occurrence of dystocia, maternal compromise.
- Auscultation: crackles, wheezes, lack of auscultable air movement in consolidated ventral areas.
- Radiography: cranioventral lung pathology, widespread peribronchiolar infiltration (early), consolidation (later).
- U/S: pulmonary consolidation, abscessation, pleuritis (Fig. 135.1).
- Transtracheal aspiration cytology and culture: meconium, inflammatory cells, bacteria and other debris.

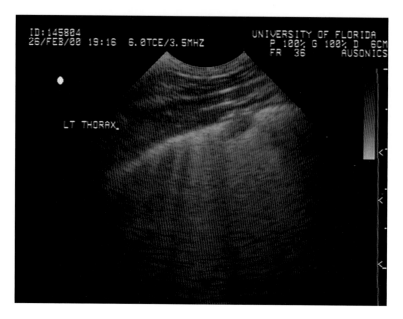

■ **Figure 135.1** Pulmonary abscessation and inflammation shown in an ultrasound.

Pathological Findings

Pulmonary tissue infiltrated by a large number of inflammatory cells. Presence of meconium and sloughed epithelial lining in the airways.

 THERAPEUTICS

- Antimicrobials: broad spectrum initially, preferably bactericidal and parenteral administration. Change according to sensitivity information, if applicable.
- Anti-inflammatories: to decrease inflammation-induced lung pathology. They also provide analgesia to improve ventilation efforts.
- General supportive therapy: intravenous fluids, adequate caloric intake.
- Positive pressure ventilation, if required.

Drug(s) of Choice

- K-penicillin: 40,000 units/kg IV, every 6 hours
- Ceftiofur sodium: 2 mg/kg IM every 12 hours, 5 to 10 mg/kg IV every 6 to 12 hours
- Amikacin: 25 mg/kg IV, every 24 hours
- Trimethoprim-sulfamethoxazole: 30 mg/kg PO, BID
- Flunixin meglumine: 1 mg/kg IV, every 12 hours
- Ketoprofen: 2 mg/kg IV, every 12 to 24 hours

Precautions/Interactions

- Be careful with the administration of bicarbonate, as this may worsen acidosis due to the buildup of carbon dioxide.
- Be careful with administering potentially nephrotoxic drugs to compromised neonates.

Appropriate Health Care

Ensure air is free from particulate irritants (e.g., dust, mold spores, and noxious gases, such as ammonia from urine decomposition).

Nursing Care

Ensure adequate caloric intake and ensure appropriate level of activity. Avoid prolonged periods of recumbency.

Activity

Encourage appropriate amount of exercise when possible.

Surgical Considerations

Affected foals are high risk anesthesia candidates due to ventilation-perfusion mismatch.

 COMMENTS

Client Education

Manage foal in environment with good air quality.

Patient Monitoring

Monitor respiratory rate and effort for deterioration.

Prevention/Avoidance

- Observe foaling to ensure timely progression.
- Consider previous parturition history of mare or any gestational abnormalities when planning for parturition.

Possible Complications

In severe or incompletely resolved cases, consolidated lung may lead to persistent pulmonary hypertension, inadequate ventilation, increased respiratory workload, and a failure to thrive.

Expected Course and Prognosis

Response to treatment is usually progressive, with rapid resolution sometimes seen. Secondary bacterial pneumonias will delay clinical response. Severe cases may succumb in spite of aggressive treatment.

Abbreviations

BID   twice a day
IM   intramuscular
IV   intravenous
MAS   meconium aspiration syndrome
PO   per os (by mouth)

See Also

- Bacterial pneumonia

Suggested Reading

Bedenice D, Heuwieser W, Brawer R, et al. 2003. Clinical and prognostic significance of radiographic pattern, distribution, and severity of thoracic radiographic changes in neonatal foals. *J Vet Intern Med* 17: 876–886.

Peek SF, Landolt G, Karasin AI, et al. 2004. Acute respiratory distress syndrome and fatal interstitial pneumonia associated with equine influenza in a neonatal foal. *J Vet Intern Med* 18: 132–134.

Wilkins PA. 2003. Lower respiratory problems of the neonate. *Vet Clin North Am Equine Pract* 19: 19–33.

Author: Peter R. Morresey

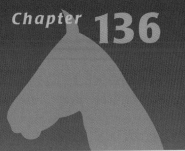

Chapter 136

Meconium Impaction

DEFINITION/OVERVIEW

Meconium is material in the terminal intestine of the term fetus. It appears as a dark pelleted to gelatinous mass and consists of cellular debris, proteinaceous intestinal gland secretions, bile, and amniotic fluid. Intestinal peristalsis normally moves meconium in the fetus. Meconium impaction is the most common cause of colic in the neonatal foal, with medical therapy alone nearly always curative.

ETIOLOGY/PATHOPHYSIOLOGY

Meconium is usually passed within the first 24 to 48 hours of life with minimal abdominal straining. Disturbances to normal gastrointestinal motility or generalized debility are most likely responsible for retention.

Systems Affected

- Gastrointestinal: distal obstruction may lead to more proximal gas and fluid accumulation. High meconium retention (colonic) leads to significant discomfort and intestinal dilation.
- Hemic/Lymphatic/Immune: sepsis if intestinal wall becomes devitalized from pressure necrosis or therapeutic interventions.
- Renal/Urologic: prerenal azotemia resulting from hypovolemia due to depressed fluid intake.
- Respiratory: elevated respiratory rate and effort due to limited diaphragmatic excursion with intestinal dilation.

SIGNALMENT/HISTORY

Passage of meconium not reported despite continued abdominal straining. Fecal color does not change to appropriate yellow-bronze-brown characteristic of milk ingestion.

Risk Factors

- Neonatal asphyxia or other disease
- Males considered to be more commonly affected due to narrower pelvic canal.

Historical Findings

Non-passage of meconium.

 CLINICAL FEATURES

- Signs usually begin within first 24 hours of delivery
- Meconium passage not observed: brown, black, greenish-brown feces are usually followed by milk feces (yellow-brown-bronze)
- Repeated tail swishing
- Repeated abdominal straining (arched back in contrast to lordosis seen with urinary problems). Rectal mucosa may be seen to evert
- Abdominal distension
- Colic
- Urachus may begin to drip urine: increased abdominal pressure
- Sepsis if intestinal wall pressure necrosis occurs

 DIFFERENTIAL DIAGNOSIS

- Rectal inflammation: repeated enema instillation
- Congenital anomaly: atresia coli, intestinal aganglionosis
- Urinary tract obstruction (distal): penile obstruction
- Ruptured bladder: abdominal distension from uroperitoneum may be present

 DIAGNOSTICS

- Abdominal radiographs: plain standing views show gas distended large intestine. Barium contrast allows delineation of high meconium retention, small colon impaction, and the presence of any congenital anomalies (i.e., stricture or atresia).
- U/S: heterogeneous large intestinal mass with regional intestinal dilation.
- Abdominal palpation: firm mass cranial to pelvic brim.

Pathological Findings

Meconium accumulation in distal large intestinal tract.

THERAPEUTICS

- Enema: soapy water, proprietary phosphate. Acetyl cysteine retention enema in intractable cases or those where meconium is retained proximally.
- Fluids: oral or intravenous
- Mineral oil: nasogastric intubation
- Restrict oral intake: intestinal and gastric distension is responsible for the foal's discomfort. Parenteral nutrition may be required.
- Analgesics: flunixin meglumine
- Sedation: relieve discomfort, straining
- Spasmolytics: N-butylscopolammonium bromide
- Surgery: caution, avoid enterotomy when possible

Drug(s) of Choice

See Table 119.1.

Precautions/Interactions

Care must be exercised with repeated enema instillation because rectal trauma is possible. Toxicity from repeated phosphate enemas has been reported.

Nursing Care

Repeated analgesia may be required until meconium has been passed.

Diet

Discontinue oral fluids and feed until the problem is resolved.

Surgical Considerations

Surgical removal by extraluminal massage or enterotomy may be required in intractable cases.

 COMMENTS

Patient Monitoring

Ensure appropriate passage of feces occurs post-resolution of the problem.

Prevention/Avoidance

Ensure freedom from or manage concurrent debilitating neonatal conditions.

Possible Complications

- Urachus opens and expels urine.
- Ruptured urinary bladder if straining is prolonged and excessive.
- Peritonitis and sepsis if intestinal wall has been compromised.

Expected Course and Prognosis

Most affected foals respond rapidly and completely to a single episode of medical therapy. Prolonged cases require more long-term medical therapy, with parenteral fluids and repeated analgesics.

Abbreviations

U/S   ultrasound, ultrasonography

See Also

- Intestinal accidents

Suggested Reading

Santschi EM, Vrotsos PD, Purdy AK, et al. 2001. Incidence of the endothelin receptor B mutation that causes lethal white foal syndrome in white-patterned horses. *AJVR* 62: 97–103.

Wilson JH, Cudd TA. 1980. Common gastrointestinal diseases. In: *Equine Clinical Neonatology*. Koterba AM, Drummond WH, Kosch PC (eds). Philadelphia: Lea & Febiger; 412–430.

Author: Peter R. Morresey

Chapter 137

Meningitis

DEFINITION/OVERVIEW

Pathogens, whether viral, bacterial, or protozoal, can cause substantial inflammation of the meninges of the CNS (pia mater, dura mater, and arachnoid membrane), whether by their own actions or the immune response to the initial infectious insult.

ETIOLOGY/PATHOPHYSIOLOGY

Organisms gain entry to the CNS by hematogenous spread (as the result of sepsis) or direct inoculation due to trauma. Often bacteria recovered from meningitis cases are the same as those responsible for the concurrent sepsis. As inflammation progresses, cerebral blood flow decreases leading to ischemic damage and further neurological dysfunction.

Systems Affected

- Hemic/Lymphatic/Immune: systemic signs of infection likely present.
- Nervous: central depression or seizure activity.
- Neuromuscular: inflammation of the meninges results in reluctance to move the neck, opisthotonus, or proprioceptive deficits.
- Ophthalmic: hypopyon, uveitis may be present.
- Respiratory: depressed ventilation efforts may be present.

SIGNALMENT/HISTORY

Risk Factors

- Sepsis: generalized sepsis leading to hematogenous spread to CNS. May be localized lesion acting as a focal source (e.g., omphalophlebitis, pneumonia, or septic arthritis).
- Trauma: direct inoculation of pathogens into the CNS.

Historical Findings

Sudden onset of neurological dysfunction. May be preceded by a period of fever or concurrent with a diagnosed septic process.

 CLINICAL FEATURES

- Fever: may have high fever in the initial stages (to 40.5°C [105°F]). As condition progresses foal may become hypothermic due to generalized depression.
- Hyperesthesia or hypertonia. Neck rigidity and pain upon manipulation may be prominent.
- Depression: centrally mediated generalized depression can occur in later stages.
- Cranial nerve dysfunction: strabismus or anisocoria.
- Seizure activity: generalized seizure activity with cerebral involvement.

 DIFFERENTIAL DIAGNOSIS

- HIE
- Trauma

 DIAGNOSTICS

- Clinical signs.
- Hematology: inflammatory leukogram.
- Cerebrospinal fluid: leukocytosis (neutrophilia or degenerative cells), increased protein, cytologic evidence of bacteria.

Pathological Findings

Presence of infected focus or widespread inflammatory changes in the meninges.

 THERAPEUTICS

- *Antimicrobials*: initially broad spectrum until culture results are available. Consideration must be given to the CNS penetrating ability of the antimicrobials used. Appropriate choices include third-generation cephalosporins, chloramphenicol, and trimethoprim potentiated sulfonamides. The inflamed blood-CNS barrier of affected patients has been shown more permeable to many drugs when compared to healthy individuals.
- *Anti-inflammatories*: NSAIDs or corticosteroids may be indicated.

- Control seizure activity, if it is present.
- *General supportive therapy*: nutrition, fluid, and electrolyte balance. Manage secondary trauma, if present.

Drug(s) of Choice

See HIE.

Precautions/Interactions

Care with potentially nephrotoxic drugs in patients with renal compromise.

Appropriate Health Care

Monitor closely for and control seizure activity.

Activity

Maintain in an environment with minimal stimulus, if seizure activity is present.

 COMMENTS

Client Education

Condition may progress to fatal outcome despite aggressive treatment.

Patient Monitoring

Observe for onset of neurological deficits and seizure activity.

Possible Complications

Secondary trauma

Expected Course and Prognosis

Guarded prognosis

Abbreviations

CNS   central nervous system
HIE   hypoxic ischemic encephalopathy
NSAID   nonsteroidal anti-inflammatory drug
PAS   perinatal asphyxia syndrome

See Also

- HIE
- PAS

Suggested Reading

Green SL, Mayhew IG. 1980. Neurologic disorders. In: *Equine Clinical Neonatology*. Koterba AM, Drummond WH, Kosch PC (eds). Philadelphia: Lea & Febiger; 496–530.

MacKay RJ. 2005. Neurologic disorders of neonatal foals. *Vet Clin North Am Equine Pract* 2: 387–406.

Author: Peter R. Morresey

Chapter 138

Microphthalmia

DEFINITION/OVERVIEW

Ocular conditions in the foal often go undiagnosed because examination is not commonly performed unless for insurance or sale purposes.

When compared to the adult horse, a number of differences are noted in the foal:

- A slight medial and ventral strabismus is present, with the adult globe position attained at approximately 1 month of age.
- The pupil is relatively round (contrast to ovoid adult pupil).
- The menace response is not present until approximately 2 weeks of age; however, it may develop at any time prior to that.
- Prominent Y sutures of the lens capsule are present and should not be confused with cataract formation.
- Comparatively low tear production.
- Corneal sensitivity to stimulation is low, predisposing to traumatic lesions.

Congenitally small globe

ETIOLOGY/PATHOPHYSIOLOGY

Idiopathic *in utero* developmental anomaly. May be secondary to uterine infection or an unknown toxicosis.

Systems Affected

Nervous: visual deficits

SIGNALMENT/HISTORY

One of the more common congenital lesions. May be unilateral or bilateral.

Risk Factors

In utero developmental anomaly

Historical Findings

Small, sunken eyes

 CLINICAL FEATURES

- Decreased palpebral fissure
- Prominent nictitans
- Affected globe may be functional
- Blindness or visual impairment may occur in severely affected globes as intraocular structures may be abnormal
- May be in association with other defects: cataracts

 DIFFERENTIAL DIAGNOSIS

- Uveitis: decreased intraocular pressure.
- Collapsed globe

 DIAGNOSTICS

Characteristic clinical findings

Pathological Findings

- Characteristic findings of small or malformed globe

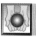 **THERAPEUTICS**

- None
- Manage complications: repair entropion or combat corneal ulceration

 COMMENTS

Client Education

Heritable component may be present. Thoroughbreds appear at increased risk.

Possible Complications

Chronic corneal ulceration and conjunctivitis may necessitate removal of affected eye if non-visual.

Expected Course and Prognosis

Prognosis good for life, guarded for vision.

Suggested Reading

Gelatt KN. 2000. Equine ophthalmology. In: *Essentials of Veterinary Ophthalmology*. Gelatt KN (ed). Philadelphia: Lippincott Williams & Wilkins; 337–376.

Turner AG. 2004. Ocular conditions of neonatal foals. *Vet Clin North Am Equine Pract* 20: 429–440.

Whitley RD. 1990. Neonatal equine ophthalmology. In: *Equine Clinical Neonatology*, vol. 1. Koterba AM, Drummond WH, Kosch PC (eds). Philadelphia: Lea & Febiger; 531–557.

Author: Peter R. Morresey

chapter 139

Necrotizing Enterocolitis

DEFINITION/OVERVIEW

Asphyxia during the perinatal period can lead to varying degrees of HIE including gastrointestinal disturbances: mild ileus, delayed gastric emptying (Fig. 139.1), and hemorrhagic diarrhea. Most severe manifestation is NE, resulting from oxidative damage and bacterial overgrowth in large intestine.

ETIOLOGY/PATHOPHYSIOLOGY

Hypoxic-ischemic insult during gestation or delivery. Disruption of gastrointestinal mucosal integrity.

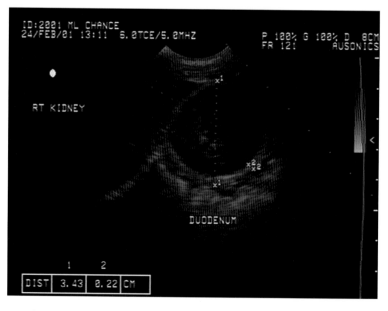

■ **Figure 139.1** Dilated duodenum, shown on ultrasound, which is indicative of delayed gastric emptying.

Systems Affected

- Hemic/Lymphatic/Immune: sepsis
- Nervous: may be part of systemic hypoxic-ischemic insult syndrome.
- Renal/Urologic: acute renal failure may be concurrent.
- Respiratory: disturbances of ventilation due to central depression or pulmonary edema.

 # SIGNALMENT/HISTORY

Foals in the early neonatal period that experienced *in utero* deprivation or dystocia.

Risk Factors

Hypoxia or hypotension

Historical Findings

Onset of depression and signs of gastrointestinal disease.

 # CLINICAL FEATURES

- Variable severity of gastrointestinal disturbance.
- Fever, then hypothermia, if advanced.
- Depression
- Sepsis
- Hemorrhagic diarrhea

 # DIFFERENTIAL DIAGNOSIS

Bacterial diarrhea: Clostridiosis, Salmonellosis

 # DIAGNOSTICS

- History: peripartum asphyxia.
- Compatible clinical signs.
- U/S: distended small intestinal loops, decreased motility, colonic gas production (may involve gut wall).

Pathological Findings

Inflammation, hemorrhage, necrosis, and possible gas infiltration of the gastrointestinal tract.

THERAPEUTICS

- Broad-spectrum antimicrobials: enteric bacterial translocation and sepsis is likely.
- Specific anticlostridial therapy: metronidazole.
- Antiulcer medication.
- Correct fluid and electrolyte abnormalities.
- Plasma transfusion.
- Anti-endotoxin therapy: polymyxin B.

Drug(s) of Choice

See Table 119.1.

Diet

Parenteral nutrition advantageous

Surgical Considerations

Resection of affected intestine may be required.

COMMENTS

Possible Complications

Death

Expected Course and Prognosis

Fatal if not treated aggressively in the early stages of disease before necrosis of intestinal wall occurs.

Abbreviations

HIE   hypoxic ischemic encephalopathy
NE   necrotizing enterocolitis
U/S   ultrasound, ultrasonography

See Also

- Bacterial diarrhea

Suggested Reading

Bueschel D, Walker R, Woods L, et al. 1998. Enterotoxigenic *Clostridium perfringens* type A necrotic enteritis in a foal. *JAVMA* 213: 1305–1307, 1280.

Byars TD. 2002. Diarrhea in foals. In: *Manual of Equine Gastroenterology*. Mair T, Divers T, Duscharme N (eds). Philadelphia: W. B. Saunders; 493–495.

East LM, Dargatz DA, Traub-Dargatz JL, et al. 2000. Foaling-management practices associated with the occurrence of enterocolitis attributed to *Clostridium perfringens* infection in the equine neonate. *Prev Vet Med* 46: 61–74.

Wilson JH, Cudd TA. 1980. Common gastrointestinal diseases. In: *Equine Clinical Neonatology*. Koterba AM, Drummond WH, Kosch PC (eds). Philadelphia: Lea & Febiger; 412–430.

Author: Peter R. Morresey

chapter 140

Neonatal Disease, Overview

DEFINITION/OVERVIEW

- Neonatal diseases are generally defined as any illness occurring in the first 2 to 4 weeks of life.
- Neonatal disease in foals is commonly subdivided into two categories.
  - Those occurring in the first week, the immediate neonatal period.
  - Those occurring in the second week and later.
- Diseases of the neonate can are also divided into:
  - Maladjustment syndromes
  - Traumatic origin
  - Infectious origin
  - Congenital or Genetic disorders
- Referral to a specialized hospital with a proper ICU should be considered before a foal becomes compromised.

ETIOLOGY/PATHOPHYSIOLOGY

- Neonatal disease can originate during pregnancy, intrapartum, or immediately postpartum.
  - Risk factors are based on an evaluation of events related to pregnancy or parturition, and evaluation of the neonate in its first 24 hours of life.
- *High-risk foal*, any foal:
  - Born to a mare that had a serious health problem during pregnancy (i.e., from a high-risk pregnancy).
  - Delivered by OB manipulation or C-section (i.e., dystocia or premature placental separation).
  - Presented with visible abnormalities that interfere with normal behavior and adjustment (e.g., trauma, twins, prematurity, or dysmaturity).
  - Combination of any of these factors place a foal in a high-risk category.
- *Moderately-at-risk foal*:
  - One for which birth and initial postpartum period were unsupervised.
  - One at risk of FPT

- *Low-risk foal*:
  - Born without complication following a normal pregnancy.
  - Has normal development and behavior.
  - Adequate passive transfer of immunoglobulin.
- Although neonatal disease can be studied by entity or body system, sick foals present with multiple system compromise if the primary disorder is not addressed rapidly.
- *Neonatal disease* is suspected based on clinical signs deviating from normal behavior, such as:
  - Depression, seizures, and respiratory distress.
  - Membrane abnormalities: petechial hemorrhage, injected, icteric, or cyanotic.
  - Fever
  - Lameness (i.e., swollen, hot, painful joints)
  - Colic (i.e., abdominal distention or pain)
  - Dysuria, stranguria
  - Milk observed in the nostrils
  - Ocular abnormalities (i.e., hyphema, hypopyon, corneal ulcers)
  - Diarrhea
  - Other obvious abnormalities (e.g., abnormal umbilicus, patent urachus, or hernias)
- *Review problems of maternal origin*:
  - Develop problem list and differential diagnoses based on mare's history.
  - Include current pregnancy, prior foaling history, foaling conditions, foal care, and her foal's condition prior to presentation.

Systems Affected

- Multiple systems may be affected
- Some abnormalities may be of genetic origin (e.g., lethal white syndrome or SCID).

 # SIGNALMENT/HISTORY

- Neonatal foal disease is a common complaint
- Foals in the first 2 to 4 weeks of life.
- Foals with predisposing factors:
  - High-risk pregnancies
  - Post-dystocia
  - Unattended foaling

Risk Factors

- See Etiology/Pathophysiology.
- Unsanitary foaling conditions
- Improper foal care
- FPT

Historical Findings

- High-risk pregnancy (i.e., placentitis, placental edema, uterine torsion, or colic surgery on the mare).
- Abnormal pregnancy length: less than or up to 320 days, or prolonged pregnancy.
- Abnormal foaling events: premature placental separation (Red Bag), dystocia.
- Abnormal events in the immediate postpartum period: severe postpartum complications, RFM, mare health emergency, agalactia, uterine artery tear or rupture (dam), or death of the dam.
- Vaccination history of the dam.

 ## CLINICAL FEATURES

Foal Behavior Evaluation

- Deviations from normal behavior (see Foal Care) should be recorded (e.g., reduction in nursing or overall activity or decreased awareness of its whereabouts, including its dam).
- Poor suckling reflex: maladjustment syndrome, HIE (i.e., PAS), septicemia, hydrocephalus.
- Any abnormal gait: lameness requires thorough evaluation.
- Inability to swallow: botulism

Clinical Signs of Importance in Sick Foals

- Scoring systems used to assess responsiveness or depression in foals in the first 2 hours of life (Table 140.1). Components include: overall appearance, pulse, responsiveness, muscle tone or activity, and respiration.
- Dam's mammary gland is found engorged.
  - Suggests a lack of nursing (full versus flattened teats, the latter being evidence of recent suckling).
- Most common abnormal clinical presentations of sick foals:
  - Conformation defects: angular limb deformities.
  - Signs of prematurity or dysmaturity (Fig. 140.1a)
    - Low birth weight
    - Disproportionate appearance (e.g., domed head, bulging eyes)
    - Tendon laxity and poor muscle development (Fig. 140.1b)
    - Weak, immature, ear cartilage (floppy ears)
    - Fine silky haircoat
    - Uncoordinated movements
    - Abnormal respiratory pattern
  - Depression or lethargy is evident in most cases of advanced neonatal disease.
  - Lameness (indicator for septic arthritis) or swollen joints may be the sole evidence of septicemia.

TABLE 140.1 Neonatal Sepsis Scoring

Equine Neonate, Sepsis Scoring

Points for item:	4	3	2	1	0	Score
I History						
1 Risk Factors		Yes			No	
2 Prematurity		<300 d	300–310 d	311–330 d	>330 d	
II Clinical Examination						
1 Depression			Marked	Mild	None	
2 Fever			>38.8°C (>102°F)	<37.7°C (<100°F)	Normal	
3 Petechiation		Marked	Moderate	Mild	None	
4 Localizing Signs		Yes				
III CBC						
1 Neutrophil count		<2000/mm³	2,000–4,000 or >12,000/mm³	8,000–12,000/mm³	Normal 4,000–8,000/mm³	
2 Band count		>200/mm³	50–200/mm³		<50 /mm³	
3 Toxic changes	Marked	Moderate	Slight		None	
4 Fibrinogen			>600 mg/dL	401–600 mg/dL	<400 mg/dL	
IV Other Lab Data						
1 Serum IgG	<200 mg/dL	200–400 mg/dL	401–800 mg/dL		>800 mg/dL	
2 Blood Glucose			<50 mg/dL	50–80 mg/dL	>80 mg/dL	
					Total:	

If foal is >12 hours old, use IgG result from lab.

If foal is <12 hours old and has nursed, assign +2

If foal is <12 hours old and has not nursed, assign +4

Sepsis score >11, Sepsis is likely

Sepsis score <10, Sepsis is unlikely

IgG, immunoglobulin G.

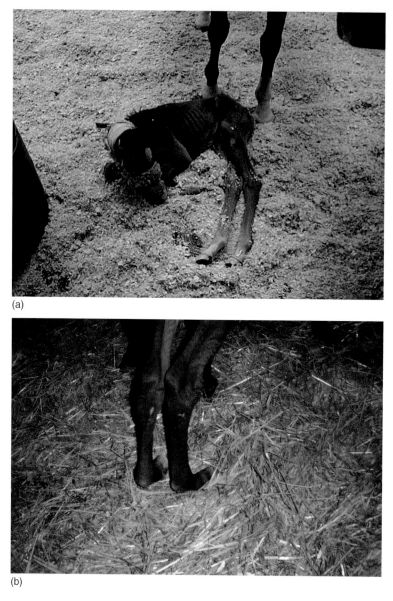

(a)

(b)

■ **Figure 140.1** *A,* Premature foal (low birth weight, silky); and *B,* Tendon laxity.

- Colic is often associated with:
  - Meconium retention (Fig. 140.2)
  - Congenital defects of the digestive tract (e.g., lethal white syndrome).
  - Uroperitoneum
  - Diarrhea (Fig. 140.3)
- Entropion is common in premature and severely ill foals.
- Mucous membrane appearance is dependent on etiology and the degree affected.

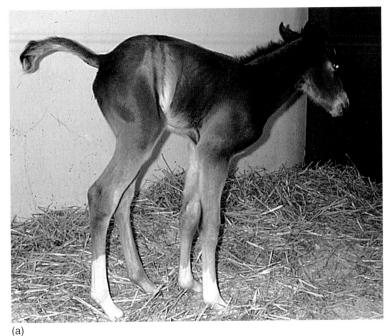

(a)

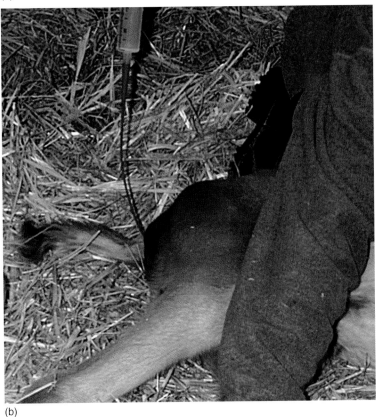

(b)

■ **Figure 140.2** Meconium retention. *A*, Straining; *B*, Administration of warm soapy enema; and *C*, Passed sticky meconium.

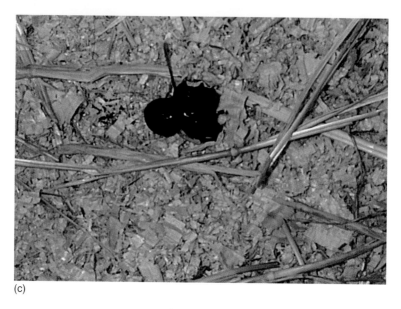

(c)

■ **Figure 140.2** continued

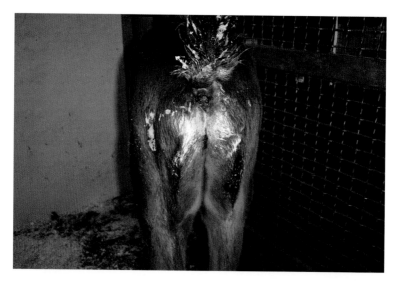

■ **Figure 140.3** Diarrhea.

- With HIE or a severely compromised foal, it may appear or be cyanotic.
- Petechial hemorrhage or hyperemia is present with sepsis.
- Icterus is obvious in advanced stages of NI (Fig. 140.4).
- Icterus is also seen in foals with HIE.
- Cardiac murmurs normally resolve in 2 weeks but are exacerbated in sick foals.
- Tachycardia and tachypnea are features of sepsis, severe trauma or painful conditions, and NI.

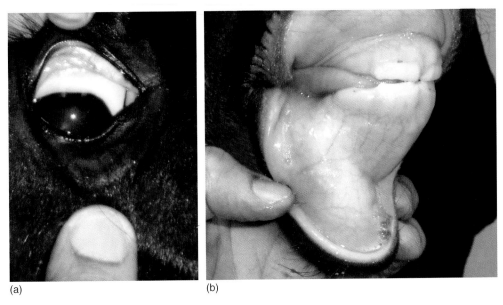

(a)   (b)

■ **Figure 140.4** Neonatal isoerythrolysis in a 3-day old foal showing icterus on the sclera *(a)* and oral mucosa *(b)*.

- Persistent pain, non-responsive to drugs, is generally associated with severe GI disease (e.g., gastroduodenal ulcers).
- Fever higher than 39°C (>102.2°F) (septic condition, may be undulating fever) or hypothermia.
  - Enlarged, painful (omphalophlebitis) (Fig. 140.5) or persistently moist umbilicus (patent urachus).
  - Milk-stained face is frequently observed in depressed foals. In the first few hours of life, dribbling of milk from the nose should warrant examination for cleft palate (Fig. 140.6).

Most Common Traumatic Disorders

- Ruptured bladder, mostly males, less than 7 days of age.
  - First diagnosis usually made by 2 or more days of age.
- Fractured ribs (location can result in pericardial and lung lacerations, Fig. 140.7).
- Traumatic injury caused by the dam or during transport.

Most Common Infectious Diseases

- Sepsis can be apparent within the first few hours of life (*in utero* infection such as placentitis).
  - Whether primary or secondary, septicemia is the most common cause of death in sick foals.
  - Predisposing factors: prematurity, FPT, *in utero* infection, perinatal asphyxia, or twinning.

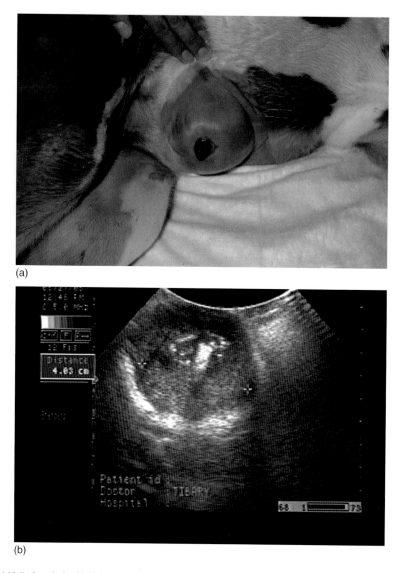

(a)

(b)

■ **Figure 140.5** Omphalophlebitis. *A*, Clinical examination; and *B*, Ultrasound of an umbilical abscess.

- ■ Generalized septicemia is a complication in more than half of foals with HIE.
- ■ Use sepsis score worksheet to establish the degree of sepsis.
- ■ Septic arthritis or osteomyelitis is a common complication of septicemia due to infections originating from GI tract, umbilical cord, pneumonia, penetrating wounds (Fig. 140.8).
- ■ Omphalophlebitis (*see* Fig. 140.5)
- ■ Enteritis/diarrhea
- ■ Pneumonia: meconium aspiration, *in utero* infection
- ■ Other uncommon infectious diseases include:
  - ■ Congenital EHV, meningitis, and botulism.

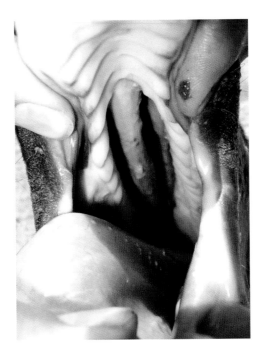

■ **Figure 140.6** Cleft palate in a 2-hour-old foal.

- Tetanus should be on list of rule outs, especially in developing countries because they have a higher percentage of unvaccinated horses, donkeys and mule foals from poor areas.
- *Rhodococcus equi* infections (endemic in some areas).

Most Common Congenital Anomalies/Genetic Disorders

- Genetic disorders of the foal should take breed incidence into account.
- NI: mares that had prior foal(s) with NI, or are known to be Aa or Qa negative.
  - NI: increased incidence in mule foals.
- SCID: from 2 days to 4 months of age, poor doer, repeated infections, common in Arabian horses.
- Angular limb deformities, contracted tendons, windswept foals are common in some areas (Fig. 140.9).
  - Associated with foal hypothyroidism, mustard toxicosis, tall fescue toxicosis.
- Patent urachus (persistently wet umbilicus): most foals are less than 14 days old and sick from other problems; this is an *emergency*.
- Congenital heart defects: VSD, PDA, patent foramen ovale, pulmonic stenosis, Tetralogy of Fallot, persistent aortic arch.
- Hydrocephalus
  - Common in miniature horses
- Persistent preputial ring (Fig. 140.10)
  - Urine scalding

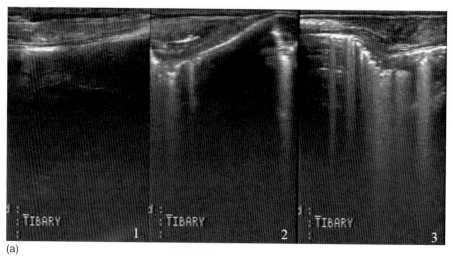

(a)

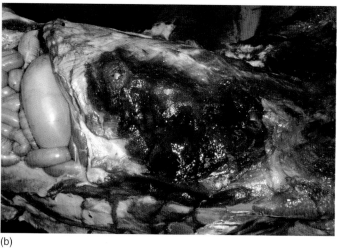

(b)

■ **Figure 140.7** Fractured ribs in a foal presenting with severe respiratory distress after dystocia. *A*, Ultrasound of normal (1) and fractured ribs (2, 3); and *B*, Postmortem findings.

- Cleft palate
  - Hernias (inguinal, umbilical) are common in some families of horses (Figs. 140.11 and 140.12).

Most Common Causes of Depression/Weakness/Lethargy

- HIE also known as PAS
- NI
- Septicemia, septic arthritis.
- Fractured ribs (*see* Fig. 140.7), lacerations of deeper tissues.
- Patent urachus
- Ruptured bladder, uroperitoneum

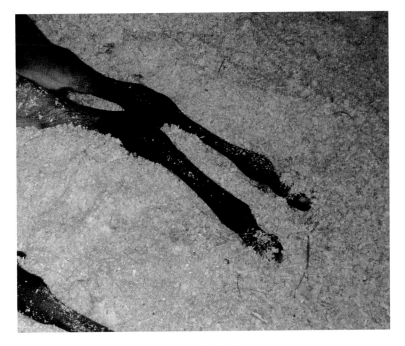

■ **Figure 140.8** An 8-day-old lame foal with septic polyarthritis.

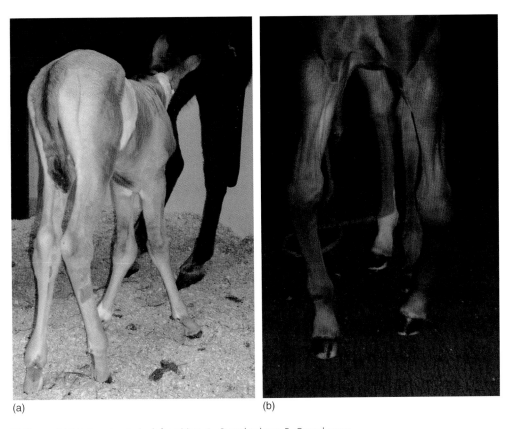

(a)   (b)

■ **Figure 140.9** Angular limb deformities: *A,* Carpal valgus; *B,* Carpal varus.

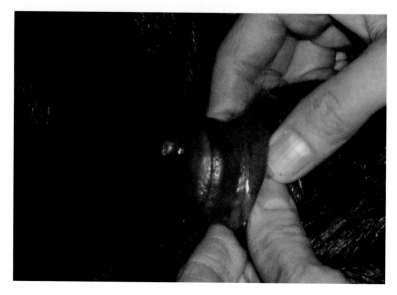

■ **Figure 140.10** Abnormal preputial ring and urethral process.

Most Common Causes of Respiratory Problems

- Perinatal asphyxia, prematurity, or dysmaturity
- Advanced septicemia
- Advanced state of NI
- Pneumonia
- Fractured ribs
- Rhodococcus equi infection
- Congenital heart defects

Most Common Causes of Colic

- Meconium retention:
  - Most common cause of colic in foals less than 24 hours old.
  - Higher prevalence in males
  - Meconium most often retained in colon or in the rectum.
- Ruptured bladder
  - Uroperitoneum can cause abdominal distension and lead to other complications, ileus, or dysuria.
- Congenital malformations if foal is less than 24 hours old (e.g., lethal white syndrome)
- Enteritis
- Strangulating hernias
- Peritonitis
- HIE, prematurity, dor ysmaturity
- Gasteroduodenal ulceration

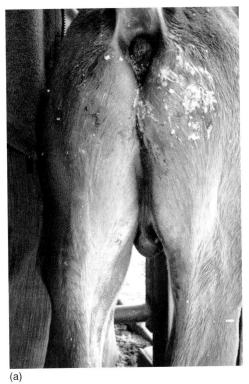

(a)

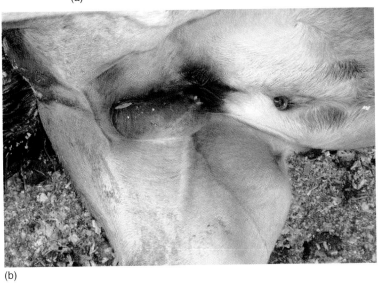

(b)

■ **Figure 140.11** Caudal *(a)* and ventral *(b)* views of inguinal hernia in an 11-day-old foal.

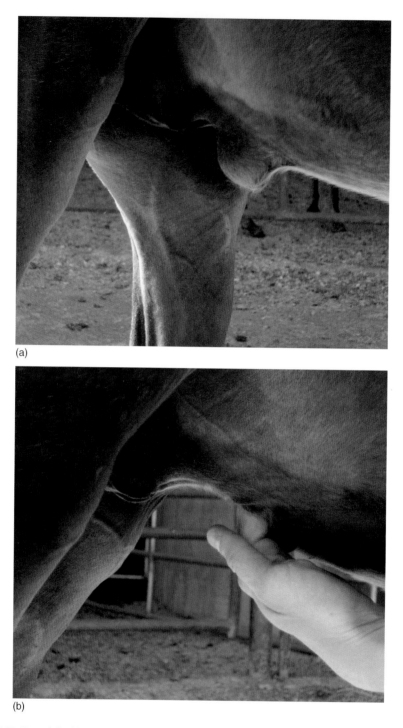

■ **Figure 140.12** Umbilical hernia before *(a)* and after *(b)* manual reduction.

- Ascarid impaction: seen earliest at 8 to 12 weeks because the prepatent period is 10 to 11 weeks.
- Miscellaneous causes: colon torsion, intussusception, volvulus of the small intestine, atresia ani, atresia coli, lethal white syndrome (ileocolonic agangliosis), enteritis, diaphragmatic hernia, ruptured bladder, and cystitis.

Most Common Causes of Seizures

- HIE
- Cranial trauma
- Metabolic disorders: electrolyte abnormalities, primarily low sodium (especially less than 120 MEq/L).
- Idiopathic epilepsy of Arabian foals

Most Common Causes of Diarrhea

- Foal-heat diarrhea occurs between 6 and 10 days of age and may last 2 to 5 days. The foal is generally bright and alert and exhibits normal behavior.
- *Salmonella* associated with sepsis (high-risk in *Salmonella* shedding mares)
- *Clostridium perfringens* type A or C, first 2 days of life.
  - Fetid hemorrhagic necrotizing enteritis.
  - Can occur as a stud farm outbreak.
- *Clostridium difficile* (less than 5 days old)
  - Severe watery diarrhea
  - Fatal hemorrhagic necrotizing enterocolitis (may be seen as a herd outbreak).
- Rotavirus (2 days to 4 months of age) outbreaks.
  - Rapid spread
  - Fever and depression
- *Strongyloides westeri* may cause diarrhea at 1 to 4 weeks of age.
  - Larvae are present in mare's milk at 4 days and peak at 10 to 12 days.
  - Incidence is region dependent.
- *Cryptosporidium* sp.: incubation 9 to 28 days.
- Giardia
- *Escherichia coli* septicemia: bloody diarrhea, septicemia.
- Lactose intolerance is usually secondary to rotavirus or *C. difficile* or *C. perfringens*.
- Gastroduodenal ulcers
  - Diarrhea, fever, and complication of stressful conditions

 # DIFFERENTIAL DIAGNOSIS

- Differential diagnosis should be based on thorough history (pregnancy, foaling and postpartum conditions) and examination of the dam and foal.
- Timing/onset of the problem and its clinical presentation may help develop differential diagnoses, however there may be several concomitant disorders in the severely ill foal.

DIAGNOSTICS

CBC/Biochemistry/Urinalysis

Laboratory

- IgG
- Hematology: assess dehydration and CBC.
- CBC
  - Leucopenia and neutropenia, *premature foal* (neutropenic).
    - The neutrophil to lymphocyte ratio is less than 1.
    - Viral infection (EHV-1) or septicemia due to *E. coli*. May also be the case with some acute salmonellosis.
  - Leucopenia, neutropenia in cases of *endotoxemia* (*C. perfringens* A and C).
  - Neutrophilia (septicemia, greater than 12,000/μL) with
    - Upper respiratory bacterial infection (*Streptococcus equi*)
    - Pneumonia (*Rhodococcus equi*)
    - Enteritis (*Salmonella*)
    - Septic umbilicus
  - Severe anemia: low RBC, hypoglobulinemia, low PCV
    - NI
  - Thrombocytosis
    - Associated with *R. equi* infections
    - Some NI cases have low platelets too.

Chemistry

- Fibrinogen is greater than 400 mg/dL.
  - Chronic infectious or parasitic disease, *if* more than 24 to 48 hours duration.
  - This impact may begin *in utero* for the fetus, if the dam has placentitis.
  - Internal abscessation
  - Gastroduodenal ulceration
- Metabolic acidosis
  - Premature foals
  - Uroperitoneum
- Hypoglycemia
  - Prematurity
  - Hypoxia
  - Septicemia
- Uroperitonium
  - Hyperkalemia, hyponatremia, hypochloremia, increased serum creatinine.
- Arterial oxygen
- Acid-base

Other Laboratory Tests

Cytology

- Synovial fluid: foals with swollen joints.
- Peritoneal fluid: colic
- CSF: foal with neurological abnormalities
  - To rule out septic meningitis

Microbiology

- Blood culture:
  - Appropriate (meticulous) technique from foal that may be septicemic.
  - Gram-negative sepsis is most common, however may be some Gram-positive bacteria.
  - Most common pathogens, *Salmonella* sp., *E. coli*, *Actinobacillus equuli*.
- Fecal culture should be performed to screen for *Salmonella* spp. Common organisms associated with diarrhea:
  - Bacterial: *C. difficile*, *Salmonella*, *C. perfringens*, *E. coli*, *R. equi* (older foals), *A. equuli*
  - Viral: Rotavirus
  - Protozoal: *Cryptosporidium parvum*
  - Parasitic: *Strongyloides westeri*
- Synovial fluid samples should be obtained from acutely inflamed and swollen joints. Etiology of septic arthritis: *E. coli*, *Actinobacillus* spp., *Salmonella* sp., *Staphylococcus* sp., *Streptococcus* sp., Rhodococcus and Corynebacterium, Mycoplasma and Chlamydial infections have been reported.

Imaging

Radiographs

- Chest radiographs may help determine the etiology of respiratory distress.
- Abdominal radiographs

U/S

- An important technique for evaluation of the sick foal.
- Of the umbilicus and abdomen: colic, abnormal appearance of the umbilicus.
- Frequent abnormalities observed are:
  - Free abdominal fluid (uroperitoneum or hemoperitoneum).
  - Increased intestinal wall thickness
  - Decreased intestinal motility
  - Intestinal intussusceptions
  - Abscesses
  - Masses
- Thoracic U/S may help diagnosis etiology of respiratory distress:
  - Fractured ribs (*see* Fig. 140.7)

- Free thoracic fluid
- Superficial consolidation/abscesses.
- Echocardiography to diagnosis congenital heart defect.

Gastroscopy

- Useful for diagnosis of gastric ulcers and pyloric outflow defects.

Other Diagnostic Procedures

Abdominocentesis

- Indications: colic, abdominal pain or distension.
- Ratio of peritoneal to serum creatinine
  - greater than 2 to 1, then it is uroperitoneum
- Colic: intestinal strangulation, peritonitis
  - increased WBC

Pathologic Findings

See with individual rule outs above.

 ## THERAPEUTICS

Appropriate Health Care

See specific diseases.

Nursing Care

- Nursing care of a sick foal is time-consuming and expensive.
- Constant (i.e., "24/7") monitoring is often required in initial treatment and care of the foal.
- Referral to a specialized hospital is often the best option. Key findings necessitating referral and intensive care:
  - Foals classified as high risk
  - Minimum conditions for foal care are unavailable on site (adequate housing, adequate light, availability of oxygen, 24/7 monitoring, ready access to lab support)
  - Foal too weak to stand or nurse
  - Foal with weak or absent suckling reflex
  - Foal with dyspnea or in respiratory distress
  - Abdominal pain failing to resolve following an enema(s), (i.e., pain unrelated to meconium retention and meconium impaction has been ruled out).
  - Lameness onset in the first week of life
  - Seizuring foal

Diet

- Need to feed a foal with a healthy GI tract, 10% to 15 % of its BW in the first 24 hours (e.g., 45-kg [100-lb] foal must get at least 4.5 kg [10 lbs] of milk in feedings divided throughout the first 24 hours).
- After 24 hours, increase intake up to 20% of BW.
  - When at "full feed," the 100-pound foal will require 9 kg (20 lbs) per day, with adjustments upward commensurate with the foal's weight gain.
  - Example: when foal weighs 63.5 kg (140 lbs), it will need to be fed approximately 13 kg (28 lbs) of milk per day, etc.
- Foal must be fed at least every 2 hours.
- If a foal won't suckle, a long-term NG tube (Mila®, a softer tube) can be placed, sutured into the nostrils, to ensure nutrition is received.

Activity

See specific condition.

Surgical Considerations

- Exploratory laparotomy
- Umbilical resection
- Ruptured bladder
- Hernia repair

 COMMENTS

Client Education

- Management of mare during pregnancy:
  - Nutrition, adjustment of needs based on stage of gestation.
  - Immunization program, minimum requirements.
- Foaling management, including frequency of observation, means of predicting date of foaling, etc.
- Care of the mare and neonate, including colostrum management (i.e., quality, frequency, quantity).
- Education regarding factors that increase the risk for neonatal disease.
- Warn client about the emotional and monetary costs of treating a sick foal.
- Advise referral to an ICU, once realistic emotional and monetary values of the neonate have been discussed.

Prevention/Avoidance

- Proper management of broodmare, foaling, and care of the mare and neonate
- Colostrum management
- Examination and monitoring of high-risk foals

Abbreviations

BW	body weight
CBC	complete blood count
CSF	cerebrospinal fluid
EHV	equine herpes virus
FPT	failure of passive transfer
GI	gastrointestinal
HIE	hypoxic ischemic encephalopathy = PAS
ICU	intensive care unit
IgG	immunoglobulin G
NG	nasogastric (tube)
NI	neonatal isoerythrolysis
OB	obstetrical
PAS	perinatal asphyxia syndrome
PCV	packed cell volume
PDA	patent ductus arteriosus
RBC	red blood cells
RFM	retained fetal membranes, retained placenta
SCID	severe combined immunodeficiency disease
U/S	ultrasound, ultrasonography
VSD	ventricular septal defect
WBC	white blood cells

See Also

- Specific foal conditions
- HIE/PAS
- Postpartum mare and foal care

Suggested Reading

Hess-Dudan F, Rossdale PD. 2003. Neonatal maladjustment syndrome and other neurological signs in the newborn foal. Part 1: Definitions, aetiopathogenesis, clinical signs and diagnosis. *Eq Vet Educ Manual* 6: 55–63.

Hess-Dudan F, Rossdale PD. 2003. Neonatal maladjustment syndrome and other neurological signs in the newborn foal. Part 2: Therapy, management and prognosis. *Eq Vet Educ Manual* 6: 64–67.

Pierce SW. 2003. Foal care from birth to 30 days: A practitioner's perspective. *Proc AAEP* 49: 13–21.

Author: Ahmed Tibary

chapter 141

Neonatal Evaluation

 ## DEFINITION/OVERVIEW

Events during gestation and those around the time of delivery profoundly affect neonatal viability and subsequent development through to adulthood.

 ## ETIOLOGY/PATHOPHYSIOLOGY

- Maternal history: illness during gestation can result in an *in utero* fetal deprivation. A previous delivery of a compromised neonate is also a risk factor for the current pregnancy.
- Prolonged gestation: may indicate degenerative endometrial change or fescue toxicosis (fetal deprivation).
- Placental pathology: placentitis leads to placental thickening or premature separation.
- Dystocia: prolonged delivery time can allow meconium aspiration and hypoxic-ischemic insult.
- Birth trauma: assisted delivery increases the likelihood of musculoskeletal injury.

 ## DIAGNOSTICS

Physical Examination

Rectal Temperature

- Appropriate neonatal range 37.2°C to 38.6°C (99°F to 101.5°F).
- Neonatal foals are unable to regulate body temperature to the same degree as older foals. This is especially evident in compromised or dysmature foals.
- A fever spike may be the first indication of sepsis; however, it can be an unreliable occurrence.
- Hypothermic extremities may indicate circulatory collapse (i.e., hypovolemia, sepsis).
- Hypoglycemia may be manifested as generalized hypothermia.

Cardiovascular System

- Appropriate neonatal range is between 70 and 120 bpm.
- HR is highly labile; however, rate and rhythm are regular. Pulses are synchronous with the heart beat and easily palpable. Deviations may indicate arrhythmia (electrolyte abnormality, congenital cardiac anomaly).
- Systolic ejection murmurs are a common finding and considered physiologic.
- A murmur associated with a PDA can occur for the first few days of life.
- Sepsis or pneumonia can result in pulmonary hypertension and right to left shunting of blood with resultant hypoxemia. A VSD, not a PDA, is most commonly responsible for the observed clinical signs. Primary valve disease is rare in the neonate.

Respiratory System

- Within the first hour of life, the RR of a normal foal can rise up to 80 bpm. The RR decreases progressively over the next few days, with a subsequent range of 30 to 40 bpm.
- An increased RR may indicate compromised pulmonary function, pain, excitement, or fever. Therefore, the RR may be an unreliable indicator of neonatal pulmonary disease.
- The thoracic excursion indicates an appropriate respiratory effort. Any decrease may indicate fatigue.
- Nostril flaring may be the only indication of increased respiratory effort.
- Air sounds are more prominent in the foal due to the decreased thoracic wall thickness.
- The absence of a cough is not a reliable indicator of the lack of respiratory compromise. This is due to a delayed maturation of airway receptors in the neonatal foal.
- Respiratory signs can occur with the presence of a congenital heart lesion. However, signs of respiratory disease are more likely the result of pathology of the tracheobronchial tree, lung parenchyma, pleural space, or pleura.

Musculoskeletal System

- Joint distension: indicative of sepsis, coagulopathy (hemarthrosis), or trauma.
- Limb contractures or tendon laxity compromise the ability of the foal to associate with the mare, obtain nutrition, or exercise appropriately.
- A minor valgus deformity is normal at birth and resolves progressively.

Integument

- Decubital ulcers: indicate trauma, unseen seizure activity, or occurrence of prolonged recumbency.
- Pitting edema: hypoproteinemia, cardiac dysfunction.
- Icterus: sepsis, neonatal isoerythrolysis, or hepatic disease. A transient total bilirubin elevation may occur during the first week of life.
- Cyanosis in the absence of respiratory distress indicates a possible congenital heart defect with right to left shunting. Pulmonary disease may not be reflected in the

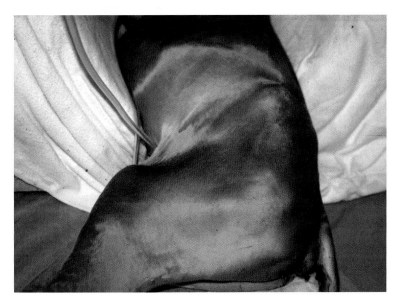

■ **Figure 141.1** Immature foal at delivery. Note short fine hair over body.

mucous membranes as very low oxygen saturation levels are necessary to effect a cyanotic color change.

■ Hemorrhage on the mucous membranes: sepsis, coagulopathy or direct trauma.
■ A silky, fine hair coat is an indicator of prematurity (Fig. 141.1).

GI Function

■ Any occurrence of colic has the potential to indicate a life-threatening episode and should thoroughly be investigated.
■ Fecal volume and consistency should be appropriate for a high volume milk diet. Following the passage of meconium (dark brown), feces should be consistently yellow-bronze in color and semi-formed in nature.
■ Abdominal distension should be monitored by regular measurement of the abdominal diameter. Distension is indicative of ileus, gastrointestinal accident or uroperitoneum.
■ The occurrence of teeth grinding and nasogastric reflux is suggestive of gastric ulceration or duodenal obstruction.

Urinary Function

■ Dysfunction is uncommon in neonates.
■ Acute renal failure: may occur as the result of decreased *in utero* blood supply or be iatrogenic from nephrotoxic drug usage.
■ Uroperitoneum: ruptured bladder, ruptured urachus, or torn ureter.
■ Urachitis: ascending infection.
■ Patent urachus: allows urine drainage and ascension of infection.
■ Congenital anomaly: ectopic ureter may lead to urinary incontinence.

Ocular Examination

- Hyperemia of the sclera: birth trauma, sepsis, or coagulopathy.
- Entropion: weight loss, dehydration leading to entophthalmia.
- Corneal opacity: ulceration, lack of tear production, or exposure keratitis.
- Ulceration: depressed blink response from general depression, decreased or absent tear production, or direct trauma.
- Anterior chamber: can reflect systemic inflammation and sepsis. Fibrin deposition (aqueous flare) and hypopyon may result.
- Cataract: a common congenital anomaly, possibly familial in some cases. Also occurs secondary to uveitis and trauma.

Mentation and Nervous Function

- General behavior of the neonate centers around feeding, investigation of the surrounding environment and association with the mare.
- Hypoxic ischemic encephalopathy: causes loss of affinity for the mare, generalized depression and a lack of vigorous suckling.
- Low level seizure activity: may appear as muscle fasciculations, chewing fits, or unexplained cutaneous trauma. Also examine the lower lip for abrasions.
- The menace response is absent from the neonate and is not an indication of vision. This reflex will take between 4 and 14 days to develop.

Bodyweight

- Thoroughbred foals should be able to increase bodyweight in the range of 1 to 2 kg/day.
- Failure to thrive or loss of bodyweight is a subtle indication of an underlying disease process causing inappetance or catabolism.

Hematology

- Normal neonatal range (birth to 1 week):
  - RBC range: 7.4 to 11.4 million cells/μL
  - WBC range: 4.9 to 13.6 thousand cells/μL.
  - Neutrophils: approximately 5500 cells/μL at birth, increasing to 8,000/μL within the first 12 hours of life.
  - Lymphocytes: may decrease to approximately 1,400 cells/μL within a few hours of birth. Increase to approximately 5,000 cells/μL by 3 months of age. Transient decreases below 1,000 cells/μL occur in some normal foals. However, this may indicate infection or immune compromise.
  - Leukopenia with a neutrophil-to-leukocyte ratio around 1 is strongly suggestive of "unreadiness for birth":
  - Noninfected premature foals with neutropenia and neutrophil-to-leukocyte ratio less than 1.5 during the first 24 hours of life have a poor prognosis when compared to normal neutrophil counts and neutrophil-to-leukocyte ratio greater than 3.

Serum Chemistry

In the absence of established parameters, normal adult equine values are often used for assessment of neonatal foal health.

- Serum electrolyte concentrations are maintained within a narrow range; do not differ substantially from established adult values.
- Glucose levels are elevated as a result of frequent suckling. Hypoglycemia is associated with sepsis.
- Foals are born with a wide range of plasma protein levels, an unreliable indicator of colostral absorption.
- Serum creatinine is unreliable as an indicator of renal performance in the neonatal foal. The placenta is primarily responsible for its elimination from the fetus and increases in creatinine reflect placental dysfunction or maternal levels.
- BUN and creatinine may be elevated for the first few days of life, with a progressive decrease to adult levels, normal at 3 to 5 days.
- Elevated total bilirubin and mild icterus are common. Consider sepsis, isoerythrolysis or hepatic disease.
- Creatine kinase may be elevated due to muscle trauma of birth origin.
- Alkaline phosphatase may be elevated due to rapid growth.
- GGT elevations may be of colostral origin.
- Fibrinogen is low in the healthy neonate (up to 200 g/dL). Elevated levels indicate *in utero* challenge and a prenatal response.
- IgG concentration: there is a strong association between an immunoglobulin concentration of less than 400 mg/dL and sepsis. Colostral intake initially may be adequate; subject to catabolism in the compromised neonate, decreasing protection.

Urinalysis

- Urine specific gravity:
  - Range for normal neonatal foal reported as 1.000 to 1.027.
  - Many foals isothenuric (1.008–1.015).
  - Specific gravity above 1.015 and below 1.008 requires intact renal tubular function.

Blood Culture

- Sepsis is an important cause of neonatal morbidity and mortality, second only to FPT.
- Infected foals initially may have vague, nonspecific signs. May progress to severe complications, multiple organ dysfunction, or death.
- Gram negative organisms are the most common pathogens, gram positive organisms are increasing in frequency.
- Anaerobic isolates are rare.

Imaging

- Radiography: assess lung fields, joints, physes, abdominal distension.
- U/S: assess lung fields, abdominal content.

 COMMENTS

Patient Monitoring

Times of Importance to the Neonate:
- Sternal recumbency: the foal should right itself and be able to maintain a sternal posture within minutes of birth.
- Standing: within 60 minutes, with a range of 15 to 165 minutes.
- Suckle reflex: usually within 20 minutes of birth, may be much sooner.
- Suckling: within 2 hours; reported range is 35 minutes to 7 hours.
- Urination: mean time to first urination is 6 hours for colts, 10 hours for fillies. Decreases in urine flow may result from decreased fluid intake, increased losses, or compromises in renal function. Obstruction of the urinary tract, or disruption due to rupture and uroperitoneum, are also possible in the compromised neonate, or one that sustained trauma during parturition.
- Defecation: most foals have abdominal straining within the first few hours, pass meconium completely within 24 hours. Ingestion of colostrum stimulates GI motility and may speed passage. Any interference with GI motility (e.g., physical obstruction, enteritis, asphyxia-related disease) will prolong the passage of meconium and increase the likelihood of an impaction.
- Milk intake: daily consumption of milk by the healthy neonate is in the order of 20% to 25% of bodyweight. For example, a 50-kg foal will ingest 10 to 12.5 L of milk. Foals ingest milk to satisfy energy requirements, and as such are forced to excrete a large volume of water.
- Scoring system: established sepsis scoring methodologies are controversial. A recent study demonstrated that sepsis scoring was the best predictor of survival. A negative blood culture increased survival when compared with foals that were blood culture positive.

Prevention/Avoidance

Prediction of the high-risk neonate: conditions associated with the high-risk neonate may conveniently be placed into the following categories:

Maternal Conditions

- Systemic illness leading to fever, gastrointestinal compromise, endotoxemia, or surgery.
- Generalized environment and social stressors including transport.

Reproductive Conditions

- History of previous neonatal compromise.
- Placental pathology: placentitis, placental insufficiency.
- Vulval discharge: placentitis.
- Loss of colostrum prepartum: placentitis.

Parturient Events

- Abnormal gestation length: endometrial degeneration, or fescue toxicosis.
- Prolonged labor: dystocia.
- Premature placental separation: placentitis.
- Premature rupture of the umbilical cord: abnormal length.
- Meconium aspiration: meconium in the amniotic fluid or amnion may be the only indication of this event.

Neonatal Conditions

- Trauma during delivery may have effects that are inapparent until a few days of age.
- Abnormal behavior
- Lack of suckle reflex
- Inability to stand
- Incomplete ossification of the cuboidal bones of the carpus and tarsus.
- Inadequate colostral intake
- Abnormal laboratory parameters: WBC count: neutropenia, band neutrophils, or toxic changes. Hypoglycemia, metabolic acidosis, or hypoxemia.

Expected Course and Prognosis

Deviations from the expected findings during any neonatal evaluation indicate the necessity for closer observation and possible medical intervention. Should referral care be required, the following should be considered (retrospective referral center information):

- Sepsis survival was significantly increased for foals that were standing, had normal appearing mucous membranes, had a respiratory rate of at least 60 bpm, and a neutrophil count greater than 4,000 cells/mL at admission.
- Septic foals born from an induced parturition or those that had a longer duration of clinical signs before admission were significantly less likely to survive (Fig. 141.2).
- No significant difference was found between neonatal ICU survivors with one race start and matched controls: in earnings, number of starts, earnings per start, and places per start over the first 2 years of a race career. Fewer affected foals had one race start, this raising the likelihood that residual deficits were present.

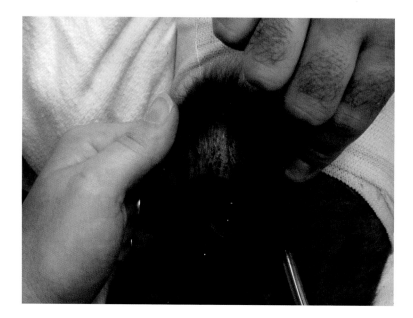

■ **Figure 141.2** Ecchymotic hemorrhages suggestive of septic process or coagulopathy.

Abbreviations

bpm	beats per minute
BUN	blood urea nitrogen
FPT	failure of passive transfer
GGT	γ-glutamyl transpeptidase
GI	gastrointestinal
HR	heart rate
ICU	intensive care unit
IgG	immunoglobulin G
PDA	patent ductus arteriosus
RBC	red blood cell
RR	respiratory rate
U/S	ultrasound, ultrasonography
VSD	ventricular septal defect
WBC	white blood cell

See Also

- Fetal evaluation
- Neonatal disease
- Neonatal isoerythrolysis
- Nutrition, foals
- Placentitis
- Placental insufficiency

Suggested Reading

Aleman M, Gillis CL, Nieto JE, et al. 2002. Ultrasonographic anatomy and biometric analysis of the thoracic and abdominal organs in healthy foals from birth to age 6 months, *Eq Vet J* 34: 649–655.

Bauer J. 1990. Normal blood chemistry. In: *Equine Clinical Neonatology*. Koterba, AM, Drummond, WH, Kosch, PC (eds). Philadelphia: Lea & Febiger; 602–614.

Bernard WV, Reimer JM. 1994. Examination of the foal. *Vet Clin North Am Equine Pract* 10: 37–66.

Harvey J. 1990. Normal hematologic values. In: *Equine Clinical Neonatology*. Koterba, AM, Drummond, WH, Kosch, PC (eds). Philadelphia: Lea & Febiger; 561–570.

Koterba A. 1990. Diagnosis and management of the normal and abnormal neonatal foal: General considerations. In: *Equine Clinical Neonatology*. Koterba, AM, Drummond, WH, Kosch, PC (eds). Philadelphia: Lea & Febiger; 3–15.

Peek SF, Darien BJ, Semrad SD, et al. 2004. A prospective study of neonatal septicemia and factors influencing survival. *Proc AAEP*, Denver, CO; 60–62.

Rossdale P. 2004. The maladjusted foal: Influences of intrauterine growth retardation and birth trauma. *Proc AAEP*, Denver, CO; 75–126.

Author: Peter R. Morresey

chapter 142

Neonatal Isoerythrolysis

DEFINITION/OVERVIEW

- First reported in newborn mules.
- Occurs after the neonate consumes colostrum containing antibodies to its own RBCs.
- Causes hemolysis of neonatal RBCs due to ingestion of maternal (colostral) antibodies to the foal's RBC antigens.

ETIOLOGY/PATHOPHYSIOLOGY

- Mare becomes sensitized to incompatible alloantigen of the foal's RBC.
- Mechanism of sensitization is not well-known but is believed to be due to placental hemorrhage or leakage.
- Most common in multiparous mares.
- Mare can become sensitized to RBCs if she had blood transfusion(s) or exposure to blood products prior to pregnancy (e.g., treatment she received).
- Antibodies accumulate prepartum in the mare's colostrum.
- Because the mare and fetal blood supplies do not mix during gestation, circulating antibodies in the mare do not affect the fetus *in utero*.
- Foals with targeted RBC antigens become affected after ingesting the colostrum containing RBC antigen antibodies.
- The severity of the clinical symptom depends on the amount of alloantibodies and the type of antigen (Aa alloantibodies are more potent hemolysins than alloantibodies against Qa).

Genetics

- RBC antigens are expressed co-dominantly.
- Factors inherited from both the stallion and the mare are expressed.
- Only a few of the more than 30 known RBC factors are commonly involved in NI.
  - Factors Aa and Qa are the predominant factors involved.
  - C, P, and U system-based cases have occurred.
- A mare cannot make antibodies against a RBC factor she possesses.
- To have an affected foal, it must inherit factors from the stallion that the mare does not possess and to which she has developed sensitivity.

Systems Affected

Hemolytic (RBC)

SIGNALMENT/HISTORY

Risk Factors

- Most often multiparous mare with high-risk blood type.
- Can be a primiparous mare with prior exposure to blood products or transfusions.

Historical Findings

Onset
- Breed predisposition: Standardbred (2% incidence), Thoroughbred (1%), but can happen in any breed of horse.
- Six to 72 hours postpartum.

CLINICAL FEATURES

Incidence/Prevalence

- Varies by breed: Standardbred (2% incidence); Thoroughbred (1%).
- Breeds with greater variability in the A and Q systems are most commonly affected:
  - Thoroughbred: 2% of mares do *not* have the Aa antigen (i.e., they are at risk of producing antibodies to that antigen). Reality: only 50% of potentially at risk Thoroughbread mares make the antibody.
  - Standardbreds: 22% of pacing mares lack the Aa antigen; only 17% of those mares produce anti-Aa antibodies.
  - Tennessee Walking Horse
- Based on Thoroughbred submissions to the laboratory in Lexington, Kentucky:
  - Most are Aad in the A system and Qabc in the Q system.
- Mares in foal to jacks may develop antibodies to the "donkey factor."
  - Have NI-affected mule foals about 10% of the time.

Physical Examination Findings

- Apparently healthy foal at birth develops lethargy after nursing.
- Some foals may show increased HR and RR.
- Pallor in severely affected foals less than 24 hours old.
- Icterus may develop at 1 to 7 days age and be the only sign in mildly affected foals.
- Anemia is confirmed by PCV.
- Severity and progression of the clinical syndrome depends on the amount of alloantibodies ingested.
- Bloodwork (CBC) consistent with RBC destruction.

DIFFERENTIAL DIAGNOSIS

- Anemia caused by blood loss due to trauma (i.e., hemoperitonium, hemothorax) or coagulopathies but does not result in icterus.
- Icterus due to sepsis or liver damage is not accompanied by anemia.
- *Isoerythrolysis is confirmed by demonstration of:*
  - Alloantibodies against the foal's RBCs either in the serum or colostrum of the dam or,
  - The presence of Abs on the foal's RBCs (Coomb's test). The Coomb's test can have false-negatives.

DIAGNOSTICS

- Knowledge of a mare's blood type provides initial evidence of whether one of the high-risk systems is involved (Q, A, C, P, U) and potentially problematic.

CBC/Biochemistry/Urinalysis

- Icterus may develop at 1 to 7 days and be the only sign in mildly affected foals.
- Anemia is confirmed by PCV.
- Bloodwork (CBC) consistent with RBC destruction.

Other Laboratory Tests

Demonstration of antibodies:
- *Cross-matching tests*: hemolytic or agglutination assays.
- *Agglutination assay*: less sensitive, may not detect all sensitizing antibodies because some act as hemolysins.
- *Hemolytic Antibody Assay*: more sensitive.
  - *Testing for hemolytic antibody*: serum from the mare is mixed with washed foal RBCs, RBC lysis occurs after addition of complement.
  - The most reliable test, but not practical in field situations.
- *JFA test*:
  - Does not require complement.
  - Serial dilutions of the colostrum are mixed with the foal's RBCs and centrifuged at low speed for several minutes and tested for agglutination.
  - The centrifuge causes colostral antibodies to agglutinate the RBCs. Agglutination is reaction that is assessed. The value assigned to the titer of the highest dilution resulting in agglutination is 3+.
  - Positive reactions are significant if: positive at or greater than 1:16 in horses or, equal to or greater than 1:64 in mules.
- Coomb's test may demonstrate the presence of antibodies on the foal's RBCs but can have false-negatives.

- Hemolytic and JFA tests are predictive for NI when performed prior to ingestion of colostrum.

Screening of Serum, Both Pre- and Postpartum Testing, to Determine NI Risk

- *Pregnant mare*: screen serum during the last 30 days of gestation for the presence of antibodies.
- *Antibody screening request*: 12 mL serum tube sent to a lab offering the service.
- Serum is tested against a panel of horses of known blood types and assessed for antibody activity.
  - Any completely lytic reaction is cause for concern if there is a possibility the foal will inherit the recognized antigen from the sire.
  - Strongly lytic is defined as complete lysis of sample RBCs with mare serum that has been diluted 1:16.
  - Activity to the Ca antigen is naturally occurring and is usually harmless to the foal unless a rare lytic reaction is observed. Most Ca antigen reactions are agglutinating and not lytic.
  - Any observed lytic reaction, even if the antigen cannot be determined, is sufficient cause for withholding the mare's colostrum from the foal.
- It may be best to manage a mare with a history of NI by breeding her only to stallions that do not possess the antigen to which she has become sensitized.
- *Stallions* can be RBC tested at any time:
  - A yellow top or purple top blood tube is required.
  - At a minimum, test the blood for Aa, Ca, Qa, and Ua antigens.
  - Other factors (small letters) in these systems (capital letters indicate the "system" designation) can be tested to generate a more thorough antigen profile even though they have a less frequent involvement in NI cases.
- *Maiden mares or mare without a known history*:
  - A blood type can also be performed.
  - Determine their susceptibility to RBC incompatibilities.
  - For example, a Thoroughbred mare negative in the A system, is at risk for developing antibodies to the Aa antigen at some point in her breeding career, due to the prevalence of Aa in the Thoroughbred population.
- Any observed lytic titer is sufficient justification to refrain from letting the foal nurse (i.e., *any expectation* that the foal could possess the antigen on its RBCs).
  - Provide the foal with a safe alternate colostrum source.
- Commercial sources of oral or intravenous IgG should be prescreened for antibody activity or be collected from horses known to possess the blood factors common in NI problems.
  - If obtaining colostrum from a bank, it should be tested for antibody activity prior to storage or come from a mare that has been screened (serum screening) for antibody activity at the time of colostrum collection.
  - The latter is preferable as colostral milk proteins can obscure test results.
- Muzzle the foal to prevent it from nursing its dam for the first 48 hours of life.

- After 48 hours the foal's gut will no longer allow the large immunoglobulin molecules to pass into the bloodstream.
- Strip the mare's colostrum from her udder several times during this period.

Pathologic Findings

- Fetal icterus develops post-suckle in the recent postpartum period.
- Fetal anemia develops during the same time frame.
- Progressive worsening of condition: lethargy to eventual collapse and death in severely affected foals, in the absence of needed care.

THERAPEUTICS

- First and foremost: Remove the foal from its dam pre-suckle and provide adequate, quality colostrum.
  - Feed an alternate, tested (safe) source of colostrum.
  - Muzzle the foal to maintain the mare-to-foal bond, but provide colostrum within first 6 hours of life and all nutrition needed for the first 48 hours.
- Management of the anemic/affected foal (in the case, the antigen-containing colostrum has been ingested):
  - Blood transfusion (whole blood from a universal donor) is often required in foals with a PCV less than 12% to 15%; severe cases may require multiple blood transfusions.
  - In case an emergency transfusion is necessary, blood from geldings is ideal.
  - The most unsatisfactory donor is the stallion.
  - The mare's RBCs can only be used if they have been washed. Absent washing, the mare's offending serum antibodies are still present.
  - Blood product transfusion and supplemental oxygen therapy should be considered in foals with severe clinical signs.
  - Intravenous concentrated source of immunoglobulins.
  - Alternate source of colostrum.
  - Oxyglobin solution is an alternative solution: a hemoglobin-based, O_2-carrying solution. This product does not require cross-matching. Delivered at a maximum rate of 10 to 30 mg/kg or 10 mL/kg per hour.

Appropriate Health Care

Refer to treatment of foal.

COMMENTS

Client Education

- See Prevention/Avoidance
- Client education for subsequent pregnancies.

Patient Monitoring

- Monitor neonate until RBC count is within normal, acceptable range.
- Muzzle to avoid the foal nursing its dam during the first 24 to 48 hours of its life.
- Provide adequate and early alternate source of colostrum to avoid the foal developing FPT.

Prevention/Avoidance

- Screen mare's serum during last 30 days of pregnancy for the presence of antibodies.
- Any lytic titer may be sufficient cause to refrain from letting the foal nurse if there is any expectation that the foal possesses the antigen on its RBCs.
- Provide the foal with a safe alternate colostrum source and muzzle the foal to prevent it from nursing its dam for 48 hours.
- Strip the mare's colostrum from her udder several times during this period.
- For future pregnancies, prevent NI by breeding the mare only to stallions lacking the offending antigens.
- Blood typing the stallion and mare is necessary in order to perform the cross-match.
- The mare will still produce a titer to the antigen as her colostrums collect, but it will be harmless to the foal if the foal's RBCs do not have or are not exposed to the antigen.

Possible Complications

- Neonatal death, if severely affected and left untreated.
- Age-related factor: most common in pluriparous mares.
- Pregnancy: NI, a postpartum condition affecting only the foal.

Synonyms

NI

Abbreviations

CBC   complete blood count
FPT   failure of passive transfer
HR   heart rate
Ig   immunoglobulin
IgG   immunoglobulin G
JFA   jaundice foal agglutination
NI   neonatal isoerythrolysis
O_2 oxygen
PCV   packed cell volume
RBC   red blood cell
RR   respiratory rate

Suggested Reading

Bailey E, Albright DG, Henney PJ. 1988. Equine neonatal isoerythrolysis: evidence for prevention by maternal antibodies to the Ca blood group antigen. *AJVR* 49(8): 1218–1222.

Boyle AG, Magdesian KG, Ruby RE. 2005. Neonatal isoerythrolysis in horse foals and a mule foal: 18 cases (1988–2003). *JAVMA* 227(8): 1276–1283.

MacLeay JM. 2001. Neonatal isoerythrolysis involving the Qc and Db antigens in a foal. *JAVMA* 219(1): 79–81.

McClure JJ. 1993. The immune system. In: *Equine Reproduction*. McKinnon AO, Voss JL (eds). Philadelphia: Lea & Febiger; 1003–1006.

Wong PL, Nickel LS, Bowling AT, et al. 1986. Clinical survey of antibodies against red blood cells in horses after homologous blood transfusion. *AJVR* 47(12): 2566–2571.

Authors: Ahmed Tibary and Kathryn Graves

chapter 143

Occipito-Atlantal-Axial Malformation

 ## DEFINITION/OVERVIEW

Affected horses usually present with the progressive onset of ataxia. Physical findings include a palpably abnormal atlas and axis, with reduced flexion and audible clicking on manipulation of the head. Confirmation requires radiological evaluation, with the presence of characteristic bony lesions.

 ## ETIOLOGY/PATHOPHYSIOLOGY

Although isolated cases occur in other breeds, OAAM is predominantly a heritable condition of newborn to juvenile Arabian foals.

Systems Affected

- Neuromuscular: progressive onset of ataxia.

 ## SIGNALMENT/HISTORY

Risk Factors

- Inherited in Arabians
- Sporadic other breeds

Historical Findings

Progressive ataxia and tetraparesis

 ## CLINICAL FEATURES

- Inapparent in many affected horses.
- Variable: symmetric ataxia, with hypometria; severity ranging from tetraparesis to tetraplegia.
- Abnormal head carriage: clicking sound may be heard.
- Stillbirth and sudden death have been reported.

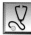

DIFFERENTIAL DIAGNOSIS

- Cervical vertebral trauma.
- Soft-tissue compressive lesion of spinal cord.

DIAGNOSTICS

- Clinical signs: progressive onset of ataxia progressing to tetraparesis
- Signalment
- Palpably abnormal atlas and axis, with reduced flexion and audible clicking on manipulation of the head
- Radiographs: congenital atlanto-occipital fusion; hypoplasia of atlas, dens; malformation of the axis; modification of the atlantoaxial joint, with frequent subluxation

Pathological Findings

Syndrome includes occipito-atlantal fusion, hypoplasia of the dens and inappropriate localized ossification of the occipito-atlantal area.

THERAPEUTICS

- None curative, however, may survive with appropriate management.
- Anti-inflammatories may decrease clinical signs during acute exacerbations.
- Euthanasia may be required in severe cases.

Activity

Confinement of severe cases in hazard free stalls may be required.

COMMENTS

Client Education

Genetic counseling

Expected Course and Prognosis

Neurologic deficits may stabilize but can progress to recumbency.

Abbreviations

OAAM   occipito-atlantal-axial malformation

Suggested Reading

Green SL, Mayhew IG. 1980. Neurologic disorders. In: *Equine Clinical Neonatology*. Koterba AM, Drummond WH, Kosch PC (eds). Philadelphia: Lea & Febiger; 496–530.

MacKay RJ. 2005. Neurologic disorders of neonatal foals. *Vet Clin North Am Equine Pract* 2: 387–406.

Author: Peter R. Morresey

chapter 144

Omphalophlebitis

DEFINITION/OVERVIEW

Infection of the umbilical remnant. The umbilical remnant consists of the urachus, the umbilical vein (coursing cranial to liver) and two umbilical arteries (flanking the urachus). The urachus itself is most commonly affected in isolation (urachitis) therefore omphalophlebitis can be considered a misnomer for this condition (Fig. 144.1).

ETIOLOGY/PATHOPHYSIOLOGY

- Ascending infection from the umbilical stump (distal to proximal) to involve the urachus and associated vascular structures.
- Localization of systemic infection (sepsis) is also possible.

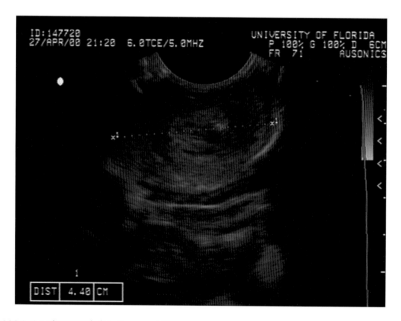

■ **Figure 144.1** An ultrasound showing urachitis.

Systems Affected

- Cardiovascular: bacteremia may cause valvular endocarditis and pericarditis.
- Gastrointestinal: adhesion of the viscera to the inflamed tissue can occur leading to strangulation and generalized peritonitis.
- Hepatobiliary: abscesses may seed to the liver via the umbilical vein.
- Ophthalmic: hypopyon can result from a systemic reaction to a localized infection of the urachus and associated structures.
- Renal/Urologic: loss of integrity of urachus can lead to uroperitoneum.
- Respiratory: seeding of abscesses to the lung.
- Skin/Exocrine: persistent umbilical discharge.

 # SIGNALMENT/HISTORY

Risk Factors

- FPT
- Environmental contamination of umbilical remnants.
- Excessive traction during parturition.
- Inappropriate placement of umbilical clamp.

Historical Findings

- Swelling of umbilical area: firm, painful.
- Purulent discharge from umbilical remnants.
- Possible urine voiding through umbilical area.
- Fever, depression, and inappetance.
- Inflammatory leukogram

 # CLINICAL FEATURES

- Umbilical swelling and discharge: painful upon palpation, purulent discharge.
- Fever
- Lethargy, weakness, and inappetance.
- Concurrent infections: septic arthritis and pulmonary and hepatic abscessation.
- Gastrointestinal accident: intestinal adhesion or strangulation.
- Peritonitis

 # DIFFERENTIAL DIAGNOSIS

Umbilical hernia

DIAGNOSTICS

- Clinical examination findings.
- Hematology: inflammatory leukogram will likely be present.
- U/S: enlargement of urachus and adjacent structures. Abscessation may be present. Accumulation of anechoic fluid or flocculent material within urachal remnants.
- Microbial culture and sensitivity: of the discharge, as well as the excised tissue.

Pathological Findings

Urachus may be thickened and inflamed. Phlebitis, thrombosis, and abscessation of regional vasculature.

THERAPEUTICS

Medical

- Antimicrobials: long-term treatment with broad-spectrum drugs likely necessary. Drug penetration into urachal structures is difficult to achieve in prolonged cases due to fibrosis.
- Anti-inflammatories: to decrease local swelling and discomfort.

Surgical

- Excision of urachal structures under general anesthesia.
- Concurrent medical treatment as above.

Drug(s) of Choice

- Antimicrobials, initially broad spectrum: K-penicillin 40,000 units/kg IV every 6 hours, amikacin 25 mg/kg IV every 24 hours, potentiated sulfonamides (e.g., trimethoprim-sulfamethoxazole 25 mg/kg PO every 12 hours). Addition of rifampin 5 to 10 mg/kg PO every 12 hours may be advantageous due to superior penetration ability.
- Select narrow spectrum drugs based on sensitivity results.
- Anti-inflammatories: flunixin meglumine 1 mg/kg IV every 12 hours, ketoprofen 2 mg/kg IV every 12 to 24 hours.

Appropriate Health Care

Monitor affected area for discharge or signs of dehiscence.

Surgical Considerations

Excision of body wall in contact with affected urachal structures may be necessary in severe cases.

COMMENTS

Client Education

Monitor umbilical area for swelling or discharge.

Prevention/Avoidance

Reassess hygiene practices pertaining to neonatal foal management.

Possible Complications

- Intra-abdominal adhesions
- Wound dehiscence
- Peritonitis

Expected Course and Prognosis

Complete resolution with appropriate treatment.

Synonyms

Navel ill

Abbreviations

FPT   failure of passive transfer
IV   intravenous
PO   per os (by mouth)
U/S   ultrasound, ultrasonography

See Also

- Sepsis
- Patent urachus

Suggested Reading

Brewer BD. 1980. The urogenital system, Section 2: Renal diease. In: *Equine Clinical Neonatology.* Koterba AM, Drummond WH, Kosch PC (eds). Philadelphia: Lea & Febiger; 446–458.
Vaala WE, Clark ES, Orsini JA. 1988. Omphalophlebitis and osteomyelitis associated with Klebsiella septicemia in a premature foal. *JAVMA* 193: 1273–1277.

Author: Peter R. Morresey

chapter 145

Osteomyelitis

DEFINITION/OVERVIEW

Disorders of the musculoskeletal system may be associated with congenital malformations, intrauterine sepsis, abnormal length of gestation, small for gestational age foals, and twinning. Trauma at delivery, neonatal bacterial sepsis, and postnatal injury can lead to additional musculoskeletal problems.

Extensive inflammation of the bone extending into or beginning in the medullary cavity. This is in contrast to osteitis which is considered only to involve the periosteum and outer cortical bone.

ETIOLOGY/PATHOPHYSIOLOGY

May be the result of hematogenous spread or local trauma.

- *Hematogenous osteomyelitis* is often associated with an infected focus elsewhere in the body, or concurrent sepsis. This condition predominantly affects the metaphyseal region due to slow blood flow in the terminal sinusoids, allowing blood-borne bacteria to localize and establish an infected focus. Thrombosis of blood vessels also occurs. Spread is via the Haversian canals and Volkmann cavities.
- *Traumatic osteomyelitis* results from direct inoculation following an open fracture or penetrating wound. Avascularity is the major factor allowing osteomyelitis to ensue. Spread of infection through the bone is by similar means to hematogenous infection. Necrotic foci resulting from blunt trauma, even without a break in the skin, can allow bacterial proliferation.

Systems Affected

- Musculoskeletal: wasting of musculature associated with the affected limb due to disuse.
- Ophthalmic: aqueous flare secondary to an infected focus.

SIGNALMENT/HISTORY

Hematogenous osteomyelitis may not be discovered early in the disease process as lameness may be the only sign.

Risk Factors

- The physeal region has increased blood delivery to enable rapid growth, but the flow rate of blood is decreased causing less aerobic conditions that favor any blood-borne pathogen.
- See Septic Arthritis.

Historical Findings

Lameness and swelling unresponsive to medical therapy.

CLINICAL FEATURES

- Fever: may be an inconsistent finding in the early stages.
- Pain on direct local palpation of the affected area of bone or physis.
- Cellulitis: may appear similar to that seen in fracture patients.
- Lameness: may be severe enough to suggest a fracture.

DIFFERENTIAL DIAGNOSIS

- Fracture
- Soft-tissue orthopedic injury
- Sepsis or other debilitating disease of the neonate

DIAGNOSTICS

- Clinical examination findings.
- Hematology: inflammatory leukogram with neutrophilia. However, this may be the result of underlying systemic disease.
- Radiographs: changes occur gradually and become evident 10 to 14 days following onset of infection. Loss of bone density in affected areas approaches 30% to 50% before radiographic signs become evident.
- U/S: adjacent soft tissue becomes reactive, with cellulitis and periostitis occurring.

Pathological Findings

- Gross evidence of lysis and purulent accumulations in bone. Regional cellulitis may be present adjacent to affected bone. May find a distant primary infected focus.

 THERAPEUTICS

- Manage concurrent causative disease or septic focus, if present.
- Systemic antimicrobials: bactericidal, ensure Gram-negative coverage. Preferably by the intravenous route initially, with oral therapy possible for prolonged treatment.
- Anti-inflammatories: analgesia, decrease fever, and debility.
- Regional limb perfusion: high local drug concentration delivered to affected area.
- Local antimicrobial deposition: PMMA beads allowing chronic regional antimicrobial elution to site of infection.
- Consider adjacent joint involvement: see Septic arthritis.

Drug(s) of Choice

See Septic Arthritis.

Precautions/Interactions

See Septic Arthritis.

Nursing Care

Ensure adequate caloric intake and ensure appropriate level of activity. Avoid prolonged periods of recumbency.

 COMMENTS

Possible Complications

Sequestrum formation. Regional spread to adjacent synovial structures. Pathological fracture of affected bone.

Expected Course and Prognosis

Early cases often respond favorably to aggressive treatment. Significant bone loss is a grave prognostic indicator.

Abbreviations

PMMA   polymethylmethacrylate
U/S   ultrasound, ultrasonography

See Also

- Neonatal evaluation
- Septic arthritis

Suggested Reading

Hardy J, Latimer F. 2003. Orthopedic disorders in the neonatal foal. *Clin Tech Eq Pract* 2: 96–119.

McIlwraith CW. 2002. Diseases of joints, tendons, ligaments and related structures. In: *Lameness in Horses*, 5th ed. Stashak TS, Adams OR (eds). Philadelphia: Lippincott Williams & Wilkins; 459–644.

Trumble TN. 2005. Orthopedic disorders in neonatal foals. *Vet Clin North Am Equine Pract* 21: 357–385.

Author: Peter R. Morresey

chapter 146

Patent Urachus

DEFINITION/OVERVIEW

Loss of urine via the urachal remnant in the neonatal foal.

ETIOLOGY/PATHOPHYSIOLOGY

Due to a congenital defect, infection of, or trauma to, the urachus, or secondary to a generalized catabolic condition, urine may be voided externally via the urachal remnants.

Systems Affected

- Renal/Urologic: ascending infection of the urinary tract is possible.
- Skin/Exocrine: urine may be deposited subcutaneously in the umbilical region leading to localized necrosis.

SIGNALMENT/HISTORY

It is usually apparent during the early neonatal period (Fig. 146.1); however, it can occur at any time before the natural closure of the urachus.

Risk Factors

- Congenital: *in utero* umbilical cord torsion or excessive traction can lead to dilation of the urachus.
- Acquired: any concurrent urachal condition (e.g., urachal remnant infection), or any medical condition leading to weight loss (e.g., diarrhea); malnutrition may lead to sufficient protein catabolism for urachal opening. Trauma at parturition resulting from excessive umbilical cord traction.

Historical Findings

Intermittent dribbling of urine with staining of the umbilical area. May progress to a complete stream passed concurrently with normal urine voiding.

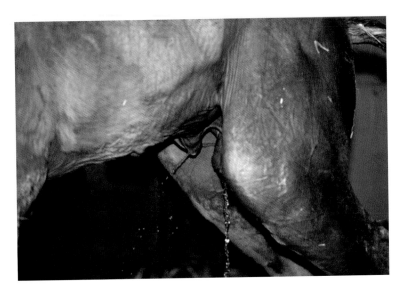

■ **Figure 146.1** Patent urachus.

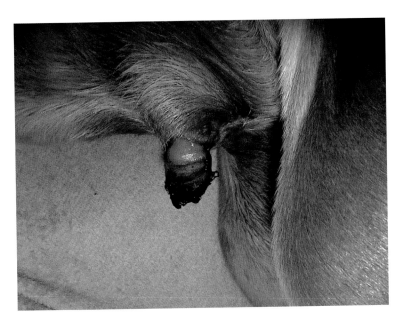

■ **Figure 146.2** Moist umbilicus.
Image courtesy of B. Ramanathan.

 CLINICAL FEATURES

- Loss of urine from the umbilicus: variable appearance, progresses from a chronically moist navel (Fig. 146.2) with occasional urine dripping to a full urine stream.

- Enlarged umbilical area that may be painful on palpation.
- Purulent discharge from urachus may be present.

DIAGNOSTICS

- Clinical signs are characteristic.
- Leukogram: inflammatory changes may not be present as septic area may be small and regionalized.
- U/S: demonstrate urachal patency and communication with bladder. Urachal structures are variably enlarged.

Pathological Findings

Urachus is dilated allowing external communication/access to the bladder.

THERAPEUTICS

Medical

- Treat concurrent medical conditions.
- Systemic antimicrobials: patent urachus is a conduit for the systemic entry of pathogens.
- Local cauterizing agents (when congenital): silver nitrate can be applied topically, however, avoid penetrating the urachal lumen or creating a necrotic focus.
- Surgical excision.
  - Remove urachal structures in their entirety under general anesthesia.

Surgical Considerations

If urachus is removed, monitor wound for normal healing.

COMMENTS

Client Education

Many cases will spontaneously resolve. This is most likely when the initiating cause is a debilitating disease that is subsequently successfully managed.

Prevention/Avoidance

- Observe good hygiene practices with neonatal foals.
- Avoid excessive umbilical cord traction during assisted delivery.

Possible Complications

- Omphalophlebitis
- Urinary tract infection
- Umbilical abscessation

Expected Course and Prognosis

Affected foals will recover completely with appropriate therapy. Long term complications are not expected.

Abbreviations

U/S   ultrasound, ultrasonography

See Also

- Neonatal evaluation
- Omphalophlebitis

Suggested Reading

Brewer BD. 1980. The urogenital system, Section 2: Renal diease. In: *Equine Clinical Neonatology*. Koterba AM, Drummond WH, Kosch PC (eds). Philadelphia: Lea & Febiger; 446–458.

Vaala WE, Clark ES, Orsini JA. 1988. Omphalophlebitis and osteomyelitis associated with Klebsiella septicemia in a premature foal. *JAVMA* 193: 1273–1277.

Author: Peter R. Morresey

chapter 147

Pericarditis/Pericardial Effusion

DEFINITION/OVERVIEW

Pericarditis and pericardial effusion may occur as a sequel to neonatal sepsis or respiratory tract infection. Infection of the pericardial structures can lead to abscessation and adhesions that potentially restricting cardiac output. Not all pericardial disease is septic in origin, with idiopathic disease also reported.

ETIOLOGY/PATHOPHYSIOLOGY

Regardless of the etiology, constriction of the heart and impairment of ventricular filling leads to decreased cardiac output. Ventricular filling may also be diminished by pericardial effusion that causes cardiac compression (tamponade).

Systems Affected

- Respiratory: restrictive pericarditis or pericardial effusion may precipitate CHF. Increased respiratory rate and effort may result.
- Hemic/Lymphatic/Immune: inflammatory leukogram if a septic process is present.
- Musculoskeletal: muscle wasting (cardiac cachexia).
- Renal/Urologic: pretenal azotemia due to poor perfusion.
- Gastrointestinal: decreased lymphatic drainage may lead to diarrhea.
- Hepatobiliary: decreased perfusion leading to hepatocellular damage.
- Ophthalmic: hypopyon due to remote septic focus.

SIGNALMENT/HISTORY

Insidious onset without having detected any precipitating disease, or secondary to a previously diagnosed sepsis. Fevers of unknown origin may have been reported.

Risk Factors

- Infectious agents:
  - Bacteria: *Streptococcus* spp., *Actinobacillus equuli*, and *Pasteurella* spp.
  - Virus: Equine arteritis virus

- Immune-mediated
- Sepsis: bacterial localization following dissemination
- Trauma: direct inoculation to pericardial sac
- Idiopathic

Historical Findings

Cardiac tamponade

 ## CLINICAL FEATURES

- Systemic illness: fever or malaise.
- Auscultation: pericardial friction rubs or muffled heart sounds.
- Cardiovascular compromise: jugular venous distension, tachycardia, reduced arterial (pulse) pressure, peripheral edema, or poor exercise tolerance.

 ## DIFFERENTIAL DIAGNOSIS

- Pulmonary disease: pneumonia or pleuritis.
- Coagulopathy: pericardial hemorrhage.
- Congenital anomaly

 ## DIAGNOSTICS

- Hematology: inflammatory leukogram.
- U/S: pericardial effusion, fibrinous pericarditis. May detect concurrent pleural or pulmonary disease.
- Radiography: assess cardiomegaly, presence of primary septic pulmonary focus, if present.
- Pericardiocentesis: determine whether exudate is inflammatory or non-inflammatory. Culture, sensitivity, and cytology of pericardial effusion is important to identify appropriate antimicrobials suitable for a prolonged treatment course. Monitor cardiac rhythm with ECG during aspiration.
- Blood culture: organism recovered is likely involved in pericardial disease.

Pathological Findings

Proliferative and fibrinous changes may be present on the pericardium and epicardium.

THERAPEUTICS

- Antimicrobials: broad spectrum initially cover known causes of sepsis. Change to narrow spectrum if indicated by sensitivity results.
- Anti-inflammatories.
- Pericardial drainage: if infective pericarditis or tamponade is present. Perform at the left fifth intercostal space above the lateral thoracic vein. Prognosis is improved with this technique. Use a large bore catheter, or preferably a chest tube, to allow repeated drainage and lavage.

Drug(s) of Choice

See Table 112.1.

Surgical Considerations

Placement of indwelling drainage tube

COMMENTS

Client Education

Long-term treatment is required.

Patient Monitoring

Repeated echocardiography to evaluate pericardial space.

Possible Complications

Chronic fibrosis and constriction of the pericardium.

Expected Course and Prognosis

Prognosis for survival and athletic function is guarded. Infective pericarditis can lead to fibrotic and constrictive chronic disease. Prognosis improved with repeated drainage and lavage.

Abbreviations

CHF   congestive heart failure
ECG   electrocardiogram
U/S   ultrasound, ultrasonography

See Also

- Neonatal evaluation

Suggested Reading

Bonagura JD, Reef VB. 2004. Disorders of the cardiovascular system. In: *Equine Internal Medicine*. Reed SM, Bayly WM, Sellon DC (eds). St. Louis: Saunders; 355–460.

Lombard CW. Cardiovascular diseases. 1980. In: *Equine Clinical Neonatology*. Koterba AM, Drummond WH, Kosch PC (eds). Philadelphia: Lea & Febiger; 240–261.

Marr CE (ed). 1999. *Cardiology of the Horse*. Philadelphia: W. B. Saunders.

Author: Peter R. Morresey

chapter 148

Pneumonia, Bacterial

DEFINITION/OVERVIEW

Infection of the lungs with bacteria. May result from overgrowth of resident flora due to compromised respiratory defenses or direct inoculation of the respiratory tract by a pathogenic organism.

ETIOLOGY/PATHOPHYSIOLOGY

Bacteria responsible for pneumonia predominantly enter the lower respiratory tract by inhalation; however, hematogenous spread from other parts of the body is possible.

Systems Affected

- Cardiovascular: increased pulmonary vascular system pressure.
- Musculoskeletal: wasting occurs due to protein catabolism. The extra energy required (beyond carbohydrates from nursing) is lacking as the foal nurses less while ill, thus cachexia is due to increased energy demands by and for immune function; some loss also due to decreased exercise while ill.
- Ophthalmic: hypopyon due to systemic reaction to infection.

SIGNALMENT/HISTORY

Foals of all ages are susceptible to bacterial pneumonia. Often a predisposing environmental factor or concurrent medical condition is present that devitalizes the pulmonary defenses allowing mucosal attachment of pathogens.

Risk Factors

- Sepsis: neonatal pneumonias often caused by the same organisms responsible for sepsis, chiefly *Escherichia coli*, *Streptococcus* spp., *Klebsiella pneumoniae*, *Pasturella* spp., and *Actinobacillus* spp. Less commonly, *Salmonella* spp., *Pseudomonas* spp., and

Staphylococcus spp. are involved. Pneumonia derived from sepsis tends to have a generalized distribution throughout the lung, with responses to sepsis exacerbating the severity of the bacterial disease.

- Aspiration: poor suckle reflex or dysphagia due to neurologic compromise.
- Generalized weakness or pharyngeal dysfunction due to concurrent condition.
- Iatrogenic: due to assisted feeding efforts.
- Transportation: stress and fluid deprivation compromise mucociliary clearance.
- Older foals most often develop bacterial pneumonia secondary to viral infection.

Historical Findings

Neonates may have few overt signs of pulmonary pathology. However, fever, depression, inappetance, increased respiratory effort, nasal discharge, and coughing may be noted.

 CLINICAL FEATURES

- Fever
- Depression
- Increased respiratory rate and effort: dyspneic foals have more extensive pulmonary infiltrates within the cranioventral lung, advanced respiratory disease, and lower survival rates
- Cough: deep, may be productive
- Nasal discharge: mucopurulent

 DIFFERENTIAL DIAGNOSIS

- Viral pneumonia
- Aspiration pneumonia
- Parasitic pneumonia
- Thoracic trauma
- Pneumothorax
- Diaphragmatic trauma

 DIAGNOSTICS

- Clinical signs: increased respiratory rate and effort may be present. Coughing.
- Auscultation: this may remain unremarkable in some foals even those with significant pulmonary disease.
- Hematology: WBC count (elevated), differential count (neutrophilic leukocytosis), and fibrinogen (elevated) support diagnosis of infection.
- Radiography: pathology has a predominantly cranioventral distribution with aspiration; however, it is more generalized secondary to sepsis. Increased caudodorsal radiographic changes have been found to be a significant indicator of nonsurvival.

- U/S: pleuritis, consolidation, and abscessation.
- Transtracheal aspiration: microbial culture and antimicrobial sensitivity, cytology allows direct visualization of bacteria and inflammatory cell population.
- Blood culture: if sepsis is suspected as the initiating cause.

Pathological Findings

Gross and microscopic evidence of pulmonary inflammation, fibrosis, and infection.

 # THERAPEUTICS

- Antimicrobials: broad spectrum initially, preferably bactericidal, and administered parenterally. Change according to sensitivity information, if applicable.
- Anti-inflammatories: decrease inflammation-induced lung pathology. Provide analgesia to improve ventilation efforts.
- General supportive therapy.
- Nebulization of antimicrobial drugs and mucolytics may be helpful in some cases.
- Ventilation: severe cases where available.

Drug(s) of Choice

- K-penicillin: 40,000 units/kg IV every 6 hours
- Ceftiofur sodium: 2 mg/kg IM every 12 hours, 5 to 10 mg/kg, IV every 6 to 12 hours
- Amikacin: 25 mg/kg IV, every 24 hours
- Trimethoprim-sulfamethoxazole: 30 mg/kg PO BID
- Flunixin meglumine: 1 mg/kg IV, every 12 hours
- Ketoprofen: 2 mg/kg IV, every 12–24 hours

Precautions/Interactions

Caution with nephrotoxic drugs in devitalized foals.

Alternative Drugs

Depending on culture and sensitivity results of the suspected pathogen, the following antimicrobials may be useful:
- Doxycycline: 10 mg/kg PO, every 12 hours
- Azithromycin: 10 mg/kg PO, every 24 hours
- Rifampin: 5 to 10 mg/kg PO, every 12 hours

Appropriate Health Care

Manage in airborne irritant free environment.

Nursing Care

Ensure appropriate activity level.

Diet

Ensure adequate caloric intake to restore and maintain body condition.

 COMMENTS

Client Education

Prolonged course of treatment may be required.

Patient Monitoring

Serial leukograms, thoracic radiographs, or thoracic U/S may be useful.

Prevention/Avoidance

Care with introduction of new horses to the farm.

Possible Complications

Pleural adhesions and abscessation.

Expected Course and Prognosis

Response to timely and appropriate therapy usually good.

Abbreviations

BID   twice a day
IM   intramuscular
IV   intravenous
PO   per os (by mouth)
U/S   ultrasound, ultrasonography
WBC   white blood cell

Suggested Reading

Bedenice D, Heuwieser W, Brawer R, et al. 2003. Clinical and prognostic significance of radiographic pattern, distribution, and severity of thoracic radiographic changes in neonatal foals. *J Vet Intern Med* 17: 876–886.
Peek SF, Landolt G, Karasin AI, et al. 2004. Acute respiratory distress syndrome and fatal interstitial pneumonia associated with equine influenza in a neonatal foal. *J Vet Intern Med* 18: 132–134.
Wilkins PA. 2003. Lower respiratory problems of the neonate. *Vet Clin North Am Equine Pract* 19: 19–33.

Author: Peter R. Morresey

chapter 149

Pneumonia, Viral

DEFINITION/OVERVIEW

Infection of the lungs with a virus capable of causing loss of mucosal integrity and cell death. Secondary infection with other pathogens can then occur.

ETIOLOGY/PATHOPHYSIOLOGY

Viral pneumonia typically reaches the lungs by inhalation of airborne virus-laden droplets. Once inoculated onto the respiratory mucosa the virus invades the cells lining the airways and the alveoli. Host cell death results from direct viral killing, virus replication, or apoptosis. The immune response to the pathogen exacerbates this damage by the production of inflammatory mediators and cytokines that recruit further immune cells to the area. Viral damage may occur in other organs and lead to extra-pulmonary disease. Loss of integrity of the respiratory defenses makes the animal more susceptible to bacterial pneumonia.

Systems Affected

- Cardiovascular: pulmonary changes may increase cardiac workload, with direct effects on cardiac muscle (immune-mediated myositis) also possible. Vasculitis also occurs in some cases.
- Hemic/Lymphatic/Immune: lymphopenia may occur due to viral-induced cell death.
- Musculoskeletal: generalized wasting due to catabolism, immune-mediated myositis.

SIGNALMENT/HISTORY

Foals of all ages are susceptible to viral pneumonia. Predisposing factors include environmental or social stresses, exposure to shedding horses or concurrent medical conditions devitalizing the pulmonary defenses.

Risk Factors

Exposure to known viral respiratory pathogens:
- EHV-1 and EHV-4

- Equine influenza
- EAV
- Equine rhinovirus
- Adenovirus: sporadic, Arabian foals with SCID.

Historical Findings

- Onset of fever, depression, nasal discharge, and deep cough.
- May occur as an outbreak in closely confined equine operations.

 CLINICAL FEATURES

- Fever
- Dry cough
- Serous (initially) to mucopurulent nasal discharge (especially if secondary bacterial infection is present).
- Upper respiratory tract inflammation causing pain and palpable swelling.
- Increased respiratory rate and effort.
- Auscultable respiratory crackles, wheezes or mucus sounds.
- EHV-1: icterus, leukopenia, neutropenia, and petechial hemorrhage prominent in neonatal cases.
- Neonates: EHV-1 or EAV almost uniformly fatal.
- Older foals: all viral pneumonia causes have similar clinical signs.

 DIFFERENTIAL DIAGNOSIS

- Bacterial pneumonia
- Aspiration pneumonia
- Parasitic pneumonia
- Thoracic trauma
- Pneumothorax

 DIAGNOSTICS

- Clinical signs as described previously.
- Hematology: initial leucopenia with left shift, differential count (lymphopenia). Later leukocytosis and fibrinogen (variably elevated) supporting diagnosis of infection.
- Radiography: diffuse radiographic changes with localized lesions due to secondary bacterial infection.
- U/S: pleuritis, consolidation and abscessation.
- Transtracheal aspiration: microbial culture may be negative initially. Cytology indicates inflammation. Viral recovery may be possible.

- Serology and PCR for virus on blood, nasal swabs and tracheal aspirates.
- Virus isolation possible on nasal swabs.
- Serology: paired samples 10 to 14 days apart useful in older foals, but unreliable in neonates due to possible maternal antibody presence.

Pathological Findings

Widespread consolidation of pulmonary tissue. Viral inclusion bodies may be present.

 # THERAPEUTICS

- Neonates: mechanical ventilation of EHV-1 and EAV cases may prolong life; however, due to the severity of the associated pulmonary pathology, death is generally inevitable. Antiviral drugs have been tried with mixed success.
- Older foals: primarily supportive care, although antimicrobial treatment of secondary bacterial infections may be required.

Drug(s) of Choice

- Neonatal EHV-1: limited success reported with acyclovir 16 mg/kg PO every 6 hours or valacyclovir 30 mg/kg PO every 12 hours
- Secondary bacterial pneumonia: see Bacterial pneumonia treatment.

Appropriate Health Care

Supportive respiratory therapies including anti-inflammatories and humidification.

Nursing Care

Foals that are suspected of having either EHV-1 or EVA should be isolated because they are generally shedding large quantities of virus and pose a threat to other neonates and any pregnant mares.

Activity

Avoid excessive exercise during clinical disease.

 # COMMENTS

Client Education

Ensure hygiene barrier procedures are in place in multi-horse facilities.

Patient Monitoring

Serial leukograms and physical examinations to monitor response to treatment.

Prevention/Avoidance

Passive immunity has large role in preventing neonatal disease therefore ensure adequate colostrum intake.

Possible Complications

Persistent pulmonary inflammation or chronic bacterial infection may result.

Expected Course and Prognosis

Uncomplicated viral pneumonias may spontaneously recover. Secondary bacterial infection prolongs course and severity of disease. Neonatal disease can be clinically severe and fatal.

Abbreviations

EAV   equine arteritis virus
EHV   equine herpes virus
EVA   equine viral arteritis
PCR   polymerase chain reaction
PO   per os (by mouth)
SCID   severe combined immunodeficiency disease
U/S   ultrasound, ultrasonography

See Also

- Pneumonia, Bacterial

Suggested Reading

Bedenice D, Heuwieser W, Brawer R, et al. 2003. Clinical and prognostic significance of radiographic pattern, distribution, and severity of thoracic radiographic changes in neonatal foals. *J Vet Intern Med* 17: 876–886.
Peek SF, Landolt G, Karasin AI, et al. 2004. Acute respiratory distress syndrome and fatal interstitial pneumonia associated with equine influenza in a neonatal foal. *J Vet Intern Med* 18: 132–134.
Wilkins PA. 2003. Lower respiratory problems of the neonate. *Vet Clin North Am Equine Pract* 19: 19–33.

Author: Peter R. Morresey

chapter 150

Pneumothorax

DEFINITION/OVERVIEW

Gas, usually air, is present free in the pleural space. This may accumulate to a level that compromises ventilation efforts.

ETIOLOGY/PATHOPHYSIOLOGY

May occur spontaneously due to exaggerated respiratory efforts or as a result of positive-pressure ventilation. Tracheal trauma may also allow air to communicate with the pleural space.

Systems Affected

- Cardiovascular: increased intrapleural pressure decreases venous return, increasing heart rate.
- Musculoskeletal: fatigue occurs due to increased respiratory efforts.

SIGNALMENT/HISTORY

Risk Factors

- Spontaneous
- Secondary to pulmonary disease
- Secondary to pulmonary laceration: direct trauma, rib fracture.
- Excessive positive-pressure ventilation during resuscitation efforts.
- Tracheostomy surgery or trauma
- Any foal being chronically mechanically ventilated

Historical Findings

Markedly increased respiratory effort. Enlarged or abnormally shaped thoracic cage.

CLINICAL FEATURES

- Respiratory distress
- Hypoxemia
- Subcutaneous emphysema
- Palpable abnormality of the thoracic wall: rib fracture(s)

 # DIFFERENTIAL DIAGNOSIS

- Any infectious or inflammatory cause of pulmonary disease
- Hemothorax
- Diaphragmatic hernia

 # DIAGNOSTICS

- Auscultation and percussion of the thorax: lack of normal lung sounds.
- U/S evaluation: loss of contact between thoracic pleura and lung.
- Radiography: standing lateral radiographs can detect lung collapse.
- Needle aspiration of air from the pleural space is confirmatory.

Pathological Findings

- Air in pleural space. Thorax is not under negative pressure when opened.

 # THERAPEUTICS

- Clinical signs: moderate to severe or progressive pneumothorax necessitates intervention.
- Closed suction of the pleural space to evacuate the air.

Appropriate Health Care

Avoid situations of stress or forced exercise.

Nursing Care

Provide oxygen supplementation to decrease work of breathing.

Surgical Considerations

- Provide closed suction of the pleural space.
- Repair thoracic wall and rib defects if present.

COMMENTS

Patient Monitoring

Monitor respiratory rate and effort in all ventilated patients.

Prevention/Avoidance

Ensure pressure valves are set and operate correctly on all resuscitation equipment.

Possible Complications

Pulmonary collapse and death

Expected Course and Prognosis

Mild cases may spontaneously resolve if pleural air intake ceases. Ventilation impairment leading to respiratory distress will not resolve without intervention.

Abbreviations

U/S ultrasound, ultrasonography

See Also

- Pneumonia, Bacterial
- Pneumonia, Viral

Suggested Reading

Bedenice D, Heuwieser W, Brawer R, et al. 2003. Clinical and prognostic significance of radiographic pattern, distribution, and severity of thoracic radiographic changes in neonatal foals. *J Vet Intern Med* 17: 876–886.

Peek SF, Landolt G, Karasin AI, et al. 2004. Acute respiratory distress syndrome and fatal interstitial pneumonia associated with equine influenza in a neonatal foal. *J Vet Intern Med* 18: 132–134.

Wilkins PA. 2003. Lower respiratory problems of the neonate. *Vet Clin North Am Equine Pract* 19: 19–33.

Author: Peter R. Morresey

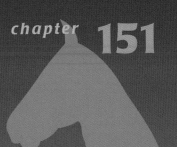
Polydactyly

Disorders of the musculoskeletal system may be associated with congenital malformations, intrauterine sepsis, abnormal length of gestation, foals that are small for gestational age, and twinning. Trauma at delivery, neonatal bacterial sepsis, and postnatal injury can lead to additional musculoskeletal problems.

DEFINITION/OVERVIEW

Presence of a supernumerary digit. The digit may be soft tissue in nature, or contain bony structures with or without joints.

ETIOLOGY/PATHOPHYSIOLOGY

Considered to be of genetic origin, whether the result of mutation of autosomal dominant genes or multifactorial in nature. A genetic component is suggested as the horse descended from animals with multiple digits (Fig. 151.1). May be part of a syndrome of multiple abnormalities.

Systems Affected

Musculoskeletal: supernumerary digits.

SIGNALMENT/HISTORY

Breed or sex predilection for polydactyly has not been established. The condition is discovered following birth.

Risk Factors

- Possible heritable cause
- Unknown gestational event

Historical Findings

- Presence of extra digits

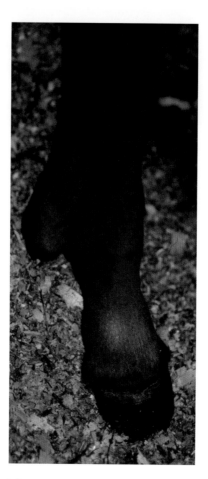

■ **Figure 151.1** Supranumerary digit.
Image courtesy of C. L. Carleton.

 CLINICAL FEATURES

- Duplication of digit: complete, partial.
- Supernumerary digits are often unilateral and predominantly medial.
- Metacarpus II and III are the most common origin of the extra digit.
- Carpal structures may be involved in the origin of the extra digit, with extra carpal bones reported.
- Flexor tendons may be present, extensor structures are usually lacking.
- Concurrent congenital anomalies in non-limb structures may occur.

DIAGNOSTICS

- Clinical appearance
- Radiography

Pathological Findings

Supernumerary digits

THERAPEUTICS

Surgical Considerations

Surgical removal of digit and associated structures.

COMMENTS

Polydactylism may be associated with other congenital abnormalities, including adactyly (lack of phalanges) and arthrogryposis. Abnormalities of the mandible and maxilla have also been associated.

Client Education

May be heritable although this is unproven.

Possible Complications

Supernumerary structures do not bear weight and may interfere with normal limb motion.

Suggested Reading

Barber SM. 1990. Unusual polydactylism in a foal. A case report. *Vet Surg* 19: 203–207.

Hardy J, Latimer F. 2003. Orthopedic disorders in the neonatal foal. *Clin Tech Eq Pract* 2: 96–119.

McIlwraith CW. 2002. Diseases of joints, tendons, ligaments and related structures. In: *Lameness in Horses*, 5th ed. Stashak TS, Adams OR (eds). Philadelphia: Lippincott Williams & Wilkins; 459–644.

Trumble TN. 2005. Orthopedic disorders in neonatal foals. *Vet Clin North Am Eq Pract* 21: 357–385.

Author: Peter R. Morresey

chapter 152

Rib Fractures

DEFINITION/OVERVIEW

Disorders of the musculoskeletal system may be associated with congenital malformations, intrauterine sepsis, abnormal length of gestation, foals that are small for gestational age, and twinning. Trauma at delivery, neonatal bacterial sepsis, and postnatal injury can lead to additional musculoskeletal problems.

Rib fractures have been recognized in 3% to 5% of all neonatal foals. Complications include respiratory distress, myocardial laceration and puncture, hemothorax, and pneumothorax. Thoracic trauma, although often present, is not always clinically significant.

ETIOLOGY/PATHOPHYSIOLOGY

Systems Affected

- Musculoskeletal: disruption of the thoracic wall. Loss of appropriate and effective thoracic ventilation excursions.
- Respiratory: potential pneumothorax due to pulmonary laceration or open fracture.
- Cardiovascular: decreased venous return. Death due to pulmonary hemorrhage or myocardial laceration/puncture.

SIGNALMENT/HISTORY

Risk Factors

- Dystocia: fetomaternal disproportion and exuberant extraction efforts.
- Foals from primiparous mares: fetomaternal disproportion.
- Filly foals have been demonstrated to have a higher incidence of birth trauma than colts.

Historical Findings

Assisted delivery, however, can occur with spontaneous birth.

CLINICAL FEATURES

- Thoracic cage asymmetry: palpable and visual.
- Paradoxical thoracic movement: depression of thoracic wall with inspiration.
- Crepitus, pain, or swelling over thorax: usually unilateral involving multiple ribs on one side of the chest. Bilateral signs occur less commonly.
- Thoracic wall hematoma: associated with arterial or intercostal muscle laceration.
- Increased thoracic respiratory effort.

 DIFFERENTIAL DIAGNOSIS

- Pneumonia
- Pleural fluid: hemothorax or pleuritis.
- Diaphragmatic abnormality: rupture or hernia.
- Trauma: subcutaneous thoracic wall hematoma.

 DIAGNOSTICS

- Palpation: crepitus over fracture site. Asymmetry.
- Auscultation over the fracture sites: crepitus.
- Radiography: thoracic cage asymmetry. Rib fractures may be difficult to see. Costochondral dislocation possible when there is no radiographic evidence of a rib fracture, but severe asymmetry is present.
- U/S: disruption of rib body. Secondary problems noted (hemothorax or hematoma).
- Hematology: anemia and hypoproteinemia due to blood loss into pleural space.

Pathological Findings

Direct visualization of rib fracture. Trauma to thoracic viscera.

 THERAPEUTICS

- Analgesia: improve demeanor and ventilation efforts.
- Anti-inflammatories: decrease soft-tissue swelling.
- Antimicrobials: broad-spectrum coverage for secondary infections at fracture site.
- Manage concurrent conditions where present: sepsis, hemothorax, or pneumothorax.
- Conservative: stall confinement, exercise restriction for 2 weeks to allow fibrous union of rib fracture ends.
- Surgical: when unstable fragments are present. Options include screws, plates, and cerclage wires. A nylon strand technique has been described.

Drug(s) of Choice

- K penicillin: 40,000 units/kg IV, every 6 hours
- Ceftiofur sodium: 2 mg/kg, IM, every 12 hours, 5 to 10 mg/kg IV, every 6 to 12 hours
- Amikacin: 25 mg/kg IV, every 24 hours
- Trimethoprim-sulfamethoxazole: 30 mg/kg PO BID
- Flunixin meglumine: 1 mg/kg IV, every 12 hours
- Ketoprofen: 2 mg/kg IV, every 24 hours

Precautions/Interactions

Care with potentially nephrotoxic drugs in compromised neonates.

Activity

Maintain in confined area free of physical hazards. Limit exercise.

Surgical Considerations

An unstable fracture site lacerates adjacent tissue; has the potential to cause fatal hemorrhage.

 COMMENTS

Patient Monitoring

Regularly assess stability of fracture site (palpation, U/S).

Possible Complications

- Hemothorax
- Cellulitis
- Death

Expected Course and Prognosis

Conservative management of nondisplaced fractures is usually uneventful. Damage to thoracic viscera and hemothorax necessitates aggressive intervention.

Abbreviations

BID   twice a day
IM   intramuscular
IV   intravenous
PO   per os (by mouth)
U/S   ultrasound, ultrasonography

Suggested Reading

Kraus BM, Richardson DW, Sheridan G, et al. 2005. Multiple rib fracture in a neonatal foal using a nylon strand suture repair technique. *Vet Surg* 34: 399–404.

Author: Peter R. Morresey

chapter 153

Septic Arthritis (Infective Arthritis)

Disorders of the musculoskeletal system may be associated with congenital malformations, intrauterine sepsis, abnormal length of gestation, foals that are small for gestational age, and twinning. Trauma at delivery, neonatal bacterial sepsis, and postnatal injury can lead to additional musculoskeletal problems.

 DEFINITION/OVERVIEW

Infection of the synovial structures of the joint (Fig. 153.1). Diagnosis of septic arthritis can be challenging in the neonate. Successful management is strongly associated with early diagnosis and aggressive, appropriate treatment.

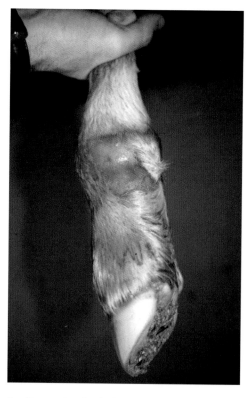

■ **Figure 153.1** Septic fetlock with associated soft-tissue swelling and devitalization.

ETIOLOGY/PATHOPHYSIOLOGY

May be the result of hematogenous spread or local trauma. Due to the relative immaturity of the neonatal foal's immune system, the joints are more susceptible to the establishment and dissemination of systemic infection. The bacteria recovered from infected joints are most often the same as those responsible for any concurrent bacteremia.

- *Hematogenous infective arthritis* is often associated with an infected focus elsewhere in the body, or concurrent sepsis. Umbilical infection is considered the most common primary focus; however, any site of infection can seed a joint (pneumonia, enteritis). Bacteria gain entry to the joint via directly penetrating the synovial membrane.
- *Traumatic infective arthritis* results from direct inoculation following a penetrating wound. Local tissue necrosis over a joint can also permit bacterial entry (decubital ulcers).

Systems Affected

- Musculoskeletal: loss of muscle mass by disuse atrophy of affected limbs.
- Ophthalmic: aqueous flare resulting from the reaction to systemic inflammation.

 # SIGNALMENT/HISTORY

Risk Factors

- Immature bones and joints experience rapid growth with high demands for blood supply. Blood oxygen tension and flow rates are low, allowing thrombosis and bacterial colonization more easily than in other areas.
- Placentitis results in sepsis of the fetus *in utero*.
- Hematogenous spread from other foci, local spread to joint(s) from adjacent osteomyelitis.
- FPT: depressed levels of maternally derived immunoglobulins increase susceptibility to infection.
- Trauma: regional bacterial colonization by direct inoculation, or anaerobic conditions allowing multiplication and spread.

Historical Findings

Depression and recumbency associated with sepsis can make infective arthritis difficult to detect due to lack of movement eliciting pain. Localized infections may not be reflected in the leukogram or other aspects of the general physical examination.

 # CLINICAL FEATURES

- Fever: may be a variable finding due to the localized nature of some infections.
- Synovial distension: associated heat and pain on palpation.

- Lameness: movement of affected joint is likely to be diminished.
- Resistance or reluctance to allow passive movement of the affected joint.
- May involve any joint, however larger joints more often affected: stifle, tarsus, carpus, or fetlock.

DIFFERENTIAL DIAGNOSIS

- Cellulitis: adjacent soft-tissue structures with no joint involvement.
- Trauma: soft tissue supporting structures or cartilaginous disruption.
- Fracture: involving articular surfaces.

DIAGNOSTICS

- Clinical examination findings: lameness or regional pain.
- Hematology: inflammatory leukogram, possibly from underlying systemic disease.
- Radiographs: bony changes delayed (may take 10–14 days). Assess for any concurrent osteomyelitis or physitis (close proximity of and communication with vasculature of the joint).
- Arthrocentesis: elevated protein content, white cell count and differential. Inflammation within the joint leads to increased permeability of the synovial membrane vasculature, allowing the entrance of increased levels of protein and

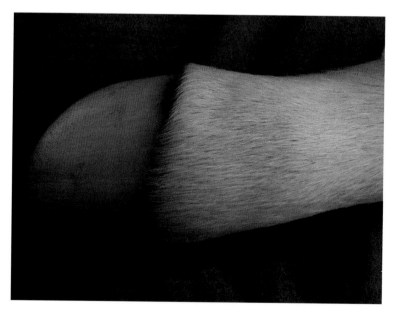

■ Figure 153.2 Inflammation visible at the coronary band (coronitis). Image courtesy of B. Ramanathan.

leukocytes. Submit aseptically collected samples for cytology, culture, and antimicrobial sensitivity.

- U/S: soft-tissue structures around joint(s) may be inflamed (Fig. 153.2). Distension of the joint capsule(s) may be present.

Pathological Findings

Septic exudate within joint(s). Cartilaginous erosions and inflammation. Inflamed periarticular tissues. Primary infected focus located in body.

 THERAPEUTICS

- Manage concurrent, causative disease.
- Medical
  - Consider the compromised state of the foal, especially the nephrotoxic potential of medications.
  - Systemic antimicrobials: begin broad spectrum therapy as soon as possible after diagnosis is confirmed or highly suspected, even prior to identification of the causative agent. Bactericidal antimicrobials are preferred due to the potential compromise of the sick neonatal foal's immune system. Consider the Gram-negative spectrum to ensure coverage of the most common pathogens. Parenteral administration (intravenous preferred as intramuscular dosage can be challenging) when possible, as drug absorption by the oral route is variable-to-poor in neonates.
  - Anti-inflammatories: analgesia, decrease fever and pain.
- Surgical
  - Joint lavage: removal of inflammatory debris and organisms.
  - Arthroscopy: debridement of fibrin and removal of bacterial reservoirs.
  - Regional limb perfusion: high local drug concentration at the site of infection.
  - PMMA beads: chronic periarticular antimicrobial instillation.

Drug(s) of Choice

- Antimicrobials
  - β-lactams: penicillins, cephalosporins. Use in conjunction with an aminoglycoside for extended Gram-negative spectrum. Penicillins have superior Gram-positive spectrum. Third-generation cephalosporins have demonstrated excellent Gram-negative spectrum and good penetration into normal bone and joints, although little is known about inflamed joints.
  - Aminoglycosides: gentamicin, amikacin. Excellent Gram-negative spectrum, with resistance seldom developing to amikacin. May be inactivated in acidic environments or where purulent material is abundant.
  - Potassium penicillin: 40,000 units/kg IV, every 6 hours
  - Ceftiofur sodium: 2 mg/kg IM, every 12 hours, 5 to 10 mg/kg IV, every 6 to 12 hours

- Amikacin: 25 mg/kg IV, every 24 hours
- Trimethoprim-sulfamethoxazole: 30 mg/kg PO BID
- Oxytetracycline: 10 mg/kg IV, every 24 hours
- Anti-inflammatories
  - NSAIDs: anti-inflammatory and analgesic. Decrease thrombosis, thus allowing better antimicrobial penetration to the synovium. They decrease the amounts of inflammatory mediators and destructive enzymes in the joint, result in preserving cartilage.
  - Flunixin meglumine: 1 mg/kg IV, every 12 hours
  - Ketoprofen: 2 mg/kg IV, every 12–24 hours
  - Phenylbutazone: 2.2 mg/kg IV, every 12 to 24 hours (Monitor closely for gastrointestinal ulceration and renal compromise).

Precautions/Interactions

- Nephrotoxicity of aminoglycosides and NSAIDs in compromised neonates.
- Provide antiulcer treatment concurrently with NSAID or when patient is stressed by pain or confinement.

Nursing Care

Ensure adequate caloric intake and appropriate level of activity. Avoid prolonged periods of recumbency that often occur with orthopedic pain.

Surgical Considerations

Multiple joint lavages may exacerbate synovial inflammation. Periarticular fluid leakage occurs from previous lavage ports.

    COMMENTS

Possible Complications

Degenerative joint disease

Expected Course and Prognosis

Loss of future athletic function is likely in cases that are already advanced at presentation. Multiple affected sites indicate a guarded prognosis for recovery.

Abbreviations

BID   twice a day
FPT   failure of passive transfer
IM   intramuscular
IV   intravenous

NSAID   nonsteroidal anti-inflammatory drug
PMMA   polymethylmethacrylate
PO   per os (by mouth)
U/S   ultrasound, ultrasonography

See Also

- Neonatal evaluation

Suggested Reading

Hardy J, Latimer F. 2003. Orthopedic disorders in the neonatal foal. *Clin Tech Eq Pract* 2: 96–119.

McIlwraith CW. 2002. Diseases of joints, tendons, ligaments and related structures. In: *Lameness in Horses*, 5th ed. Stashak TS, Adams OR (eds). Philadelphia: Lippincott Williams & Wilkins; 459–644.

Trumble TN. 2005. Orthopedic disorders in neonatal foals. *Vet Clin North Am Equine Pract* 21: 357–385.

Author: Peter R. Morresey

chapter 154

Small Intestinal Accident

DEFINITION/OVERVIEW

Entrapment, volvulus, or intussusception leading to ischemia and necrosis of the small intestine. The large intestine may become displaced, obstructed, or suffer from torsion leading to devitalization.

ETIOLOGY/PATHOPHYSIOLOGY

Factors predisposing to intestinal tract accidents necessitating surgical correction are largely unknown. Sudden feed changes, general debility, and periods of recumbency have all been associated.

Systems Affected

- Cardiovascular: elevated heart rate due to decreased venous return resulting from increased intra-abdominal pressure and splanchnic pooling.
- Hemic/Lymphatic/Immune: signs of sepsis develop once devitalization of intestinal tissue occurs.
- Renal/Urologic: hypovolemia may precipitate prerenal azotemia.
- Respiratory: elevated respiratory rate and effort due to diminished diaphragmatic excursion resulting from dilated abdominal viscera.

SIGNALMENT/HISTORY

Sudden onset of abdominal discomfort. May be associated with overt distension and loss of appropriate borborygmus.

Risk Factors

- Herniation: umbilical or inguinal.
- Intra-abdominal adhesions: resulting from previous abdominal surgery or peritonitis.
- Mesenteric rents: allow intra-abdominal entrapment of viscera.
- Concurrent medical conditions: sepsis, illness leading to recumbency, ileus.

Historical Findings

Sudden onset of colic or abdominal distension. May be found dead with signs of struggle.

 CLINICAL FEATURES

- Acute abdominal pain: may be intermittent or chronic in nature.
- Abdominal distension: increasing in magnitude as condition progresses.
- Elevated heart rate: non-responsive or poorly responsive to therapy.
- Dehydration: splanchnic pooling of fluid.
- Electrolyte disturbances.
- Endotoxemia: loss of mucosal integrity allows systemic endotoxin dissemination.
- Chronic duration: recumbency or moribund.

 DIFFERENTIAL DIAGNOSIS

- Enterocolitis: fluid pooling in the intestinal tract due to mucosal leakage; disturbed motility may lead to marked and painful distension.
- Congenital abnormality: atresia coli or intestinal aganglionosis.

 DIAGNOSTICS

- Hematology/serum chemistry: hemoconcentration or leukopenia. Electrolyte abnormalities.
- Nasogastric intubation and reflux: persistently elevated heart rate, continuing pain post-reflux indicates gastric distension alone is not responsible for clinical signs. Surgical exploration is usually indicated in these cases.
- U/S: dilated hypomotile small intestine, thickened intestinal wall may be present (Fig. 154.1).
  - Increased peritoneal fluid volume, may be turbid or have fibrin strands with intra-abdominal sepsis (peritonitis).
  - Enlarged stomach indicates outflow obstruction (may be due to compression distally).
  - Characteristic "target lesion" (concentric small intestinal walls) may be observed with intussusception (Fig. 154.2).
- Radiography: dilated small intestine, gas distended colon.
- Abdominocentesis: peritoneal white cell count, red cell count, and protein elevated; degree dependent on duration of clinical signs. Normal values do not rule out intestinal compromise.

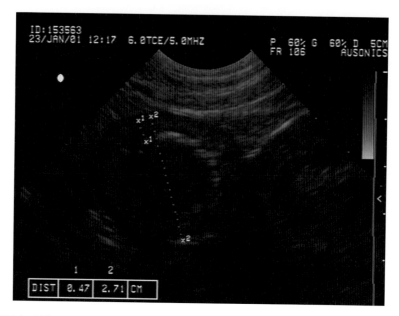

■ **Figure 154.1** Thick-walled small intestine indicative of vascular compromise.

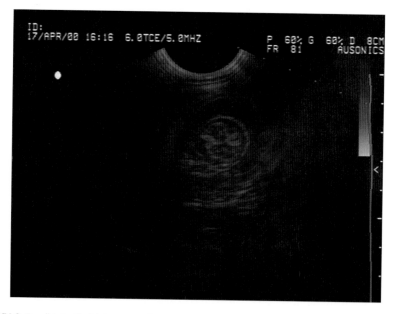

■ **Figure 154.2** Small intestinal intussusception.

Pathological Findings

Abnormal disposition or entrapment of intestinal tract. Devitalization of associated viscera.

 THERAPEUTICS

- Exploratory celiotomy: allows direct visualization to assess the integrity of the intestine. Correction of intestinal displacement or entrapment. Resection and anastomosis of devitalized areas.
- Peritonitis management: antimicrobials, anti-inflammatories, fibrinolytics (heparin), or peritoneal lavage.
- Supportive care: normalize fluid and electrolyte balances. Nutritional support.

Drug(s) of Choice

See Table 119.1.

Nursing Care

Routine postsurgical care

Diet

Progressive reintroduction to regular feeding program

Surgical Considerations

Exploratory celiotomy: allows correction of problem, with assessment of intestinal and peritoneal health. Requires considerable financial commitment.

 COMMENTS

Prevention/Avoidance

Difficult because its occurrence is sporadic

Possible Complications

- Intra-abdominal adhesions
- Breakdown of surgical site
- Recurrence of lesion

Expected Course and Prognosis

Rapid diagnosis and appropriate treatment usually gives good results. Pre-existing adhesions or peritonitis at time of surgical correction increases likelihood of chronic problem.

Abbreviations

U/S   ultrasound, ultrasonography

See Also

- Diarrhea
- Congenital lesions

Suggested Reading

Bueschel D, Walker R, Woods L, et al. 1998. Enterotoxigenic *Clostridium perfringens* type A necrotic enteritis in a foal. *JAVMA* 213: 1305–1307, 1280.

Santschi EM, Vrotsos PD, Purdy AK, et al. 2001. Incidence of the endothelin receptor B mutation that causes lethal white foal syndrome in white-patterned horses. *AJVR* 62: 97–103.

Wilson JH, Cudd TA. 1980. Common gastrointestinal diseases. In: *Equine Clinical Neonatology.* Koterba AM, Drummond WH, Kosch PC (eds). Philadelphia: Lea & Febiger; 412–430.

Author: Peter R. Morresey

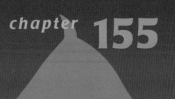

chapter 155

Trauma

DEFINITION/OVERVIEW

The skull and vertebral column may suffer from exogenous or self-inflicted damage. Clinical signs may be immediately apparent, or be evident once soft-tissue inflammation and infection have ensued.

ETIOLOGY/PATHOPHYSIOLOGY

Trauma to the horse may result in stretching and tearing of the neural tissue in response to shearing forces. Absence of neurological signs in the initial postinjury period does not rule out future neurological dysfunction as CNS injury has a complex and progressive pathophysiology. Swelling of neural tissue and hemorrhage within the bony confinements of the cranium and vertebral column, bony displacement along fracture lines, and blood pressure alterations can occur rapidly resulting in sudden changes to the neurologic status of a trauma patient.

Systems Affected

- Musculoskeletal: loss of function may lead to muscle wasting.
- Neuromuscular: spastic paralysis may occur in the areas supplied by the damaged nervous tissue.
- Respiratory: central respiratory depression may decrease ventilation and lead to respiratory acidosis further exacerbating generalized depression.

SIGNALMENT/HISTORY

Risk Factors

- Aggression by in-contact horse.
- Misadventure or collision with another horse or object.
- Iatrogenic as a result of resistance to handling.

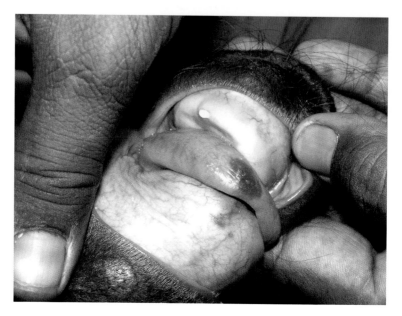

■ **Figure 155.1** Unobserved trauma may be the only indication of seizure activity. Image courtesy of B. Ramanathan.

Historical Findings

Trauma to horse may be witnessed or suspected with the occurrence of cutaneous lesions or palpable bony damage (Fig. 155.1). There may be a sudden onset of seizure activity or loss of musculoskeletal function.

 CLINICAL FEATURES

- External trauma: swelling, localized pain, hemorrhage, or crepitus over sites of suspected bony damage.
- Hemorrhage: blood at nares or ears is highly suggestive of a skull fracture.
- Skull: frontal bone or occipital bone visually displaced.
- Neurological dysfunction: cerebral signs (i.e., depression, stupor, coma, or seizure), cranial nerves (i.e., facial muscle deformity, strabismus, anisocoria, or head tilt), spinal ataxia.

 DIFFERENTIAL DIAGNOSIS

- Cerebral mass: abscess, hematoma, or tumor.
- Meningitis: focal or generalized, central or spinal cord.
- Hypoxic insult
- Idiopathic cerebral dysfunction: epilepsy.

DIAGNOSTICS

- Clinical signs: neuroanatomic localization of the presenting neurologic deficit. Is the lesion focal or diffuse or multifocal in nature?
- Radiography: determine the presence of a fracture. Note integrity of the skull base.
- U/S: periosteal lifting and hemorrhage visible in areas of nondisplaced fractures.
- Endoscopy: examine guttural pouches for hemorrhage, degenerative lesions.
- Cerebrospinal fluid: hemorrhage, meningitis.

Pathological Findings

Bony displacement, hemorrhage or necrosis of neural tissue at site of lesion. May detect infected focus.

THERAPEUTICS

- Treat as for HIE.
- Antimicrobials, anti-inflammatories, and general supportive therapies.
- Surgical stabilization of bony fragments (if found to be present and technically feasible) allowing decompression of adjacent soft tissue.

Drug(s) of Choice

See HIE.

Precautions/Interactions

See HIE/PAS.

Appropriate Health Care

Monitor closely for and control seizure activity.

Nursing Care

Decubital ulcers common with unsteady or recumbent patients.

Diet

Ensure adequate caloric intake.

Activity

Maintain in environment with minimal stimulus if seizure activity present.

Surgical Considerations

Stabilize fracture sites where practicable.

COMMENTS

Client Education

Recovery may be prolonged and residual deficits likely.

Patient Monitoring

Regularly assess neurological status.

Possible Complications

Chronic neurological dysfunction

Expected Course and Prognosis

Recovery may be uneventful in cases where trauma is minimal and appropriate early treatment is instituted. Significant neural disruption or delayed treatment increase chance of residual deficits.

Abbreviations

CNS central nervous system
HIE hypoxic ischemic encephalopathy (alternate: PAS)
PAS perinatal asphyxia syndrome
U/S ultrasound, ultrasonography

Suggested Reading

Green SL, Mayhew IG. 1980. Neurologic disorders. In: *Equine Clinical Neonatology*. Koterba AM, Drummond WH, Kosch PC (eds). Philadelphia: Lea & Febiger; 496–530.
MacKay RJ. 2005. Neurologic disorders of neonatal foals. *Vet Clin North Am Equine Pract* 2: 387–406.

Author: Peter R. Morresey

Ultrasound Assessment of Feto-Placental Well-Being, Mid- to Late Gestation

DEFINITION/OVERVIEW

- Assessed by serial U/S examinations of the gravid uterus, from mid-gestation to term.
- Parameters evaluated include:
  - Number of fetuses
  - Fetal presentation and position
  - FHR
  - Activity
  - Size
  - Tone
  - Fetal fluid depth and quality
  - Utero-placental contact and combined thickness
- Feto-placental parameters by stage of gestation.
- Normal measurements have been reported for light breed mares from 4 months to term.
- U/S examination from mid-gestation to term may identify fetal congenital abnormalities, fetal distress, abnormal fetal growth patterns, abnormal presentation, placental pathology, and abnormal volumes of fetal fluids, all of which may cause fetal compromise.
- Fetal compromise may result in abortion, perinatal complications, stillbirth or neonatal disease.

DIAGNOSTICS

Transrectal U/S

Equipment

- U/S: B-mode, real-time
- Transducer: linear-array, transrectal, 5 to 10 MHz.

Procedure for Transrectal Examination

- Restrain mare
- Evacuate feces from rectum and evaluate cervical tone and length.
- Place U/S transducer over gravid uterus.

- Assess fetal presentation (Fig. 156.1).
- Measure orbital diameters and record the sum (anterior presentation) (Fig. 156.2).
- Record fetal peripheral pulses, when they can be visualized (i.e., fetal carotid pulse from 6 months gestation to term).
- Measure CTUP unit at the cervical pole and assess contact (Fig. 156.3).

Beware: under normal circumstances, no distinction should be appreciated between uterine wall and allantochorion, except in late term, when a diffuse loss of allantochorial echotexture is commonly observed (Fig. 156.4).

Transabdominal U/S

Equipment

- U/S: B-mode, real-time.
- Transducer: Sector or convex technology, 2.5 to 5.0 MHz.
- Selection of transducer frequency is dependent on gestational age, size of mare, and subcutaneous fat.
- Linear-array may be used, but linear transducers are less adaptable to the curvilinear abdominal contour.

Procedure for Transabdominal Examination

- Restrain mare
- Clip abdomen, if needed; spray or sponge alcohol onto clean skin; apply coupling gel to the transducer foot.
- Scan the ventral abdomen from the mammary gland to the sternum to localize the fetus.
- Assess fetal presentation and position (Fig. 156.5).
- Locate cardiac area (Fig. 156.6).
- Record FHR, both at rest and during activity, through an M-mode ultrasound tracing (Fig. 156.7).
- Assess FHR variability between rest and activity tracings.
- An average of 10 FHR recordings are usually registered during the course of a 45- to 60-minute examination.
- Aortic diameter is measured in systole, close to the base of the heart (Fig. 156.8). Make several recordings.
- Measure orbital diameters and record sum of them.
- Assess and record stomach size (*see* Fig. 156.5).
- Assess fetal tone.
- Record episodes of major activity and fine tuned movements.
  - Major activity: decreases as gestation advances; includes:
    - Rotations over short and long axis.
    - Whole body shifting (cranio-caudal, ventro-dorsal and vice versa).
  - Fine-tuned movements:
    - Limbs and neck and head flexion/extensions.
    - Blinking, suckling, lip smacking, and so on.

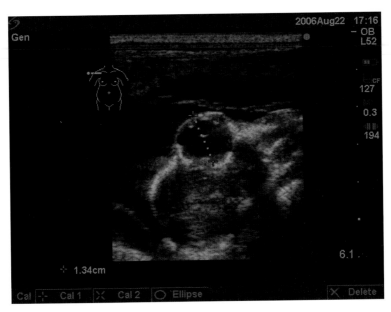

■ **Figure 156.1** Transrectal sonogram of a 5-month old fetus in anterior presentation. Skull and fetal eye are visible. Mare's caudal right of sonogram.

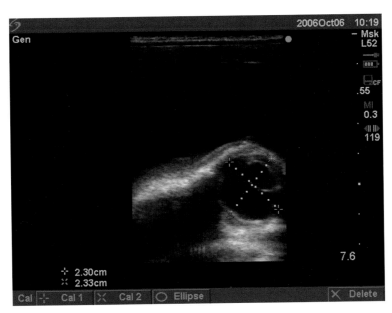

■ **Figure 156.2** Transrectal sonogram of a 7-month old fetus in anterior presentation. Fetal orbital/eye measurements are calculated by the sum of 2 perpendicular diameters, drawn on a still image of the eye, where the lens is visualized. Mare's caudal right of sonogram.

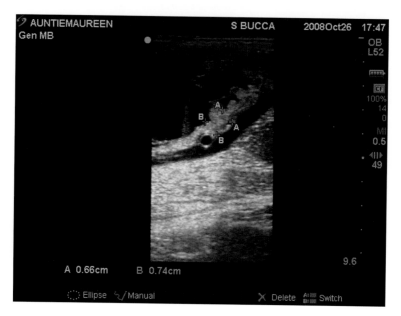

■ **Figure 156.3** Transrectal sonogram of a 5-month utero-placental unit at the cervical pole. Measurements should be consistently taken from the ventral aspect of the cervical pole, just cranial to the cervix, where the uterine artery is visualized. Several measurements should be obtained and the mean calculated. Mare's caudal right of sonogram.

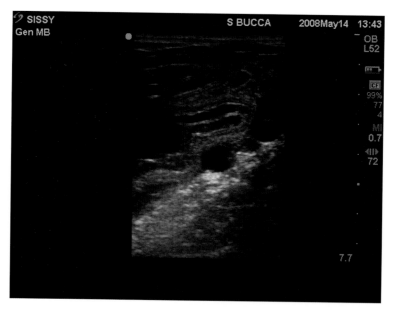

■ **Figure 156.4** Transrectal sonogram of a term utero-placental unit at the cervical pole, displaying loss of allantochorial echotexture (edema). Mare's caudal right of sonogram.

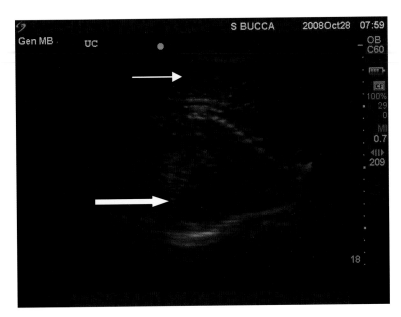

■ **Figure 156.5** Transabdominal sonogram of a 4-month old fetus in posterior presentation. Stomach location *(larger arrow)*, away from the transducer's foot, indicates fetus to be in right lateral recumbency. A thick layer of fat *(small arrow)* is visible on the mare's abdominal wall. Mare's caudal left of sonogram.

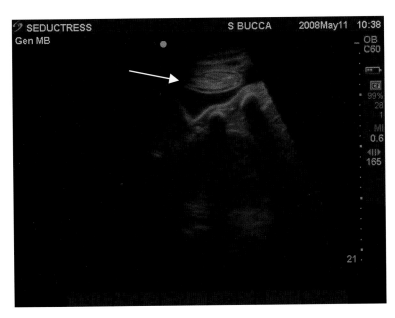

■ **Figure 156.6** Transabdominal sonogram of a term fetus, in anterior presentation. The cardiac area is visualized, with a cross-sectional view of both ventricles. Acoustic shadowing artifacts, caused by bone density (ribs), partly obscure the cardiac silhouette. The hippomane *(arrow)* is imaged between the fetal chest and the ventral utero-placental unit. Mare's caudal left of sonogram.

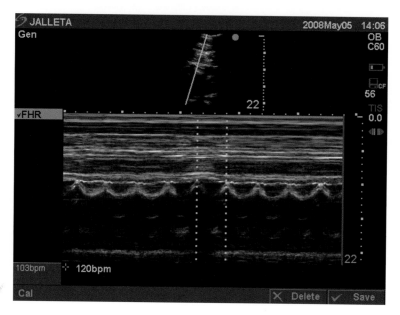

■ Figure 156.7 Transabdominal sonogram of a fetal echocardiogram, obtained by M-mode from an 8-month old fetus in activity phase, showing a cardiac frequency of 120 beats per minute.

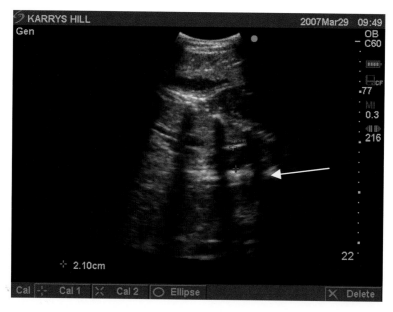

■ Figure 156.8 Transabdominal sonogram of the chest of an 8-month old fetus in anterior presentation, demonstrating measurement of the aortic diameter. Measurements are taken in systole, close to the base of the heart, as the aorta runs along the spinal cord *(arrow)*. Mare's caudal right of the sonogram.

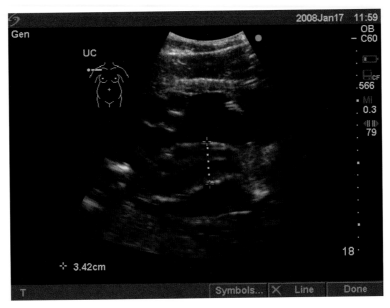

■ **Figure 156.9** Transabdominal sonogram of a 7-month old fetus in transverse presentation, showing measurement of the umbilical cord, close to the umbilicus. A cross-sectional view of the amniotic tract of the umbilical cord is also visible top left of the sonogram, typically showing one vein and two umbilical arteries.

- Evaluate fetal fluid depth and quality.
- Assess utero-placental contact at all accessible areas.
- Localize, measure and record areas of placental detachment.
- Record CTUP measurements on different sections of the mare ventral abdomen.
- If accessible, take measurements of the fetal bladder and U/C (Fig. 156.9).

Pathological Findings

Number of Fetuses

- Multiple fetuses are undesirable.

Presentation

- Posterior or transverse after day 270 of gestation.

Cardiac Activity

- Tachycardia for gestational age.
- Bradycardia for gestational age.
- Arrhythmias
- Lack of FHR reactivity.

Size

- Small aortic diameter for gestational age.
- Small combined orbital diameters for gestational age.
- May be suggestive of IUGR.

Tone

- Lack of fetal tone.

Stomach Size

- Small size may indicate impaired swallowing (risk of hydramnios).

Activity

- Decreased for gestational age.
- Increased for gestational age.
  Beware: dormant, non-active, phases up to 60 minutes duration may occur in normal pregnancies.

Fetal Fluid Depth

- Decreased for gestational age (chronic fetal hypoxia).
- Increased for gestational age (hydramnios/hydroallantois).

Utero-placental Contact

- Large areas of contact loss.
- Nonhomogeneous echotexture; caused by edema (unless close to term).
- Appreciable distinction (separation) between uterine wall and chorioallantois.

CTUP

- Increased for gestational age.
- Decreased for gestational age.

Fetal Bladder-Umbilical Cord

- Increased size may indicate impaired urachal flow or U/C pathology.

 ## COMMENTS

Synonyms

- Fetal Monitoring

Abbreviations

CTUP   combined thickness of the uterus and placenta
FHR   fetal heart rate

IUGR   intrauterine growth retardation
U/C   umbilical cord
U/S   ultrasound, ultrasonography

Suggested Reading

Bocca S, Carli A, Fogarty U. 2007. How to assess equine fetal viability by transrectal ultrasound evaluation of fetal peripheral pulses. *Proc AAEP* 335–338.

Bucca S, Fogarty U, Collins A, et al. 2005. Assessment of feto-placental well-being in the mare from mid-gestation to term: Transrectal and transabdominal ultrasonographic features. *Therio* 64: 542–557.

Reef VB, Vaala WE, Worth LT, et al. 1996. Ultrasonographic assessment of fetal well-being during late gestation: development of an equine biophysical profile. *Eq Vet J* 28: 200–208.

Renaudin CD, Gillis CL, Tarantal AF, et al. 2000. Evaluation of equine fetal growth from day 100 of gestation to parturition, by ultrasonography. *J Reprod Fertil* (Suppl) 56: 651–660.

Authors: Stefania Bucca and Andrea Carli

chapter 157

Uroperitoneum

DEFINITION/OVERVIEW

Urine free in the peritoneal cavity

ETIOLOGY/PATHOPHYSIOLOGY

The most common cause is a traumatic defect in the urinary bladder. Disruption of ureters and urethra is reported to be rare. Congenital defects in the bladder wall are similarly rarely seen. A compromised urachus can also lead to urine leakage into the peritoneum.

Systems Affected

- Cardiovascular: electrolyte derangements (hyponatremia or hyperkalemia) lead to aberrant cardiac rhythms and death.
- Nervous: seizure activity due to neuronal cell swelling (hyponatremia).
- Respiratory: compromised diaphragmatic excursion leads to depressed ventilation.

SIGNALMENT/HISTORY

A sex predilection has been reported, with males more likely affected; however variable retrospective study results exist.

Risk Factors

- Abdominal trauma: parturient or in the early neonatal period.
- Traumatic umbilical cord separation: excessive traction on the umbilical cord at birth may lead to urachal tearing.
- Strenuous exercise
- Prematurity: generalized debility and absence of normal tissue maturity.
- FPT: increased likelihood of sepsis, depression, and recumbency increase the likelihood of inoculation of infection to the urachus.

- Sepsis: debilitation of the foal may allow bacterial dissemination and establishment of localized infection.
- Cystitis: focal necrosis of the bladder wall or urachus.
- Urachal infection: urachal necrosis and rupture allow urine leakage.

Historical Findings

- Depression and lethargy
- Muscular weakness progressing to recumbency
- Variable history regarding urination or urination may be absent (dysuria, anuria).
- Abdominal straining (accompanying lordosis) may be confused with straining to pass a meconium impaction (accompanying kyphosis).
- Abdominal distension with palpable fluid wave upon ballottement.
- May have reports of colic-like activity.
- Seizure activity possible in protracted cases.

 # CLINICAL FEATURES

- Anuria, pollakiuria, or stranguria
- Abdominal discomfort
- Abdominal distention
- Tachycardia
- Tachypnea
- Dehydration
- Depression
- Neurological dysfunction progressing to seizure activity

 # DIFFERENTIAL DIAGNOSIS

- Intestinal accident: abdominal distension and pain
- Enterocolitis: abdominal distension, pain, electrolyte derangements
- Sepsis: weakness or depression
- HIE: depression or seizure activity

 # DIAGNOSTICS

- Electrolyte derangements: hyponatremia, hypochloremia, or hyperkalemia.
- Metabolic acidosis
- Creatinine: elevated serum creatinine. Peritoneal fluid to serum ratio at least 2:1 is considered confirmatory of uroperitoneum.
- U/S: large quantity of hypoechoic peritoneal fluid is present. Bladder may be difficult to visualize or appear partially collapsed if disruption is small or dorsally located

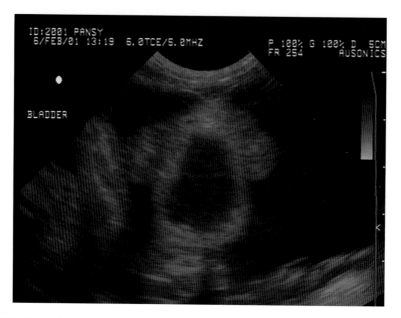

■ **Figure 157.1** Uroperitoneum. A collapsed bladder with attached umbilical artery remnants is visible on this ultrasound.

(Fig. 157.1). Bladder wall disruption may be visualized. Abnormal urachal architecture may be present (i.e., wall disruption or abscessation).

■ Contrast radiography: retrograde cystogram may show location of bladder/urachal defect. Intravenous pyelography may show location of ureteral rent if bladder and urachus appear intact.

Pathological Findings

■ Physical evidence of defect in wall of bladder, urachus, or disruption of ureter or urethra.
■ Free urine in peritoneal cavity with yellow staining of viscera.

THERAPEUTICS

Medical/Non-Surgical

■ Metabolic stabilization and correct electrolyte derangements.
  ■ Correct hypovolemia if present: administer potassium-deficient intravenous fluids.
  ■ Correct hyponatremia, hypochloremia: administer sodium-containing fluids (normal not hypertonic saline).
  ■ Correct hyperkalemia: insulin, glucose/dextrose, or sodium bicarbonate.
  ■ Myocardial stabilization: calcium administration.

- Peritoneal lavage and drainage: avoid rapid decompression because hypovolemic shock may ensue. Lavage with isotonic potassium-deficient fluids.
- Antimicrobials: broad spectrum. Assess renal function when possible and exercise care with potentially nephrotoxic drugs (e.g., aminoglycosides or NSAIDs).
- Chronic urethral catheterization: nonsurgical option that may allow small bladder wall defects to heal over. Useful as a postsurgical management to minimize pressure on the bladder repair and when bladder integrity remains suspect.

Surgical

- Cystorrhaphy: dorsal defects of the bladder wall are the predominant site of leakage.
- Removal of urachal remnants: may be the site of infection or loss of integrity of the urinary tract.
- Nephrectomy: unilateral removal may be required in cases with irreparable ureteral tears.
- Surgical risks: anesthetic cardiotoxicity associated with electrolyte derangements makes it prudent to address metabolic derangements prior to induction of anesthesia.

Drug(s) of Choice

- Potassium-deficient intravenous fluids.
- Sodium containing fluids: normal saline, 0.45% sodium chloride with 2.5% dextrose.
- Sodium bicarbonate: calculate deficit and administer half in the short term. Further administration may not be necessary.
- Urethral spasmolytics: phenazopyridine 5 mg/kg PO, every 24 hours. May decrease intravesicular pressure by aiding passage of urine stream, especially in cases when catheterization has occurred.

Precautions/Interactions

- Avoid postassium-containing drugs (potassium-penicillin).
- Avoid nephrotoxic drugs if renal function is severely compromised (aminoglycosides or NSAIDs).

Appropriate Health Care

- Manage concurrent conditions: sepsis or hypoxic insult.
- Manage surgical wound site.
- Aseptic technique with urinary catheter placement and maintenance.

Nursing Care

Ensure adequate caloric intake.

Surgical Considerations

- Ensure the patient is hemodynamically stable and electrolyte levels are within normal range to minimize anesthetic death risk.
- Avoid rapid decompression of peritoneal cavity.

 COMMENTS

Client Education

- Monitor abdominal wound in surgical cases.
- Monitor urinary catheter placement (if present).

Patient Monitoring

Monitor urination frequency.

Possible Complications

- Wound dehiscence
- Depression
- Death

Expected Course and Prognosis

Prognosis for recovery is good in cases that are identified and treated early. Surgical repair of urinary tract defects is the preferred option; however, cost and potential for peritoneal adhesions must be considered. Nonsurgical management has less success and is dependent on the presence of a small, solitary lesion without secondary complications.

Synonyms

Ruptured bladder (however, a bladder defect may be present along with defects of the ureter, urethra, or urachus).

Abbreviations

FPT   failure of passive transfer
HIE   hypoxic ischemic encephalopathy
NSAID nonsteroidal anti-inflammatory drug
PO   per os (by mouth)
U/S   ultrasound, ultrasonography

See Also

- Neonatal evaluation

Suggested Reading

Brewer BD. 1980. The urogenital system, Section 2: Renal disease. In: *Equine Clinical Neonatology.* Koterba AM, Drummond WH, Kosch PC (eds). Philadelphia: Lea & Febiger; 446–458.

Morisset S, Hawkins JF, Frank N, et al. 2002. Surgical management of a ureteral defect with ureterorrhaphy and of ureteritis with ureteroneocystostomy in a foal. *JAVMA* 220: 354–358, 323.

Vaala WE, Clark ES, Orsini JA. 1988. Omphalophlebitis and osteomyelitis associated with Klebsiella septicemia in a premature foal. *JAVMA* 193: 1273–1277.

Author: Peter R. Morresey

chapter 158

Uveitis

DEFINITION/OVERVIEW

Ocular conditions in the foal often go undiagnosed because examination is not commonly performed unless for insurance or sale purposes.

When compared to the adult horse, a number of differences are noted in the foal:

- A slight medial and ventral strabismus is present, with the adult globe position attained at approximately 1 month of age.
- The pupil is relatively round (contrast to ovoid adult pupil).
- The menace response is not present until approximately 2 weeks of age; however, it may develop at any time prior to that.
- Prominent Y sutures of the lens capsule are present and should not be confused with cataract formation.
- Comparatively low tear production
- Corneal sensitivity to stimulation is low, predisposing to traumatic lesions.

Inflammation of the iris. May be further differentiated into anterior (involving the ciliary body) and posterior (involving the choroid). Uveitis is a common manifestation of a wide range of inflammatory conditions, both ocular and systemic.

ETIOLOGY/PATHOPHYSIOLOGY

Primary ophthalmic diseases that result in uveitis include trauma to the eye, corneal ulceration, and neoplasia. Systemic diseases resulting in uveitis include sepsis and those with the potential for immune-complex deposition (Fig. 158.1).

Systems Affected

Nervous: impaired vision

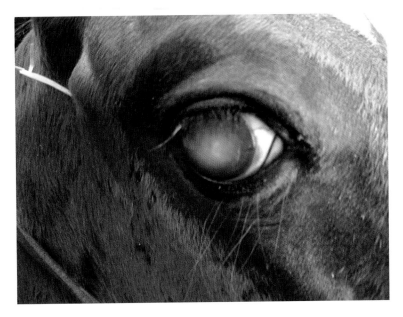

■ Figure 158.1 Aqueous flare secondary to systemic disease (Salmonellosis).

SIGNALMENT/HISTORY

Risk Factors

- Trauma
- Corneal ulceration
- Systemic disease: sepsis or inflammatory focus
- Immune-mediated diseases

CLINICAL FEATURES

- Epiphora
- Blepharospasm
- Conjunctivitis
- Photophobia
- Pupillary constriction
- Corneal edema
- Anterior chamber: hyphema, hemorrhage, fibrin, or hypopyon.

DIFFERENTIAL DIAGNOSIS

- Conjunctivitis
- Corneal ulceration
- Glaucoma

DIAGNOSTICS

- Clinical signs
- Determine presence or absence of corneal ulceration (fluorescein uptake) or abscessation.

THERAPEUTICS

Preserve vision, manage pain:
- Diagnose and manage underlying systemic disease, if present. If secondary to neo-natal sepsis, uveitis is most often sterile.
- Manage corneal ulceration if present.
- Systemic antimicrobials: broad spectrum, good penetration.
- Systemic anti-inflammatories: NSAID or corticosteroids (no ulcer).
- Topical antimicrobials: broad spectrum, good penetration.
- Topical anti-inflammatories: NSAID or corticosteroids (no ulcer).
- Topical mydriatics: atropine.

Drug(s) of Choice

See Table 116.1.

Appropriate Health Care

Strict adherence to recommended treatment schedule

Nursing Care

Discourage and prevent self-trauma to affected eye.

COMMENTS

Client Education

Recurrent episodes are possible, especially if the result of trauma (leakage of lens protein) or if systemically derived antigen intraocular deposition has occurred.

Patient Monitoring

Repeated ophthalmological evaluations required to monitor response to treatment.

Possible Complications

- Synechiae: anterior (to cornea), posterior (to lens capsule)
- Cataracts
- Loss of vision or removal of globe required in chronic cases.

Expected Course and Prognosis

Prognosis guarded in recurrent cases.

Abbreviations

NSAID   nonsteroidal anti-inflammatory drug

See Also

Corneal ulceration

Suggested Reading

Gelatt KN. 2000. Equine ophthalmology. In: *Essentials of Veterinary Ophthalmology*. Gelatt KN (ed). Philadelphia: Lippincott Williams & Wilkins; 337–376.

Turner AG. 2004. Ocular conditions of neonatal foals. *Vet Clin North Am Equine Pract* 20: 429–440.

Whitley RD. 1990. Neonatal equine ophthalmology. In: *Equine Clinical Neonatology*, vol. 1. Koterba AM, Drummond WH, Kosch PC (eds). Philadelphia: Lea & Febiger; 531–557.

Author: Peter R. Morresey

Index

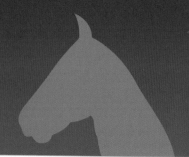

Note: Italicized page locators indicate photos/figures; tables noted with a *t*.